CANCER

AND ITS MANAGEMENT

To Jessica and Gabriela

CANCER

AND ITS MANAGEMENT

ROBERT SOUHAMI
MD FRCP FRCR
Kathleen Ferrier Professor of
Clinical Oncology,
University College London
Medical School
AND
JEFFREY TOBIAS
MA (Cantab) MD FRCP FRCR
Clinical Director,
The Meyerstein Institute
of Oncology,
Middlesex Hospital,
London

SECOND EDITION

Blackwell
Science

© 1986, 1995 by
Blackwell Science Ltd
Editorial Offices:
Osney Mead, Oxford OX2 0EL
25 John Street, London WC1N 2BL
23 Ainslie Place, Edinburgh EH3 6AJ
238 Main Street, Cambridge
   Massachusetts 02142, USA
54 University Street, Carlton
   Victoria 3053, Australia

Other Editorial Offices:
Arnette Blackwell SA
1, rue de Lille, 75007 Paris
France

Blackwell Wissenschafts-Verlag GmbH
Kurfürstendamm 57
10707 Berlin
Germany

Blackwell MZV
Feldgasse 13, A-1238 Wien
Austria

First published 1986
Reprinted 1987, 1988
Second edition 1995

Set by Setrite Typesetters, Hong Kong
Printed and bound in Great Britain
by the Bath Press, Bath, Avon

DISTRIBUTORS

Marston Book Services Ltd
PO Box 87
Oxford OX2 0DT
(*Orders*: Tel: 01865 791155
            Fax: 01865 791927
            Telex: 837515)

North America
Blackwell Science, Inc.
238 Main Street
Cambridge, MA 02142
(*Orders*: Tel: 800 215-1000
            617 876-7000
            Fax: 617 492-5263)

Australia
Blackwell Science Pty Ltd
54 University Street
Carlton, Victoria 3053
(*Orders*: Tel: 03 347-5552)

A catalogue record for this title
is available from the British Library

ISBN 0-632-03371-1

Library of Congress
Cataloging in Publication Data

Souhami, Robert L.
    Cancer and its management/Robert Souhami,
   Jeffrey Tobias. — [2nd ed.]
        p.   cm.
    Includes bibliographical references
    and index.
    ISBN 0-632-03371-1
    1. Cancer — Treatment.
    I. Tobias, Jeffrey S.   II. Title.
    [DNLM: 1. Neoplasms — diagnosis.
    2. Neoplasms — therapy.   QZ 200
S721c 1994]
RC270.8.S68   1995
616.99'4 — dc20
DNLM/DLC   94-21772
                                                CIP

Contents

Preface, vii

List of Abbreviations, ix

1 The Modern Management of Cancer: An Introductory Note, 1

2 Epidemiology; Cure; Treatment Trials; Screening, 7

3 Biology of Cancer, 27

4 Staging of Tumours, 47

5 Radiotherapy, 63

6 Systemic Treatment for Cancer, 85

7 Supportive Care and Symptom Relief, 121

8 Medical Problems and Radiotherapy Emergencies, 139

9 Hormonal and Paraneoplastic Syndromes, 159

10 Cancer of the Head and Neck, 171

11 Tumours of the Nervous System, 201

12 Tumours of the Lung and Mediastinum, 227

13 Breast Cancer, 251

14 Cancer of the Oesophagus and Stomach, 273

15 Cancer of the Liver, Biliary Tract and Pancreas, 289

16 Tumours of the Small and Large Bowel, 305

17 Gynaecological Cancer, 317

18 Genito-urinary Cancer, 351

19 Testicular Cancer, 377

20 Thyroid and Adrenal Cancer, 393

21 Metastases from an Unknown Primary Site, 407

22 Skin Cancer, 413

23 Bone and Soft Tissue Sarcomas, 433

24 Paediatric Malignancies, 453

25 Hodgkin's Disease, 479

26 Non-Hodgkin's Lymphomas, 503

27 Myeloma and Other Paraproteinaemias, 531

28 Leukaemia, 547

Index, 567

Preface

We were encouraged by the reception of the first edition of this book which seemed to be welcome as an introductory text for doctors, other medical workers and scientists interested in the problems of cancer. In this second edition we have attempted a thorough revision without greatly lengthening the book.

Cancer medicine is one of the most rapidly changing of all medical specialties. Not long ago most cancers were treated either by surgery or local radiotherapy, with almost no hope of success if the cancer had spread to involve local lymph nodes, or if distant metastases were present. Recent advances in chemotherapy, hormone therapy, radiotherapy and diagnostic imaging have transformed our clinical practice; and progress in cell biology has led to a far greater understanding of the process of malignant transformation.

We wrote this book because we were aware that many busy physicians, surgeons and gynaecologists, who are not themselves cancer specialists, may find it difficult to keep abreast of areas which are of considerable importance to them. General surgeons, for example, spend a substantial portion of their time dealing with gastro-intestinal and abdominal tumours, yet have little working knowledge of non-surgical treatment of these conditions. Similarly, gynaecological surgeons need to know more about what the radiotherapist and medical oncologist can offer for gynaecological tumours.

Many medical schools still do not provide any integrated teaching in cancer medicine, and student knowledge of the management of malignant disease is often acquired from specialists whose main interest may not be related to cancer. Medical students should know more about the disease which is the second largest cause of mortality in the Western world. We hope that trainees in medicine, surgery and gynaecology will also find the book of value, and that it will be of help to postgraduates beginning a career in radiotherapy or medical oncology. Finally, we hope that general practitioners, all of whom look after cancer patients and who have an important role in management and in terminal care, will find this book helpful. If specialists in cancer medicine feel it is a useful digest of current thought in cancer management, so much the better. However, this book is not primarily intended for them. There are several very large texts which give specialist advice. Although some of these details necessarily appear in our book, we do not regard it as a handbook of chemotherapy or radiotherapy. To some extent it is a personal view of cancer and its management today and, as such, it will differ in some details from the attitudes and approaches of our colleagues.

We have attempted to give a thorough working knowledge of the principles of diagnosis, staging and treatment of tumours and to do so at a level which brings the reader up to date. We have tried to indicate where the subject is growing, where controversies lie, and from which direction future advances might come. In the first nine chapters we have provided a review of some of the mechanisms of tumour development, cancer treatment and supportive care. In the remaining chapters we have given an account of the principles of management of the major cancers. For each tumour we have given details of the pathology, mode of spread, clinical presentation, and staging and treatment with radiotherapy and chemotherapy. The role of surgery is outlined, but details of surgical procedure are beyond the scope of this book. The references which we have included for further reading have been chosen because they are clear reviews or representative of many similar articles, and sometimes because they are historical landmarks or represent important recent work.

ACKNOWLEDGEMENTS

We are well aware that no two people can be expert in all branches of cancer, but we wished to achieve a uniformity of style and approach which is not possible in multi-author books. It is a great pleasure to record our grateful thanks to the following colleagues who kindly read parts of the manuscript, invariably adding valuable comments which have greatly improved the final result: Dr Thurston Brewin; Professor John Cawley; Professor Alan Craft; Dr Michael Cullen; Professor Alfred Cuschieri; Dr Gillian Duchesne; Professor Adrian Eddlestone; Dr Charles Edmonds; Dr Anthony Goldstone; Mr Henry Grant; Dr John Hartley; Professor Peter Isaacson; Professor David Linch; Dr David Machin; Dr John Richards; Dr Marjorie Ridley; Mr Anthony Silverstone; Dr Maurice Slevin; Dr Stephen Spiro; Professor David Thomas; Dr Colin Trask; Dr Christopher Williams; Mr Alan Wilson and Mr Peter Worth. Professor Peter Isaacson and Dr Meryl Griffiths helped us with the pathology illustrations.

The major revision of the text required considerable reorganization and we are greatly indebted to Caroline Christian for her invaluable help. We were greatly helped by Lorna Dickson of Blackwell Science; and Clare Williams drew the excellent line drawings.

R.S., J.T.

List of Abbreviations

ABCM   doxorubicin, BCNU,
       cyclophosphamide and melphalan
ABMT   autologous bone marrow
       transplantation
ACh   acetylcholine
ACTH   adrenocorticotrophic hormone
ADH   antidiuretic hormone
AFP   α-fetoprotein
AHA   autoimmune haemolytic anaemia
AIDS   acquired immune deficiency
       syndrome
ALL   acute lymphoblastic leukaemia
AML   acute myeloblastic (myelogenous)
       leukaemia
AMML   acute myelomonocytic leukaemia
ANL   acute non-lymphocytic leukaemia
APC   adenomatous polyposis coli
APUD   amine precursors uptake and
       decarboxylation
ATRA   all-*trans*-retinoic-acid

BACOP bleomycin, A-doxorubicin,
       cyclophosphamide, O-vincristine
       and prednisone
BCG   bacille Calmette−Guérin
BCNU   bis-chloroethyl nitrosourea
BEP   bleomycin, etoposide and
       cisplatin
BIP   bleomycin, ifosfamide and
       cisplatin
BJP   Bence-Jones protein
BMT   bone marrow transplantation
BOLD   bleomycin, lomustine, vincristine
       and dacarbazine
BUdR   bromodeoxyuridine
BSO   buthionine sulfoximine

CALLA common acute lymphoblastic
       leukaemia antigen
CCNU   cis-chloroethyl nitrosourea
CEA   carcinoembryonic antigen
CGL   chronic granulocytic leukaemia
ChLVPP chlorambucil, vinblastine,
       procarbazine and prednisone
CHOP   cyclophosphamide,
       H-doxorubicin, O-vincristine and
       prednisolone
CIN   cervical intraepithelial neoplasia
CIS   carcinoma *in situ*
CLL   chronic lymphocytic (lymphatic)
       leukaemia
CMF   cyclophosphamide, methotrexate
       and 5-FU
CMI   cell-mediated immunity
CML   chronic myeloblastic
       (myelogenous) leukaemia
CMV   cytomegalovirus
COMP   cyclophosphamide, vincristine,
       methotrexate and prednisolone
CR   complete response
CRC   Cancer Research Campaign
CSF   cerebrospinal fluid
CSF   colony stimulating factor

DCC   deleted in colorectal carcinoma
DIC   disseminated intravascular
       coagulation
DNCB   dinitrochlorobenzene
DTIC   dimethyltriazenoimidazole
       carboxamide (dacarbazine)
DTPA   diethylene triamine penta ascitic
       acid

EBV   Epstein−Barr virus

ix

EBVNA	Epstein–Barr virus associated nuclear antigens	HLA	human leucocyte antigen
ECOG	Eastern co-operative oncology group	HPV	human papilloma virus
		HSV	herpes simplex virus
ED	extensive disease	5HT	5-hydroxytryptamine
EF	extended field	HVA	homovanillic acid
EGF	epidermal growth factor		
EGFR	epidermal growth factor receptor	ICRF	Imperial Cancer Research Fund
EM	electron microscope	IF	involved field
EMG	electromyogram	IFN	interferon
EORTC	European Organisation for Research and Treatment of Cancer	IG	immunoglobulin
		IL-2	interleukin-2 (etc.)
EPO	erythropoietin	IPSID	immune proliferative small intestine disease
ER	oestrogen receptor		
ERCP	endoscopic retrograde cholangiopancreatography	IVC	inferior vena cava
		IVU	intravenous urography
ESR	erythrocyte sedimentation rate	KS	Kaposi's sarcoma
FAM	5-FU, doxorubicin and mitomycin	LAK	lymphokine-activated killer
FdUMP	5-fluoro-2 deoxyuridine monophosphate	LD	limited disease
		LDH	lactate dehydrogenase
FEV_1	forced expiratory volume/second	LET	linear energy transfer
FIGO	International Federation of Gynaecology and Obstetrics	LHRH	luteinizing hormone releasing hormone
FPC	familial polyposis coli	LTR	long terminal repeat
FSH	follicle stimulating hormone		
5-FU	5-fluorouracil	mAb	monoclonal antibody
		M-BACOD	methotrexate, bleomycin, A-doxorubicin, cyclophosphamide, O-vincristine, dexamethasone
G6PD	glucose 6-phosphate dehydrogenase		
G-CSF	granulocyte colony stimulating factors		
		M-CSF	macrophage colony stimulating factor
GH	growth hormone	MDR	multi-drug resistance
GSH	glutathione	MDS	myelodysplastic syndromes
GVHD	graft-versus-host disease	MEN	multiple endocrine neoplasia
		MGUS	monoclonal gammopathy of unknown significance
HBI	half body irradiation		
HBLV	human B cell lymphotrophic virus	MIBG	meta-iodo-benzylguanidine
HBV	hepatitis B virus	MMC	major histocompatibility
HCG	human chorionic gonadotrophin	MMP	matrix metalloproteinase
HCL	hairy cell leukaemia	MOPP	mustine, vincristine (oncovin), prednisone and procarbazine
HDMTX	high-dose methotrexate		
HGPRT	hypoxanthine-guanine phosphoribosyltransferase	6MPRP	6-mercaptopurine ribose phosphate
		MRC	Medical Research Council
HHM	humoral hypercalcaemia of malignancy	mRNA	messenger ribonucleic acid
5HIAA	5-hydroxyindoleacetic acid		

MSH	melanocyte-stimulating hormone	RS cells	Reed–Sternberg cells
MTI	malignant teratoma intermediate	RSV	Rous sarcoma virus
MTT	malignant teratoma trophoblastic		
MTU	malignant teratoma undifferentiated	SCLC	small-cell lung cancer
		SIADH	syndrome of inappropriate ADH secretion
MVPP	mustine, vinblastine, prednisone and procarbazine	SVCO	superior vena caval obstruction
NCAM	neural-cell adhesion molecule	TBI	total body irradiation
NHL	non-Hodgkin's lymphomas	TCC	transitional cell carcinoma
NK	natural killer	TD	teratoma differentiated
NSABP	National Surgical Adjuvant Breast Project (USA)	6TG	6-thioguanine
		TGF	transforming growth factor
NSCLC	non-small-cell lung cancer	TIBC	total iron binding capacity
NSD	nominal standard dose	TIMPS	tissue inhibitors of metalloproteinases
OAF	osteoclast activating factor	TLI	total lymphoid irradiation
		TNF	tumour necrosis factor
PAS	periodic acid-Schiff	TNI	total nodal irradiation
PBSC	peripheral blood stem cell	TNM	tumour node metastases staging
PCI	prophylactic cranial irradiation	TSH	thyroid-stimulating hormone
PCR	polymerase chain reaction	TSTA	tumour specific transplantation antigens
PCV	procarbazine, CCNU and vincristine	TUR	transurethral resection
PDT	photodynamic therapy		
PLAP	placental alkaline phosphatase	UICC	Union Internationale Contre le Cancer
PNET	primitive neuroectodermal tumour		
PR	partial response	VAD	vincristine, infused doxorubicin and high-dose dexamethasone
PR	progesterone receptor	VAIN	vaginal intraepithelial neoplasia
PSA	prostate-specific antigen		
PTHrP	parathyroid hormone-related protein	VCA	viral capsid antigen
		VIN	vulval intraepithelial neoplasia
pUVA	psoralens and ultraviolet light 'A'	VIP	vasoactive intestinal peptide
PVB	cisplatin, vinblastine and bleomycin	VMA	vanillyl mandelic acid
PVC	polyvinylchloride	WBC	white blood count

Chapter 1
The Modern Management of Cancer:
An Introductory Note

Cancer is a vast medical problem. As a cause of mortality it is second only to cardiovascular disease. It is diagnosed each year in 1 in every 250 men and 1 in every 300 women. The incidence rises steeply so that over the age of 60, 3 in 100 men develop the disease each year (Fig. 1.1). It is often a costly disease to diagnose and investigate, and treatment is time-consuming, labour intensive and usually requires hospital care. In the Western world the commonest cancers are of the lung, breast, skin, gut and prostate gland (Fig. 1.2). The life-time risk of developing a cancer is shown in Fig. 1.3.

In the past the main methods of treating cancer have been by surgery and radiotherapy. The control of the primary tumour has been seen as the major problem, since it is this which is usually responsible for the patient's symptoms. There may be exceedingly unpleasant symptoms due to local spread, and a failure to control the disease locally means certain death. For many tumours, breast cancer for example, the energies of those treating the disease have been directed towards defining the optimum methods of eradication of the primary tumour. This is a worthwhile and important aim, but it is perhaps not surprising that these efforts, while improving management, have not greatly improved the prognosis because the most important cause of mortality is metastatic spread. Although prompt and effective treatment of the primary cancer diminishes the likelihood of recurrence, metastases have often developed before diagnosis and treatment have begun. The prognosis is not then altered by treatment of the primary cancer even though the presenting symptoms may be alleviated.

Every medical specialty has its own types of cancer which are the concern of the specialist in that area. Cancer is a diagnosis to which every clinician is alerted whatever his field and, because malignant disease is common, specialists acquire great expertise in diagnosis, often with the aid of techniques such as bronchoscopy and other forms of endoscopy. On the other hand the management of cancer once the diagnosis has been made, especially the non-surgical management, is not part of the training or interest of many specialists and the patient is often transferred to other hands at this point. While this is in some respects desirable, especially as cancer treatments become more complicated, it presents serious problems. For example, radiotherapists and medical oncologists are often asked to see patients who have had a laparotomy at which a tumour such as an ovarian cancer or a lymphoma has been found but the abdomen has been closed without the surgeon having made an attempt to stage the disease properly, or where appropriate, to remove the main mass of tumour. This poses considerable problems for the further management of the patient. At a more general level, lack of familiarity with the principles of cancer management and of what treatment can achieve, leads to a low level of recruitment into clinical trials. An understanding of the principles of investigation and treatment of cancer has become essential for every physician and surgeon if the best results for their patients are to be achieved.

Recent advances in the chemotherapy and radiotherapy of uncommon tumours such as Hodgkin's disease and teratoma of the testis

Fig. 1.1 Age-specific cancer incidence in England and Wales.

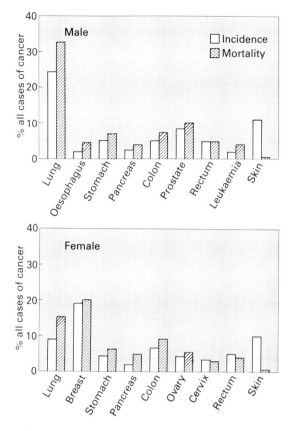

Fig. 1.2 Incidence and mortality of cancer in men and women in the United Kingdom.

have led to a more general awareness of the importance of a planned approach to the management of patients. This has been true not only for the problems of individual patients but also in the planning of clinical trials of treatment. It has become clear that for every cancer, an understanding of which patients can be helped, or even cured, can only come by attention to the details of disease stage and types. Patients in whom these details are unknown are at risk from inappropriate overtreatment or from inadequate treatment, resulting in the chance of cure being missed. Even though chemotherapy has not been of great benefit to patients with diseases such as squamous lung cancer or adenocarcinoma of the pancreas, it is now clearly essential that clinicians with a detailed and specialized knowledge of the risks and dangers of chemotherapy in these and other

diseases are part of the staff of every oncology department. Knowing when not to treat is as important as knowing when to do so.

The improvement in chemotherapy of some cancers has greatly increased the complexity of management. Cancer specialists have a particular responsibility to validate the treatment which they give, since the toxicity and dangers of some regimens mean that the indications for treatment have to be established precisely. In a few cases an imaginative step forward has dramatically improved results and the need for controlled comparison with previous treatment is scarcely necessary. Examples are the use of combination chemotherapy in the management of advanced Hodgkin's disease and prevention

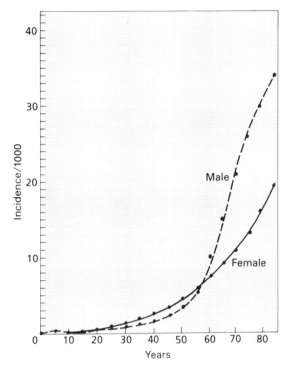

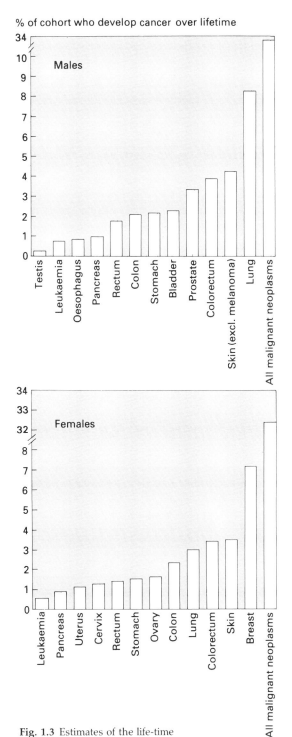

% of cohort who develop cancer over lifetime

Males

Testis · Leukaemia · Oesophagus · Pancreas · Rectum · Colon · Stomach · Bladder · Prostate · Colorectum · Skin (excl. melanoma) · Lung · All malignant neoplasms

Females

Leukaemia · Pancreas · Uterus · Cervix · Rectum · Stomach · Ovary · Colon · Lung · Colorectum · Skin · Breast · All malignant neoplasms

Fig. 1.3 Estimates of the life-time risk of developing cancer in England and Wales.

of central nervous system relapse of leukaemia by prophylactic treatment. However, such clear-cut advances are seldom made. In the main, improvement in treatment is made slowly in a piecemeal fashion and prospective trials of treatment must be undertaken in order to validate each step in management. Modest advances are none the less numerically important for such common diseases. Only large-scale trials can detect these small differences reliably. National and international collaboration has become increasingly important and the result of these studies has had a major impact on management — for example in operable breast cancer. There is always a tendency in dealing with cancer to want to believe good news and for early, uncontrolled but promising results to be seized upon and over-interpreted. Although understandable, uncritical enthusiasm for a particular form of treatment is greatly to be deplored, since it leads to a clamour for the treatment and the establishment of patterns of treatment which are improperly validated. An example is the widespread and uncritical acceptance of chemotherapy in the treatment of advanced lung cancer. The benefits of this approach are not proven, yet in some countries comparisons of such treatment with untreated control groups is regarded as unethical. The toxicity of cancer treatments is considerable and can only be justified if it is unequivocally clear that the end results are worthwhile either by increasing the cure rate or by improving the quality of life.

The increasing complexity of management has brought with it a recognition that in many areas it is necessary to establish an effective working collaboration between specialists. Joint planning of management in specialized clinics is now widely practised for diseases such as lymphomas, head and neck and gynaecological cancer. Some surgeons and gynaecologists are beginning to concentrate on the oncological aspects of their specialty. In this way patients can benefit from a co-ordinated and planned approach to their individual problems.

Before a patient can be treated not only must

it be established that he or she has cancer, but the pathological nature of the tumour must be defined and the extent of the local and systemic disease determined. For each of these goals to be attained the oncologist must rely on colleagues in departments of histopathology, diagnostic imaging, haematology and chemical pathology. Every oncologist has patients referred where the diagnosis of cancer has not been definitely made pathologically but is based on a very strong clinical suspicion with suggestive pathological evidence, or where a pathological diagnosis of cancer has been made which, on review, proves to be incorrect. It is essential for the oncologist to be in close contact with histopathologists and cytologists so that diagnoses can be reviewed regularly. Many departments of oncology have regular pathology review meetings so that the clinician can learn of the difficulties which pathologists have with diagnosis and vice versa. Similarly, modern imaging techniques have led to a previously unattainable accuracy in pre-operative and post-operative staging, although many of these techniques are only as reliable as those using them (e.g. abdominal or pelvic ultrasound). The cancer specialist must be fully conversant with the uses and limitations of imaging methods. The techniques are expensive and the results must be interpreted in the light of other clinical information. The practice of holding regular meetings to review cases with specialists from the imaging departments has much to commend it.

Modern cancer treatment often carries a substantial risk of toxicity. Complex and difficult treatments are best managed in a specialized unit with skilled personnel. The centralization of high-dependency care allows staff to become particularly aware of the physical and emotional problems of patients undergoing treatments of this kind. Additionally, colleagues from other departments such as haematology, biochemistry and bacteriology can more easily help in the investigation and management of some of the very difficult problems which occur, for example in the immunosuppressed patient.

The increasingly intensive investigative and treatment policies which have been adopted in the last 20 years impose on clinicians the additional responsibility of having to stand back from the treatment of their patients, and decide at each stage what the aim of treatment is. Clearly radical and aggressive therapy is essential if the patient has a reasonable chance of being cured. However, palliative treatment will be used if the case is quite clearly beyond any prospect of cure. What is more difficult is to know when the intention of treatment must move from the radical to the palliative, with avoidance of toxicity as a major priority. For example, while many patients with advanced lymphomas will be cured by intensive combination chemotherapy, there is no prospect of cure in advanced breast cancer by these means, and chemotherapy must in this case be regarded as palliative therapy: a situation in which it makes little sense to press treatment to the point of toxicity. The judgement of what is tolerable and acceptable is a major task in cancer management. Such judgement can only come from considerable experience of the treatments in question and of the natural history of individual tumours.

Modern cancer management often involves highly technological and intensive medical care. It is expensive, time-consuming and sometimes dangerous. Nowadays patients should seldom be in total ignorance of what is wrong with them or what the treatment involves. The increasingly technical nature of cancer management, and the change in public and professional attitudes towards malignant disease, has altered the way in which doctors who are experienced in cancer treatment approach their patients. There has been a decisive swing towards honest and careful discussion with patients about the disease and its treatment. This does not mean that a bald statement should be made to the patient about the diagnosis and its outcome, since doctors must sustain the patient with hope and encouragement through what is obviously a frightening and depressing period. One of the most difficult and rewarding aspects of the management of malignant disease lies in the judgement of how much information to give to each particular patient, at what speed, and how to incorporate the patient's own wishes into a rational treatment plan.

The emotional impact of the diagnosis and treatment can be considerable for both patients and relatives. Above everything else, treating patients with cancer involves an awareness of how patients think and feel. All doctors dealing with cancer patients must be prepared to devote time to talking to patients and their families, to answer questions and explain what is happening and what can be achieved. Because many patients will die from their disease the doctor must learn to cope with the emotional and physical needs of dying patients and the effects of grief and bereavement on their family.

The care and support of patients with advanced malignant disease and the control of symptoms such as pain and nausea have greatly improved in the last 10 years. This aspect of cancer management has been improved by the collaboration of many medical workers. Nurses who specialize in the control of symptoms of malignancy are now attached to many cancer units and social workers skilled in dealing with the problems of malignant disease and bereavement are an essential part of the team. The development of hospices has led to a much greater appreciation of the way in which symp-toms might be controlled and to a considerable improvement in the standards of the care of the dying in general hospitals. Many cancer departments now have a symptom support team based in the hospital, but able to undertake the care of patients in their own homes, giving advice on control of symptoms such as pain and nausea and providing support to the patient's family.

There have been dramatic advances in cell and molecular biology in the last 10 years with the result that our understanding of the nature of malignant transformation has increased. This trend will continue and places an additional demand on the oncologist, namely to keep abreast both of advances in management and the scientific foundations on which they are based. The power of modern techniques to explore some of the fundamental processes in malignant transformation has meant that cancer is at the heart of many aspects of medical research and has led to an increased academic interest in malignancy. This in turn has led to a more critical approach to many aspects of cancer treatment. Cancer and its management is now one of the most complex and demanding aspects of medicine. More health care workers are seeing that cancer medicine is rewarding and interesting, and standards of patient care are improving as a result of these welcome changes.

Chapter 2
Epidemiology; Cure;
Treatment Trials; Screening

The epidemiology of cancer, which concerns the study of the frequency of the disease in populations living under different conditions, has been illuminating in several ways. It has allowed the testing of theories about the cause of a cancer by relating a particular characteristic, for example cigarette smoking, to the occurrence of disease. It has suggested ways in which cancer might be prevented by changing the prevalence of a postulated aetiological agent, as shown by the decline of lung cancer in doctors who have given up smoking. Finally, epidemiological evidence has proved invaluable in planning cancer services.

TERMINOLOGY AND METHODS IN EPIDEMIOLOGY

When epidemiologists use the word *prevalence* they mean the proportion of a defined group having a condition at a single point in time. By *incidence* they mean the proportion of a defined population developing the disease within a stated time period. When they talk of *crude incidence* or *prevalence rates* they are talking of whole population. *Specific rates* refer to selected groups, for example a higher crude fatality rate from breast cancer in one population might be due to more postmenopausal women being in the population in question. *Standardized populations* should, therefore, be used when comparing incidence and prevalence.

In trying to find connections between a disease and a postulated causal factor, epidemiologists may construct either *case–control* or *cohort* studies. Take, for example, a study to determine if there is a connection between dietary fat and breast cancer. A *case–control study* would compare the dietary intake of people with the disease (cases) and those without (controls). Choosing appropriate controls is vital to the study design. Case–control studies are also suitable for studies of rare tumours in which a group of people who are exposed to the putative aetiological agent are followed and the frequency of the disease is measured. The control group is unexposed, or exposed to a lesser extent. In the case of dietary fat and breast cancer a *cohort study* would compare the incidence of the disease in those with, say, a high-fat and a low-fat diet. If the cancer incidence is low, as it usually is, large numbers of women will be followed over many years before an answer is obtained. Other variables must be allowed for since eating habits, for example, are influenced by social class and ethnic origin and these may in turn be independently linked to the likelihood of developing breast cancer. Cohort studies take a long time, are very expensive, and are unsuitable for rare tumour studies.

There are considerable problems in the interpretation of data obtained from epidemiological studies. A possible relationship between a characteristic and a cancer may be discovered but there are several considerations which should influence us in deciding whether a causal connection really exists. First, is the relationship between the characteristic and the disease specific, or can a similar association be found with other diseases? An association with other diseases does not necessarily invalidate a causal connection but may suggest that both the characteristic and the cancer are themselves associated with another factor. For example, both lung cancer and coronary artery disease are more common in social classes 4 and 5. The problem is then to decide if these diseases are due to social class itself or to the higher frequency of cigarette smoking in these social groups. Second, is the relationship a strong one? The likelihood of a causal connection is strengthened if, for example, the risk of cancer in the population showing the characteristic is increased 10-fold rather than doubled. Third, is there a gradation of risk with differing exposure? This is the situation with lung cancer and cigarette smoking. Such a gradation greatly increases the likelihood of a causal connection. Fourth, is the association biologically plausible? For example, it appears intuitively reasonable to accept an association between smoking and lung cancer, but the relationship between smoking and bladder cancer is at first more surprising (see p. 357). It is, however, difficult to assess the biological basis for an association since often we do not know the explanation for these events until further investigation, perhaps prompted by the discovery of an association, reveals it. Finally, is there an alternative explanation for what has been found and do the findings fit in with other epidemiological data? The nature of epidemiological evidence is such that absolute proof that an association is causal is impossible to obtain except by randomized intervention studies in which the suspected factor is altered or removed to see if the incidence of cancer then falls. Such studies are difficult, expensive and time-consuming. In some circumstances randomized intervention may be impossible (we cannot randomize to give up smoking!) and the epidemiological data provide the only possible information.

GEOGRAPHICAL DISTRIBUTION OF CANCER

Clues to the aetiology of cancer have been obtained from studies of the difference in incidence of cancers in different countries, races and cultures, although there are obvious difficulties in obtaining reliable data in many countries. Problems of different age distributions can to some extent be overcome by using age-standardized incidence and by restricting the comparison to the mature adult population aged 35–64 years. This age-range excludes the ages where the figures are likely to be least reliable. A further difficulty lies in incomplete documentation of histological type. Sometimes the registration refers to the whole organ, for example 'bone cancer' without specification of histological type and may combine several different histologies.

Even allowing for some uncertainty in the reliability of the data, huge differences in incidence of various tumours between one country and another have been disclosed (Table 2.1). The very high incidence of liver cancer in Mozambique may be related to aflatoxin mould on stored peanuts, and the incidence is now falling since steps have been taken to store the peanuts under different conditions. In the Ghurjev region of Kazakhstan, carcinoma of the oesophagus is 200 times more common than in Holland, and the same is true for the Transkei region where the incidence of the disease appears to have increased greatly in the last 30 years. The high incidence of carcinoma of the stomach in Japan is in contrast to Britain and the United States where the incidence of the disease is falling [1]. The dietary factors which may be responsible are not understood.

Table 2.1 Geographical variation in cancer incidence

Cancer type	Ratio high : low rate	High incidence	Low incidence
Oesophagus	200 : 1	Kazakhstan	Holland
Skin	200 : 1	Queensland	India
Liver	100 : 1	Mozambique	Birmingham
Nasopharynx	100 : 1	China	Uganda
Lung	40 : 1	Birmingham	Ibadan (Nigeria)
Stomach	30 : 1	Japan	Birmingham
Cervix	20 : 1	Hawaii Colombia	Israel
Rectum	20 : 1	Denmark	Nigeria

Studies such as these provide strong evidence for environmental factors causing cancer, but of course an interaction with possible genetic predisposition is also possible. An analysis of the relative contributions of the environmental and genetic components can be made by studying cancer incidence in people who have settled in a new country and who have taken on a new way of life. Japanese immigrants in the United States, for example, have a similar incidence of colon cancer to native Americans but five times that of Japanese in Japan [2] (see also Table 2.2) and it is therefore clear that this difference in rates is not primarily genetic.

TEMPORAL DISTRIBUTION OF CANCER

The incidence of cancer in a given community may change with time providing further clues to aetiology. With rare tumours, this may be more dramatically apparent when a disease appears as a cluster in a given place at a given time. An example would be several cases of acute leukaemia occurring in close proximity in a town within a short space of time. Such clustering has indeed been observed in acute leukaemia and has been suggested for Hodgkin's disease. Chance effects make analysis difficult. However, in the case of Burkitt's lymphoma, outbreaks in Uganda have been shown to spread from one part of a district to another in a way

which cannot be attributed to chance but which fits well with an infective aetiology widespread in the community while producing cancer in only a few. More dramatic evidence of environmental factors comes from the change in cancer incidence with time. The dramatic rise in lung cancer can be attributed to smoking but the fall in stomach cancer is of unknown cause.

CAUSES OF CANCER SUGGESTED BY EPIDEMIOLOGICAL STUDIES

The idea that cancer might largely be preventable has gained more widespread acceptance in recent years [3]. While many substances present in the environment or in the diet have been shown to be carcinogenic in animals this does not mean that they will be so in humans. One contribution of the epidemiological approach has been to try to verify the link between human cancers and substances which in animals are known to be carcinogens. Another has been to identify unsuspected carcinogens by observations on human populations without reference to previous animal experiments. Some of the factors which are known or strongly suspected to be carcinogenic in humans are shown in Table 2.3.

Inhaled carcinogens

Cigarette smoking has been the subject of intense epidemiological investigation since the early work of Doll and Hill demonstrated the relationship between smoking and lung cancer [4]. All studies have shown a higher mortality for lung cancer in smokers. This mortality has a dose−response relationship with the numbers of cigarettes smoked and diminishes with time after stopping smoking. This relationship is discussed further in Chapter 12. Cigarette smoking has also been implicated in the development of carcinoma of the bladder, larynx, pancreas and kidney and may be responsible for 35% of all cancer deaths.

Cigarette smoking is the major known cause of cancer; all other causes are vastly less import-

Table 2.2 Cancer incidence* in Japanese immigrants compared with country of origin and residents of adopted country

Cancer	Japanese in Japan	United States (mostly Hawaii)	
		Japanese	White
Stomach	130	40	21
Breast	31	120	190
Colon	8.4	37	37
Ovary	5.2	17	27
Prostate	1.5	15	35

* Incidence : cases per year per 100 000

Table 2.3 Some aetiological factors

Ionizing irradiation	
Atomic bomb and nuclear accidents	Acute leukaemia
(Nagasaki, Hiroshima, Chernobyl)	Breast cancer
X-rays	
for ankylosing spondylitis	Acute leukaemia
in diagnostic and therapeutic radiologists	Squamous cell carcinoma of skin
Ultraviolet irradiation	Basal cell carcinoma Squamous cell carcinomas of skin Melanoma
Background irradiation	?Acute leukaemia
Inhaled or ingested carcinogens	
Cigarette smoking	Lung cancer Laryngeal cancer Bladder cancer
Atmospheric pollution with polycyclic hydrocarbons	Lung cancer
Asbestos	Mesothelioma Bronchial carcinoma
Nickel	Lung cancer and paranasal sinuses
Chromates	Lung cancer
Arsenic	Lung cancer Skin cancer
Aluminium	Bladder
Aromatic amines	Bladder
Benzene	Erythroleukaemia
Polyvinylchloride	Angiosarcoma of the liver

ant. It is calculated that cigarette smoking-related diseases will kill 500 000 000 of the world's population alive in 1990. Reversal of this public health hazard will do more to improve health than any other preventive measure.

Atmosphere pollutants such as chimney smoke and exhaust fumes have been widely suspected as a cause of lung cancer. Polycyclic hydrocarbons, such as 3:4-benzpyrene, are present in these fumes and are known to be carcinogenic in humans (see pp. 27, 228). Several large-scale studies have shown that the incidence of lung cancer in men in large cities is two or three times greater than those living in the country. This increase, which may or may not be attributable to air pollution, is probably present at all levels of cigarette smoking but is very small compared with the increase in incidence in smokers compared with non-smokers.

Ionizing irradiation

Ionizing irradiation has been well established as a human carcinogen. There has been an increased incidence of leukaemia [5] and breast cancer [6] in the survivors of the Nagasaki and Hiroshima atom bombs. Skin cancer frequently occurred on the hands of radiologists in the days before the significance of radiation exposure was understood. There is also an increased incidence of leukaemia in patients treated by irradiation for ankylosing spondylitis [7]. Ultraviolet irradiation is probably responsible for the increased incidence of skin cancer on exposed sites in those who work out of doors in strong sunshine, for example in Australia.

The level of background radiation in the environment is of course much smaller than that received in the examples given above. The doses are not only smaller in total, but are received at a much slower rate (<100 millionth) than that of diagnostic X-rays. While there is no safe lower limit to radiation dose it is possible to calculate the approximate risk, and it is generally accepted that for most cancers background radioactivity constitutes a small risk at present; this may not be true, however, of leukaemia where background radiation may be responsible for a slight increase in incidence.

Occupational factors (Table 2.3)

Asbestos inhalation has been shown to be associated with two types of cancer: mesothelioma of the pleura and peritoneum, and bronchogenic carcinoma. Prolonged and heavy exposure is needed in the case of bronchogenic cancer, and cigarette smoking further increases the risk [8]. Mesothelioma is a rare tumour and there is often a clear history of asbestos exposure. Although the duration and intensity of the exposure is very variable, the relationship with this tumour is not in doubt. There is also an increased risk of lung cancer in workers in nickel refining and the manufacture of chromates and a possible association with haematite mining and gold mining. Lung cancer has also been described in workers in a sheep dip factory where there was a very high exposure to inhaled arsenic. These workers had signs of chronic arsenicalism and the risk of lung cancer with lower levels of exposure is probably very small.

Other human carcinogens have been identified as a result of industrial epidemiological evidence (see p. 27). Aniline dye workers were shown to have a greatly increased incidence of bladder cancer, and this observation led to the demonstration, in animals, of the carcinogenic effect of 2-naphthylamine. Benzidine and 2-naphthylamine have also been implicated in the pathogenesis of bladder cancer in these workers and those in the rubber industry who are also exposed.

Workers in the aluminium industry have been shown to have an increased incidence of bladder cancer. It has been estimated that about 4% of all cancers can be related to occupational factors.

Life-style and diet

What other factors in our environment or life-style might contribute to the development of cancer? Some American epidemiologists attribute a large proportion of cancers to as yet unspecified industrial poisons and claim that cancer incidence has increased in the last decade in the United States, an increase which is unrelated to tobacco consumption [9]. The figures are disputed, however, since there are the confounding variables of improved diagnosis and registration among the poorer sections of American society during this period (see below). The issue is intensely political and

the prevention and control of industrial pollution potentially involves large sums of money. The truth becomes obscured in a mass of conflicting epidemiological data.

The place of dietary factors in cancer causation is equally poorly understood. Recent studies have shown that in countries where there is a high average daily fat intake the age-adjusted death rate of breast cancer is also high and that the converse is true for populations consuming low-fat diets. The problem here is of course that those countries where dietary fat intake is high also tend to be the most heavily industrialized. Furthermore, the total caloric intake is higher in these nations and a similar association exists for levels of dietary protein. Overnutrition has been shown to increase the incidence of spontaneous tumours in animals. Obesity appears to be an aetiological factor in cancers of the endometrium and gall bladder. Case–control studies relating dietary fat to cancer incidence have given conflicting results. Rather than being causally linked to the cancer, it may be that these dietary constituents are associated with other factors which are themselves causal. Other dietary factors which may be associated with the development of cancer are dietary fibre, which may protect against the development of cancer of the large bowel, and vitamin A analogues (retinoids). The incidence of many types of cancer appears to have an inverse relationship with serum vitamin A levels.

An appreciation of the difficulties involved in analysing the relative contributions of diet, life-style and occupational risk can be gained by reading the contradictory accounts of Epstein [9] and Peto [10].

Viral causes

Although many animal cancers are caused by viruses (feline leukaemia, murine sarcoma, polyoma) there is no epidemiological evidence to implicate viruses as a direct cause of the vast majority of human cancers. Nevertheless, viral infections may be a very important co-factor in producing cancer and this is discussed in more detail in Chapter 3. There is an undoubted association between HIV infection and cancer (lymphoma, Kaposi's sarcoma and other malignancies). There is a clear epidemiological association between Epstein–Barr virus (EBV) and Burkitt's lymphoma (see Chapter 3) and the epidemiological evidence suggesting an infective aetiology preceded the demonstration of the association with EBV infection. The disease mainly occurs in Africa and New Guinea in areas where the temperatures are above 16°C and the rainfall is over 50 cm a year. Furthermore, in affected areas, cases occur in a non-random pattern moving from one district to another, presumably to susceptible populations.

Other possible viral causes are discussed in Chapter 3, but it may be noted here that chronic infection with hepatitis B virus is associated with an increased risk of hepatoma and that the viral genome has been demonstrated both in hepatoma cells and also in normal areas of the affected liver. It is of great interest that there is an increased risk of cancer in patients who are chronically immunosuppressed [11]. These cancers are squamous carcinoma of the skin and cervix, lymphoma of B cell type (especially intracerebral), Kaposi's sarcoma and melanoma.

CANCER STATISTICS

In recent years a number of registries have been established in Britain and in other industrialized countries to record the number of patients developing cancer. The registry is usually notified of new cancer cases by the hospital where the diagnosis is made. In addition, it receives copies of all death certificates of patients within the region, where the diagnosis of cancer appears on a certificate. The quality of the data collected varies greatly from registry to registry and between countries. Incomplete information; changing patterns of registration and diagnosis; introduction of screening programmes and improved treatment, may all alter the number of patients being registered as dying of the disease in a given

area in a given time. Minor fluctuations in incidence should, therefore, be viewed with caution. Consistent trends over several years require investigation before it can be accepted that a change in the incidence or mortality of a disease is occurring.

Still more caution must be attached to any report which seeks to determine the impact of a *treatment* by examining cancer registry data. The nature of the registry data is such that only relatively crude statements about survival can be made and the merits of one treatment over another has to be decided by prospective randomized trials (see p. 17).

Even the most complete registries may have histological confirmation of the diagnosis in less than 60% of cases although the completeness of the records with respect to primary site of the tumour is much greater. The incidence figures for tumours of a defined histological type are, therefore, usually much less reliable than those which describe its site of origin.

In spite of these reservations a glance at the age-specific incidence of various tumours is interesting and revealing. For example, the figures for female genital cancer (Fig. 2.1) show that cancer of the ovary and uterus follow a very similar pattern, the incidence rising sharply towards the end of the child-bearing years, reaching a peak postmenopause. An understanding of the causes of these cancers must clearly take into account these dramatic changes. This is not the pattern seen with all adenocarcinomas in women (Fig. 2.2). Indeed cancer of the ovary and uterus stand out as not showing the typical huge increase in incidence from the age of 60 onwards which characterizes other adenocarcinomas such as bowel, stomach and pancreas.

Cancer of the cervix and of the vagina, chiefly squamous cell cancers, are quite unlike each other in age of onset, that of the cervix being a disease of young and middle-aged women, and that of the vagina a disease of elderly women (Fig. 2.1). There is an obvious problem in interpreting these data. The impact of screening programmes for cervical cancer has meant that

Fig. 2.1 Age-specific incidence of female genital cancer. The figures for cervical cancer include carcinoma *in situ*, diagnosed by screening examination, which accounts for the majority of cases in young patients.

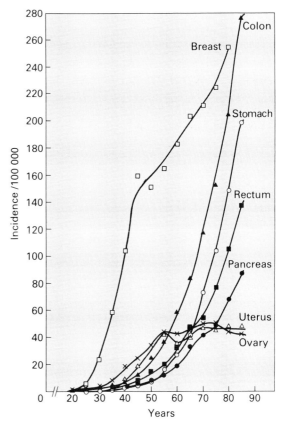

Fig. 2.2 Age-specific incidence of female adeno-carcinoma. The incidence of cancer of the breast increases rapidly in premenopausal women and then slows. This change is more marked with ovarian and uterine adenocarcinoma. By contrast, the incidence of gastro-intestinal cancers shows no relation to menopause but increases markedly over the age of 60.

many of these cases are diagnosed at a very early stage and study of the histology shows a large percentage of cases diagnosed *in situ*. Should we therefore conclude that the higher incidence of cervical cancer in young women is an artefact of early diagnosis and that these cancers would only have been clinically apparent, if at all, many years later? This problem is discussed in more detail in Chapter 17 but it serves to illustrate how cancer statistics may be dramatically altered by early diagnosis.

The figures for other adenocarcinomas in women (Fig. 2.2) are revealing in another respect. The onset of cancer of the uterus and ovary is earlier than that of the gut and stomach, and does not increase in incidence with old age. Cancer of the breast, on the other hand, rises rapidly in incidence in early middle age, and then continues to rise in incidence post-menopause but at a somewhat slower rate compared to colonic cancer, so that the incidence over 80 years of age is less than that of the colon while at 40 years of age, breast cancer occurs

14 times more frequently. The factors responsible for the origin and growth of breast cancer clearly differ from those giving rise to gastro-intestinal malignancy.

SURVIVAL DATA AND DETERMINATION OF CURE IN CANCER

When results of cancer treatment are presented, a graph of survival is often shown, or the proportion of patients alive at, say, 5 or 10 years is stated. It is often difficult to decide whether the results mean that some patients are cured, and unfortunately claims are often made on the basis of figures that are incomplete. An understanding of how survival figures are derived is therefore essential for judging the effectiveness of treatment.

A *survival curve* is a plot of the proportion of patients surviving as a function of time (Fig. 2.3), curve A gives the survival up to 20 years for all cases of cancer of the ovary. A *disease-free survival curve* is displayed in a similar manner but the *x*-axis represents the length of time before the disease reappears. Since some patients may be effectively treated on relapse the information is not the same as with a survival curve. This is especially true in a disease such as Hodgkin's disease where many patients can be cured on relapse.

Can we judge whether patients are cured by looking at survival curves? The general answer is that cure can be assumed if the group of

patients returns to a normal pattern of survival similar to those who have not had that cancer. In the case of ovarian cancer the comparison would be made with a large population of women with the same age distribution. The survival curve expected in such a population is the *age-adjusted expected survival curve*. In Fig. 2.3 the data for ovarian cancer are shown for a 20-year follow-up period. Curve A is the observed survival of the patients, curve E is the age-adjusted expected survival curve and it can be seen that A is approximately parallel to E at 15–20 years. The age-adjusted relative survival curve (R) is constructed by dividing the observed survival curve (A) by the expected curve (E). If there is no increased risk of dying due to the cancer this curve will run parallel to the abscissa. A difficulty might arise if the ability to cure the cancer were dependent on age, for example if young women were more easily cured than elderly women. The age distribution of survivors would then change with time and the age distribution of the control population would, therefore, have to be adjusted accordingly.

Survival does depend on age for many tumours: Fig. 2.4 shows *age-related survival rates* at 1 and 3 years for a variety of common tumours. For most cancers survival is worse in the elderly population at both 1 and 3 years. Curves C and D give the age-related survival rates for all cancers for 3 successive years. During this period there was no improvement except in young men, due to better treatment of teratoma of the testis, which is a common cause of cancer at this age.

In Figs 2.3 and 2.7 the survival curves are given for all cases of cancer of the ovary but of course they could be plotted for individual ages at presentation, or stages of the disease. In this way one may investigate whether cure is being achieved only for certain age groups or stages of disease. In practice, however, data on very large groups of patients (thousands) is needed to demonstrate cure with confidence.

A linear scale plot of survival figures may suggest that a small proportion of patients

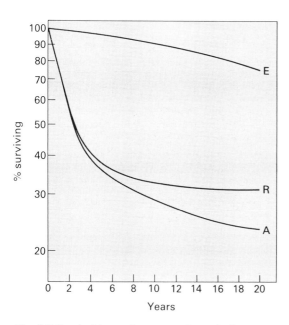

Fig. 2.3 Survival in ovarian cancer. Curve A shows observed survival, Curve E shows age-adjusted expected survival and Curve R shows relative survival. (From Bush *et al.* In Stoll B.A., ed. *Prolonged Arrest of Cancer.* Chichester: John Wylie & Sons Ltd., 1982. With permission.)

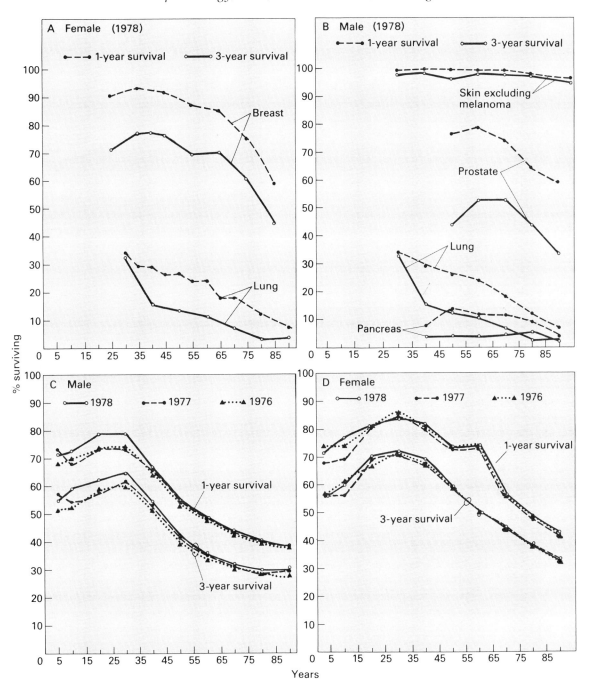

Fig. 2.4 Age-related relative survival rates. (A) Cancer of breast and lung in women; (B) cancer of skin, prostate, lung and pancreas in men. Figures are given for survival at 1 year and at 3 years; (C) cancer at all sites in men (resident in England and Wales) for 3 consecutive years; (D) cancer at all sites in women for 3 consecutive years.

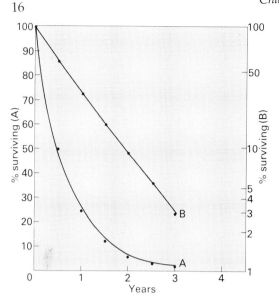

Fig. 2.5 Survival in advanced small cell carcinoma of the bronchus. There appears to be a flattening of the survival curve (Curve A) but the rate of death is in fact exponential (Curve B).

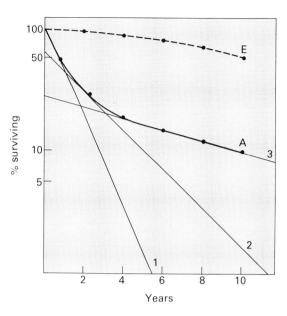

Fig. 2.6 Survival following gastrectomy for carcinoma of the stomach. Curve A can be considered to be a composite of three separate populations (1, 2 and 3) one of which is cured of the disease (3). Age-adjusted expected survival of a control population is shown by Curve E.

are going to be long survivors. In Fig. 2.5, for example, the survival figures for a large trial in small cell bronchogenic cancer are shown on the linear scale. Curve A seems to flatten out at 2 years which might be interpreted as showing that a proportion of patients are cured. However, on a logarithmic scale the curve (B) is shown to be a straight line, that is, exponential, indicating that the rate of death has remained constant with time; the slope of the line giving the rate. This shows that up to this point there is no evidence of cure in the group in question. Many survival curves do not, however, show an exponential shape on a logarithmic scale. Figure 2.6 shows the survival after gastrectomy for carcinoma of the stomach (curve A) and the age-adjusted expected survival (curve E). The survival curve is not exponential. We might speculate that the curve consists of three separate components, a group (line 1) dying rapidly, another (line 2) whose rate of death is lower and a third group (line 3) who appeared to be cured.

In constructing a survival curve a number of

statistical methods may have been used. If, for example, the cases of ovarian cancer in Fig. 2.7 were all diagnosed between 1960 and 1970 and the results were analysed in 1980, all the cases would have been followed for at least 10 years, that is, a 10-year follow-up would be complete. If the cases had been diagnosed between 1965 and 1975 then, in 1980, some cases would have been followed for more than 10 years and other cases for 5—10 years. The curve can none the less be constructed by dividing the follow-up period into fixed intervals, calculating the probability of surviving through each interval and combining these into an overall survival probability which is plotted as a function of time. This is an *actuarial survival curve* and may be thought of as a prediction of how the final survival curve will look if all the cases have similar survival characteristics to those which have been followed longest. These curves are less reliable in the 'tails' when the follow-up period for many patients is short and the num-

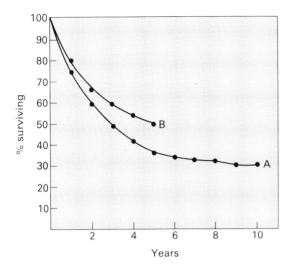

Fig. 2.7 Survival in ovarian cancer (all stages). Curve A represents survival of a group of patients where all patients had been diagnosed at least 10 years previously. Curve B is an actuarial survival curve: none of these patients had been diagnosed more than 5 years previously and some had been diagnosed only 2 years previously.

ber of late survivors is correspondingly small. Figure 2.7 curve B is a hypothetical survival curve, for similar cases to curve A, of 40 patients where only 30 have been followed for 2 or more years and five for 4 or more years. The curve is similar in shape to curve A for the first 2 years (when there are most observations) but appears to show improved survival thereafter. Such a conclusion would be unwise, however, because of the small number of observations between 2 and 4 years on which the curve is based. It would not need many deaths to occur to alter the shape of curve B to that of curve A.

ASSESSMENT OF RESULTS: TRIALS OF TREATMENT

Many of the basic methods and techniques of treatment in cancer have been developed by experienced physicians and surgeons using their common sense. When the treatment has resulted in a clear improvement, as was the case, for example, when mastectomy was first introduced to treat patients with breast cancer, this approach has worked satisfactorily. When differences in treatment results have been less obvious, for example in the case of simple versus radical mastectomy, the results are harder to evaluate.

The problem of assessment is made more complex by changing criteria for diagnosis and treatment during the period in question. For example, refined methods of detection of metastases at presentation (e.g. CT scanning) may result in patients being rejected for a treatment which in earlier days they would have received. This means survival may alter as a result of a *change in selection* in the characteristics of the patients being included in the series being analysed. This hidden change might then be falsely attributed to a recently introduced treatment.

Randomized trials

It is now generally accepted that the only way to avoid bias is to carry out a randomized prospective comparison of the new treatment with the best standard regimen, or in some cases with no treatment. In this way hidden factors in case selection such as histological subtypes, presence of occult metastases and site of tumour, will be randomly distributed in the two groups. Similarly factors which are not known to be associated with prognosis at the start of the trial but which are later shown to be so, do not bias the results since these factors should be equally represented in each of the randomly allocated groups, especially if the number of patients is large.

When an analysis of the effect of different treatments is made, the data may be examined for effect on survival or disease-free survival. The results are typically presented as in Fig. 2.8 which illustrates the disease-free survival curves from a controlled trial of two treatments in breast cancer. Patient group A had received adjuvant chemotherapy and group B had not. There are several points to notice. Firstly, the curves are actuarial curves, that is, not all the

Fig. 2.8 Actuarial relapse-free survival in operable breast cancer. Curve A: treated with adjuvant chemotherapy. Curve B: no adjuvant chemotherapy. (From Rossi *et al. British Medical Journal* 1981; **282**: 1427. With permission.)

Fig. 2.9 Actuarial survival in operable breast cancer. Curve A: treated with adjuvant chemotherapy. Curve B: no adjuvant chemotherapy. (From Rossi *et al. British Medical Journal* 1981; **282**: 1427. With permission.)

patients have been followed for 5 years. If the numbers of long-term survivors are small the tails of the curves may be misleading. Secondly, a difference in favour of chemotherapy is apparent. The probability of this happening purely by chance can be assessed by statistical methods. The log-rank test is a convenient and commonly used method of comparing survival and disease-free survival curves. The test is sensitive to curves which separate to reveal a consistent survival difference. Other tests are more sensitive to early differences which are less apparent later. Thirdly, if the difference is genuine, it represents a delay in onset of recurrence. This may not be reflected in improved *survival*. The survival curves for the groups are shown in Fig. 2.9; it can be seen that the difference is much less striking. This apparent discrepancy may be due to a delay in onset of metastases in the chemotherapy treated group leading to an improved disease-free survival. Once metasta-

ses have appeared, the patients in the control group, who have not received chemotherapy, might benefit from its use so that the overall survival curves are less divergent. Early effects of this type on disease-free survival are often seen in cancer treatment. Delay of recurrence is certainly desirable, but one should bear in mind that for most treatments improved survival is the real objective.

A commonly used method of presentation of results is to quote *median* survival, that is, the time from randomization at which 50% of the patients will be alive. These figures are very unreliable unless the death rate in the 25–75% range is high and the numbers of patients in the study is large (Fig. 2.10). Average or *mean* survival times are often misleading because they can be greatly affected by one or two long-term survivors. Analysis of the proportion surviving at a single point in time makes use of only part of the data available. A survival curve

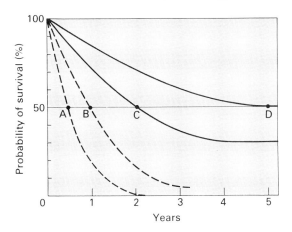

Fig. 2.10 Median survival in cancer trials. Trial 1 (dotted lines) median survival: A, 6 months; B, 1 year. Trial 2 (continuous lines) median survival: C, 2 years; D, 5 years. The differences are reliable in Trial 1 but less so in Trial 2.

analysis is preferred because it makes use of the whole time span of the study.

It should also be remembered that tests of significance merely provide estimates of the probability that an observed difference (or a more extreme one) could have arisen by chance. There are many considerations besides the probability level which should affect one's judgement about whether the difference is interesting or important and whether or not it is solely the result of the treatment.

In designing a prospective randomized trial of treatment many factors must be taken into account, some of which may affect the value of the study:

1 *Can a single question be asked?* Wherever possible the hypothesis being tested should be as simple as possible. For example, can the study ask the question 'Is treatment "A" better than no treatment at all?' A simple study design is always preferable but sometimes not possible. Is it ethically justified to give no treatment? If, for example, the effect of adjuvant chemotherapy on survival following mastectomy is being compared with no postoperative treatment, how will the 'no chemotherapy' group be treated on relapse? A policy for treatment at

each stage of the disease must be devised and agreed before the trial begins. Studies in which there is a 'cross-over' from one treatment to another are usually hard to interpret. Studies which include several randomized groups will usually have to be very large if they are to detect realistic differences between the groups.

2 *Which patients will be included?* A precise statement must be made of the type of patient in which the treatments are to be tested.

3 *Are there known prognostic factors?* Patients with 'limited' stage small cell lung cancer (SCLC) have a better prognosis than those with 'extensive' disease. In trials of treatment in SCLC it is advisable to randomize limited and extensive category patients separately to ensure balanced numbers of each group in each arm of the study. This is termed *stratification*. Major prognostic criteria should be stratified, but too many stratifications can cause confusion and are unnecessary in a large trial.

4 *What is the end-point?* Some trials will be concerned with differences in survival, others with disease-free interval, others with local recurrence. In some studies differences in median survival may be shown without any change in the final long-term survival. An example is a trial of the treatment of advanced or metastatic cancer with cytotoxic drugs. Although all patients may die of the disease, in both treated and untreated groups, death might be delayed by treatment. For example, in the treated groups the death rate at 1, 2 and 5 years might be 50%, 75% and 100%, while in the untreated it might be 85%, 95% and 100%. Such differences may be clinically worthwhile especially if associated with symptomatic relief and minimal toxicity.

5 *Is the difference between the treatments in question likely to be large?* This is seldom the case in cancer where, if the effect of the therapy is dramatic, the trial would probably not be considered necessary or justified. To detect absolute differences in survival of 10% with a significance level of 0.05, between 160 and 500 patients will be needed per patient group, the numbers varying with the proportion surviving. It requires fewer patients to show a 10% survival difference between 10% and 20% than a difference between 40% and 50% (20/10 = 2 (a doubling of survival) while 50/40 = 1.25). Because of the very large numbers of patients necessary to detect even smaller small differences with confidence, many cancer trials are collaborative efforts between different centres. Indeed for rare diseases such as leukaemia or osteosarcoma, treatment trials are almost impossible without such collaboration. Those responsible have to decide what sort of difference they will consider clinically worthwhile.

6 *The difficulties of collaboration are considerable.* Doctors participating in the study must agree on what is the most important question to be asked; how the treatment should be administered (including details of surgery, radiotherapy and chemotherapy); what the documentation should be and how it should be organized; who will pay for the study; who will analyse the data and so on. In a disease like breast cancer where the rate of death is low, the answers may not be available for 10 years or more. Doctors are usually, to put it kindly, 'individualistic' in their approach to treatment and large-scale trials sometimes acquire a design which proves an unsatisfactory compromise. Exceptionally intensive treatments cannot be carried out in every hospital and may not be of the same quality as when undertaken by a few specialized units. Such treatments may be 'watered down' in order to include more centres, possibly weakening the intention of the study.

7 *Even if the differences in survival are small they may be clinically worthwhile.* Dramatic advances in treatment are rare and come from an imaginative step forward by a few individuals, for example, CNS prophylaxis in acute leukaemia or combination chemotherapy in Hodgkin's disease. Large randomized studies are usually carried out where it is not clear if one treatment is better than another and differences are therefore likely to be small. A small difference may, however, lead to a change in clinical practice. If in breast cancer following local therapy, treat-

ment with a drug such as tamoxifen led to a 5% improvement in long-term survival, this would be a major contribution to management because in 20 000 women this could mean 1000 lives saved with negligible toxicity. On the other hand some might regard a 5% improvement achieved with cytotoxic chemotherapy as less compelling, due to the greater toxicity of the treatment. In Europe a 5% improvement in mortality would save 40 000 lives each year. This is a greater saving than that achieved by the successful treatment of diseases such as lymphoma or leukaemia.

There is a growing awareness that our expectations of likely improvements in survival with cancer treatments need to be revised downwards. We cannot expect 20% absolute improvements in survival. We might expect 10–20% improvements in *relative* survival (from 40% to 44–48%) but such improvements require trials vastly greater than those which we have been accustomed to perform. The reason is shown in Fig. 2.12A. The failure to achieve these numbers leads to false-negative results. Figure 2.12B shows the results of treatment trials of adjuvant chemotherapy and/or tamoxifen in breast cancer. The trials were usually small so the 95% confidence intervals overlapped with 'no effect' (see Table 13.6, p. 269). The combined data set shows a

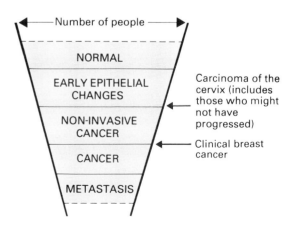

Fig. 2.11 The later in the natural history the fewer 'false-positives', but there is less chance to alter the outcome.

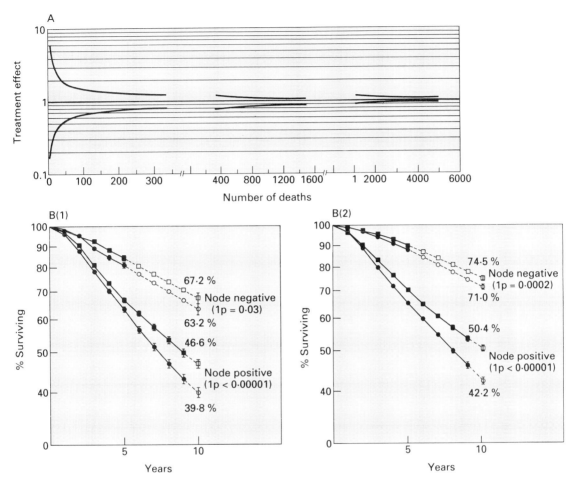

Fig. 2.12 (A) In a comparison between treatments A and B the darker line at 1 is the line of equivalence between the treatments. The curves represent the 95% confidence intervals of this line. For a result to be significantly different it must lie outside this line. Each horizontal line represents a relative difference of 10% between treatments. A difference of 30% in favour of B will only be seen if there are more than 300 deaths in the study; a difference of 10% will require several thousands of deaths to be observed. (B) Results of treatment trials of (1) adjuvant chemotherapy and (2) adjuvant tamoxifen in operable breast cancer. An overview of analysis of many thousands of randomized patients allows a significant survival benefit to be demonstrated.

clear difference with a reduction of relative risk of 22% (7% increase in 5-year survival) and the confidence intervals are separated from the point where no effect is observed. Trials designed to recruit thousands of patients need to be of simple design and execution, with flexible entry criteria and must concern a widely practicable treatment [12]. The organization and execution of these studies is a major task for cancer specialists.

ANALYSIS OF THE RESULTS
OF RANDOMIZED TRIALS

Just as it is essential not to be over-impressed by dramatic results from uncontrolled studies, it is important not to be intimidated by the authority which randomized clinical trials appear to possess. A critical approach is needed. Some points to watch out for are:

1 *Is it likely that a false-positive result (type 1 or α* error) or false-negative (type 2 or β error) has occured? False-positive errors are uncommon. False-negative errors are commoner, but negative trials are not published as frequently as positive ones because journal editors tend to prefer 'positive' results. Does the trial accord with other studies addressing the same point?

2 *Were the treatments genuinely randomized?* Authors sometimes claim their study was randomized but a closer inspection of the method reveals it was not. These studies are nearly always misleading.

3 *Did one particular group of patients benefit?* This is an important matter because it allows treatment to be offered selectively and suggests future directions for study. However, it is almost impossible to draw firm conclusions about subgroups from a single study unless it contains thousands of patients.

4 *Have all the patients been included in the analysis, and if not, why not?* Sometimes patients who are not able to be evaluated are discarded from the report. One should beware of this, particularly if it occurs for large numbers of patients. One reason sometimes given is that the patient only completed one part of the treatment before deteriorating. The patient is discarded as not having had a fair trial of treatment. This practice will of course greatly improve the apparent results because early failures are not included.

5 *Has the trial run for sufficient time to allow enough events (deaths, relapses) to have occurred?* What are the confidence intervals for the treatment difference? A statement of the 95% confidence limits for the treatment difference allows the reader to judge the result being presented and is more informative than a 'p' value from a significance test. A p value indicates the level of statistical significance. What the clinician also needs to know is the *degree* of likely difference. If the confidence intervals of the difference in survival between 2 treatments is -4% to $+15\%$ with a point estimate of 7% this will be judged differently from an outcome where the confidence interval ranges from $+4\%$ to $+20\%$ with a point estimate of 11%. Although both results may be 'significant' the latter is more

compelling because the difference is larger and the certainty of benefit greater.

INFORMED CONSENT

Before starting any treatment most doctors will want to discuss the benefits and problems of treatment and the possible different approaches which might be used. In a clinical trial doctors also have to discuss the reason for the study, the meaning of randomization and the right of the patient not to be involved. This creates problems for both doctors and patient. Their relationship may be upset by these disclosures, especially the admission that the results of the treatments are not known with certainty. There may have to be discussion of failure rates in the disease. The patient may become confused, and this, and the time necessary for explanation, may deter many doctors from becoming involved in trials.

In most studies the patient is asked if he or she will take part. If he declines, he is not entered into the study but if he agrees randomization proceeds. In order to avoid some of the difficulties posed by this procedure Zelen [13] has proposed a randomized consent design. In this system patients are randomized to A (conventional treatment) or B (new treatment). No consent is sought for A. For those randomized to B, consent is sought. If it is not given, the patient undergoes treatment A.

Several problems are posed with Zelen's system. Is this really informed consent? What if those patients randomized to B accept or refuse for reasons relating to their illness? For example, more patients with large tumours might opt for radical surgery than those with small ones. This would bias the distribution of cases. To meet these objections the method has been further modified. It is too soon to judge the usefulness of this approach. One problem is that if many patients drop out of the study the trial efficiency is considerably weakened.

Non-randomized studies of treatment

The difficulties of controlled trials of treatment have led many investigators to perform uncontrolled studies and to report survival with a given treatment in the hope that a clear advantage over the best current methods of treatment will be shown. The result has been a plethora of sometimes misleading small-scale studies. There is an important role for well conducted pilot studies but the results must be interpreted cautiously.

A compromise has been sought between the cumbersome controlled trial and the unreliable uncontrolled study. This has involved the use of *historical control* which compares present treatment to patients treated in the past. An attempt is normally, but not always, made to match the controls for age, sex, site and stage of tumour and other known prognostic factors such as histological grade and menopausal status. The problems are of course that staging methods are changing continually, that selection of control cases may not be impartial, and that not all prognostic factors will be known.

These studies may sometimes point the way in management and indicate which questions should be asked in large-scale prospective studies. Another variant is the use of 'data bases' containing results of treatment of very large numbers of patients. Such analyses have the same problems of selection bias and thus the same unreliability in deciding on the value of a treatment.

SCREENING FOR CANCER

The aim of screening a population for cancer is to make the diagnosis early and thereby increase the cure rate. So far, the practical benefits have been small or non-existent, with the exception of carcinoma of the cervix. Recent studies in breast cancer screening (see p. 256) have shown some benefit for the screened population compared with the control (unscreened) population but the cost per patient cured is formidable. The problem is simply summarized in Fig. 2.11. The objective of screening is simple yet there are many problems and assumptions involved:

1 *What is the sensitivity of the test used?* Highly sensitive tests are essential if the disease is curable early and if the consequences of a false-positive test are not serious for the patients physically or psychologically. The Papanicolaou smear is a sensitive test for cervical cancer and the diagnosis can be easily confirmed on biopsy. By contrast, abdominal ultrasound is an insensitive test for carcinoma of the pancreas and the diagnosis is difficult to confirm. This test is therefore of no value as a screening investigation. Self-examination for breast cancer is relatively insensitive but the finding of a lump can lead to early confirmation of the diagnosis. However, it does not improve results of treatment and is not a useful screening method.

2 *Is the disease curable if diagnosed early?* Carcinoma *in situ* or locally invasive carcinoma of the cervix are curable diseases. It remains to be proven, however, whether earlier diagnosis of colorectal cancer using screening by sigmoidoscopy or faecal occult blood testing will increase cure rate. Tumours such as colorectal cancer present late in their natural history and the limit of detection by screening may be only one or two doublings earlier than when the tumour would be clinically apparent. The question is whether the potential for metastasis is significantly less at the time when such a tumour is detectable by screening methods compared with the stage at which it is clinically apparent. It is true that, in breast cancer for example, small tumours have a better prognosis than large ones. This may, however, be partly due to the biological behaviour of small tumours rather than the tumour being detected earlier in its natural history. There is nothing to suggest that carcinoma of the head of the pancreas carries a better prognosis if diagnosed early since the results of treatment are poor at any stage.

3 *Is the disease common?* Cancer of the breast, cervix and lung are so common at certain ages

and in certain groups that screening is a practical proposition. Screening a general population for a disease such as gastric carcinoma is less practicable in Britain, but it is in Japan where the disease is much more common. Clearly the incidence of the tumour has to be high enough to justify the screening programme.
4 *How frequently should the examination be undertaken, and in which population?* In some countries cervical smears are recommended every 3 years in women aged 20–65 years. In Britain the recommendation is for all sexually active women to be screened and the recommended frequency is 5-yearly. Breast self-examination can be carried out frequently but has not been shown to be of value in screening. It is not clear what recommendations should be made for other investigations such as pelvic examination (for ovarian and uterine cancer) and sigmoidoscopy. The group at greatest risk from ovarian cancer includes nulliparous women over the age of 40 years; and for colorectal cancer, men and women over 50 years. Routine chest X-rays, even in smokers, have failed to show any benefit from early detection of lung cancer. Patients with a greatly increased genetic predisposition to certain cancers (e.g. polyposis coli (Chapter 16, p. 308) should have regular checks by the appropriate specialist.
5 *What are the disadvantages of screening?* Routine screening examinations can produce anxiety in the mind of the public at large and in certain individuals in particular. If applied to the whole population they would require a great expenditure of time and money. The benefits may be small and achieved at great expense. If the yearly incidence of breast cancer in women aged 50–70 years is taken at 2 per 1000, by screening 10 000 women every two years, 40 new cases may be expected. If this is done by mammography and trained nurses in a clinic the cost might be in the region of £20 per visit. Even if the cure rate were improved from 30% to 60% by this procedure then six women would have been saved at a cost of £200 000. Screening of this type is, therefore, more expensive than much 'high technology' medicine.

The longest established screening procedure in the Western world is the cervical smear for carcinoma of the cervix. Breast cancer screening has now been introduced in the United Kingdom and other European countries. There remain considerable doubts as to its cost-effectiveness, and difficulties over the treatment to be recommended when early breast cancer is diagnosed (e.g. ductal carcinoma *in situ*). Screening procedures which have been proposed, but not always convincingly validated, are listed below and are discussed in the appropriate chapters:

Breast cancer (Chapter 13)	Self-examination Nurse or doctor examination Mammography
Colorectal cancer (Chapter 16)	Occult blood testing Rectal examination Sigmoidoscopy
Ovarian and uterine cancer (Chapter 17)	Pelvic examination Pelvic ultrasound CA-125
Skin cancers (Chapter 22)	Self-examination
Gastric cancer — Japan (Chapter 14)	Radiological and endoscopic examination

The most important outcome measure in a screening programme is *mortality*, which may require prolonged follow-up (for example, in the case of breast cancer). The efficacy of the screening programme should also be reflected in a shift towards diagnosis at an earlier stage of the tumour.

SECONDARY PREVENTION OF CANCER

Some cancers arise in a 'field' of malignant change in which the tissue adjacent to a cancer has been subject to the same carcinogenic process which gave rise to the initial tumour. The clearest example of this is the squamous carcinoma of the upper aerodigestive tract —

mouth, pharynx, oesophagus and bronchi — which have been exposed to cigarette smoke. After development and treatment of one such cancer could a second be prevented? In the case of head and neck cancer, after successful therapy, 30–50% of patients develop local or regional recurrence and 10–40% a second primary tumour.

In recent years it has been shown that vitamin A analogues are able to modulate the differentiation of epithelial cells, can cause the regression of the lesions of leucoplakia, and diminish the likelihood of developing squamous cancer as long as treatment continues. A recent trial [14] has now shown that isotretinoin (13-*cis*-retinoic acid), given as an adjuvant following treatment of head and neck cancer, greatly diminishes the risk of second cancers developing but does not diminish the likelihood of recurrence. This interesting finding will open the way to other secondary prevention trials (for example in squamous lung cancer) as well as primary prevention in high-risk groups.

REFERENCES

1 Devesa S.S., Silverman D.T. Cancer incidence and mortality trends in the United States: 1935–1974. *Journal of the National Cancer Institute* 1978; **60**: 545–71.

2 Haenszel W., Kurihera M. Studies of Japanese migrants: 1 Mortality from cancer and other diseases among Japanese in the United States. *Journal of the National Cancer Institute* 1968; **40**: 43–68.

3 Doll R. The epidemiology of cancer. *Cancer* 1980; **45**: 2475–85.

4 Doll R., Hill A.B. Study of aetiology of carcinoma of the lung. *British Medical Journal* 1952; ii: 1271–86.

5 Bizzoreo O.J., Johnson K.G., Ciocco A. Leukaemia in Hiroshima and Nagasaki. *New England Journal of Medicine* 1966; **274**: 1095–1101.

6 Tokunaga M., Land C.E., Yamanisho T., Asano M., Tokuokas Ezaki H., Nishimori I. Breast cancer in Japanese A-bomb survivors. *Lancet* 1982; ii: 924.

7 Court-Brown W.M., Doll R. *Leukaemia and aplastic anaemia in patients treated for ankylosing spondylitis* (Medical Research Council Special Report Series, No. 295), London, HMSO, 1957.

8 Doll R. An epidemiological perspective of the biology of cancer. *Cancer Research* 1978; **38**: 3573–83.

9 Epstein S.S., Swartz J.B. Fallacies of life-style cancer theories. *Nature* 1981; **289**: 127–30.

10 Peto R. Distorting the epidemiology of cancer: the need for a more balanced overview. *Nature* 1980; **284**: 297–300.

11 Sheil A.G.R. Cancer in organ transplant recipients: part of an induced immune deficiency syndrome. *British Medical Journal* 1984; **288**, 659–61.

12 Yusuf S., Collins R., Peto R. Why do we need some large, simple randomized trials? *Statistics in Medicine* 1984; **3**: 409–22.

13 Zelen M. A new design for randomized clinical trials. *New England Journal of Medicine* 1979; **300**: 1242–50.

14 Hong W.K., Lippman S.M., Itri L.M. *et al.* Prevention of second primary tumours with isotretinoin in squamous-cell carcinoma of the head and neck. *New England Journal of Medicine* 1990; **323**: 795–801.

FURTHER READING

Peto R., Pike M.C., Armitage P. *et al.* Design and analysis of randomized clinical trials requiring prolonged observation of each patient. *British Journal of Cancer* **34**, 585 (1976); **35**, 1–29 (1977).

Pocock S.J. *Clinical trials.* Chichester: Wiley, 1983.

Spodick D.H. The randomised controlled clinical trial: scientific and ethical bases. *American Journal of Medicine* 1982; **73**: 420–25.

Chapter 3
Biology of Cancer

INTRODUCTION

When thinking about cancer many scientists and physicians, and members of the public, perceive cancer as being 'foreign' to the body. Analogies with infections caused by parasites and germs are often drawn, and many infectious agents have been proposed as aetiological agents. As knowledge has progressed it has, however, become apparent that in many respects cancer cells are similar to normal cells and that there is considerable diversity of function and structure within a single neoplasm. Even greater diversity exists between tumours of the same type in different individuals and between tumours of different types. The fundamental property of cancer which distinguishes the disease from normal tissues, and which makes treatment so difficult, is metastasis. We are still ignorant of the mechanisms which underlie this remarkable process.

In this chapter some of the mechanisms of oncogenesis, growth and spread of tumours are briefly reviewed.

PHYSICOCHEMICAL CAUSES OF CANCER

Chemical carcinogens

It has long been suspected that cancers might have a chemical cause. In 1775, Sir Percival Pott noticed an unusually large number of cases of cancer of the scrotum in chimney sweeps and in 1895, Rehn pointed out the high frequency of bladder cancer in dye factory workers. A wide variety of carcinogens has been described and some of these are shown in Table 3.1.

Some of the mechanisms of chemical carcinogenesis have now been elucidated. There are several types of carcinogen which are candidates for causing cancer in humans (see below). For a more detailed account the reader is referred to references [1] and [2].

POLYCYCLIC HYDROCARBONS

These chemicals are among the products of combustion of carbon-containing materials. They are present in coal tar (from soot), cigarette smoke, car exhaust fumes and some cooked foods. One of the major developments in understanding the relationship between cancer and

Table 3.1 Some chemical carcinogens

Polycyclic hydrocarbons:	3:4-benzpyrene 1:2, 5:6-dibenzpyrene
Nitrosamines:	Dimethylnitrosamine
Aromatic amines and azo dyes:	Beta-naphthylamine Dimethylamino azobenzene Benzidine
Plant products:	Aflatoxin Senecis (producing pyrrolozidium)
Alkylating agents:	Nitrogen mustard Melphalan Nitrosourea Etoposide
Inorganic chemicals:	Arsenic Nickel Asbestos Cadmium

the environment was when Kennaway and his co-workers showed that benzanthracene was present in coal tar and subsequently that it was carcinogenic. Later 3:4-benzpyrene was isolated from coal tar and was also shown to be carcinogenic and capable of inducing skin cancers in animals. Not all polycyclic hydrocarbons are carcinogens. It appears that the carcinogenic property resides in one region of the molecule, the K-region, to which oxygen is added in a reaction catalysed by cellular enzymes (e.g. aryl hydrocarbon hydroxylase). This epoxide portion of the molecule reacts with cellular DNA, especially with guanine bases. It is this reaction with DNA which is thought to be responsible for its carcinogenic effect.

NITROSAMINES

Dimethylnitrosamine was shown to cause liver cancer in animals when added to their food. Nitrites, which are present in many foods, are converted to nitrous acid in the stomach and may then react with amines in food to produce nitrosamines. Thus a mechanism exists for the formation of a potential carcinogen from food. However, there is no definite evidence that the formation of nitrosamines is important in carcinogenesis in humans.

AROMATIC AMINES AND AZO DYES

Following Rehn's original observation of the increased frequency of bladder cancer in aniline dye workers, the aniline derivatives β-naphthylamine and benzidine were shown to be carcinogens. Later azo dye derivatives were also found to be carcinogenic including dimethylamino azobenzene (butter yellow) which was used to add colour to margarine (Table 3.1). When ingested these substances produce cancers at sites remote from the gut. They are first metabolized to an active form which is the carcinogen. For example, β-naphthylamine is hydroxylated to a carcinogen which is then glucuronated to an inactive water-soluble form in the liver and excreted in the urine. Glucuronidases in the bladder mucosa liberate active carcinogen (an aminophenol) again and the cancers develop only in those species which possess this bladder enzyme.

The aminophenol reacts directly with guanine bases on DNA and, as with polycyclic hydrocarbons, this is presumed to be the basis of their carcinogenic action. In humans there is a 20-year latent period between exposure and the development of bladder cancer. Cigarette smoke also contains β-naphthylamine (see Chapter 12) and bladder cancer is associated with smoking

AFLATOXIN

This toxin is produced by *Aspergillus flavus* which may contaminate staple foods. It may be a carcinogen in hepatic cancer and there is an association between dietary aflatoxin and the high frequency of hepatic cancers in Mozambique, although direct proof is lacking. The hepatitis B virus is involved in the development of a hepatoma, aflatoxin perhaps acting as a promoter (see below). The toxin is a complex molecule which is metabolized by the same pathway as polycyclic hydrocarbons and the hydroxy product reacts with DNA.

ALKYLATING AGENTS

Drugs used in the treatment of cancer are also carcinogens. Alkylating agents bind directly to DNA (see pp. 94—97) and their use has been associated with the development of second malignancies, for example acute leukaemia in patients successfully treated for Hodgkin's disease or ovarian cancer.

Ionizing and ultraviolet irradiation

The effects of ionizing irradiation on the cell are discussed in Chapter 5. Irradiation produces breaks in DNA strands and chromosomal abnormalities such as fragmentations, deletions and translocations. These abnormalities lead to cell death in dividing cells. The mechanisms of carcinogenesis are, however, poorly understood. There is no doubt that cancers can be caused by ionizing radiation. Skin cancers developed on the hands of the early radiologists, and there is a significant and dose-related increase in acute and chronic myeloid leukaemia and in breast and thyroid cancer in the survivors of the atom bomb explosions at Hiroshima and Nagasaki.

It is difficult to extrapolate from the high dose received after the atom bomb explosions, to an assessment of the risks from the much smaller levels of background radiation. The average exposure as a result of toxic waste is 0.001 mSv (millisievert) with a maximum of 0.3 mSv. 0.3 mSv is the average dose from clinical X-rays, and the same as cosmic rays. The average annual total dose in the United Kingdom from all sources is about 2.5 mSv. The best estimates now place the death rate at about 3 to 5 cases per 100000 per millisievert of prolonged exposure. This would account for perhaps 2000 cancer deaths per year out of 160000 annually in the United Kingdom. Radiation exposure is a vastly less important cause of cancer than cigarette smoking, and industrial exposure is the least important source of background radiation [3].

Ultraviolet (UV) light increases the likelihood of development of skin cancer (see Chapter 22). DNA absorbs photons and alterations in thymine bases occur with the formation of dimers. In normal individuals these pyrimidine dimers are rapidly repaired by nucleotide excision repair. Faulty repair leads to base mismatch mutations. UV damage to the p53 gene (see p. 35) may be inefficiently repaired and the resulting mutation may lead to an impaired function of the p53 protein. This, in turn, leads to disordered cell growth (see p. 38). In xeroderma pigmentosum the DNA repair process is faulty, leading to an excess of skin cancers (though not cancers at other sites).

Initiators and promoters in carcinogenesis

Some agents appear to act as 'initiators' (Fig. 3.1): they produce a permanent change in the cells with which they come in contact but do not themselves cause cancer. This contact may result in a gene mutation. Other agents act as 'promoters' producing *transient* changes and only causing cancer when they are repeatedly in contact with cells which have been 'initiated' by another compound [2]. Promoters work over a long period of time and do not appear to be mutagenic themselves, while initiators may only require a brief exposure. The distinction is, however, not clear-cut since some initiators can themselves cause cancer. Mutagenic agents tend to act as initiators; and other factors, such as hormones or dietary constituents (e.g. cholesterol), as promoters. From a clinical point of view, cancers are more likely to arise as a result of long-continued exposure to an agent and removal of the agent may result in stabilization or even diminution of the increased risk. Cessation of cigarette smoking is an example of how the risk of developing cancer can be reduced by removal of the stimulus.

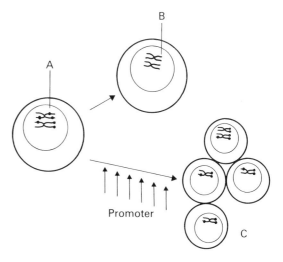

Fig. 3.1 Initiators and promoters in carcinogenesis. A: chromosomal damage is caused by an initiator. This might be repaired, as in B, or, under the influence of a promoter, give rise to neoplastic growth, stage C.

Repair of damage to DNA [4]

Cells are able to repair damage to DNA. The process of repair is through two general mechanisms. In base excision repair the abnormal piece of DNA is excised enzymatically, firstly by endonucleases which cleave the DNA strand, then by exonucleases which remove the abnormal segment, followed by the action of a polymerase which resynthesizes the missing segment which is then joined to the strand by a ligase. More complex lesions are repaired by *nucleotide excision repair* in which there is excision of a longer strand of DNA, the strand being then resynthesized by polymerase. These repair processes are essential mechanisms for all living cells. Actively transcribed genes are repaired more efficiently than inactive genes. After the cell has undergone division, if any unrepaired lesions remain on the DNA, the DNA is replicated up to the point of damage and this damaged segment is then resynthesized using the other strand as a template.

DNA repair therefore depends on complex mechanisms in which many repair enzymes are involved. The ability of the cells of an individual to repair DNA damage varies and may itself be under genetic control. Thus susceptibility to cancer may depend on the genetic control of enzymes which convert carcinogens to their active form and on regulation of other enzymes which are responsible for the repair process.

VIRAL CAUSES OF CANCER

Some animal cancers are known to be virally induced, and the possibility that human cancers might also be caused by a virus has led to research to find candidate viruses and evidence of infection.

Viruses causing tumours in animals were discovered at the turn of the century. In 1910, Peyton Rous showed that a cell-free filtrate made from avian sarcomas could induce new sarcomas in chickens, and at the same time the disease avian myeloblastosis was shown to be viral in origin. Much later it was realized that

viruses might require a long latent period before the tumour appeared. However, it was not until the 1960s that it was appreciated that incorporation of viral DNA into the host genome was usually a prerequisite of malignant transformation, and that infectious virus might not be isolated from the cancer cell.

Two patterns of viral oncogenesis have been described. In both instances the viral genome is incorporated into the cellular DNA. In the first, the virus has a gene, *oncogene*, which quickly 'transforms' the cell in culture and causes tumours *in vivo*. The action of the oncogene dominates the cell. In the second, the virus acts slowly and tumours take longer to appear. These viruses do not transform cells in culture.

RNA viruses

RNA viruses are implicated in the production of a wide variety of tumours in animals, notably lymphomas, leukaemias and sarcomas. In the virus there are two identical RNA molecules within a glycoprotein envelope together with the duplex enzyme reverse transcriptase. Through the action of this enzyme the viruses are able to make the cell synthesize a sequence of DNA, complementary to their RNA, which is incorporated into host DNA. The action of the DNA leads to the manufacture of new viral proteins, envelope and reverse transcriptase (Fig. 3.2). They are therefore sometimes called *retroviruses*. They are of similar appearance on electron microscopy and are the smallest of the tumour viruses.

Some retroviruses (e.g. avian leukosis, feline and murine leukaemia) have only three genes and have a long incubation period before producing the tumour in animals. Others rapidly transform cells and are usually isolated from tumours in culture. They produce tumours quickly after inoculation, an example being the Rous sarcoma virus (RSV). RSV has been shown to contain a gene (now called V-*src*) which appears to be the gene responsible for transformation of fibroblasts in culture. This gene appears to code for a protein kinase which

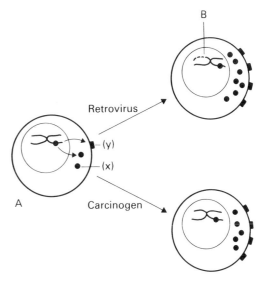

Fig. 3.2 The process of retrovirus multiplication.

Fig. 3.3 Oncogenes and malignant transformation. In stage A, a normal cell has a low level of proto-oncogene activity producing a growth factor (x), or a differentiation protein or a receptor (y). Carcinogens increase the activity of the proto-oncogene and give rise to neoplastic transformation. Infection with a retrovirus leads to insertion of viral promoter sequences or oncogenes, stage B, and excess oncogene activity, also resulting in neoplastic transformation.

phosphorylates tyrosine, but it is not clear how this enzyme might be involved in malignant transformation.

It has become apparent that normal and malignant cells contain DNA sequences which are similar or identical to the oncogenic sequences of RNA tumour viruses. These are known as *cellular proto-oncogenes*, as distinct from viral oncogenes. It is postulated that it is these cellular oncogenes which, when activated by carcinogens, cause the events which lead to malignant transformation (Fig. 3.3). It has been suggested that retroviruses have incorporated these cellular genes into the viral genome during evolution.

The products of gene activation are now receiving increasing attention. As mentioned above, a phosphokinase is produced by *src* and other viral oncogenes; epidermal growth factor receptor by the v-*erb* B gene; a platelet-derived growth factor fragment by the v-*sis* gene and a variety of nuclear-binding proteins by avian leukaemia virus. The connection between these viral gene products and malignant transformation remains to be determined. Viral oncogene products may differ from their cellular counterparts (from which they may originally have been derived). They lack introns and may have structural differences. For example, the v-*erb* product is the homologue of the cellular receptor for epidermal growth factor (EGF) but lacks part of the extracellular domain including the EGF binding site. Together with loss of a cytoplasmic site for autophosphorylation the receptor is permanently 'switched on' (see Fig. 3.5).

In other cases the virus may activate cellular processes by inserting a promoter or enhancer sequence adjacent to a region of an oncogene, disturbing its normal process of control of transcription. This process of insertional muta-genesis may be very complex. An example is the insertion of the viral long terminal repeat (LTR) sequence which may allow transcription of both viral and cellular genes since the LTR may be able to initiate transcription in either direction on the DNA strand. This occurs with the avian leukosis virus which is integrated next to c-*myc* thereby activating it.

The first retrovirus to be definitely associated with malignancy was HTLV-1 (human T cell leukaemia/lymphoma virus) isolated from the T cell cancer mycosis fungoides. The virus is widely distributed, transmitted sexually, by intravenous drug abuse, and perinatally. It is prevalent in tropical countries, but in the United States seropositivity is 1 in 4000. In addition to the association with T cell leukaemia it is the cause of tropical spastic paraplegia. The risk of disease over 20 years of seropositivity is about 5%.

The greatest impetus to research in this area has undoubtedly come from analysis of the structure and function of the human immuno-deficiency virus-1 (HIV-1) which is the cause of AIDS. A simplified structure of the HIV-1 virus is shown in Fig. 3.4. The envelope protein (gp120) binds to the CD4 protein on helper T cells and monocytoid cells, fuses with the cell membrane and enters the cell. A single strand of DNA is synthesized from viral RNA by the enzyme reverse transcriptase (a duplex of ribonuclease and polymerase). The DNA is integrated into host DNA and more virus is produced. Mutations in the HIV genome occur rapidly and make vaccine development difficult.

HIV-1 infection is associated with cancers [5] which are mainly of three types: intermediate or high-grade B cell lymphoma, Kaposi's sarcoma (KS) and cervical carcinoma. About 40% of all patients infected will develop a can-cer. The relationship between the viral infec-tion and the different cancers is, however, complex. In AIDS patients it is six times more common in homosexual or bisexual men or their contacts. KS may not be an autonomous

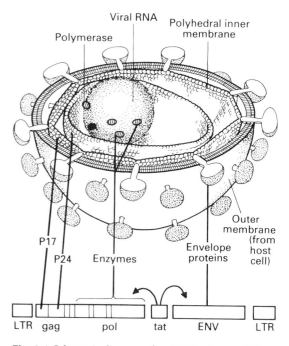

Fig. 3.4 Schematic diagram of an HIV-1 virus particle and its genetic structure. At the centre of the particle, the viral RNA is surrounded by a bullet-shaped core. The core, in turn, is surrounded by a polyhedral-shaped inner membrane. The virion's outer envelope, formed from the host cell membrane, is coated with 72 'spikes' of envelope proteins, which enable the virion to bind to a new host cell surface.

monoclonal tumour but an autocrine or para-crine driven proliferation. The lymphomas also have a complex pathogenesis since they are usually tumours of B cells which are not infected by HIV-1. Other viruses such as Epstein–Barr virus (EBV) may be involved on a background of chronic immunosuppression. Similarly, cer-vical cancer may be due to a second virus (such as human papilloma virus) in women who are immunosuppressed by HIV-1. The tumour appears particularly aggressive clinically.

DNA viruses

DNA viruses have also been implicated in the production of cancer. The largest in size is the herpes group which can cause malignancies in animals. EBV was first demonstrated in cultured cells from a patient with Burkitt's lymphoma. Virally coded proteins are present on the surface of Burkitt's lymphoma cell lines in tissue culture, and EBV will cause proliferation of human B cells *in vitro*. Antibody titres to viral capsid antigen and membrane antigen are higher in patients than in controls. Nevertheless, many African children are infected with EBV at some time although Burkitt's lymphoma develops in very few, so its role in oncogenesis is not clear. In addition, some non-African cases of Burkitt's lymphoma are not associated with the virus. EBV has been implicated in the pathogenesis of nasopharyngeal carcinoma.

Cytomegalovirus (CMV) is another DNA virus of the herpes group which may be implicated in the pathogenesis of Kaposi's sarcoma. AIDS patients have a high incidence of infection with CMV.

The DNA virus herpes simplex (HSV) type 2 causes recurrent ulceration of the genital tract. Recent seroepidemiological data have linked HSV2 with cervical carcinoma, and viral antigens have been shown in the cytoplasm of carcinoma *in situ*. However, a direct causal connection has not been established. Infection with HSV may be necessary, but not sufficient, to cause malignant transformation.

Other viruses

Human papilloma viruses are associated with *in situ* carcinoma of the cervix (see Chapter 17), and also cause benign papillomas.

Hepatitis B is associated with the development of hepatocellular carcinoma (see Chapter 15). It is not clear if the virus is a cause of malignant transformation; whether the viral infected cells are more susceptible to other carcinogens, for example, aflatoxin; or whether the association exists because the virus can cause cirrhosis which is associated with the development of hepatocellular cancer.

Cellular oncogenes [6]

The discovery of the sequence homologies between viral oncogenes and DNA found in normal and cancer cells has led to a greater understanding of growth regulatory mechanisms which may be abnormal in malignant cells. The term 'oncogene' may perhaps be a misnomer since, in malignancy, there may be abnormal activation of a normal gene or an abnormality in the gene leading to abnormal expression. In this sense these are not cancer genes but proliferation genes whose regulation may be disturbed in cancer.

Genes have been identified by homology with retroviral genes by DNA transfer and by gene rearrangements. The mechanisms of activation of the gene are varied.

In Burkitt's lymphoma there is reciprocal translocation of part of chromosome 8 with chromosomes 2, 14 or 22. The 8;14 translocation is commonest. The C-*myc* oncogene is adjacent to the part of chromosome 8 which is translocated, and the translocation is accompanied by reorganization of the C-*myc* gene. In chronic granulocytic leukaemia the C-*abl* oncogene is adjacent to the site of the chromosomal translocation (the Philadelphia chromosome, see Chapter 28, p. 551).

Although it is by no means clear that activation of a single proto-oncogene can lead to malignancy, increased expression of cellular oncogenes has been found in many human cancer cell lines, for example, C-*myc* in small cell lung cancer and Burkitt's lymphoma, and N-*myc* in neuroblastoma.

Examples are numerous and one or two will serve to illustrate some of the mechanisms.

Figure 3.5 shows a simplified scheme of the events which occur following binding of a growth factor to a membrane associated receptor. The receptor activates a signal transducing protein which may in turn bind other molecules such as guanine nucleotides (when the signal transducer is then called a G protein). These molecules in turn may stimulate the activity of a second messenger such as cAMP. Alternatively the internal component of the receptor may have tyrosine kinase activity leading to phosphorylation of tyrosines on intracellular proteins which results in activation.

Some of the best described 'oncogenes' and their products are shown in Table 3.2. The oncoprotein C-*erb* B1 is the receptor for epidermal growth factor (EGF). Binding of EGF (the ligand) to the receptor activates its tyrosine kinase activity which leads to protein phosphorylation in the cell. Altered expression or mutation of C-*erb* B1 in cancer (or by viral homologue v-*erb*) may lead to overactivation of receptor activity.

As previously mentioned, nine proteins bind GTP and also have GTPase activity which terminates the signal. Abnormal G proteins may be produced by mutated *ras* oncogenes, which have deficient GTPase activity and consequently lead to defective signal termination. The *ras* family consists of 3 members (H-*ras*-1, K-*ras*-2, N-*ras*) and other proteins which show partial homology (*rho*, R-*ras*, *ras*, *rab*). Activating

ras mutations have been found in 40% of human colon cancers, and 95% of pancreatic cancers. Excess production of the *ras* protein has been found in these cancers. The *ras* protein is capable of transforming fibroblasts in tissue culture, and its expression is associated with various stages of differentiation in embryonic life.

Recessive genetic mechanisms in cancer development [7,8]

The previous brief account of oncogenes has dwelt on genes which, when over-expressed, produce a transforming or growth-enhancing effect. It is now clear that some genes result in abnormal growth regulation when they are deleted, i.e. they act in a recessive manner. Usually both alleles must be affected and for this reason these recessive mechanisms have been most clearly defined in inherited cancer syndromes where there is a germ-line mutation or deletion of one allele and the tumour is associated with deletion or mutation of the remaining allele in childhood or adult life. Chromosome loss has been studied by using cell–cell hybrids and it has been shown that introduction of single chromosomes can suppress the tumorigenicity of cultured cells which lack a particular chromosome. Table 3.3 lists some of the features distinguishing oncogenes and 'anti-oncogenes'.

Retinoblastoma (p. 470), the Li–Fraumeni syndrome (p. 434) and Wilms' tumour (p. 461) are among the best studied tumours where recessive mechanisms have been shown. Knudson suggested that retinoblastoma would arise as a two-step process in which a germline allele loss would be followed by loss of the other allele. It seems that loss of the second allele is usually by recombination or mitotic non-disjunction. Survivors of retinoblastoma have a greatly increased (500×) risk of osteosarcoma but, curiously, the tumours are restricted to these sites (bone and eye). The Rb gene is located at chromosome 13q14. Its function is unknown but it might be to suppress other genes whose action leads to cell growth.

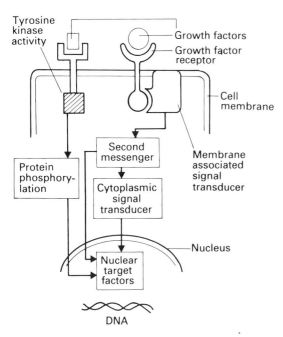

Fig. 3.5 Mechanisms of signal transduction of lay membrane-associated receptors for a growth factor. The normal events are shown in this simplified diagram. Abnormal activation may contribute to tumour growth.

Table 3.2 Some oncogenes and their products associated with cancer in humans and animals

Oncogene	Activity	Association with human tumour	Association with animal tumour
src	Membrane Tyrosine Kinase		Chicken sarcoma
abl	Membrane Tyrosine Kinase	Chronic myeloid leukaemia, acute leukaemias	Murine leukaemia
erb B1	EGF receptor	Breast cancer	Chicken erythroblastosis
erb B2	EGF receptor activity Ligand unknown	Increased oppression in breast cancer (comedo and *in situ*)	
sis	Platelet derived growth factor	? Breast cancer	Simian sarcoma
ras	G protein	Adenocarcinoma of lung, prostate, large bowel	Rat sarcoma

The Wilms' tumour gene is located at 11p13 and, like retinoblastoma, loss of this region of the gene is found sporadically in non-inherited cancers such as osteosarcoma. Hereditary forms of Wilms' tumour are rare and 50% of people with the abnormal gene do not develop the tumour (see p. 461). The non-inherited tumour does, however, sometimes show a deleted 11p13 band and polymorphism studies have shown chromosome loss at this site in almost 50% of tumours.

Table 3.3 The distinguishing features of 'anti-oncogenes' and oncogenes

'Anti-oncogenes' or tumour suppressor genes	Oncogenes
Recessive in effect	Dominant in effect
Often tissue specific tumours, e.g. retinoblastoma	Tends to be broad specificity
Deletions promote cancer	Translocations increase activity
Germ line inheritance in some cases	Both hereditary and non-hereditary forms
Solid tumours	Often lymphomas and leukaemias

In the Li—Fraumeni syndrome there is a germ-line mutation in the p53 gene. Affected families are characterized by the proband having sarcoma in childhood, early-onset breast cancer in the mother or female siblings, and increased likelihood of cancer of the brain, adrenal gland or of leukaemia in other members. The p53 protein is a cell cycle regulatory nuclear phosphoprotein. It is frequently mutated in sporadic cancers of many types (p. 38).

INHERITANCE OF CANCER [9]

There are numerous inherited genetic abnormalities which predispose to the development of malignancy. The major syndromes are shown in Table 3.4. There has been great progress in the isolation and cloning of some of the genes involved in familial cancer syndromes. This is leading to an understanding of the molecular mechanisms of oncogenesis which has a wider significance than the inherited disorder itself. For example, in xeroderma pigmentosum the inherited abnormality appears to be in a DNA-repair protein. Furthermore, it is now apparent that there is a major genetic component in some common cancers such as cancer of the breast, ovary and colon. Isolation of genes

Table 3.4 Constitutional (inherited) genetic factors in cancer

Abnormality	Cancer	Abnormality	Cancer
Chromosomal abnormalities		*Immune deficiency disorders*	
Trisomy 21 (Down's syndrome)	Acute leukaemia	X-linked	Lymphoma
47 XXY (Klinefelter's syndrome)	Breast cancer	lymphoproliferative	
Mosaicism (45X0/46XY)	Gonadoblastoma	syndrome (XLR)	
11p−(aniridia−Wilms'	Wilms' tumour	Ataxia-telangiectasia (AR)	Lymphoma
syndrome)			Gastric cancer
13q−(multiple malformations)	Retinoblastoma	Sex-linked	Lymphoma
		agammaglobulinaemia	
Inherited bowel disorders		(Bruton) (XLR)	
Polyposis coli (AD)	Carcinoma of colon	Wiskott−Aldrich syndrome	Lymphoma
Gardner's syndrome (AD)	Carcinoma of colon	(XLR)	
Peutz−Jeghers syndrome (AD)	Duodenal cancer	IgA deficiency (S, AD, AR)	Adenocarcinomas
Tylosis palmaris (AD)	Oesophageal cancer		
		Miscellaneous syndromes	
Neurological−cutaneous disorders		Hemihypertrophy (AR)	Wilms' tumour
Von Recklinghausen's	Sarcomas		Hepatoblastoma
neurofibromatosis (AD)	Glioma	Beckwith's syndrome	Wilms' tumour
	Acoustic neuroma	(gigantism, macroglossia,	Hepatoblastoma
	Medullary thyroid cancer	mental retardation,	
Retinal/cerebellar angiomatosis	Phaeochromocytoma	visceromegaly) (S)	
(Von-Hippel−Lindau	Hypernephroma	Multiple enchondromas	Chrondrosarcoma
syndrome) (AD)	Ependymoma	(Ollier's syndrome) (S)	
Tuberous sclerosis (AD)		Bloom's syndrome	Leukaemias
	Gliomas	(telangiectasia, short	Numerous other cancers
Skin disorders		stature, chromosome	
(see Chapter 9, Table 9.2)		fragility) (AR)	
		Fanconi's anaemia	Acute leukaemia
		(skeletal abnormalities,	
		mental retardation,	
		pigmented patches)	

AD, autosomal dominant; AR, autosomal recessive; XLR, X-linked recessive; S, sporadic.

predicting for an increased likelihood of developing cancer will have major implications for cancer screening and for counselling services. At present we have little to guide us in approaching families of affected patients, either in helping them decide if they would wish to be screened for carrier status or in helping them cope with the knowledge that they may have inherited a susceptibility gene.

CLONAL ORIGIN, PROGRESSION AND GROWTH OF A CANCER

The three major characteristics of malignant neoplasms in humans are first, that growth is not subject to the normal constraints of the parent tissue. Second, that cancers always show a degree of anaplasia, which is a loss of cellular differentiation. This is associated with a lack of some of the functions of the normal, differentiated parent tissue. Third, that cancers have the property of metastasis, that is the ability to spread from the site of origin to distant tissues.

While these features are present in most human malignant neoplasms, some of these properties are not absolutely distinct from normal tissues. Thus it is true that the normal regulatory mechanisms controlling growth are defective in cancer, but that is not to say that there is no check or constraint on the pattern of growth of human neoplasms (see below). Similarly, although we regard the most anaplastic of cancers as 'undifferentiated' in the sense that they seem to have arisen from the more primitive precursors of the differentiated tissue; many cancers none the less do retain some of the functions of the mature tissues. Metastasis is, however, a property unique to cancer. Furthermore, it is metastasis which in most instances kills the patient and understanding the biology of metastasis is one of the central problems of cancer research.

In previous sections we have considered stimuli to the development of cancer either by viruses or chemical agents. This section is concerned with the events which follow the carcinogenic event and which lead to the development of an invasive, metastasizing malignancy.

Monoclonality and heterogeneity in cancer

There is now a considerable body of evidence that most human neoplasms are monoclonal in origin. This means that the original oncogenic event affected a single cell, and that the tumour is the result of growth from that one cell. There are two major lines of evidence which have led to this conclusion. First, certain women are heterozygotes for two forms of the enzyme glucose 6-phosphate dehydrogenase (G6PD). These forms can be recognized by their different electrophoretic mobilities. The gene for the enzyme is carried on the X chromosome and, in female heterozygotes, either the maternal or paternal form is present on either one of the X chromosomes. In a female, each cell loses activity of one or other X chromosome and therefore, in a heterozygote for this enzyme, every cell in the body will either have one form of the enzyme or the other. In studies on haematological malignancies arising in heterozygotes for G6PD, the cancers are found either to contain the maternal form of the enzyme or the paternal form is present, implying that the original cancer arose from one cell which either had one form of the enzyme or the other.

In chronic granulocytic leukaemia the restriction of the enzyme expression is found in cells of the granulocyte series and, importantly, in red cells and platelets as well as implying that a stem cell is affected by the malignant process.

In Burkitt's lymphoma the lymphoid cells are also restricted in enzyme expression. If a remission is induced and the patient relapses quickly the same isoenzyme will be present indicating a failure to eradicate the disease. With later relapse the other form of the isoenzyme may be present alone, implying that the 'relapse' is really a new malignant clone.

The technique is much harder to apply to carcinomas and the results in solid tumours may prove to be different from those in haematological malignancies. It is still possible that some carcinomas arise from a 'field of change' in a tissue with many clones arising at the same time. An interesting analysis of bladder cancer in women [10] has shown that in bladder cancer cells arising in different areas of the bladder there was the same pattern of suppression ('Lyonization') of the X chromosome in all cells from a given tumour, while the normal bladder cells showed random suppression of one or other of the two chromosomes. This strongly suggests a single clonal origin. In addition there was the same pattern of allele deletion on 9q, while losses on 17p and 18q were variable, suggesting these were later events in the evolution of the tumour.

The second line of evidence pointing towards the monoclonal origin of human neoplasms comes from lymphomas and other lymphoid malignancies in which it can be shown that the immunoglobulin produced by the lymphoid neoplasm (on its surface, or exported into the blood in the case of myeloma) is nearly always monoclonal, being of a single class and showing light chain restriction (see Chapter 27).

One problem with the concept of monoclonality is that it has sometimes led investigators to believe that there is a far greater uniformity of behaviour of cancer than is in fact the case. In spite of the monoclonal origin of neoplasms, significant heterogeneity appears to arise during the course of development of the tumours. This has important implications for treatment and for understanding the nature of metastases.

How does heterogeneity arise? If the tumour is *polyclonal* in origin then diversity can be explained on this basis. If *monoclonal*, other explanations are needed. It has been postulated that the occurrence of malignancy confers an inherent genetic instability on the clonogenic cells and that, during the course of the growth of the tumour, phenotypic differences in clonogenic cells develop. Thus there is the development of mutants, some of which survive and undergo still further changes, whereas others, depending on their ability to survive hormonal, biochemical or immunological adversity, die. The mature tumour can therefore be envisaged as being composed of cells which are monoclonal in origin, but diverse in capacity to metastasize and to resist cytotoxic drugs and immune attack.

We now have a much greater insight into the genetic events which are associated with some of the generation of diversity within the tumour. A sequence of defined chromosomal alteration during the progression from colonic polyp to colonic cancer is illustrated in Fig. 16.3. As the tumour progresses increasing genetic instability occurs with different cells within the same tumour showing a wide variety of chromosome breaks, deletions and reduplications. Morphologically, this is accompanied by change in nuclear appearance and increasingly bizarre and pleomorphic cytological forms.

Great interest has been aroused by the finding that many cancers acquire mutations in the p53 gene [11]. This gene encodes a nuclear phosphoprotein which appears to act as a check to the cell cycle, arresting the cell in G_1 as a result of DNA damage. UV light and cytotoxic drugs induce a rapid increase in p53 in normal cells due to a stabilization of the protein after translation (not due to increased transcription). Loss of p53 function (by mutation of the gene) means that mitosis can begin with damaged DNA.

The stimulus to p53 stabilization may be DNA double-strand breaks, but we do not yet know how the normal cell relays the signal or how the stabilization is produced. The mutations in cancer result in a conformational change in the protein making it inactive. It is known that normal p53 binds to DNA as a tetramer after an activation step. Mutant forms of the protein may be exceptionally stable and unable to bind to DNA. p53 mutation may thus be an important step on the pathway of tumour progression where an already malignant cell is permitted to move into cell cycle without time to repair damaged DNA. The scene may in this way be set for further unstable mutants to develop.

Diversities within the cells of a single tumour in both humans and in animals have been described with regard to growth rate, cytoplasmic constituents, hormone receptor status, radiosensitivity and susceptibility to killing by cytotoxic agents. For example, in the case of small cell carcinoma of the bronchus, different levels of cytoplasmic calcitonin, histaminase and L-dopa decarboxylase have been found in the primary tumour compared with a metastasis. Primary and secondary tumours may also show karyotypic differences.

Heterogeneity of neoplasms presents a formidable problem for the cancer therapist. If a single tumour shows diversity in cell phenotype and antigenic expression, it becomes hard to imagine how immunological attack can be successful. Likewise, a single tumour may contain cells with a wide variation in susceptibility to cytotoxic agents, thus providing the means for drug resistance to become clinically evident with repeated drug treatment.

The growth of cancer

Following mitosis (see Chapter 6, Fig. 6.1) cells may rest in the early growth phase (G_1) for a long period of time, but then enter a phase of DNA synthesis (S phase) and subsequently a later, shorter, G_2 phase. This is a prelude to mitosis which then takes place over a period of 30–90 minutes. The two daughter cells then enter G_1. Some cells of both normal tissues and cancer are not in cycle, and the term G_0 has been used to describe these cells.

Normal tissues vary greatly in both the rate of cell division and the numbers of cells which are actively proliferating. Examples of rapidly proliferating cells are the intestinal mucosa, the bone marrow, the hair follicle cells, and normal tissue regenerating after injury, for example after surgical resection or infections.

An idealized representation of the way in which proliferation occurs in a normal tissue is shown in Fig. 3.6. This figure shows the stem or progenitor cell supplying a proliferating pool of cells which follow a particular differentiation pathway. These become mature cells which are held to be incapable of further division and subsequently die. While this model may apply to human cancers, it is possibly an over-simplification. Tumours probably do contain progenitor and mature cells but it is not clear whether cell renewal in a tumour comes from a small progenitor fraction. Nevertheless the model is useful in explaining many aspects of tumour growth. In Fig. 3.7 the stem cell is shown as self-renewing. While the progeny of stem cell division go through successive divisions their number increases, but the number of further divisions they are 'programmed' to make declines concomitantly. Cell death is now the subject of intense investigation. It is apparent that the stimulus to death, and its mechanism is a programmed process under genetic control. Programmed cell death has been termed *apoptosis*. The morphological changes are condensation of the nucleus followed by pitting and explosion of the cytoplasm. The cell density rises, there is endo-nuclease activation and the DNA is cleaved. The bcl 2, *ras*, and LMP-1 genes appear to permit population expansion while p53 may prevent this. The cell may thus be switched to growth arrest, cell death or division by an active process. Explanation of these events may help us to understand more about the killing effects of cytotoxic drugs and radiation.

When a tumour is treated with radiation or

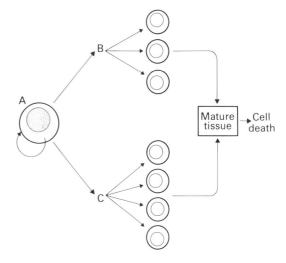

Fig. 3.6 Normal tissue renewal. The self-renewing stem cell (A) produces cells committed to differentiation path B or C. Cellular proliferation leads to mature tissue and then to cell death.

cytotoxic drugs it may shrink in size. This response may be entirely at the expense of later, non-self-renewing cells, in which case the tumour will regrow. To prevent regrowth it is probably essential to kill the progenitor or stem cells responsible for tumour growth. The growth fraction of a tumour is the proportion of cells in active proliferation. Many cancer cells have long cycle times and calculations of the growth fraction may underestimate the proliferative capacity of the tumour. These slow growing cells are probably less susceptible to chemo-therapy, particularly using cycle active agents. It is possible that the cell cycle time in these cells may shorten as a result of cytoreductive treatment.

A normal tissue grows and develops to a point when cell proliferation is balanced by cell loss and the tissue remains static in size, unless subjected to a changing environment, for example the normal breast ductular tissue during the menstrual cycle or during pregnancy. In a cancer, on the other hand, the regulatory mechanisms appear to be defective and the tumour gradually increases in size. Nevertheless, it must be emphasized that this

Fig. 3.7 A model of tumour growth. The progeny of the stem cells divide, increasing the tumour size but gradually losing their proliferative capacity.

more than 150 μm from a nutrient capillary. Sometimes the centres of human cancers are grossly necrotic where the tumour has clearly outstripped its blood supply. Other possible causes of cell loss are unsuccessful mitosis (possibly due to chromosomal aberrations), and death of tumours by immune or inflammatory attack as a result of both specific immunity and non-specific processes excited by the tumour.

Doubling times of human tumours are enormously variable and Table 6.1 shows some of the measured volume doubling times in common human cancers. It is not clear whether tumours exhibit a consistent rate of growth from the origin of the cancer to the time when the patient has a massive tumour and is about to die. Certainly one can observe exponential growth (Fig. 3.8) in some human malignancies. In the case shown, if one were to extrapolate back to the origin of the tumour, it would prove to have arisen some 30 doublings (30 years) before the clinical presentation if the growth had been

Fig. 3.8 Growth of a squamous carcinoma. The patient had a peripheral squamous carcinoma, untreated because of dementia and hypertension. Over 4 years this almost spherical tumour increased slowly in size exhibiting exponential growth with a doubling time of just over 1 year.

does not necessarily mean a rapid growth. Figure 3.8 shows the volume doubling time of an almost spherical squamous carcinoma from one of our patients observed, untreated, over 4 years. Slow exponential growth can be seen with a volume doubling time of 1 year. During their growth, tumours undergo cell loss as well as cell renewal. This cell loss is partly due to the vascularization of tumours being somewhat defective. It appears that there is inadequate nutrition in the centre of tissues when they are may involve a complex interplay between MMPs, produced by the endothelial cells, and their natural inhibitors (see below).

One of the results of local invasion is that tumour cells can enter vascular and other channels of the body and metastasize. The sequence of events is shown in Fig. 3.11. Lymphatic spread, which is particularly common with carcinomas, follows invasion of lymphatic channels and the tumour cells grow in cords and clumps in the lymphatic vessels and lymph nodes. From there spread to distal lymph nodes readily occurs. Haematogenous spread occurs after tumour cells have entered the vessels near the primary tumour or have been shed into the blood from the thoracic duct. Tumour cells are then trapped in the next capillary network, that is, in the lung or liver. Certain tumours characteristically spread to some structures while others do not; for example, sarcomas typically metastasize to lungs, and breast cancer to the axial skeleton. Local anatomy is often important, for example, gastro-intestinal cancers typically spread via the portal venous system to the liver. Tumours may also metastasize via a tissue space, for example those arising in the peritoneal cavity may seed widely over the peritoneal space, and lung cancer may spread over the pleura.

Regional lymph nodes may form a barrier to further metastases from the primary site. It is not clear whether lymph nodes create a barrier to spread of tumour by virtue of specific immune mechanisms.

Having penetrated the vascular compartment, tumour cells must withstand the process of arrest in the capillary bed of an organ and then start to divide. At this site the tumour cell must leave the capillary bed of the new tissue. To do this the tumour cell must pass through the capillary endothelium and survive attack by host defence mechanisms such as phagocytic cells and so-called *natural killer* (NK) cells.

The capacity for invasion and colonization of distant tissues varies with different classes of tumour. Likewise, a given tumour type has a different tendency to metastasize in different

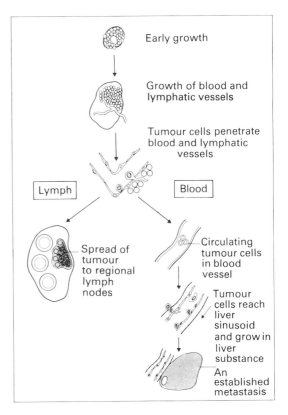

Fig. 3.11 Tissue invasion and the development of metastasis.

individuals. More disconcertingly, there may be heterogeneity in the metastatic potential of its constituent cells, even within a single tumour in an individual. In experiments using the B16 melanoma, it has been shown that cloned sublines from a single tumour differ markedly in their ability to metastasize. This suggests that the parent tumour is heterogenous in this respect. The basis of this variability is not known but it is possible that it may reflect differences in the surface properties of the neoplastic cells.

It is apparent that the problems of tissue invasion, metastatic spread and tumour heterogeneity are amongst the most fundamental in cancer research and clinical management of cancer patients. The lack of homogeneity of tumours, the similarities between tumours and their parent tissue and the lack of a single identifiable lesion in cancer cells which distinguishes them from normal, means that many of our simple assumptions about tumour immunity and the mode of action of cytotoxic drugs must be looked at critically, particularly if they are derived from experiments using homogeneous tumours.

TUMOUR IMMUNOLOGY

The idea that human tumours might be recognized as foreign to the host has obvious attractions, since if an immune response to the tumour occurred as part of the disease, or could be provoked artificially, there would be opportunities for using such an immune response diagnostically or therapeutically.

Methylcholanthrene-induced tumours, when transplanted to identical mice, sometimes regress and 'regressor' mice have resistance to further tumour transplants. This was shown to be tumour specific, i.e. resistance was only to the original tumour and not to an unrelated one. The antigens responsible were called tumour specific transplantation antigens (TSTA). Similar regression has been seen in virus-induced sarcomas in mice and here the antigen being recognized is a virally coded product on the tumour surface.

T cell cytotoxicity

T lymphocyte reactivity against human tumours is being reinvestigated now that it is possible to identify types of lymphocytes reliably, using antibodies (usually monoclonal — see below) to lymphocyte surface antigens which relate to function. Thus subpopulations of T cell with cytotoxic, helper and suppressor function can be identified in blood, lymph nodes and the infiltrates in tumours. T cells can be separated from natural killer cells in cytotoxicity experiments. It has now become clear that, in many cytotoxic systems, T cell killing will only take place if there is genetic identity between the effector T cells and the targets. This leads to

difficulty in demonstrating specific T cell anti-tumour cytotoxicity in humans, because the effector and target cells need to be derived from either the same individual, or one identical with respect to histocompatibility antigens.

This problem can be surmounted by techniques whereby antigen-specific T cells can be grown and multiplied in culture using a growth factor (IL-2) which allows T cells with both specific and defined functions to be propagated for long periods of time *in vitro*. If T cells from blood, draining lymph nodes or better still, from tumours, can be isolated, expanded in number and cloned, then a precise definition of their properties and target specificity should become possible. Carcinoma cells usually express class I major histocompatibility (MHC) antigens on their surface, but not class II. Some cancers also show loss of class I. It is now apparent that cellular proteins can be degraded in the cell to peptides which can bind to class I MHC and be potential recognition targets for CD4 T cells. Oligopeptides from exogenous proteins are, on the other hand, processed differently in the cell and are subsequently presented with class II MHC.

The questions now being addressed are therefore the nature of the peptides which are potentially tumour derived, whether they differ from cellular peptides of normal cells and whether they can be presented in such a way as to provoke a CD8 (cytotoxic) response [13].

Monoclonal antibodies

The development of somatic cell hybridization has allowed a serological definition of the tumour cell surface with a hitherto unattainable precision. Monoclonal antibodies are now prepared by this technique. The B-cell fusion partner is usually a murine myeloma. Some of the potential uses of monoclonal antibodies are listed in Table 3.5.

So far, monoclonal antibodies to human tumours have not been shown to define an antigen exclusively associated with malignant proliferation. Other antigens may be expressed as a result of rapid cell division and while they may be demonstrable in some cancers, using monoclonal reagents, they may also be present on some normal tissues such as bone marrow cells. The 'anti-cancer' monoclonals thus far produced appear to be identifying antigens which are expressed at a particular stage of differentiation of the cell type and it remains to be seen whether a truly cancer-associated antigen will be identified.

It is already clear that monoclonal reagents will be very useful in helping in the classification of cancer, in the diagnosis of undifferentiated tumours (Fig. 3.12) and possibly of therapeutic value in clearing sites such as the bone marrow of unwanted cells as part of the technique of autologous or allogeneic bone marrow. Coupling radioisotopes to these antibodies may be of value in tumour localization and treatment, while coupling of a cytotoxic agent to the monoclonal may provide a means of specific immunotherapy if the antibody can be shown not to identify vital host cells such as gut or marrow stem cells.

Immunotherapy of cancer

Until tumour antigens are defined and the nature of the immune response to them, if any, is elucidated, active specific immunity to cancer remains an elusive goal. In the absence of

knowledge of the antigens to which a specific and effective immune response could be generated attempts have been made to provoke immunity by altered widely distributed substances such as mucins, epithelial membrane antigen, the NCAM, and glycolipids. A related approach is to generate antibodies to the idiotype (the specific binding region) of other antibodies which recognize cell surface antigens. The anti-idiotype antibodies act as if they were

Table 3.5 Potential uses of monoclonal antibodies in cancer

Classification of tumours in tissue sections
Identification of 'undifferentiated' tumours in tissue sections
Diagnosis and classification of leukaemias
Diagnosis of metastatic tumour cells in low frequency, e.g. in bone marrow
Elimination of unwanted cells from bone marrow, e.g. metastatic tumour cells, residual leukaemic cells
Tumour localization by isotopically labelled antibody
Measurement of tumour products and 'markers', e.g. α-fetoprotein, CEA, peptide hormones
Coupling with cytotoxic agents or isotopes to kill tumour cells

---

Fig. 3.12 Use of monoclonal antibodies for immunocytochemical diagnosis. (A) Undifferentiated nasopharyngeal tumour. Differential diagnosis would include anaplastic carcinoma, lymphoma and melanoma. (B) Same tumour as in A, stained for common leucocyte antigen using a monoclonal antibody. The tumour cells show dark membrane staining indicating that the tumour is a lymphoma.

the 'tumour antigen' itself and may be more effective in provoking an immune response in which the actual tumour is damaged. Vaccines to viral antigens of hepatitis B, Epstein–Barr virus, or human papilloma virus may prove to be a practical approach for immunization to prevent cancer in high-risk groups, but tumour associated antigens are not sufficiently defined for this to be a practical proposition.

Treatment with non-specific immune or inflammatory mediators has not been generally effective (Table 3.5). These cytokine treatments are discussed in Chapter 6 (p. 117). Expansion of autologous lymphokine-activated killer (LAK) cells *in vitro*, by using IL-2, followed by reinfusion of the expanded and activated cell population has been extensively investigated. The aim is to divert a large number of activated non-specific cytotoxic lymphocytes to the tumour. There is little evidence that there is an increase in response over that achieved by the lymphokine (IL-2) alone. Curiously with most of these immunologically non-specific approaches to cancer treatment (BCG, IL-2, interferon, LAK cells) responses are confined to the same tumour types, namely melanoma and renal cell carcinoma. It is clear that there is something exceptional about these two tumours which renders them occasionally responsive to mediators of inflammation.

REFERENCES

1 Miller E.C., Miller J.A. Mechanisms of chemical carcinogenesis. *Cancer* 1981; **47**: 1055–64.

2 Farber E. Chemical carcinogenesis. *New England Journal of Medicine* 1981; **305**: 1379–89.

3 Dunster H.J. The appreciation of radiation risks. *Journal of the Royal College of Physicians* 1990; **24**: 154–55.

4 Barnes D.E., Lindahl T., Sedgwick B. DNA repair. *Current Opinion in Cell Biology* 1993; **5**: 15–20.

5 Levine A.M. AIDS-related malignancies: the emerging epidemic. *Journal of the National Cancer Institute* 1993; **85**: 1382–97.

6 Glover D.M., Hames B.D. *Oncogenes*. Oxford: Oxford University Press (IRL Press), 1989.

7 Knudson A.G. Hereditary cancer oncogenes and antioncogenes. *Cancer Research* 1985; **45**: 1437–43.

8 Green A.R. Recessive mechanisms of malignancy. *British Journal of Cancer* 1988; **58**: 115–21.

9 Li F.P. Cancer families: Human models of susceptibility to cancer. *Cancer Research* 1988; **48**: 5381–86.

10 Sidransky D., Frost P., von Eschenbach A. *et al.* Clonal origin of bladder cancer. *New England Journal of Medicine* 1992; **326**: 737–40.

11 Harris C.C., Hollstein M. Clinical implications of the p53 tumour-suppressor gene. *New England Journal of Medicine* 1993; **329**: 1318–28.

12 Hart I.R., Saini A. Biology of tumour metastasis. *Lancet* 1992; **339**: 1453–58.

13 Cerottini J.C., von Fliedner V., Boon T. Recognition of tumour-associated antigens by T lymphocytes: from basic concepts to new approaches. *Annals of Oncology* 1992; **3**: 11–16.

Chapter 4
Staging of Tumours

Although the overall prognosis of malignant tumours is often summarized by stating the proportion of patients alive at 5 or 10 years, such figures usually conceal a wide variation in survival, ranging from cures to deaths within a few months of diagnosis. The search for indicators of prognosis has occupied the attention of oncologists for many years. The object is to identify those patients for whom a treatment strategy (e.g. surgery alone) is likely to be successful and those in whom it will fail and for whom another approach must be adopted.

Staging the extent of the disease at presentation is one aspect of the identification of factors which will influence prognosis in any individual patient. The purposes of careful staging of tumour spread are:

1 To give appropriately planned treatment to the individual patient.

2 To be able to give the best estimate of prognosis.

3 To compare similar cases in assessing and designing trials of treatment (see Chapter 2).

4 To impose discipline in the accurate documentation of the initial tumour.

5 To assist our understanding of tumour biology.

STAGING NOTATION

For many tumours a useful staging notation is the TNM system developed by the American Joint Committee on Cancer Staging and End Result Reporting [1]. This system has the virtue of simplicity, drawing attention to the prognostic relevance of the size or local invasiveness of the primary tumour (T), lymph node spread (N) and the presence of distant metastases (M). Although widely used for solid tumours, and initially developed as an essentially surgical approach, it has obvious drawbacks for disorders such as diffuse lymphoma where the disease is often generalized, and is clearly inappropriate for leukaemias. Even in some solid tumours, such as small cell carcinoma of the bronchus and ovarian cancer, the practicality and usefulness of the system is limited. In these diseases different approaches must be used for staging, which are described in the appropriate chapters. For many gynaecological tumours the FIGO system (International Federation of Gynaecologists and Obstetricians) is often preferred (see, for example, p. 320). However, in the majority of solid tumours including cancers of the breast, head and neck, non-small cell lung cancer and genito-urinary system, the TNM system has found wide acceptance.

The primary tumour (T)

In some cancers the *size* of the primary tumour relates to prognosis. This is well illustrated by many cancers of the head and neck, such as oropharynx and oral cavity (see Chapter 10). In other tumours the T stage relates not to size but to *depth of invasion*, for example in melanoma, colon and bladder cancer (Fig. 4.1A). In squamous lung cancer the *size and site* of the primary tumour are both factors of prognostic importance (see Fig. 4.18). In some diseases the mode of spread is such as to make T status largely irrelevant. Examples are ovarian cancer, soft tissue sarcoma and small cell carcinoma of the lung. In such tumours 'stages of spread' are

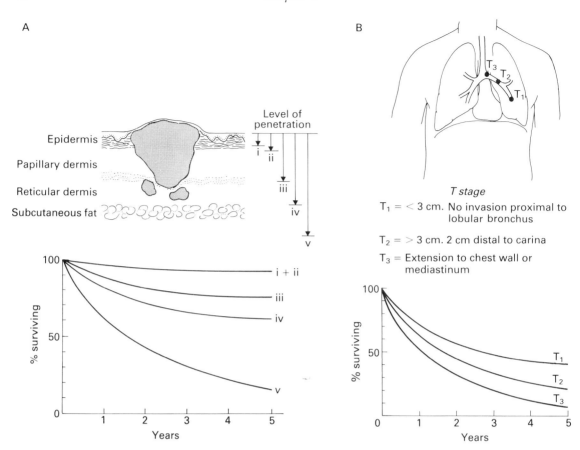

Fig. 4.1 Prognosis related to local extent of primary tumour. (A) Melanoma; (B) squamous carcinoma of the lung.

used which are often composites of tumour size and local or distant invasion. In melanoma, the depth of involvement in millimetres is probably a better predictor of prognosis than any other simple measure. In contrast, in squamous lung cancer local invasiveness and tumour site are more important than tumour size *per se* (p. 234).

Lymph node involvement (N)

Nodal involvement has profoundly important prognostic influence in many solid tumours (Fig. 4.2). In head and neck, bladder and large bowel cancers, for example, it is probably the most important determinant of survival. In most types of cancer, fixed (N_3) lymph nodes, which are surgically inaccessible, carry a far worse prognosis than mobile ipsilateral (N_1) nodes. Nodal involvement may strongly reflect a high probability of widespread haematogenous metastases, as for example in breast carcinoma. However, in other diseases, particularly cancers of the head and neck, it appears to carry considerable prognostic importance because of a higher local failure rate in such cases, often with fatal results.

Presence of metastases (M)

This clearly defines a group of patients who are surgically incurable. With very few exceptions (notably testicular tumours) the presence of distant metastatic disease has considerable prognostic implications, usually proving fatal

Prognosis related to N stage (all cases)

N_0 = No palpable nodes
N_1 = Mobile ipsilateral nodes
N_2 = Fixed ipsilateral nodes
N_3 = Supra- and infra-clavicular nodes

Prognosis related to tumour size and number of involved nodes

Fig. 4.2 Breast cancer. Prognosis related to N stage and to number of involved nodes and tumour size.

within months or a few years of diagnosis. Metastases may have been detected by clinical examination alone, or may have been found by meticulous investigation using specialized techniques.

STAGING TECHNIQUES

Many techniques are available for determining the extent of spread of a tumour at the time when a patient first presents. Much information can be obtained by investigations such as chest X-ray, full blood count and liver enzyme tests. Many of these investigations are performed routinely in a patient who has been diagnosed as having cancer or where the diagnosis is suspected.

A chest X-ray may show metastases in the lungs or the bones or extension of a bronchogenic carcinoma into the pleura or overlying ribs. Hilar or paratracheal lymph node enlargement may also be present. These findings indicate that the tumour has spread beyond its site of origin, and will considerably alter the approach to management.

A full blood count may show anaemia of an iron deficient type, or a normochromic anaemia typical of the anaemia of chronic diseases, and commonly found in patients with advanced cancer. More specifically the blood count may show leuco-erythroblastic anaemia in which there are immature white cells and red cell precursors present in the blood. This finding is typical of widespread bone marrow infiltration with cancer and is most frequently caused by adenocarcinomas, particularly adenocarcinoma of the breast. Further haematological investigation may include bone marrow examination if infiltration is suspected. In some tumours, for example small cell carcinoma of the bronchus, marrow examination is sometimes part of the staging if there is no other evidence of spread and if localized treatment with radiotherapy is considered in addition to chemotherapy. Occult marrow involvement is detected by aspiration and trephine biopsy in 5–10% of cases but in 20–30% if staining with monoclonal antibodies is used (p. 45). In other diseases such as cancer of the ovary or colorectal cancer, marrow examination is not routinely performed. It is essential in patients with newly diagnosed non-Hodgkin's lymphoma, in which the probability of marrow involvement is higher.

Measurement of the liver enzymes may support a clinical suspicion of liver metastases, but more precise methods are now available and are discussed below. A raised plasma calcium may indicate bone metastases but isotope scanning (see p. 56) is the most sensitive investigative technique.

In recent years diagnostic imaging has been revolutionized by technical advances and has led to a previously unattainable degree of precision in staging of the extent of the primary tumour and in assessing whether there has been metastatic spread. Many of these investigations are time-consuming and expensive, and should therefore be used judiciously in order to answer specific questions which are designed to alter management. It must also be remembered that some investigations, including both ultrasound examination and CT scanning, are very much dependent on the skill and enthusiasm of the radiologist and it is important to have a healthy degree of scepticism about equivocal or uncertain findings, especially if these are not in accordance with the clinical circumstances.

Ultrasound investigation

Diagnostic ultrasound has been greatly refined in the last 15 years [2]. It was first introduced into clinical practice in the 1950s and relies on the differing echo patterns which tissues create when bombarded by sound from an ultrasonic transducer. The echoes are generated at interfaces of tissues whose density differs, then recorded, interpreted and presented as a two-dimensional display. The orientation of the slice or 'cut' is determined by the operator who places the probe in the position most appropriate for demonstrating the organ and abnormality suspected (Fig. 4.3). This flexibility allows images to be obtained in many planes. Ultrasound echoes cannot be obtained if the organ is shielded by an area of bone or gas since these reflect all the sound from the beam and no echoes can be obtained from beyond these structures. For this reason ultrasound has its main diagnostic use in the abdomen and soft tissues. A great advantage of ultrasound is that it is cheap, quick and non-invasive. It can therefore be used to monitor the responses to

treatment with measurements being made between chemotherapy cycles. Other techniques, such as CT scanning, which are more accurate, are too expensive to be used in this way and the dose of radiation is too high.

Ultrasound is particularly useful for diagnosis of liver metastases (Fig. 4.3). The type of echo obtained varies depending on the kind of metastases which are present. Thus echo-poor areas are often associated with lymphomas and sarcomas, while gastro-intestinal metastases produce a more echo-dense appearance. In colorectal cancer the accuracy of ultrasound approaches that of CT scanning. Ultrasound is also useful in visualizing lesions in the pancreas, but it is usually only able to define a relatively large tumour. It is of value in the investigation of patients with obstructive jaundice, although the ability of ultrasound to define intra-abdominal metastases, for example in retroperitoneal nodes, is fairly limited. If it is important to know whether there is node involvement in the abdomen, CT scanning and lymphography are better techniques.

In the kidney ultrasound examination is frequently able to detect a renal carcinoma and distinguish this from cysts. The accuracy in this differential diagnosis is said to be of the order of 90% and the resolving power is approximately 2−3 cm. Ultrasound of the thyroid is useful in making the distinction between solid and cystic lesions, and in the testis it can sometimes demonstrate an occult or doubtfully palpable tumour. It is also increasingly used in distinguishing solid and cystic masses within the breast. Endoscopic ultrasound is increasingly used, for example by the trans-rectal route. The latter is particularly valuable for the assessment of prostatic carcinomas.

Computed tomography (CT)

Modern CT scanners are able to demonstrate normal anatomy in detail which would have been thought impossible in the early 1970s. The accuracy of the technique has been greatly improved and its use in staging continues to be

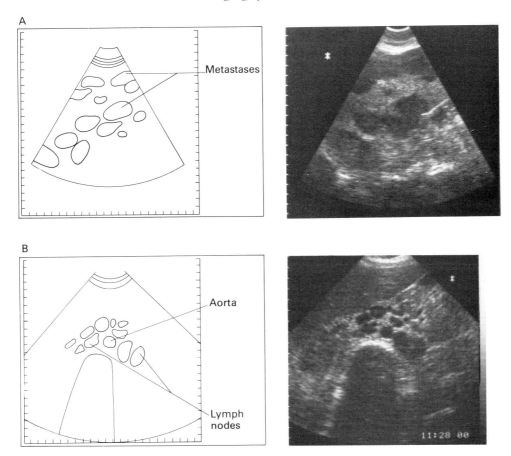

Fig. 4.3 Diagnosis of hepatic metastases and lymph node enlargement by ultrasound. (A) Hepatic metastases. Several large metastases are shown in this transverse scan of the liver; (B) para-aortic lymph nodes. These are demonstrated lying in front of and behind the aorta. (We are grateful to Dr K. Walmsley, UCH, London, for providing these scans.)

defined. There are, however, limitations to the use and interpretation of CT scans, and it is important to be aware that they can give both false-positive and false-negative results. For example, in the abdomen, false-positive results are usually due to confusion with non-specified bowel loops and false-negatives due to the inability of CT to detect malignant infiltration of normal-sized nodes. Clarity of the CT scan image depends partly on the presence of the normal fat planes which surround anatomical structures. If these are lost, alteration of the anatomy is less easily detected and the investigation loses reliability. The tomographic technique can demonstrate a tumour by showing distortion or enlargement of an organ, or a change in its density. In cancer the CT scan is of use in demonstrating both the extent of infiltration of the primary tumour (T staging) and to delineate metastatic spread to adjacent lymph nodes and to other structures such as liver or lung (N and M staging).

CT scanning is of great importance in the definition of the spread of tumours within the chest [3]. Several studies have shown that chest X-ray and conventional tomography greatly underestimate the extent of infiltration of lung cancer within the chest, particularly in the mediastinum (Fig. 4.4). The CT scan has also been valuable in demonstrating the true extent

Fig. 4.4 CT scan of thorax. Left-sided bronchogenic carcinoma behind the heart. The tumour extends to the pleura. The chest X-ray was normal.

Fig. 4.5 CT scan (coronal plane) through the nose and maxillary antrum. A large tumour fills the left maxillary antrum, destroying its walls and extending medially into the nasal fossa.

of infiltration of tumours arising in the head and neck, particularly in the paranasal sinuses (Fig. 4.5). For retroperitoneal structures, CT scanning remains the most reliable pre-operative investigation and is particularly useful in demonstrating both lymph node enlargement and abnormalities of the adrenal and pancreas. Using fine flexible needles CT-guided aspiration may help in the distinction between a benign and malignant neoplasm (Fig. 4.6), or between an inflammatory mass and a carcinoma, for example in the pancreas. The extent of retroperitoneal tumours such as sarcomas and lymphomas can be assessed with CT scanning, as can the size of malignant tumours of the kidney. In the pelvis, CT scanning frequently demonstrates the extent of advanced carcinomas of the cervix, bladder, prostate and rectum (Fig. 4.7). However, interpretation requires considerable expertise. CT scanning is also used to determine the degree of lymph node involvement. In the chest, the CT scan is much more reliable than chest X-ray or lung tomography in demonstrating mediastinal and hilar node involvement. In the abdomen, CT scanning delineates pelvic

Fig. 4.6 CT scan of the abdomen, showing a large para-aortic mass. The track of a CT scan-guided biopsy needle is shown.

and abdominal lymph nodes. The nodes are less clearly outlined than in the chest and must usually be enlarged to more than twice their normal size before they can be confidently assessed as pathological.

Fig. 4.7 CT scan of the pelvis, showing a large central mass (arrowed) anterior to the rectum. This was an advanced carcinoma of the cervix.

examination, but is very much more expensive. The technique is made more accurate by using intravenous contrast material which may also clearly distinguish benign from malignant hepatic lesions. CT scanning is also the most widely used method of demonstrating brain metastases (see below).

A CT scan is of little practical value in the search for an occult primary tumour presenting with distant metastases. Similarly, it is not employed for detecting bone metastases — isotope scanning is much better for this purpose. Occasionally, CT scanning may be helpful in showing the extent of destruction in a bone lesion which is causing pain. This is particularly likely to be the case in vertebral deposits where infiltration of the soft tissues and surrounding structure is difficult to demonstrate on conventional X-rays (Fig. 4.9).

Magnetic resonance (MR) imaging

Magnetic resonance scanning has taken a further step forward in imaging particular areas

In the pelvis lymphography may sometimes prove more sensitive, since it demonstrates the fine anatomical detail of the lymph node, while CT scanning merely shows enlargement. However, lymphography does not outline upper para-aortic nodes and CT scanning is therefore of more value at this site. Although CT scanning has largely replaced lymphography as the primary imaging procedure in the lymphomas, the two techniques can give complementary information and lymphography is valuable when CT is equivocal, occasionally demonstrating involvement of normal sized nodes.

CT scanning is the most sensitive method available to assess pulmonary metastases [4]. It is used for this purpose in testicular germ cell tumours and osteosarcomas, where occult pulmonary metastases are frequently demonstrated in patients whose chest X-ray is normal (Fig. 4.8). The technique is particularly valuable in demonstrating metastases which lie in front of and behind the heart or subpleurally, which are not visible on plain X-ray. In the liver CT scanning is now more sensitive than ultrasound

Fig. 4.8 CT scan of thorax, showing a solitary metastasis (arrowed) behind the heart. In this patient with osteosarcoma, the chest X-ray was normal.

Fig. 4.9 CT scan of thoracic vertebra at level of carina. The vertebra and rib are largely destroyed by local extension of a bronchogenic carcinoma.

of the body, especially the brain and spinal cord and in sarcomas [5]. In this technique the patient lies within an intense magnetic field which produces magnetization of atomic nuclei in the patient, in the direction of the field. Electromagnetic pulses are then applied to the patient to change the direction of this nuclear magnetization. Following the cessation of the pulse the nuclei return to their orientation within the static field. This recovery time, which is measured by the scanner, depends on exchange of energy between protons and surrounding atoms and molecules. The recovery time is different in tumours compared with normal tissues. The technique has proved particularly valuable in the brain where deep-seated primary tumours can be visualized (Fig. 4.10). MR scanning has been able to detect tumours in the brain stem, cerebellum and deep midline structures when CT scanning has been inconclusive. The use of gadolinium contrast techniques has refined the role of MR scanning still further.

In the spine, MR scanning has largely replaced myelography since it often demonstrates secondary deposits without the need for lumbar puncture. Use of gadolinium contrast further increases the diagnostic range. In bone and soft tissue sarcomas, MR provides unsurpassed detail of the extent of the primary site, which greatly assists the surgeon and radiotherapist in operative and planning technique (Fig. 4.11A). Abdominopelvic MR scanning is also superior to CT, at least in definition of cervical anatomy and pelvic node assessment (Fig. 4.11B).

Lymphography

Contrast material is injected into lymphatics in the dorsum of the feet, and nodes are opacified in the pelvic, iliac and para-aortic regions.

Fig. 4.10 (A) MRI scan (sagittal view) showing large brain-stem tumour. The CT scan was normal. (B) MRI scan of brain showing deep-seated thalamic tumour which was not clearly shown on the CT scan.

Fig. 4.11 (A) MR scan of soft tissue sarcoma in the lower half of the femur. The tumour mass (arrowed) is seen to be closely applied to the femur and the femoral artery is clearly seen passing through the substance of the tumour. (B) MR scan of the brain showing a very large metastasis. An area of haemorrhage is shown as a dense, black, central opacity. The midline structures are displaced from right to left.

Occasionally, lymphography of the arm and neck has been carried out, but such techniques are now rarely used, having been replaced by other less invasive investigations. One advantage of lymphography over CT scanning is that it may allow abnormal internal anatomy of the lymph nodes to be shown at a time when overall enlargement has not taken place. There are two 'classical' patterns of abnormality. In lymphomas the nodes are often very large with a lace-like texture (Fig. 4.12), whereas in carcinomas the appearances are usually those of a filling defect in a moderately enlarged node.

The disadvantages of lymphography are that it is invasive; that many nodes are not outlined in the abdomen (particularly mesenteric, high para-aortic, splenic and porta hepatic nodes); that false-positive filling defects or equivocal abnormalities occur, and that lymph nodes which are totally replaced by tumour sometimes

Fig. 4.12 (A) Lymphogram showing bilateral para-aortic lymphadenopathy, with the typical lace-like structure often seen in lymphoma; (B) After treatment the appearance returns to normal.

do not opacify at all. In lymphomas the overall accuracy of the technique is in the region of 80% with a false-positive rate of approximately 15%. With other tumours the accuracy is less. With increasing availability of CT and MR scanning, lymphography is now less widely used.

Isotope scanning

Scanning with radioactive isotopes is a simple and widely available technique for assessing metastatic spread. In certain sites it has a rather poor accuracy, that is, a low percentage of correct results. This is due to both a poor *sensitivity* of detection (the percentage of positive tests in abnormal tissues) and poor *specificity* (percentage of negative tests in normal tissues). However, the dose of radiation is small, the technique is safe and reproducible and it is relatively inexpensive.

Skeletal metastases are best demonstrated by isotope scanning and bone scans are now the most frequent test requested in most service departments [3]. Technetium-labelled phosphate compounds are usually used. The isotope is rapidly taken up into bone, rate of uptake being related to both blood flow through the bone and the amount of new bone formation. Metastases cause increase in blood flow and an increase in osteoblastic activity, usually sufficient to be demonstrable as areas of increased uptake of isotope (Fig. 4.13). An exception to this is in multiple myeloma where osteoblastic activity is minimal.

Because of the non-specific nature of the uptake, a variety of other conditions will cause increased uptake. Rib fractures, arthritis and vertebral collapse from osteoporosis may all give rise to increased uptake and be misinterpreted as due to metastases in a patient with a malignancy. Single areas of increased uptake in an otherwise fit patient should therefore be interpreted with extreme caution. X-rays of the affected region should be taken and if necessary a CT scan should be obtained if the presence of a metastasis would materially alter the therapeutic decision. This is especially important if

Fig. 4.13 Isotope bone scan, showing multiple bone metastases in the ribs, pelvis, spine and left femur.

the single site is in the vertebral column, since degenerative disease is common at this site. In spite of these problems an area of increased uptake in a patient with cancer is likely to be due to a secondary deposit and should be carefully evaluated. Multiple areas of increased uptake are almost certainly due to disseminated tumour. An isotope bone scan is generally regarded as an important staging investigation in all patients with newly diagnosed carcinoma of the breast.

In the liver, scanning is performed with ^{99m}technetium-labelled sulphur colloid. Metastases appear as areas of diminished uptake. Isotope liver scan is less accurate than ultrasound or CT scanning, and hepatic isotope scanning has now been largely eclipsed.

Similarly, in the brain, isotope scanning has been almost completely replaced by CT scanning as the most accurate method of demonstrating metastases.

DIAGNOSIS OF SPECIFIC METASTATIC SITES

Pulmonary metastases

A chest X-ray is the most widely used method of screening. CT scanning greatly increases diagnostic accuracy with an overall sensitivity up to 60–65%. Doubtful lesions such as subpleural deposits and isolated opacities can be examined by percutaneous needle aspiration. Small pleural effusions, not apparent on chest X-ray, may also be demonstrated.

Bone metastases

Bone scanning is the most accurate and rapid means of screening for bone metastases. Skeletal X-rays are used to demonstrate the degree of bone erosion at a site of metastasis if an alternative explanation for increased isotope uptake such as trauma or infection is possible. Percutaneous needle aspiration of bone can be undertaken safely at many sites and is helpful when the diagnosis is uncertain. MR scanning is useful to demonstrate intramedullary metastasis.

Hepatic metastases

Biochemical tests of liver function are the most widely used screening procedure. For imaging the liver, ultrasound and CT scanning are useful not only for diagnosis of hepatic metastases but also adrenal, mesenteric and other sites of abdominal disease [6]. These investigations may confirm metastatic liver disease even if the liver function tests are normal. In lymphomas (particularly Hodgkin's disease), abdominal CT scanning is now the most widely performed staging procedure, useful both for hepatic deposits and also (more commonly) to demonstrate intra-abdominal lymph node involvement.

Brain metastases

CT scanning is widely available and is the usual preliminary investigation, although it is seldom positive in neurologically normal patients. MR scanning is more sensitive and can show leptomeningeal spread when CT scans are normal.

THE ROLE OF SURGERY IN DIAGNOSIS AND STAGING

Traditionally, surgery has been the most effective local treatment for patients with cancer. The importance of surgery was based not only on the uniqueness of the cancer operation for controlling the primary tumour, but also on the general view that most cancers tended to recur at the original site making wide local excision essential.

In the past, the surgical roles of diagnosis, staging and cure have been understandably confused. For example, a patient with a carcinoma of the large bowel might present with constipation, rectal bleeding and abdominal mass; at laparotomy, the diagnosis would be confirmed and the appropriate operation carried out. This has led to the common practice of surgical removal of the primary tumour before consultation with a non-surgical specialist, which can certainly lead to difficulties where there are competing approaches for control of the primary tumour; breast cancer is a good example. With the increasing precision of simpler diagnostic techniques, such as aspiration cytology, percutaneous needle biopsy and CT-guided fine needle biopsy, major surgical procedures are sometimes unnecessary simply to establish the diagnosis. In carcinoma of the pancreas, for example, it has been difficult in the past to obtain histological confirmation without laparotomy. The increasing use of non-surgical techniques often leads to a pre-operative tissue diagnosis. This may allow new therapeutic approaches to be considered in the future, in which planned surgery might be undertaken following pre-operative radio-therapy or chemotherapy. With the emphasis on tailoring of treatment to the extent of the disease, the cancer surgeon sometimes performs staging procedures which are not in themselves therapeutic but are intended to assist radio-therapists and medical oncologists in deciding their therapeutic strategy. In ovarian cancer, for example, an important part of the initial procedure is the careful examination of the peritoneal cavity with particular attention to subdiaphragmatic spaces, which have been shown to harbour secondary deposits in patients otherwise thought to have only pelvic disease. In carcinoma of the colon, excision of the tu-mour should be accompanied by surgical staging since the presence of lymph nodes and hep-atic metastases have considerable prognostic significance.

Surgical procedures may also be performed for reassessment of patients who have under-gone treatment, particularly with intensive drug and irradiation schedules. The aim is to deter-mine if treatment can be discontinued if there is no evidence of disease, or changed if disease persists. In advanced ovarian cancer, laparos-copy has been widely employed as a means of confirming a complete response following treat-ment with chemotherapy or irradiation (see Chapter 17). Based on these findings, it may sometimes be appropriate to proceed to lapar-otomy and resection of residual tumour deposits.

THE EFFECT OF STAGING ON TREATMENT AND PROGNOSIS

It is self-evident that the results of staging investigations will alter management. Radical operations are clearly inappropriate in patients with disseminated disease and attempts to cure these patients with local radiotherapy will also fail. What may be less apparent is that the introduction of staging investigations as a rou-tine will appear to alter the results of treatment and invalidate historical comparisons.

If we consider a tumour diagnosed and treated in the 1950s when many staging inves-tigations were not available we might find the results shown in Table 4.1. Many patients with Stage I disease had occult Stage II or III disease (i.e. they were 'understaged'). The 5-year sur-vival is only 50%. Similarly patients with Stage II disease have occult Stage III disease and 5-year survival is poor (20%). Only patients with clinically obvious metastases are included in Stage III with a dismal prognosis (2%). By introducing staging investigations but keeping the treatment the same, Stage I patients have a better prognosis (because investigation has placed many into Stage II or Stage III) and the same is true for Stage II. Even Stage III now has a better prognosis because patients with small,

Table 4.1 Effects of staging on survival ('stage–shift' effect)

	(a) Tumour diagnosed in 1950s, but with only clinical staging; treated with surgery for Stages I and II.		(b) Same tumour diagnosed and carefully staged in 1980s; treated with surgery for Stages I and II as in 1950s.	
	all cases (%)	5-year survival (%)	all cases (%)	5-year survival (%)
Stage I: Local disease	40	50	10	80
Stage II: Nodes involved	40	20	40	40
Stage III: Distant metastasis	20	2	50	10
Overall 5-year survival (%)		28.5		29

clinically inapparent metastases are now in this category and more of them (10%) survive for 5 years. However, the overall prognosis of the tumour has not changed. The 5-year survival was 28.5% in 1950 and 29% in 1980. All that has happened is that patients have been reassigned to different categories, but each stage now has a better prognosis!

TUMOUR MARKERS

Some malignant tumours produce substances which can be detected in the blood and which may serve as a marker both of the presence of the tumour and sometimes of its size. Measurement of these tumour markers has become an important part of the management of testicular and ovarian germ cell tumours, choriocarcinoma and hepatoma [7]. The ideal requirements for a tumour marker are as follows:

1 *The markers should always be produced by the tumour type.* This is not the case for the great majority of markers (Table 4.2). In teratoma, α-fetoprotein (AFP) and human chorionic gonadotrophin (HCG) are present in serum in 75% of cases and HCG is present in almost all choriocarcinomas. Apart from carcinoembryonic antigen (CEA) and acid phosphatase, most other markers are of little value in diagnosis or staging.

2 *The marker should give an accurate and sensitive indication of tumour mass.* This is the case with the β subunit of HCG and AFP in germ cell tumours. In other tumours the marker is inconsistently produced or is too insensitive to be a useful guide to treatment although acid phosphatase is of value in monitoring progress in prostatic cancers and CEA in colorectal cancer.

3 *The marker should be produced by recurrent and metastatic disease.* One of the major uses of markers is to diagnose recurrence early. Occasionally in teratomas recurrent disease is associated with a rise in either HCG or AFP, even though the original tumour produced both. Marker negative recurrences (from a

Table 4.2 Circulating tumour markers

Marker	Tumour
Placental products	
Human chorionic gonadotrophin	Choriocarcinoma, teratoma
Placental alkaline phosphatase	Ovarian cancer, seminoma
Placental lactogen	Choriocarcinoma
Oncofetal antigens	
Carcinoembryonic antigen	Gut cancer, breast, pancreas
α-fetoprotein	Germ cell tumours, hepatoma
Pancreatic oncofetal antigen	Pancreatic carcinoma
Ca-125	Ovarian cancer
Tissue or organ antigens	
Thyroglobulin	Thyroid cancer
Ectopic hormones	
Calcitonin	Medullary carcinoma of thyroid
ACTH	Small cell carcinoma of bronchus
ADH	Small cell carcinoma of bronchus
Isoenzymes	
Alkaline phosphatase	Osteosarcoma and variety of other cancers
Lactic dehydrogenase	Neuroblastoma
Prostatic acid phosphatase	Cancer of prostate

previously positive tumour) are rare. Similarly a rise in CEA, acid phosphatase or Ca-125 may precede clinical evidence of recurrence in bowel, prostate or ovarian cancer respectively.

4 *The tumour should be amenable to therapy.* There is little value in detecting recurrence early if no treatment is available. For example, recurrence of colorectal or pancreatic cancer is seldom curable and early diagnosis of metastasis may serve only to alarm the patient. In teratoma on the other hand, a rise in AFP or HCG is a firm indication for full investigation since curative treatment is available.

5 *The marker should be specific for the disease*

and easy to measure. Some markers, for example AFP and HCG (β subunit), are seldom present unless there is a tumour. However, AFP may be raised in pregnancy and with liver disease. CEA can be produced in inflammatory bowel disease as well as in colorectal and pancreatic cancer, and raised levels are found in smokers. The advent of sensitive radioimmunoassay techniques has led to the measurement of AFP and HCG as a routine in germ cell tumours and hepatoma. Some peptide hormones, for example antidiuretic hormone (ADH) are extremely difficult to measure accurately.

Examples of tumour markers are given in Table 4.2. Some of these are in daily clinical use and justify more detailed consideration.

Human chorionic gonadotrophin (HCG). The β subunit is measured to avoid cross reactivity with luteinizing hormone. HCG is measured by radioimmunoassay. It is used to detect and monitor therapy in choriocarcinoma and testicular and other germ cell tumours. The half-life ($t_{1/2}$) is 24−36 hours, and it is measurable in both blood and urine (where it gives a positive pregnancy test).

α-Fetoprotein (AFP). This protein is similar in size to albumin and is a major serum component before birth. It may cross the placenta and be detected in maternal blood. It is produced during liver regeneration and is elevated in viral hepatitis and cirrhosis. AFP is produced by malignant yolk-sac elements in germ cell tumours (see Chapter 19) and by the malignant hepatocytes in hepatomas. It is present in small amounts in some patients with pancreatic carcinoma and occasionally in gastric carcinoma. The plasma half-life is 5−7 days.

Carcinoembryonic antigen (CEA). CEA refers to a family of glycoproteins produced by many epithelial tumours, the molecule usually being demonstrable at the cell surface rather than at the cytoplasm. It is produced by normal colonic epithelium but is not usually present in the blood unless there is inflammation or neoplasia involving the epithelium. It is also found in plasma in pancreatitis, heavy smokers, ulcerative colitis and gastritis, thus limiting its usefulness in diagnosis. It is of little value in early diagnosis of bowel cancer and its value in early diagnosis of recurrent disease is limited by the lack of successful therapy in the majority of patients. CEA is elevated in approximately 60% of cases of advanced ovarian cancer and 40−70% of advanced breast cancers. It is therefore of little value in diagnosis of metastasis from an unknown primary site. On the other hand, early surgical exploration of potential local anastomotic recurrences are increasingly undertaken in patients in whom CT scanning coupled with a rise in CEA level has aided the diagnosis while the patient is still asymptomatic. The increasing use of surgical resection, radiation and chemotherapy in patients with advanced colorectal cancer has led to an increased use of this tumour marker.

CA-125 is a complex antigen which is a high molecular weight glycoprotein produced in coelomic epithelium and re-expressed in epithelial ovarian, pancreatic and breast cancer. 80% of ovarian cancers are associated with antigenaemia and rising or falling levels correlate with disease in 93%. Levels above the upper limit of normal (35 U/ml) are not specific for ovarian cancer (being found in endometriosis, hepatitis and benign ovarian lesions) and are thus of limited value for screening. During treatment, CA-125 levels fall, but persistent disease is often found even when plasma levels are normal. However, elevated or rising levels can be used to detect early response to chemotherapy.

CA-19−9. This is a mucin-like antigen which is a polysialated Lewis blood group antigen. It is found particularly in pancreatic cancers and in pancreatitis. Its value is limited by non-specificity and the lack of effective treatment of pancreatic cancer.

Placental alkaline phosphatase is frequently present in the serum of men with testicular and mediastinal seminoma and in dysgerminoma in women. If raised it is useful for monitoring response to therapy and recurrence.

REFERENCES

1 UICC (Union Internationale Contre le Cancer) *TNM Atlas: Classification of malignant tumours*, 3rd edn. Berlin: Springer-Verlag, 1989.
2 Bragg D.G., Rubin P., Youker J.E., eds. *Oncologic Imaging*. New York: Pergamon Press, 1985.
3 Epstein D.M., Stephenson L.W., Gefter W.B. *et al.* The value of CT in the preoperative assessment of lung cancer. *Radiology* 1986; **161**: 423–27.
4 Siegelman S.S., Zerhouni E.A., Leo F.P. *et al.* CT of the solitary pulmonary nodule. *American Journal of Roentgenology* 1980; **135**: 1–13.
5 Brant-Zawadski M., Norman D., eds. *Magnetic Resonance Imaging of the Central Nervous System*. New York: Raven Press, 1987.
6 Zeman R.K., Paushter D.M., Schiebler M.L. *et al.* Hepatic imaging: current status. *Radiological Clinics of North America* 1985; **23**: 473–87.
7 Bosl G.J., Geller N.L., Cirricione C. *et al.* Serum tumor markers in patients with metastatic germ cell tumors of the testis: a 10 year experience. *American Journal of Medicine* 1983; **75**: 29–35.

Chapter 5
Radiotherapy

Ever since the discovery of X-rays by Roentgen in 1895, attempts have been made not only to understand their physical nature but also to use them both in the biological sciences and in a variety of human illnesses. The development of the X-ray tube rapidly led to clinical applications, first as a diagnostic tool and later for therapy in patients with malignant disease. The discovery of radium by Marie and Pierre Curie in 1898 also resulted in the use of radioactive materials for the approach of cancer, since surgery was the only alternative approach available at that time. Over the past 80 years our understanding of the physical characteristics, biological effects and clinical roles of ionizing radiation has greatly increased.

To understand the nature of radioactivity and radioactive decay, it is important to grasp the concept of a natural spectrum of electromagnetic waves whose energy varies widely, in inverse proportion to the length of the wave itself. This spectrum (Fig. 5.1) includes X-rays (very high energy and very short wavelength), visible light rays (of intermediate wavelength and energy) and also radiowaves (of generally longer wavelength and lower energy) which are responsible for modern telecommunications and include the transmission signals for radio and television. Of these various types of electromagnetic waves, only X-rays and gamma rays (the terms are almost interchangeable) are of sufficiently high energy to produce the ionization of atoms which occurs when a beam of radiation passes through biological tissue.

In the process of ionization, the essential event is the displacement of an electron from its orbital path around the nucleus of the atom.

This creates an unstable or ionized atom, and a free electron which is normally 'captured' by a neighbouring atom, which then becomes equally unstable because of its possession of an extra negative electric charge. When radiation beams pass through living tissue, the intensity, duration and site of these ionization events can be controlled by varying the characteristics of the radiation source. This permits a deliberate and controlled cellular destruction in the case of therapeutic radiation (radiotherapy), whereas with diagnostic radiation, trivial and short-lived alterations occur, which usually have no permanent biological effect. The creation of the radiographic image is due to the differential alteration of the X-ray beam by biological tissues containing atoms of differing atomic weights.

SOURCES AND PRODUCTION OF IONIZING RADIATION

Radioactive isotopes

Radioactivity is an unalterable property of many naturally occurring atoms which exist in a relatively unstable state. Although the identity of any given atom is defined by the number of protons and electrons it possesses, the atoms of any one element may contain differing numbers of nuclear neutrons, so that their atomic weights (as determined by the proton and neutron component) differ. Such atoms or *isotopes* occur naturally in fixed proportions, and most pure substances (particularly metals such as iron, manganese or cobalt) consist of mixtures of these isotopes. Emission of radioactivity is

Fig. 5.1 The electromagnetic spectrum.

one of the consequences of physical decay of unstable atoms resulting in a final and more stable state. The rate and intensity of these emissions varies with each element.

There is a wide variety of naturally occurring radioactive materials, whose chief characteristic is the emission of electromagnetic waves of a frequency which can produce ionization within biological materials. Historically, these emissions have been divided into alpha, beta or gamma waves, depending on the characteristics of the emission. Alpha particles are no more than helium nuclei, emitted from unstable or decaying radionuclides. It is worth remembering that although many of the properties of radioactive emission are better understood in terms of their characteristic wave forms, the 'wave' also has features of a particle. Alpha and beta emission are best understood in terms of these features since alpha particles are positively charged helium nuclei, with a substantial mass, and beta particles are no more than electrons,

with a negative charge but almost no mass. Gamma rays, on the other hand, are uncharged.

Although alpha, beta and gamma rays can all produce ionization in tissues it is the gamma rays which have the greatest application in radiation therapy. For example, in a reaction of great clinical importance, the unstable isotope of cobalt, with an atomic number of 60, disintegrates to a more stable isotope (atomic number 59) by discharging one of its nuclear neutrons, together with gamma rays. The characteristics of the emitted gamma radiation are constant for this particular reaction, and the rate of the nuclear disintegration is unalterable, such that after 5.33 years, exactly half of the original radioactive material still remains, thus defining the radioactive 'half-life' of ^{60}Co. The half-life is an important concept in theoretical and clinical work, and varies between a fraction of a second, and hundreds or thousands of years (Table 5.1). Radium, widely used before the introduction of more suitable radioactive materials, has a half-life of 1620 years, which meant that radioactive sources for therapeutic use never needed replacing. Beta particles, or electrons, however, are now increasingly used as their characteristics are more suitable in certain clinical situations. In addition, other atomic fragments are being studied since they have theoretical advantages as a result of their different biological effects. These include neutrons, protons and pi-mesons (see p. 68).

Although the early radioactive substances discovered by the Curies and others were all naturally occurring, modern high energy physics has provided ready access to many new materials, or artificially manufactured isotopes. These substances, *radionuclides*, are generally manufactured in nuclear reactors by heavy particle bombardment of natural materials. The chief advantage is that their properties more closely resemble the theoretical ideal for radioactive half-life, gamma ray characteristics and intensity, than any natural substance. The changing demands of both diagnosis, for example in radioisotope imaging, and therapy have led to ever-increasing attempts at produc-

Table 5.1 Therapeutically useful isotopes

Isotope	Type of radiation	Energy (MeV)	Half-life
^{60}Co	β,γ	0.31 (β), 1.17 and 1.33 (γ)	5.3 years
^{137}Cs	β,γ	0.51 (β) and 0.66 (γ)	30 years
^{131}I	β,γ	0.61 (β) and 0.36 (γ)	8 days
^{198}Au	β,γ	0.96 (β) and 0.41 (γ)	2.7 days
^{32}P	β	1.71 (β)	14 days
^{192}Ir	γ	0.36−0.6 (γ)	74 days
^{226}Ra (decays to radon, then Ra A,B,C)	α then β,γ	1.0 (γ)	1620 years for radium but 3−27 mins for Ra A,B,C

ing new radioactive isotopes with differing radiation characteristics. For therapeutic work, this includes the production of both sealed and unsealed sources. For sealed sources, the radioactive material is physically enclosed by an impenetrable barrier such as the platinum casing of a typical radium or caesium needle (Fig. 5.2), so that the radioactive material can be inserted into the tissue to be irradiated, and then removed at some predetermined time. With unsealed sources, such as ^{131}I, the isotope is physically ingested either by mouth or injection, passing via the bloodstream to the end organ and taken up (in this case, by the thyroid), where the effects of the radioactive emission cause local damage to both the normal thyroid gland and the cancer within it. The isotope cannot then be recovered.

Unsealed sources are widely used in diagnostic work such as the radioactive technetium bone or brain scan. In therapeutic work, the most specific and ideal application is for carcinoma of the thyroid, where radioactive isotopes of iodine (usually ^{131}I) are given by mouth, and selectively taken up by the thyroid gland and thyroid cancer cells providing 'internal' irradiation to a high intensity without compromising other organs by the delivery of an unacceptable dose of radiation at an unwanted site. Use of injectable radioactive phosphorus (^{32}P) for bone marrow irradiation in polycythaemia rubra vera is another well known example. Other less specific instances of the therapeutic use of unsealed sources include the intraperitoneal or intrapleural use of radioactive gold colloids for malignant ascites or pleural effusions.

For use in clinical work, the choice of either naturally occurring or artificially produced radioactive isotopes will depend on the clinical requirement. For example, in interstitial implantation work where radioactive needles are directly placed adjacent to or even within the malignant tissue, caesium needles have increasingly been employed in preference to radium, because of the more suitable characteristics of the emitted radiation from this material. This is because the specific activity (number of radioactive disintegrations per second) is so high with radium that protection for doctors, radiographers, nurses and other staff has always been a major problem. With caesium, however, the specific activity is substantially lower, making protection easier.

Radioactive isotopes are also used as a source of external radiation (teletherapy). All clinical departments place a heavy clinical reliance on

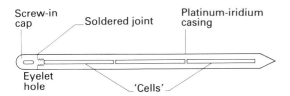

Fig. 5.2 A radium needle. (From Meredith W.J., Massey J.B. *Fundamental Physics of Radiology*. Baltimore: Williams & Wilkins, 1972. With permission.)

their external therapy techniques since the majority of tumours are deeply situated and inaccessible to irradiation by direct implantation (brachytherapy). Nowadays when gamma irradiation from a major radioactive source is employed, the most common choice of material is ^{60}Co, a material which emits a high-energy gamma ray (mean energy 1.2 MeV) of sufficient penetration to allow for treatment of deeply situated tumours. ^{60}Co has a reasonably satisfactory half-life of 5.3 years so that major source replacement will not be required more than every 3−4 years.

A traditional cobalt unit is in essence no more than a cylindrical source of ^{60}Co produced artificially within a nuclear fission pile, placed in a protective shell made of lead, and supplied with a simple mechanism for moving the source into the treatment position when required (Fig. 5.3). In this position, the radioactive cobalt source is still protected by a lead sphere, though a cone of the protective material has been removed and moveable jaws fitted allowing the beam of gamma rays to be altered in size to suit the clinical requirements. This extremely simple piece of equipment is still the most widely used high energy apparatus in the world today, and

has the advantage of reliability, simplicity, and longevity, as well as being relatively inexpensive both to purchase and to maintain. Its disadvantages are that there is a substantial 'penumbra' of scattered radiation, which forms a significant part of the edge of the beam and that treatment times can be lengthy. This is particularly the case when the source has started to age, since radioactive decay results in a loss of residual radioactive material and treatment time increases proportionately.

Artificial production of X-rays and particles

Shortly after the discovery of radium by the Curies, Roentgen constructed the first X-ray apparatus, consisting of a sealed glass vacuum tube containing an electrode at one end and a target at the other. Heating the electrode resulted in a discharge of electrons which travelled relatively easily through the vacuum, to bombard the target at the other end of the tube. This produced characteristic rays which, like those of radium, could create an image on a photographic plate. The nature of these rays was uncertain; *X-rays* therefore seemed the most suitable title. It gradually became clear that X-rays and gamma rays were fundamentally similar although their method of production is quite different. Unlike the gamma irradiation from radioactive materials whose characteristics cannot be changed other than by altering either the choice or the purity of the material, X-rays of quite different properties can be produced simply by varying the voltage input to the cathode of the X-ray tube.

For instance the X-rays used in diagnostic radiology are generated in a low voltage machine (e.g. 50 kV), have a longer wavelength and less penetrating power. In contrast, therapeutic X-rays are produced by equipment of higher voltage varying from 50 kV up to 30 MeV, a 600-fold increase. As voltage is increased, X-rays of shorter wavelength are produced, which have far greater penetrating power.

For therapeutic use, one of the chief criteria for successful treatment is the availability of

Fig. 5.3 Schematic representation of a typical ^{60}Co treatment unit. The treatment unit is usually mounted on a counterbalanced gantry capable of rotation through 360° permitting treatment from underneath the patient where necessary. (From Meredith W.J., Massey J.B. *Fundamental Physics of Radiology*. Baltimore: Williams & Wilkins, 1972. With permission.)

X-rays of sufficient penetrating power, or depth dose, to deal effectively with deep-seated tumours. For this reason, departments of radiotherapy need a range of equipment with a wide spectrum of clinically useful X-ray beams available to deal with both superficial tumours such as skin cancers and those more deeply situated, such as tumours of the mediastinum or pelvis. With conventional or *orthovoltage* X-ray equipment, the maximum deposition of radiation energy is in the superficial tissues, with a steep fall-off (Fig. 5.4), such that the dosage received by a deep tumour which may be 10 cm or more below the skin surface is low, and limited by the skin reaction that this treatment will inevitably cause. The physical and electromagnetic problems of safely applying a very high tension (voltage) input had to be overcome before further progress could be made.

Fortunately, most of these technical difficulties were solved in the 1960s with the advent of an entirely fresh approach to the generation of high-energy megavoltage beams, and the development of the modern linear accelerator. Instead of the traditional X-ray tube, with its cumbersome, fragile construction and somewhat unpredictable emission, a new means of X-ray production was developed, which depended on the acceleration of electrons down a cylindrical 'wave guide' terminating in the deliberate bombardment of a fixed target by electrons travelling almost at the speed of light and resulting in a harder beam of much higher intensity (Fig. 5.5). As well as possessing much greater depth-dose, these beams typically have far less in the way of scattered radiation, leading to a much cleaner, more precise beam with a narrower penumbra than with traditional cobalt apparatus. In addition, the output (or dose rate) is considerably greater, leading to shorter treatment times. Unfortunately, the drawbacks of very high initial expenditure and maintenance costs combined with slightly lower reliability than cobalt equipment, have yet to be fully overcome. Nevertheless, the linear accelerator has become the standard work-horse of most sophisticated radiotherapy departments. A further important advantage of this equipment is that the target can be moved out of position, yielding a beam of high-velocity electrons

Fig. 5.4 Typical depth-dose curves for radiotherapy equipment (kilovoltage, megavoltage and 30 MeV electron beam). There is skin 'build-up' over the first centimetre for megavoltage therapy but not for kilovoltage or electron treatment. Depth-dose for both megavoltage and electron beam therapy is much superior to kilovoltage treatment and the 'skin-sparing' effect has great clinical benefit.

Fig. 5.5 Schematic representation of an isocentrically mounted 4–8 MeV linear accelerator. (From Meredith W.J., Massey J.B. *Fundamental Physics of Radiology*. Baltimore: Williams & Wilkins, 1972. With permission.)

(instead of X-rays) of up to 30 MeV energy or more which can be useful therapeutically in certain clinical situations (see below).

To the clinician, the fundamental difference between X-ray and electron therapy lies in their entirely different depth-dose characteristics (Fig. 5.4). With X-ray or gamma ray therapy, the amount of radiation energy deposited at any given depth of tissue (the depth-dose) falls off exponentially which means that however powerful the source and whatever the distance, unwanted areas of tissue will be irradiated, both superficial to the tumour area, and also beyond it. The entrance and exit dose will irradiate a substantial volume of normal host tissue, and this unavoidable characteristic is usually the limiting factor in a course of treatment. With electron therapy this disadvantage is at least partly overcome, since the beam decays completely at a depth entirely dependent on the energy of the electron beam.

With low and medium voltage X-rays, the energy deposited in the tissues is critically dependent on the mean atomic number of the tissue in which this deposition is occurring. With high voltage X-rays, gamma rays and electrons, the energy absorbed by the tissue is much less dependent on the atomic number, so that the drawbacks of very high bone absorption (with its twin problems of dosage inhomogeneity and radionecrosis) is largely avoided. Radiotherapists are therefore very careful when irradiating superficial lesions situated over bone or cartilage, which require treatment with low voltage (superficial) beams. For this reason, electron therapy is often preferred in these cases, particularly for skin tumours which overlie an area of cartilage. Common examples include basal cell carcinomas on the nose or pinna of the ear.

A further intriguing possibility under active clinical trial at present, is the use of heavy charged and uncharged particles, including neutrons, protons and pi-mesons. All of these beams have theoretical advantages, although the capital expenditure required for the development and building of neutron and charged particle generators is substantially greater than the cost of more conventional equipment. Only a few centres throughout the world have these resources available at present. With neutron beam therapy the major theoretical advantage is that the radiosensitivity of tumour cells is much less dependent on their state of oxygenation than when X-rays are used, a critically important characteristic since local tumour recurrence after conventional radiotherapy is thought to be largely due to the relative ineffectiveness of X-ray treatment on hypoxic malignant cells (see below). If this is so, then treatment by neutron therapy could perhaps prove curative with localized but relatively radio-insensitive tumours such as glioma, sarcoma, salivary tumours and malignant melanoma.

Preliminary work in the 1970s was encouraging, but further clinical trials have largely failed to confirm any advantage, particularly in pelvic tumours in which a large-scale Medical Research Council sponsored trial, using conventional X-ray treatment as the 'control' arm of the study, was recently discontinued because of the failure of neutron therapy to offer superior treatment, coupled with an increase in the normal tissue damage to surrounding areas. In neutron therapy for head-and-neck cases, there appears unequivocally to have been an increase in major (sometimes life-threatening) side-effects including a dramatically worse capacity for surgical healing, making surgical management for local recurrences almost impossible. The final report of the important Edinburgh study confirmed equivalent local control rates for both photon (or conventional X-ray) and neutron therapy (44% versus 45%) but better 5-year and 10-year survival with photons, due to increased fatalities from treatment morbidity in the neutron group. Seven of the 85 patients in the neutron group died from local tissue necrosis compared with none (out of 80) in the conventionally treated group. Neutron therapy appears to have few if any clinical applications at present, although the results of continuing head-and-neck trials of neutron therapy are awaited.

Irradiation with protons or pi-mesons requires even more expensive equipment and is not currently available in Britain, although there are centres both in the United States and Europe which are carrying out clinical trials. The particular theoretical advantage with these beams is that the energy is deposited at a defined narrow level in tissue, which is determined by the energy of the beam. Very little of the beam energy is lost in superficial tissues, and virtually none in tissue deep to the chosen volume. This phenomenon, known as the Bragg effect after its discoverer, naturally makes the concept of heavy charged particle irradiation attractive to the radiotherapist, since it might perhaps be possible to irradiate a given tumour to a very high dosage without compromising host tissues. With increasingly sophisticated methods of tumour imaging and localization, the precision use of this kind of beam would seem to approach an ideal form of radiation therapy.

BIOLOGICAL PROPERTIES OF IONIZING RADIATION

Tumour sensitivity

Ever since the turn of the century, clinical scientists have been fascinated by the extraordinary cellular events which occur when living tissue is exposed to a beam of ionizing radiation. It is now clear that radiation-induced damage may be lethal, resulting in cell death, or sublethal, in which case the cellular damage can be partially or completely repaired. In general the degree of radiosensitivity of any given tumour type will depend not only on the immediate damage sustained by the cell (a measure of its true 'intrinsic' sensitivity) but also on its ability to repair the sublethal damage that has been caused. Although a high degree of radiosensitivity is generally required if there is to be any hope of a radiation cure, other factors may prevent the realization of this aim; radiosensitivity is not in itself sufficient. Acute lymphoblastic leukaemia, for instance, is highly radiosensitive, since small malignant lympho-blasts are permanently damaged by a relatively low dose of radiation. However, the widespread nature of this disease, which by definition affects the whole of the bone marrow and therefore every organ supplied by the peripheral bloodstream, made it impossible until recently to deliver curative radiotherapy without fatal over-irradiation. The modern technique of allogeneic bone marrow transplantation has resulted in safe delivery of total body irradiation to a sufficiently high dosage for total irreversible ablation of the malignant marrow elements. It is not the bone marrow transplant itself which is the therapeutic event, but the lethal radiation damage inflicted on the leukaemic cell population.

The physicochemical events which take place within the radiation-damaged cells are far from understood. Although there is little doubt that the important target site is the nuclear DNA, it is less common for the damage to be inflicted as a result of a 'direct hit', though this mechanism will certainly produce irreversible cleavage of the DNA strands. More commonly the effects are indirect, resulting in the production of unstable, highly reactive and short-lived free radicals which in turn produce destruction of the normal DNA molecule with which they rapidly react. The probability of a lethal cell injury varies not only with the quantity of radiation energy deposited in the tissues (a function of the output of the radiation beam) but also with the intensity of the beam and with its 'type', that is whether the radiation is produced by gamma rays, electrons, neutrons or other particles. These differences give rise to the concept of linear energy transfer (LET) which refers to the amount of radiation energy transferred to the tissue per unit track length by the particular beam. In general, kilovoltage beams of X-rays have a higher LET than megavoltage beams, and neutron beams have a very much higher LET than X-rays or gamma rays. Thus appropriate adjustments in total doses will have to be made if neutron therapy, for example, is offered as an alternative to conventional treatment. Another important principle is that the relatively protective effect of hypoxia (on tumour cells) is particularly apparent with beams of relatively low LET. This is one of the reasons why neutron therapy was long thought to be more effective regardless of the state of oxygenation of the malignant tissues and should prove superior to X-ray therapy if, indeed, anoxia is genuinely as critical as it appears to be from the mass of radiobiological literature that has accumulated during the last 50 years.

The clinical failure of neutron therapy, though at odds with this theoretical understanding of cellular resistance, might be explained on the grounds of the technically poor quality of neutron beams presently available.

Experimental studies have shown that human tumour cells have markedly different intrinsic radiosensitivities which closely parallel clinical experience. Our present understanding of this correlation postulates two components to cell kill, the α-component which is log−linear (exponential) and therefore appears as a straight line in dose−survival curves (Fig. 5.6); and a bending or β-component which occurs over a shorter dose-range and at low dose-levels. Intrinsic differences in sensitivity are most marked in the low-dose region (clinically of greatest importance) below 2 Gy per treatment fraction, and low dose-rate irradiation is likely to exaggerate these differences. Indeed, at low dose rates, less sensitive cells become relatively more resistant. This is often forwarded as an argument for larger fractions in less sensitive tumours. In the linear quadratic mathematical model, using an α-component which is the linear dose-function and β the square of the dose, cell survival is the common end-point. Fractionation tends to spare late responding tissues more than early responding tissues and tumours.

In other clinical circumstances, failure of radiation therapy may occur because of the recurrence of disease after apparently successful radiation treatment. This is a frequent event, for example in squamous cell carcinoma of the bronchus, where careful assessment by chest X-ray and even bronchoscopy may well demonstrate an apparently satisfactory response to treatment. When relapse occurs, often 1−2 years after primary treatment, what can we suggest by way of explanation? One widely held view, for which there is a good deal of experimental evidence, is that at the time of the initial treatment, there is a spectrum of cellular sensitivity to the radiation, and that the degree of oxygenation of each cell is the key determining factor. A great deal of radiobiological work has gone into defining and characterizing this phenomenon, and almost all studies (both with experimental animals and *in vitro* tissue culture systems) have shown that well oxygenated cells are substantially more radiosensitive than those which are anoxic.

This difference in sensitivity may be reflected in a 2- or 3-fold increase in the dosage required for tumour eradication in an anoxic environment (Fig. 5.6), and the clinical importance of this observation is thought by many to be critical, since cells far removed from a good arterial supply will inevitably be relatively anoxic. In large tumours with a relatively rapid

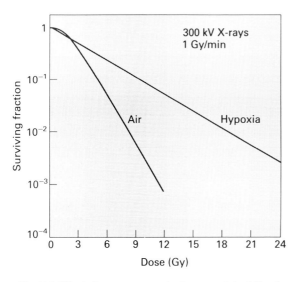

Fig. 5.6 Effect of oxygen concentration on cytotoxicity of X-rays. The survival of Hela cells are shown under conditions of hypoxia and in air. (From Duncan W., Nias A.H.W. *Clinical Radiology*. Edinburgh: Churchill Livingstone, 1977. With permission.)

growth rate and in areas of necrosis where vascularization is poor, anoxia may be a major cause of radioresistance, and experiments using microelectrodes for measurement of oxygen tension have confirmed these theoretical predictions.

Quite apart from the oxygen effect, the progenitor cells will not be equally radiosensitive so that recurrence after apparently successful treatment may be due to repopulation through regeneration of the radioresistant stem cells within the tumour. This can take place either after a complete course of radiotherapy, or rapidly, even between fractions given, say, on a daily basis. There is at least some evidence that regrowth through repopulation may be more delayed with malignant tissues than with normal host cells, and that this may be an important basis for the difference between the relatively adequate regenerative capability of many normal tissues, in contrast to the more permanent destructive effects on malignant tumours. This is analogous to the effects of chemotherapy on normal and malignant tissue (see Chapter 6).

Fractionation and cell death

Fractionation, the use of repeated dosage of radiation within a course of treatment, has been the subject of considerable interest. Early radiation workers rapidly realized that repeated use of modest radiation doses seemed to be the best method of safely delivering a higher total dose of radiation than would be possible with a single large treatment, and that this, in general, led to a greater likelihood of cure. Interest in fractionation has developed not only because of a natural desire to understand the mechanisms of radiation-induced cell damage, but also to learn how best to exploit this phenomenon and to advise the clinician as to the optimal choice of fraction size and overall treatment time. These are important details which might make the difference between success and failure. In most single-dose experiments, the degree of damage to the malignant cell (usually measured

by inhibition of cell division) is directly proportional to the radiation dose, in a log–linear fashion (Fig. 5.6). The important additional feature is that at low dosage, the steep curve is flattened to form a characteristic 'shoulder'. With relatively more radioresistant cells (such as malignant melanoma) the shoulder will be broader, and the rest of the curve less steep.

Most theorists agree that the shoulder region represents an area of sublethal damage, from which repair is possible. With repeated or fractionated treatment, further radiation damage can be inflicted before completion of this repair, although naturally the degree of cell recovery between fractions will depend on the interval and intensity of each fraction of treatment. If recovery outweighs the degree of newly inflicted damage by each succeeding fraction of radiation, then the total effect might well be less satisfactory than treatment employing a single large fraction. Although most experimental work suggests that with each daily fraction of treatment, the shoulder region is reproduced (Fig. 5.7), the clinical superiority of fractionated treatment may, in large part, be due to the relatively slow rate of recovery in malignant cells.

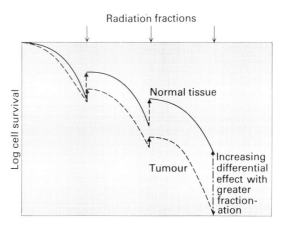

Radiation fractions

Log cell survival

Normal tissue

Tumour

Increasing differential effect with greater fractionation

Fig. 5.7 Fractionation: the effect of repeated doses of radiation. Fractionation increases the differential cytotoxic effect on normal and malignant tissue. (From Duncan W., Nias A.H.W. *Clinical Radiology*. Edinburgh: Churchill Livingstone, 1977. With permission.)

Other possible advantages of fractionated treatment relate to the rapid improvement in oxygenation of the tissues following early treatments, which, by reduction of the tumour mass, leads to relief of vascular obstruction, a more effective blood supply and greater sensitivity to subsequent doses of irradiation, again due to the oxygen effect. In addition to these theoretical advantages, fractionated treatment has other benefits since the earlier fractions may produce a significant improvement in clinical well-being, allowing better tolerance of the total course. Radiation sickness is often much less pronounced with fractionated treatments than with a single large radiation dose. This allows much greater flexibility from a course rather than a single treatment, permitting, for example, for a change in radiation volume and/or dose rate, which may well be called for as the tumour begins to resolve.

On the other hand, lengthy periods of fractionated treatment — often up to 6 weeks in current practice — carry the potential disadvantage of tumour cell repopulation during the course of therapy, with acceleration of repopulating clonogenic cells as little as 1 week after initiation of treatment. For this and other reasons there is increasing interest in the concept of continuous hyperfractionated treatment, using two or three treatment fractions in a single day and treating the patient within a much shorter period of time, even including weekends, for say 2–3 weeks rather than the conventional 6-week period. This approach appears extremely promising in certain clinical situations but remains to be proven in prospectively randomized trials [8,10,13].

Despite these general comments, there have been few satisfactory studies comparing different fractionation regimens. Most radiotherapists rely on approaches which have been empirically tested and found acceptable in terms of both effectiveness and toxicity. For example, lengthy fractionation regimens of 6 weeks of daily treatment are often used for squamous carcinomas, while other radiotherapists offer treatment which takes no more than 3 or 4 weeks. Very careful estimates of dose equivalence have to be employed when comparing treatment regimens since all radiotherapists know that, for example, the radiobiological effect of a single dose of 10 Gy (1000 rad) is greatly in excess of the effect produced by 10 daily doses of 1 Gy (100 rad). A yardstick for measurement of dose equivalence is therefore essential, not only for prospective trials of fractionation regimens but also for the radiotherapist who may sometimes need to deviate from his standard regimen for a whole host of reasons. Unexpected machine breakdown, pressures on equipment and staff shortages can all occur unpredictably from time to time.

Although no system can accurately predict absolute dose equivalence, the most satisfactory approach remains that of Ellis, who introduced the concept of a *nominal standard dose* (NSD), or single dose which produces a clinical reaction as close as possible to that produced by any given fractionation regimen. The important parameters of this NSD equation were the total dose of radiation, the number of fractions and the length of the treatment from first to last fraction. Use of the NSD concept has at least permitted an attempt at comparing the clinical effectiveness of differing treatment approaches, and has been helpful in confirming the importance of the dose response concept for optimal tumour control at a variety of sites.

RESPONSE OF TISSUES TO RADIATION

Normal tissues

Since the adverse effects of radiation limit the clinician in choice of dosage, an understanding of the radiation tolerance of normal host tissues is an important facet of the radiotherapist's training and practice. The study of radiation response in normal tissues has become a major area of specialized research, and very wide discrepancies of the radiation tolerance of different organs have been demonstrated (Table 5.2). In general, the most radiosensitive tissues are those with a rapid cell

Table 5.2 Radiosensitivity of normal and malignant tissue

Radiosensitivity	Normal	Malignant
Highly sensitive	Marrow Gonad Gut (mucosa) Lymphatic tissue Eye (lens)	Lymphoma Leukaemia Seminoma Ewing's sarcoma Many embryonal tumours

Moderately sensitive	Liver
	Kidney
	Lung
	Skin
	Breast
	Gut wall
	Nervous tissue
		Small cell lung cancer
		Breast cancer
		Squamous carcinomas (including
		   gynaecological, head and neck, and
		   skin tumours)
		Adenocarcinomas of the bowel
		Glioma

Relatively insensitive	Bone Connective tissue Muscle	Sarcoma of bone and connective tissue Melanoma

division which include the bone marrow, the stem cells of the gonads and the epithelial lining of the alimentary tract, all of which are damaged by relatively low doses of radiation.

A particularly tragic and clear-cut illustration of the critical importance of radiation dose for long-term damage was provided by the unintended over-irradiation of over 200 cancer patients treated in the United Kingdom at a single centre in 1988. Due to the miscalibration of a radiocobalt source, most of these patients received doses of 25% above the recommended prescribed level, with varying effects dependent upon the site. Many patients treated for breast carcinoma suffered profound local effects in the breast itself, together with local chest wall damage (including rib fracture) and in some cases a brachial plexus radioneuropathy. It seems clear that relatively small dose excesses ('small' at least in comparison with current drug therapy) can for the radiotherapist result in disastrous and in many cases irreversible consequences.

Clinically, there is an important distinction to be drawn between early, *acute*, effects and later, *chronic*, damage. It is not necessarily the intensity of the acute reaction which determines the probability and duration of the long-term effects. Even where recovery from acute irradiation appears complete, the 'reserve' of stem cells in these organs is often permanently depleted, so that further treatment either with radiation therapy or cytotoxic drugs may well produce a surprising degree of tissue damage including, for example, marrow suppression. Understanding of this long-term but latent (invisible) damage is of great importance since increasing numbers of cancer patients are likely to be offered both these forms of therapy.

Highly radiosensitive tissues

HAEMOPOIETIC TISSUES

The bone marrow is exceedingly sensitive to irradiation. In humans, a single total body dose of 4 Gy (400 rad) would prove lethal to about half of all patients, the majority of these deaths due to early myelosuppression producing anaemia, neutropenia and thrombocytopenia. With localized treatment at high dose (a much more common clinical situation), long-lasting inhibition of myelopoiesis occurs, but usually without appreciable effect on the blood count. Lymphopenia is a well recognized complication of localized radiotherapy at any site, resulting from irradiation of the blood as it passes through the beam—a consequence of the extreme radiosensitivity of the small lymphocyte. Allogeneic bone marrow transplantation has permitted total body irradiation to a higher dose (often up to 10 Gy, 1000 rad) as part of the therapy for acute leukaemia and other diseases, including non-Hodgkin's lymphoma and myeloma. In addition, large areas of the body can now be treated with therapeutic irradiation for widespread and painful bony metastases (e.g. from myeloma or carcinoma of the prostate) without recourse to marrow transplantation techniques since the unirradiated marrow is able to compensate by increased production. This is the basis of so-called 'hemi-body irradiation', an increasingly used method of simple palliation for patients with widespread metastatic disease, which can be repeated to the opposite half of the body providing a suitable gap of 6–8 weeks is allowed between the two fractions of treatment.

THE GONADS

In the testes and ovary, small single doses of radiotherapy can permanently damage reproductive function, although the testis is undoubtedly more sensitive. It is likely that some of the primitive spermatogonia (the precursors of the spermatocytes) may be sensitive to a dose of as little as 1 Gy (100 rad) although a dose as low as this would be unlikely to reduce the human sperm count to zero. The radiation sensitivity of the hormone-producing testicular Leydig cell is very much less, so that large doses of radiotherapy to the human testis do not result in loss of secondary sexual characteristics. In the female, single doses of 4–5 Gy (4–500 rad) have been used to induce artificial menopause, although some 30% of women appear to continue regular menstruation following this single fraction of radiation. Fractionated treatment to 10–12 Gy (1000–1200 rad) results in complete cessation of menses in virtually every patient.

Moderately radiosensitive tissues

This group is characterized by relatively low cell turnover rates which are paralleled by a relative, but by no means complete insensitivity to radiation; these include nerve cells, including the brain itself, as well as the spinal cord and peripheral nervous system, skin, kidney, gut and other sites (Table 5.2).

NERVOUS TISSUE

The nervous system is of great concern partly because the sequelae of damage to the central nervous system can be both profound and irreversible, and also because for the large majority of malignant brain tumours, radiation therapy is much the most valuable non-surgical modality available (see Chapter 11). During the early acute phase of radiation response, the blood vessels, nerve cells and supporting glial structures are all injured directly; sufficiently large doses may result in acute cerebral oedema and a sudden rise in intracranial pressure. These changes will gradually subside, but chronic effects include demyelination, vascular damage with proliferation of subendothelial fibrous tissue, and, eventually, brain necrosis if the dose is sufficiently high. It is generally accepted that the hypothalamus, brain stem and upper cervical spine are rather more sensitive to radiation than other parts of the brain and it is also thought that concurrent administration of chemotherapy (chiefly methotrexate and vincristine) may also reduce radiation tolerance.

Irradiation of the spinal cord may pose even more problems, particularly since this may be unavoidable in, for example, the palliation of painful bony metastases of the spine. The radiation tolerance of the spinal cord is governed by a variety of important details such as the length of cord irradiated, the fractionation employed, and the total dose given. It is widely held that for a 10 cm length of cord, a total dose of 40 Gy (4000 rad) in 4 weeks is safe although many clinicians err on the side of great caution since radiation myelitis, leading to irreversible paraparesis, is such an appalling complication. Recent work with total body irradiation has shown that a single dose of about 10 Gy (1000 rad) delivered to the whole length of the spinal cord very rarely produces significant neurological sequelae, although the mildest (reversible) late complication, that of Lhermitte's syndrome of paraesthesiae in the extremities on flexion of the neck, is often encountered. Moreover, with prophylactic spinal cord irradiation in children with medulloblastoma, the risk of clinically significant neurological sequelae, after doses as high as 30 Gy (3000 rad) applied over 5–6 weeks to the whole of the spinal cord, seems acceptably low. In general, careful fractionation should be employed wherever a significant length of cord is likely to be irradiated in a patient whose survival may be prolonged. For palliative radiation treatment it seems prudent to recommend the lowest effective dose which is compatible with durable pain relief, particularly since further treatment may well be required, inevitably adding to the possibility of cord damage.

THE SKIN

A portion of skin will be irradiated in all patients treated by external methods of X-ray therapy. Historically, the skin reaction was the chief guide in determining the total radiation dose. With modern high-energy (megavoltage) equipment, far fewer severe skin reactions are seen, since the scattered radiation component of these beams is almost exclusively in the forward direction so that maximum energy deposition takes place well beneath the skin surface (Fig. 5.4). None the less, clinically important skin reactions can still pose major problems both with orthovoltage and even with megavoltage beams (Table 5.3). Typically, the changes consist of an erythema of increasing severity, leading to dry and then moist desquamation, followed (if the radiation therapy is discontinued) by a repair process associated with progressive fibrosis, hyperplasia of vascular elements (sometimes resulting in telangiectasia much later on) and

Table 5.3 Skin reactions to radiotherapy

Early changes	Later changes
Erythema	Fibrosis
Dry and moist desquamation	Loss of pigment
Pigmentation	Telangiectasia
Epilation	Loss of skin appendages
Loss of sweat gland function	Loss of connective
Tissue oedema	tissue

also by excessive pigmentation which may be permanent, although depigmentation can also occur. If the skin is further irradiated at a time when moist desquamation is evident, then extensive skin and subcutaneous necrosis may occur; this takes place when the treatment is separated by months or even years. It is therefore unwise to attempt re-irradiation of recurrent skin carcinomas, since the risk of necrosis is ever present and such cases are usually better treated by surgery. It is also worth remembering that the skin 'appendages' such as sweat glands, sebaceous glands and hair follicles are also damaged directly by radiation. Radiation-induced epilation of the scalp is an inevitable drawback of whole brain irradiation for cerebral metastases, which is in other respects an effective technique with few side-effects. Both single doses (as in total body irradiation) and fractionated treatment will cause complete epilation of the scalp if the dose is high enough, although hair regrowth will usually occur, given time, even when a radical dose has been used as, for example, in children with medulloblastoma.

THE EYE

The eye is frequently irradiated, particularly during the treatment of carcinomas of the maxillary antrum and paranasal sinuses, and of course in the definitive radiation therapy of orbital lymphomas, rhabdomyosarcomas, retinoblastomas and other orbital tumours. It is often not appreciated that for the most part, the eye is relatively radioresistant, particularly its more posterior structures. Careful attention to detail can result in a healthy eye with very adequate vision even after whole orbital irradiation. However, there are two important points to remember. Firstly, the greatest danger to the eye is posed by dryness of the cornea, leading to keratoconjunctivitis sicca. This generally results from lack of tear formation, following irradiation of the lacrymal gland which can be avoided in most instances by the use of a small lead shield. Second, the most radiosensitive structure of the eye is the lens, which is particularly sensitive to large single fractions of irradiation. Cataract formation can often be prevented by the use of a pencil-shaped corneal shield, although there is always the danger of under-irradiation of important structures deep to the protected cornea and lens. Fortunately, radiation-induced cataracts can be removed without difficulty; only a small proportion give rise to significant visual symptoms.

THE KIDNEY

The kidney is frequently irradiated during treatment of abdominal or retroperitoneal tumours, and is a relatively radiosensitive structure. Both glomerular filtration rate and renal plasma flow are reduced after modest radiation doses, and it is often a year or more before recovery begins. Acute radiation nephritis can occur when the dose to both kidneys is no greater than about 25 Gy (2500 rad) in 5 weeks. The acute clinical syndrome includes proteinuria, uraemia and hypertension which can be irreversible and even fatal. More chronic changes include persistent albuminuria and poor glomerular and tubular function, which may be life-long even in patients who recover from the acute syndrome. These complications are particularly likely to occur after whole abdominal irradiation.

THE GUT

Although both small and large bowel tissues are sensitive to radiation, the rectum deserves special mention since this is frequently the organ of limiting tolerance when treating carcinomas of the cervix and other pelvic tumours. Acute radiation reactions, accompanied by diarrhoea, tenesmus and occasional rectal haemorrhage, are encountered both with external irradiation of the pelvis and also with intracavitary treatment. When intracavitary sources are used, careful attempts must be made to reduce the rectal dose by packing the vagina in order to keep the rectum well away from the high doses of radiation. The later radiation effects are of even greater importance, and include oedema and fibrosis of the bowel, which once again may be responsible for diarrhoea, painful proctitis and rectal bleeding, sometimes progressing to stricture, abscess or fistula formation. Occasionally these complications are severe enough to warrant temporary or even permanent colostomy or may cause difficult diagnostic problems by mimicking symptoms of recurrence of the cancer. Fortunately these severe sequelae have become less frequent with better understanding of radiation dosimetry within the pelvis, coupled with increased attention to technical details. Radiation damage to the small bowel is pathologically similar to that of the rectum and may limit treatment of intraabdominal tumours. Late sequelae include stricture formation which may cause intestinal obstruction.

Less radiosensitive tissues

BONE

Therapeutic radiation of bone is a particular problem in children since normal growth may be interrupted, especially when the epiphyseal plate is included in volumes taken to radical dosage, as this area is responsible for the increase in length of any growing long bone. Direct irradiation of the epiphysis interferes with the high mitotic rate of the cartilaginous cells adjacent to the shaft. Radiation damage to the metaphysis may also be severe, though apparently fully reversible provided that the radiation dose is moderate.

The severity of radiation-induced deformity

and/or growth disturbance is much greater with high dosage, most particularly with large radiation volumes. The advent of megavoltage irradiation has been particularly helpful in this respect. None the less in children treated for medulloblastoma, where the whole spine is irradiated to a minimum dose of 30 Gy (3000 rad) in 5–6 weeks, the majority of survivors have some deficit in the sitting height. As many as one-third remain persistently below the 3rd centile for height. Younger children are at particular risk but this has to be accepted when radiotherapy is essential for cure, as in medulloblastoma. The late sequelae of radiotherapy and chemotherapy following treatment of childhood cancer are discussed in Chapter 24. Modern treatment with growth hormone replacement has greatly reduced the severity of these problems.

OTHER CONNECTIVE TISSUES

Muscle, tendon and connective tissue are all relatively insensitive to radiation and do not usually limit dosage. Fibrosis may occur when high or repeated doses are used, sometimes leading to loss of joint mobility and contractures.

LATE SEQUELAE OF RADIATION

In addition to the specific effects on the various organs as described above, there are a number of important long-term hazards following the use of radiotherapy. These include carcinogenicity, mutagenicity and teratogenicity, and are all attributable to a fundamental property of ionizing radiation, namely its biological effect on nuclear DNA with consequent permanent damage to genetic material.

Carcinogenesis

This is a well documented phenomenon. Survivors from Hiroshima have an increased incidence of neoplasia, particularly leukaemia. Recently an increased incidence of breast cancer has been reported, 35 years after the acute radiation damage was inflicted. Analysis of a large series of patients with ankylosing spondylitis treated by low doses of radiotherapy, has demonstrated a 10-fold increase in the incidence of leukaemia. Occasionally malignant change develops at the site of previous localized irradiation, for example osteosarcoma of the scapula following radiation for carcinoma of the breast. In children treated for retinoblastoma, late orbital neoplasms may occur (see Chapter 24).

These studies illustrate the general points that neoplasia tends to occur within an organ directly affected by the radiation beam, that there is usually a latent period of at least 10 years before neoplasia develops, and that even moderate doses of irradiation such as those which used to be employed for benign disease during childhood or young adult life may lead to a radiation-induced malignancy later on. Much higher doses of radiation are usually given to patients with cancer but the patients are usually older and with a far smaller likelihood of long survival, so that the true risk of late radiation carcinogenesis is much less amenable to study. In addition it is now widely accepted that patients with cancer have a higher probability of developing a second neoplasm. This is sometimes due to common risk factors, for example, patients cured of early laryngeal carcinomas who continue to smoke and then succumb to carcinoma of the bronchus. Patients with cancer also have an inherent increased probability of developing a second malignancy for reasons which are currently unclear (see p. 35). Increasingly, patients are nowadays treated with radiation and cytotoxic chemotherapy, the latter adding to the risk of carcinogenesis. This is well demonstrated by the higher risk of acute leukaemia following treatment of Hodgkin's disease (see Chapters 6 and 25). As more patients are treated with, and cured by, the combination of radiation and chemotherapy, we must expect the incidence of second neoplasms to rise. Although the risk of radiation carcinogenesis is low, it should certainly deter radiotherapists from treating benign skin and other disorders, particularly in children, which could be better and more safely dealt with by other means.

Teratogenicity

The teratogenic effects of ionizing radiation are well known. Minimal exposure, even to 'soft' X-rays in pregnant women is hazardous because of the risk of growth retardation and serious malformation in the developing embryo. Irradiation during the last trimester, well after organogenesis is complete, is safer although growth retardation may still occur. Radiation treatment of pregnant women must be avoided wherever possible. This may well lead to difficult points of judgement especially when the diagnosis of malignancy is made early in the pregnancy. For example, in patients with pelvic tumours (usually carcinoma of the cervix which has become increasingly common in the child-bearing age group) there is general agreement that during the first trimester of pregnancy, treatment should be given as if the patient were not pregnant. Spontaneous abortion will always occur but few would feel justified in delaying therapy for perhaps 6 months until the pregnancy is over (see p. 327).

Mutagenicity

This refers to genetic alteration in somatic or germ cells resulting from their direct irradiation. In somatic cells these mutations may be the basis of radiation-induced carcinogenesis. In germ cells mutation may lead to fetal death or abnormality although in humans, most germ cell mutations are thought to be non-viable. For these reasons abnormal births following scattered irradiation to the testis are very uncommon.

THE RADIOTHERAPY DEPARTMENT

In order to deal adequately with both surface and deep-seated tumours, departments of radiotherapy must possess a suitable range of equipment, comprising superficial (low energy), orthovoltage (medium energy) and supervoltage (high energy) machines. In general, a department will need to draw on a population of at least half a million in order to have a sufficient throughput of new cases. At least 40% of cancer patients require treatment with radiotherapy at some point. Important additional features of the modern department include facilities for planning the radiation treatment, closely liaising with departments of medical physics. For many patients, multifield techniques are used and the physics staff, in conjunction with the radiotherapist, will decide (usually with the aid of a planning computer) on the most appropriate field arrangement. Modern computing techniques have enormously improved the tasks of defining and comparing the alternative plans; drawing out the isodose curves (similar to contour lines on an ordnance survey map) defining points of equal radiation depth-dose and making suitable corrections for tissues of unusual density such as lung or bone (Fig. 5.8). In many departments, a treatment simulator is available. This is able to mimic the radiation therapy apparatus in its geometry, capability and limitations, and is useful in 'setting-up' patients without actually delivering any treatment, allowing the careful appraisal of both the tumour volume to be irradiated and the best alternative techniques. In addition, a mould room, often separately staffed, will be necessary if there is a sizeable demand for treatment immobilization devices such as individually manufactured perspex head shells for use in head and neck or brain tumour work. Mould room staff are often responsible for manufacturing templates which might be necessary either for superficial irradiation of irregularly shaped skin cancers, or when individualized shaped fields are used such as the 'mantle' or 'inverted-Y' fields for irradiation of patients with Hodgkin's disease.

As recently pointed out by Horwich, 'since the birth of radiotherapy at the beginning of this century it has been apparent that the radio-

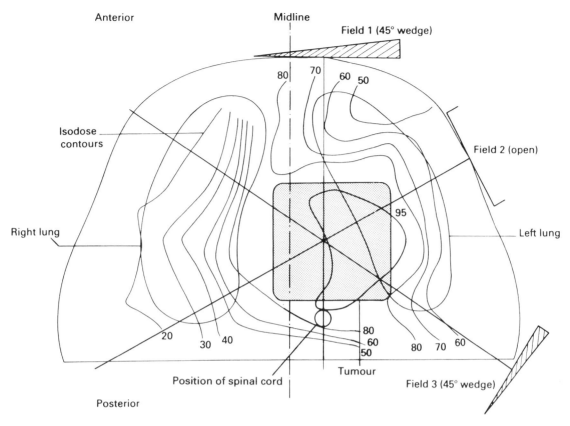

Fig. 5.8 Typical plan for multifield irradiation of carcinoma of left main bronchus showing site of tumour, position of lungs and isodose contours.

therapist must be fully conversant with the physics of ionizing radiation and with technical aspects of radiation delivery systems, including machine design, dosimetry, treatment planning and simulation, fixation and beam alignment.' Clearly, it is the radiotherapist's responsibility not only to judge whether radiotherapeutic treatment is indicated but also to decide upon the best technique, field arrangement, choice of therapy unit, total dose and fractionation. Although these technical aspects of radiotherapy are often thought to be synonomous with the total workload of the radiotherapist, they in fact form a limited part of the task. Perhaps even more important is his continuing and ever-present role as the clinician respon-

sible for diagnosis, management and follow-up of patients with cancer. In Britain, where the division of radiotherapy from diagnostic radiology occurred early, departments of radiotherapy have been entirely clinical (i.e. non-diagnostic) for well over 30 years, and have assumed the complete care of cancer patients.

RADIOTHERAPY PLANNING AND TREATMENT TECHNIQUES

Non-radiotherapists are often puzzled by the technical vocabulary which radiotherapists use, making it difficult for them to understand the intentions, achievements and limitations of the techniques employed. A short glossary follows:

Treatment prescription. The total dose and treatment time are normally prescribed at the outset of treatment, though in certain circumstances the radiotherapist may prefer to prescribe, say, the first week's treatment and then make a further decision as to whether to continue or not. Total absorbed dose is given in rad, Gray (Gy) or centiGray (cGy). 1 rad = 100 ergs/g and 1 Gy = 1 J/kg of absorber. The Gray is increasingly preferred as it is the S.I. unit of dose; 1 Gy = 100 rad and some radiotherapists prefer centiGrays to Grays since 1 centiGray = 1 rad, so that total dose in cGy is identical to total dose in rad. For most treatments, the total dose is split into a number of equal fractions given either on a daily basis or intermittently. The number of fractions of treatment is also prescribed by the radiotherapist. The *treatment volume*, that is the volume of tissue to be covered by the prescribed radiation dose, is determined by the radiotherapist using whatever radiological and imaging aids he feels to be necessary.

Maximum, minimum and modal dose. Since it is impossible to achieve homogeneous irradiation of the desired volume without irradiation of surrounding normal tissue, the radiotherapist must decide on the appropriate compromise. One traditional approach was to prescribe to a *maximum* dose, that is, a dose which would not be exceeded, even if this particular dose level was reached only in a small part of the tumour. The opposite approach, to prescribe to a *minimum* dose which represented the lowest possible dose level was also commonly used. The problem with prescriptions of this kind is that neither maximum nor minimum dosage is necessarily representative as a reference dose. A more satisfactory recommendation is to the *modal* dose, that is, the particular dose level occurring with the greatest frequency in the prescribed volume — by definition a more representative dose level. The *applied dose* is used where the radiotherapist wishes to prescribe the dose at the surface of the skin. If he wishes to state more precisely what the dose at a certain depth should be (e.g. when treating

spinal metastases where the dosage at a certain depth is of greater interest than the surface dose) a *depth-dose* prescription may be preferable. The radiotherapist may specify a certain dose at, say, 4 cm depth for metastases in the upper spine, but at 7 cm depth for those in the lower spine, following the expected normal anatomy.

Open (direct) and wedged fields. An open or direct field is usually applied perpendicular to the patient's skin surface and the beam emerging from the treatment machine is not modified in any way. In treatments using several fields (multifield techniques), a number of fields, usually two to four, are used and, by inserting wedges of various dimensions into the beam and using radiation fields applied obliquely, the tumour volume can be irradiated to a more homogeneous level (Fig. 5.8). The use of multifield arrangements, often employing wedged fields, has permitted safer megavoltage irradiation of deeply seated tumours to a high dose level.

Parallel opposed fields. The simplest type of multifield technique is provided by a two-field arrangement where the fields are opposed in opposite directions, usually applied to the anterior and posterior skin surface (Fig. 5.9) and irradiating the block of tissue in between. This technique is widely used and if necessary, the fields can be shaped so that important structures are avoided, for example, the use of the 'mantle' irradiation technique for patients with supradiaphragmatic Hodgkin's disease where the lungs are protected from over-irradiation (see p. 493). For parallel opposed pairs of fields, the dose normally prescribed is the *midplane dose* since this will define the dose achieved at a point midway between the two fields and indeed midway between the anterior and posterior skin surface of the patient.

Shrinking field technique. During a course of treatment it is sometimes desirable to reduce the treatment volume so that part of the initial

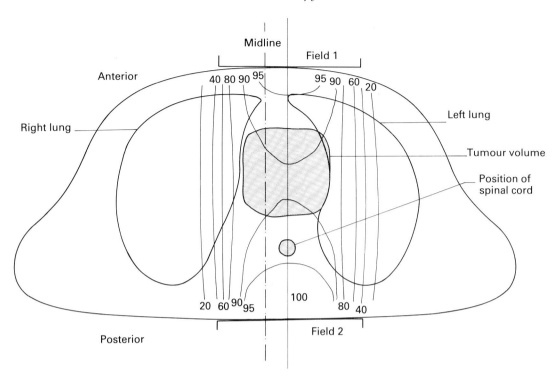

Fig. 5.9 Typical antero-posterior parallel pair field arrangement. This is often used for treating thoracic or pelvic tumours. In this instance the patient had an inoperable carcinoma of the bronchus and the tumour position and size were determined by CT scanning. The spinal cord is also shown since irradiation of this structure is often dose-limiting with this set-up.

treatment volume is treated to a certain dose level and a smaller area then taken to a higher dose. This is often done, for example, in pelvic tumours such as carcinomas of the bladder or prostate where the original treatment volume might include pelvic lymph nodes with the intention to treat these to a 'prophylactic' dose of irradiation to deal with microscopic disease, whilst the primary site requires a higher dosage. A further good example is the irradiation technique often employed in a primary bone sarcoma such as Ewing's tumour where the whole of the long bone might be irradiated to a moderate dose, the field being reduced during treatment so that the primary tumour site receives the full total dose.

Systemic irradiation. This refers to the use of radiotherapy not as traditionally used for speci-

fic local sites but throughout the whole body or substantial parts of it. Total body irradiation is well established as a means of eradicating leukaemia or lymphoma cells prior to allogeneic or autologous bone marrow transplantation (it is this irradiation which kills the tumour cells — not the transplant itself!) Hemi-body irradiation, usually to the upper or lower half of the body, is increasingly used as an excellent palliative technique for multiple painful bone metastases and in multiple myeloma (see Chapter 27).

Immobilization devices. For precision work, particularly treatment of head and neck cancers, it is essential that the patient be absolutely still, and in a reproducible position throughout the whole of the lengthy treatment period. The best means of achieving this is to use an immobilization device such as a perspex headcast (Fig.

5.10) which is individually made by obtaining a plaster impression, which is then used to produce a perspex shell which fits the patient snugly and can be screwed to the treatment couch. Use of these devices also carries the advantage that field markings can be made on the cast rather than the patient, thereby avoiding unsightly ink marks or tattoos, and ensuring accurate reproduction for each day's treatment.

There have been numerous attempts to enhance the local and regional control of cancer by means of novel approaches using particle beams (see above,) radiosensitivity drugs, photodynamic therapy and other techniques. Few of these approaches are yet established as standard therapy, indeed most, after promising theoretical preclinical data, have failed to withstand the rigours of the prospectively randomized clinical trial — nitroimidazole radio-sensitizers are perhaps the best example. Hyperfractionation, already referred to, and hypofractionation are also areas of major research efforts at present. Photodynamic therapy (PDT) has been increasingly used in certain tumours, and is a form of treatment dependent on the excitation of a number of photoactive compounds by laser-generated light of the appropriate wavelength. Haematoporphyrin derivatives are synthetic haemoglobulin compounds which when administered systematically may localize in human tumour tissue. When exposed to laser light of the correct wavelength, dose derivatives react with oxygen to form a highly reactive fragment which appears to be locally cytotoxic. Such treatment has now been attempted in head and neck, genito-urinary and gynaecological cancers as well as melanoma and endobronchial tumours.

Conformational therapy is a new and as yet experimental technique in which the high-dose volume is made to conform closely with the target volume. The intention, of course, is to use external beam therapy to better effect by excluding more normal tissue than was previously possible, thereby increasing the dose which can safely be applied to the tumour volume. Evaluation of these techniques is under active study at present, increasingly using customized field shaping designed from three-dimensional 'beam's eye view' planning, although no clear-cut benefits have yet been reported. These and other novel aspects of radiotherapy are well reviewed by Ruckdeschel.

INTEGRATION OF RADIOTHERAPY AND CHEMOTHERAPY

Remarkable changes in the therapy of cancer have occurred over the past 25 years. Whereas it was once unusual for patients to be treated both with radiotherapy and also with cytotoxic chemotherapy, it has now become commonplace. This trend is almost certain to continue for at least two reasons. First, radiation therapy is now increasingly used as an alternative to surgery for treatment of the primary tumour, particularly with carcinoma of the larynx and other head-and-neck sites, carcinoma of the cervix, and, over the past few years, with many carcinomas of the breast, bladder and prostate. Second, there is increasing use of chemotherapy both for palliation and, in some tumours, as

Fig. 5.10 Perspex head shell. Shells are individually made to ensure accurate positioning. These are widely used in treatment of tumours of the head and neck, and for pituitary tumours.

adjuvant therapy immediately preceding or succeeding the initial local treatment.

There are important disadvantages and even risks in the simultaneous use of both treatments. Some cytotoxic agents act as radiation sensitizers, increasing the local reactions from radiotherapy and occasionally producing 'recall' of previous skin reactions. The most important example is actinomycin D, although there is evidence that other drugs such as doxorubicin may also interact with radiotherapy in this way. For example, oesophageal stricture has been documented in patients undergoing mediastinal irradiation and concurrent treatment with this drug. The danger of doxorubicin-induced cardiomyopathy occurs at a lower dosage in patients who have undergone mediastinal or chest wall radiation, if a significant volume of cardiac muscle has been included. For patients undergoing wide-field irradiation, particularly if a substantial volume of bone marrow is involved (such as in children with medulloblastoma), the use of adjuvant chemotherapy may lead to more troublesome myelosuppression than with the radiation alone. In general it is true that the synchronous use of chemotherapy and radiotherapy (particularly with radiation-sensitizing drugs) leads to greater toxicity. The combination should be avoided particularly when treatment is palliative or large areas of mucosa are being irradiated. There is, however, increasing interest in the use of concurrent chemo−radiation regimens in order to improve local control (in tumours such as Ewing's sarcoma or small cell lung cancer), and at the same time to treat micrometastatic disease.

Despite these drawbacks, there are many theoretical and actual advantages to combined use of radiotherapy and chemotherapy as initial treatment, even if not administered synchronously. Radiotherapy as a powerful local tool is often able to produce tumour control with minimal physiological disturbance, though without effect on occult metastases. It may not be possible to ensure satisfactory irradiation of the primary tumour and its lymph node drainage area if nodal metastases are known to be present, for example, in gynaecological, testicular or bladder tumours with known para-aortic involvement. Chemotherapy, on the other hand, can seldom be relied upon to deal adequately with the primary tumour, though it does at least offer hope in dealing with occult metastatic disease. Combined therapy should then represent a logical approach in a disease which by its very nature has often spread widely.

Use of chemotherapy with curative intent after radiation failure represents a different form of combined therapy, since the treatments are separated in time. This approach is only likely to be successful in highly chemosensitive tumours such as Hodgkin's disease, in which chemotherapy for radiation failure is probably as successful as it is for primary therapy. A newer concept, as yet relatively unexplored, is the use of 'adjuvant' radiotherapy in patients treated primarily by chemotherapy. In small cell carcinoma of the bronchus, for example, chemotherapy is now widely employed as the mainstay of treatment. We now have to ask whether mediastinal irradiation, formerly the most widely used method of treatment, still has a role to play (see Chapter 12). Radiotherapy may also be valuable in a slightly different adjuvant fashion as, for example, in the use of cranial irradiation as prophylaxis for children with acute lymphoblastic leukaemia in whom meningeal relapse is substantially reduced by routine irradiation, since the CSF is poorly penetrated by the drugs used for systemic control.

Because many radiotherapists in Britain have no access to specialist medical oncologists, most regard themselves as specialists in chemotherapy as well, although there is substantial local variation. It is probably fair to say that with the advent of more specialist medical oncologists, and increasingly complex and taxing regimens often including new and hazardous drugs, many radiotherapists are increasingly prepared to pass this aspect of their work to those more thoroughly trained in cancer chemotherapy, although most would be unhappy to forego this role entirely.

In our view, boundary disputes between these specialties are for the most part pointless and are best solved by the radiotherapist and medical oncologist working closely together, preferably from within a single department. It seems increasingly counterproductive to maintain distinct departments of radiotherapy and medical oncology often with an uneasy relationship, rather than to create a single unified department of Clinical Oncology which is responsible for all non-surgical aspects of cancer treatment.

FURTHER READING

Abulafi A.M., Williams N.S. Photodynamic therapy for cancer. *British Medical Journal* 1992; **304**: 589–90.

Dische S., Saunders M.I. The rationale for continuous, hyperfractionated accelerated radiotherapy. *International Journal of Radiation Oncology, Biology and Physics* 1990; **19**: 1317–20.

Dobbs J., Barrett A., Ash D.V. *Practical Radiotherapy Planning*, 2nd edn. London: Edward Arnold, 1992.

Dutreix A. When and how can we improve precision in radiotherapy? *Radiation and Oncology* 1984; **2**: 275–92.

Fowler J. La Ronde — Radiation Sciences and Medical Radiology. *Radiotherapy and Oncology* 1983; **1**: 1–22.

Gilbert H.A., Kagan A.R. *Modern Radiation Oncology: Classic Literature and Current Management*, vol. 1 (1978); vol. 2 (1983). New York: Harper & Row.

Hall E.J. *Radiobiology for the Radiologist*, 3rd edn. Philadelphia: J.B. Lippincott, 1988.

Horiot J.C., Le Fur R., N'Guyen T. *et al*. Hyperfractionation versus conventional fractionation in osopharyngeal carcinoma: final analysis of a randomized trial of the EORTC cooperative group of radiotherapy. *Radiotherapy and Oncology* 1992; **25**: 229–32.

Horwich A. *Combined Radiotherapy and Chemotherapy in Clinical Oncology*. London: Edward Arnold, 1992.

Horwich A. The future of radiotherapy. *Radiotherapy and Oncology* 1990; **19**: 353–56.

Perez C.A., Brady L.W. *Principles and Practice of Radiation Oncology*. Philadelphia: J.B. Lippincott, 1987.

Peters L.J. Inherent radiosensitivity of tumor and normal tissue cells as a predictor of human tumor response. *Radiotherapy and Oncology* 1990; **17**: 177–90.

Price P. Radiotherapy in the 21st century. In Tobias J.S., Thomas P.R.M. (eds) *Current Radiation Oncology*, vol. 1. London: Edward Arnold, 1994.

Ruckdeschel J.C. Attempts to enhance locoregional control of cancer by radiotherapy, phototherapy and combined modality therapy. *Current Opinion in Oncology* 1989; **1**: 231–35.

Scalliet P. The trouble with neutrons. *European Journal of Cancer* 1991; **27**: 225–30.

Tobias J.S. Clinical practice of radiotherapy. *Lancet* 1992; **339**: 159–63.

Withers H.R. Biological basis of radiation therapy for cancers. *Lancet* 1992; **339**: 156–59.

Chapter 6
Systemic Treatment for Cancer

Over the past 30 years there has been little change in the 5-year survival rate for some common cancers. There has been a modest improvement in some tumours, for example in bladder cancer and cancer of the rectum, which is related in part to earlier diagnosis, but other tumours such as lung and pancreatic carcinoma have nearly as bad a prognosis now as in 1950. While there have been advances in the surgical and radiotherapeutic control of the primary tumour during this period, failure to improve survival is due to the fact that the major cause of death is lymphatic and blood-borne metastasis. Better control of the primary site has in general a modest effect on metastatic spread, which has often occurred by the time of surgery.

For this reason hopes of improvement in survival lie mainly in the development of better methods of treatment of metastases. The systemic treatment of cancer has, in the last 20 years, become an important part of cancer management. In some uncommon tumours such as childhood cancers, lymphomas and teratomas great progress has been made with the use of cytotoxic drugs. In other, more common cancers, the results have been less impressive, although modest improvements in survival have been obtained with chemotherapy and endocrine therapy in breast cancer. Since the treatments are sometimes toxic, a clear understanding of the uses and limitations of chemotherapy and other forms of medical treatment is essential. If there is a reasonable chance of cure, toxicity and expense can usually be accepted. If there is not, then the potential benefits of palliative treatment with cytotoxic agents must be carefully weighed against unwanted effects.

CHEMOTHERAPY [1]

In 1946 Gilman and Philips published a review of their data on the use of nitrogen mustard. The effectiveness of this class of compound in producing regression in lymphomas was rapidly established, as was the gastro-intestinal and haematological toxicity they produced, and they became the first cytotoxic agents to be introduced into clinical practice. In 1947 Farber introduced the antifolates and showed that aminopterin could produce remissions in acute leukaemia. This was followed by the production of the closely related drug methotrexate in 1949. Development of other drugs followed swiftly: 6-mercaptopurine in 1952, and the antitumour antibiotic actinomycin D in 1954. Since 1965, numerous new antimetabolites, alkylating agents and antibiotics with significant activity have been developed, many of which are related to the parent molecules discovered over 20 years ago. Examples of important drugs introduced into clinical practice in the last 15 years are epipodophyllotoxins (germ cell tumours and small cell lung cancer) and platinum analogues (lung cancer, germ cell tumours, ovarian cancer and bone sarcomas).

Recent new agents such as taxanes are now under evaluation in a variety of tumours. The process of discovery, preclinical testing and clinical evaluation is slow. The final definition of the value of a new drug may take 10 years or more following its original discovery.

The development of an anticancer drug

Before an agent is introduced into practice it

undergoes evaluation on human tumour cells in culture, on animals and then in early clinical trials. The preclinical screening is now largely using panels of human tumour cell lines. Evidence is sought for efficacy and of particular efficiency of killing against particular tumour types. These assays use growth inhibition techniques such as the sulphor-rhadamine B assay and have largely replaced screening on murine systems.

Animal toxicological studies are then performed together with assessment of responsiveness of human cancers grown as xenografts in nude mice. Using larger animals, data on pharmacokinetics, optimum schedule and toxicity are obtained, including dose, absorption, tissue distribution, plasma half-life and pathways of metabolism and excretion. Drugs showing activity are then taken forward to early (Phase 1) clinical studies. The patients selected have cancers which are widespread and usually resistant to a wide variety of cytotoxic agents. The aims are to determine optimum dosage, schedule, pharmacokinetics and metabolism. Any tumour response or toxicity is noted. It has long been recognized that previously treated ill patients have a much lower tumour response rate than well patients who have not previously been treated. Phase 1 studies are therefore not optimal for determining efficacy. In the next phase (Phase 2) a more detailed study is made on patients with tumours of defined categories, both previously treated and untreated. Here an assessment of tumour responsiveness is made. If no responses are observed in the first 15 patients there is only a 1 in 20 chance that a response rate of 20% will have been missed. In subsequent studies the drug will be assessed in combination with other agents active in a particular disease. This process usually consists of several different types of study. The simplest is a non-randomized single agent study in which a more precise definition of response and toxicity is made in a single tumour type. Occasionally such studies are a randomized comparison against another single, well established agent. When evidence of activity has been confirmed

the new agent is combined with other, established, drugs and again used in a chosen tumour type and stage. Here the aim is to assess efficacy and tolerability of the combination regimen. Such studies carry more weight if a randomized comparison is made with a standard regimen of generally accepted value.

Once the process of establishing the value of the drug, alone and in combination, is complete the agent may be used in very large-scale studies, such as those outlined in Chapter 2, in which the value of chemotherapy in improving survival in a given tumour is assessed as precisely as possible.

Principles of cancer chemotherapy

Many of the recent advances in cancer chemotherapy have come from a greater understanding of the best way to use cytotoxic agents rather than the appearance of new agents with superior efficacy. A knowledge of the way in which normal cells and tumours grow is important in order to understand the way in which cancer chemotherapy is used.

THE CELL CYCLE (see also pp. 38–42)

After cell division each cell enters a growth phase, G_1 (Fig. 6.1), which lasts for a variable period of time in different tissues. Cells which are not dividing at all are said to be in G_0 phase. After G_1 the cells move into the phase of DNA synthesis, S phase, in which the amount of chromosomal material is doubled. The cell then passes through a premitotic phase, G_2, and then into mitosis, M, in which the pairs of chromosomes separate and the cell divides.

As with other tissues, tumours are heterogeneous with respect to cell division; some cells proliferating, others dying or dormant. The tumours probably contain progenitor or 'stem' cells which are capable of cell division, continuously renewing and increasing the tumour mass. The rate of cell division in human tumours, and the speed with which their size increases, varies considerably from one disease

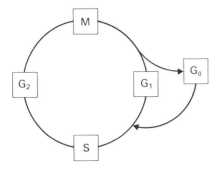

M = Mitosis (prophase→ metaphase→ anaphase→
  telophase)
G₀ = Resting phase
G₁ = Early growth phase
S = DNA synthesis
G₂ = Later growth phase

Fig. 6.1 The cell cycle.

to another as is shown in Table 6.1. The majority of common cancers increase in size very slowly in comparison with sensitive normal tissues such as bone marrow and gastro-intestinal epithelium. Even rapidly dividing tumours, such as acute myeloblastic leukaemia, do not divide as rapidly as normal myelopoietic precursors.

Vascularization of large tumour masses is

often defective and the rate of cell death is high in those areas of tumour more than 150 μ from a capillary. The tumour growth rate also depends on the proportion of cells dividing at any given time, called the *growth fraction*. In experimental tumours the growth fraction falls as the tumour becomes larger, but in humans, direct proof that small tumours have a higher growth fraction is lacking.

The potential importance of these considerations lies in the fact that some cytotoxic drugs are thought to be effective only against cells which divide. If the growth fraction is indeed higher for small tumours, these would be more susceptible to chemotherapy and this concept is often used as a rationale for adjuvant chemotherapy. Similarly if surgical removal of massive disease led to increased cell division in the remaining cells, this might also be exploited therapeutically.

Cytotoxic drugs produce their effect by damaging the reproductive integrity of cells. In general the more rapidly growing tumours with a high growth fraction are more likely to respond to drug treatment. This, however, is a generalization. The explanation of why some types of cancer (lymphoma, testicular cancer, leukaemia) are sensitive to cytotoxic drugs and other types are not (pancreatic, colonic cancer) is almost certainly not solely a matter of cell kinetics. Most cytotoxic regimens have been derived empirically, not on the basis of cell kinetics. Some drugs (for example methotrexate) are only effective at a particular phase of the cell cycle such as DNA synthesis, while others, such as alkylating agents, exhibit some action even against resting cells. Table 6.2 shows the phase specificity of some anticancer drugs.

The relationship between cell cycle and cell death is modified by repair mechanisms. For example, in a resting cell, DNA damage by an alkylating agent may be repaired before the cell moves into cycle, if the repair mechanisms are efficient and if the interval between drug exposure and onset of DNA synthesis is long. In a previously treated slowly growing tumour, damage to resting cells from alkylating agents

Table 6.1 Approximate volume doubling times of human tumours

Tumour	Doubling time (days)	
	mean	range
Burkitt's lymphoma	—	2–5
Acute lymphoblastic leukaemia	—	3–5
Small cell lung cancer	50	20–100
Squamous carcinoma of lung	90	30–300
Adenocarcinoma of lung	130	25–350
Colon cancer	100	50–250
Late breast cancer	150	25–500
Lymphoma	25	10–200
Seminoma	20	10–100

Table 6.2 Phase specificity of anticancer drugs

Phase of cell cycle	Effective agents
S phase	Cytosine arabinoside, methotrexate, 6MP, hydroxyurea
Mitosis	Vinca alkaloids
Phase non-specific	Alkylating agents, nitrosoureas, antibiotics, procarbazine, cisplatin

will be repaired before cell division occurs, so the drug will prove ineffective.

Attempts have been made with human cancers to time drug administration in such a way that the cells are synchronized into a phase of the cell cycle which renders them especially sensitive to the cytotoxic agent. For example, in experimental systems, vinblastine can be used to arrest cells in mitosis. These 'synchronized' cells enter cycle together and can be killed by a cycle active S phase specific agent, such as cytosine arabinoside. Other mechanisms of synergy between drugs may be important, for example cyclophosphamide depletes intracellular glutathione which may lead to increased sensitivity to agents normally detoxified by glutathione such as other alkylating agents. Cells arrested in S phase by cytosine arabinoside are more susceptible to etoposide-induced DNA damage. It must be stated, however, that most drug schedules are not devised on the basis of cell kinetics or synergy but on the knowledge of toxicity and practicability.

KINETICS OF CELL KILLING
BY CYTOTOXIC DRUGS

Some of the principles on which modern methods of chemotherapy are based stem from an understanding of the kinetics of killing of tumour cells by cytotoxic agents. A given dose of a cytotoxic drug kills a given proportion of cells and not a given number. The fractional cell kill hypothesis is shown diagrammatically in Fig. 6.2. A single dose of a drug might, for example, kill 99% of cells and will do so whether 10^{12} cells are treated (leaving 10^{10} cells) or 10^4 cells (leaving 10^2 cells). If true for solid human cancers, the implications are that a small tumour will be killed by fewer chemotherapy cycles than a large one. Because fewer exposures to drugs will be needed there will be less chance of resistance emerging. Drugs should then be scheduled in such a way as to produce maximum killing. This will depend on the rate of regrowth of the tumour and on the rate of recovery of the normal tissues which have been most damaged by the drug. In humans these tissues are usually the gut and marrow which

Fig. 6.2 The fractional cell kill hypothesis. In part 1 of the figure a given dose of a drug is shown killing 99% of cells in both case A and case B. In case A the tumour is reduced from 10^{12} cells to 10^{10} cells and in case B from 10^4 to 10^2 cells. In part 2 of the figure, T shows the effect of repeated drug administration (arrowed) on tumour growth. With repeated doses there is less killing of tumour, indicating the emergence of drug resistance. M shows the effect of drug administration on marrow progenitor cells. The marrow recovers quickly but with repeated doses this is less complete and myelosuppression becomes clinically evident.

regenerate quickly in comparison with most cancer tissue (Fig. 6.2). For this reason pulsed intermittent therapy, with time for normal tissues to recover, is the usual method of drug administration.

This approach has both theoretical and practical limitations: (a) the fractional cell kill hypothesis was validated in homogeneous rapidly growing (doubling time less than 1 day) experimental tumours. Extrapolation to slowly growing human cancers (doubling times up to 1 year) has obvious weakness; (b) experimental tumours grown as ascites or in body fluids (such as leukaemias) can be assumed to have uniform exposure to a drug. This is obviously not the case for poorly vascularized solid neoplasms, so that the kinetics of killing will be a much more complex function than the first order kinetics of experimental systems; (c) the proportion of inherently insensitive tumour cells may be a function of size of the tumour (see drug resistance, below), being greater with large tumours; (d) the rate of regrowth of the tumour may change with repeated chemotherapy. Although this does not appear to occur with tumours such as L1210 the situation may be different for solid tumours; (e) the recovery of normal tissues as judged, for example, by blood count, may appear complete after the first few cycles, but becomes less so as treatment proceeds (Fig. 6.2), which limits dosage in successive cycles; (f) there is very little clinical data on the dose–response relationship for a given cytotoxic drug in a particular tumour. The clinical pharmacology of cytotoxic drugs is extremely complex and varies from drug to drug. There is clinical evidence that an antitumour effect of a drug will only be seen if a maximum dose is given and in practice the range from ineffective to maximum tolerated dose may be quite small.

These considerations notwithstanding, pulsed intermittent therapy is the schedule of drug administration most widely employed in cancer chemotherapy.

THE USE OF DRUGS IN COMBINATION

Even in sensitive tumours, such as Hodgkin's disease, single-agent chemotherapy is rarely curative. It is, therefore, logical to try and improve response rate and duration by the use of drugs in combination. The intention behind the combined therapy is to circumvent as many resistance mechanisms as possible. This approach soon proved effective in childhood leukaemia and adult lymphomas and has been adopted for a wide variety of other tumours.

The development of a combination chemotherapy schedule should follow a number of general principles.

1 Only drugs which are known to be effective as single agents should be used.

2 Wherever possible it is preferable to use drugs of non-overlapping toxicity.

3 Pulsed intermittent treatment should be used, to allow gut and marrow recovery.

4 Ideally, each drug should be used in its optimal dose and schedule.

5 Where possible, drugs with synergistic killing effects should be used (normally not known in practice).

6 Drugs which work at different phases of the cell cycle are used if practicable.

7 Most schedules are derived from an informed empiricism.

The improved efficacy of these combination regimens has several possible explanations, for example:

1 the tumour is exposed to a wider variety of agents, and the chances of complete resistance are smaller;

2 a maximal killing effect is achieved without undue toxicity; and

3 there may be less opportunity for the early emergence of a resistant cell population.

DRUG RESISTANCE

The cells in a solid tumour are not uniformly sensitive to a cytotoxic drug before treatment starts. Nowell [2] suggested that genetic instability increases as cancers grow and that greater heterogeneity develops accordingly, due to somatic cell mutation, both with respect to cell surface properties and resistance to drugs. This concept provides a partial explanation for greater drug resistance in large tumours (as judged by diminished extent and duration of response).

As the tumour grows in size the frequency of development of resistant cells increases so that large tumours have a greater number of intrinsically resistant cells. This resistance is produced by one or more of the mechanisms shown in Table 6.3 and discussed below. Its fundamental cause is an alteration in control of enzyme concentration or transport proteins. Host defence mechanisms and the use of cytotoxic drugs exert a selection pressure encouraging the survival of the resistant cells, which grow and multiply.

In addition to this type of cellular resistance at least two other mechanisms are important. The first is diminished vascularity of parts of the tumour as it becomes larger resulting in hypoxia and decreased drug penetration. There is also evidence to suggest that, as with radio-

therapy (see Chapter 5) cellular hypoxia may be a determinant of resistance to cytotoxic agents. The second is that only a small proportion of cells may be in cycle, allowing time for repair from cytotoxic damage before cell division.

CELLULAR MECHANISMS OF RESISTANCE TO CYTOTOXIC DRUGS [3,4]

Somatic mutation and the survival advantage of resistant cells means that a distinction between 'intrinsic' and 'acquired' cannot be made. The cellular mechanisms are a combination of genetic alteration and selection of cells which have the resistance mechanisms found in normal cells. These resistance mechanisms may be found singly in some cells, or more than one mechanism may co-exist in a cell. In the entire tumour we can expect that numerous mechanisms will be present, unevenly distributed in the cellular population.

One of the unexplained phenomena of cancer chemotherapy is that some tumours are generally sensitive to drugs and others are resistant. This inherent sensitivity or resistance extends to drugs of many different classes and mechanisms of action. Thus lymphomas and germ cell tumours show extreme sensitivity (and chemocurability) while pancreatic cancer and melanoma are highly resistant. This general susceptibility is not easily explained by any of the individual mechanisms detailed below, except possibly in the induction of cell death (apoptosis) more easily in some cell types than in others as a result of exposure to cytotoxic agents. Cell death is now known to be a programmed, multi-step process under genetic control. In the past much research has concentrated on drug resistance, by analogy with antibiotic resistance in bacteria. Attention is now turning to drug sensitivity as perhaps the more remarkable phenomenon since normal tissues are not permanently damaged by cytotoxic agents, yet some cancers can be eliminated. The basis of this susceptibility may lie in the events which drive the cell to die rather than to repair damage.

Table 6.3 Cellular mechanisms of resistance to anticancer drugs

Mechanism	Drug (examples)
Efficient repair to damaged DNA	Alkylating agents
Decreased uptake by cell	Methotrexate Doxorubicin
Increased drug efflux (p-glycoprotein)	Epipodophyllotoxin Vinca alkaloids Anthracyclines
Decreased intracellular activation	6MP, 5-FU
Increased intracellular breakdown	Cytosine arabinoside
Bypass biochemical pathways	Methotrexate 6MP Asparaginase
Gene amplification or over-production of blocked enzyme	Methotrexate Nitrosoureas

Some of the mechanisms of resistance are summarized in Table 6.3 and are outlined briefly below. It must be emphasized that these mechanisms are the properties of normal as well as malignant cells.

Multi-drug resistance (MDR) [5]

A membrane of glycoprotein (p-glycoprotein, pgp, gp170) has been characterized, of molecular weight 170 kDa, which acts as a drug efflux pump reducing the intracellular concentration of some, but not all, cytotoxic agents. This protein has a homology with a bacterial cell wall transport protein and is widely distributed in nature. In normal tissues it is found in the endothelium of the upper gastrointestinal tract, in the adrenal and kidney. It may act as a detoxifying mechanism. Its presence confers relative resistance to a series of cytotoxic agents such as vinca alkaloids, anthracyclines and epipodophyllotoxin. There is some clinical evidence that pgp expression in tumours correlates with worse prognosis (for example, in childhood soft tissue sarcoma) but it is not clear whether this is directly due to an adverse response to cytotoxic agents. The effect of pgp can be reversed *in vitro* by calcium-channel blocking drugs (such as verapamil), but with this drug it is difficult to attain appropriate plasma concentrations clinically and thus far there has been little clinical success in reversing the MDR mechanism. Other drugs besides verapamil are being evaluated. The MDR genes are part of a family of genes which produce proteins important in drug efflux.

Glutathione (GSH)

This small tri-peptide is an -SH containing reducing agent which also acts as a general intracellular detoxifying agent. In the cytosol it is kept in the highly reduced -SH form and serves to prevent unwanted S−S linkages in proteins which might result in incorrect folding. GSH is kept in its reduced form by glutathione reductase. These are a series of transferases which facilitate the reaction of GSH with a toxin. Much interest has been shown in the π isozyme but the transferase specificity of many cytotoxic agents is not yet clear.

For alkylating agents in particular, the GSH concentration and glutathione transferase activity appear to be important determinants of cellular sensitivity. Concentrations vary widely in different normal tissues and in tumours. It may be possible to alter cellular sensitivity by agents which deplete intracellular glutathione, such as buthionine sulfoximine (BSO), or by agents which inhibit transferases, such as ethacrynic acid. In cells made resistant to nitrogen mustard the increase in transferase activity is due to gene amplification (see below) but it is not clear if this mechanism is important in spontaneous tumours.

Gene amplification

In tumour cell cultures, cells showing resistance to some cytotoxic agents exhibit amplification of genes responsible for mediating resistance. Marked degrees of amplification can be demonstrated in karyotypes as homogeneously staining regions. The mechanism of gene amplification is not completely understood, but it appears to be hereditable during successive cell divisions. An example is amplification of the dihydrofolate reductase gene, leading to increased intracellular levels of this enzyme which confers relative resistance to methotrexate (see p. 99). Other examples include amplification of glutathione-S-transferase isozymes (important in resistance to alkylating agents) and O_6 alkyltransferase (which confers resistance to nitrosoureas).

Increase in DNA repair

Covalent adducts between alkylating agents (and other drugs) and DNA bases are excised by enzymes. The reactions are complex, involving DNA glycosylases and polymerases. Repair mechanisms include base excision repair in which glyosylases excise the damaged base from the sugar, and nucleotide excision repair in which larger portions of the DNA strand are excised and re-ligated. Until recently it has been technically very difficult to study the precise mechanisms of repair of individual drug/DNA adducts. We know very little both about DNA repair in cancer cells, compared with normal cells, and whether drug resistance is related to increased efficiency of repair of cytotoxic drug-induced DNA damage. The repair mechanisms differ with lesions at chemically distinct sites on the bases, and may vary in efficiency at different sites in the gene and depending on whether the gene is being transcribed or not.

Decreased drug activation

Agents such as cytosine arabinoside and 5-flourouracil are converted in the cell to an active form before exerting antitumour effect. Low levels of converting enzymes or competing enzyme pathways may decrease intracellular concentrations of active drug.

Drugs such as cyclophosphamide are converted to the active form in normal tissues (in this case the liver). Heritable differences in efficiency of activation will lead to variation in the amount, and rate of formation, of active drug. These are not intracellular mechanisms in the tumour but may account for diminished drug efficacy. The cellular concentration of a reducing enzyme such as DT-diaphorase may be critical in conversion of bioreductive drugs, such as quinones, to their active form.

Other mechanisms

Increased intracellular drug breakdown (e.g. deamination of cytosine arabinoside, inefficient membrane transport (methotrexate), competing enzyme pathways such as asparagine production by asparagine synthetase decreasing the efficacy of asparaginase) are among the numerous biochemical pathways subverting drug effect. Many of these are discussed in relation to individual drugs (see below).

REMISSION INDUCTION AND MAINTENANCE

In Chapter 3 it has been pointed out that the 'remission' or 'complete response' of a tumour in response to chemotherapy treatment is a clinical description which is compatible with up to 10^{10} cells still being present. If treatment stops, relapse-free interval is dependent on the size of the residual tumour and the growth rate of the surviving cells. Mathematical models show that these two variables can adequately account for the shape of the curves of remission duration. The aim of initial chemotherapy is to induce clinical remission.

'Maintenance' therapy was a term introduced in treatment of acute leukaemia where, following the induction of a remission, chemotherapy of a less intensive type is used to 'maintain' the remission. In acute lymphoblastic leukaemia this has been shown to contribute to survival. The improvement is due to continued cytotoxic effect on the tumour when the induction therapy has not completely eradicated the disease. In this sense the treatment is not really 'maintenance' but continued treatment.

In most tumours 'maintenance' therapy has not been shown to improve the results of cyclical combination chemotherapy given over a period of several months. In Hodgkin's disease, for example, survival is not improved by treating the patient with further cycles of MOPP chemotherapy after six cycles have been given. A similar lack of effect has been found in small cell lung cancer and testicular tumours. In these diseases the patient is cured (or not) during the early phase of treatment. There are strong arguments (discussed above) for ensuring that this initial treatment is as intense as possible.

ADJUVANT CHEMOTHERAPY

Following resection of an operable cancer (for example of the breast or stomach) many patients will develop local or distant recurrence even if no evidence of spread was found at operation or during pre-operative investigations. It is therefore logical to consider the use of cytotoxic chemotherapy as an adjuvant to surgery. The aim is to eradicate micrometastases at this early stage. As discussed above there are reasons to believe that chemotherapy may be more effective on small tumours than when they have become clinically detectable.

There is little doubt that this approach has been very effective in sensitive paediatric tumours such as Wilms' tumour, Ewing's sarcoma and rhabdomyosarcoma. For many years it has not been clear whether chemotherapy given as an adjuvant to surgery or radiotherapy would be effective in the much more common tumours of adults. It is now becoming clear that modest benefits may be obtained, but that the degree of benefit can only be determined in trials of considerable size to exclude moderate biases which distort results of smaller trials (discussed in Chapter 2, p. 19). Adjuvant chemotherapy is of proven value in premenopausal women with breast cancer, may be of value in colorectal cancer, and is under investigation in loco-regional inoperable non small-cell lung cancer, inoperable head and neck cancer, and advanced bladder cancer. These important uses of chemotherapy (and hormone and biological therapy) will become clearer over the next decade as the necessary studies are completed. It is highly probable that adjuvant chemotherapy will improve survival to a small degree in these common cancers.

Predicting sensitivity to anticancer drugs

A wide variety of techniques has been used to attempt to assess the activity of a drug against the patient's own tumour. These have included: (a) measurement of inhibition of cell growth or metabolism in cell suspension or short-term culture; (b) inhibition of the formation of clones of cells grown in soft agar; and (c) growth inhibition in longer-term cell cultures.

The problems, both technical and in inter-

pretation, are formidable. Cell suspensions may not be representative of the whole tumour; not all tumours will form clones in soft agar; longer-term cultures often cannot be established; the pharmacology and exposure of the drug is different in culture than *in vivo*. These difficulties are increased by the methodological problems of proving that there is a benefit in selecting drugs for an individual patient rather than using a standard combination. Drug combinations usually contain many or most of the active drugs so that selection in the assay may be only to predict which drugs to leave out. It will be difficult to show survival benefit by this means although toxicity may be reduced. It seems probable that the current *in vitro* tests can predict clinical resistance fairly reliably. They are less accurate in predicting sensitivity. At present they do not have a place as a routine procedure in cancer chemotherapy [6].

What cancer chemotherapy has achieved

The majority of curable cancers are uncommon tumours such as childhood cancers, leukaemias, lymphomas and testicular tumours. Other cancers are partially responsive but the impact of chemotherapy on survival is small or unproven. These other cancers include cancer of the breast, small cell lung cancer, ovarian cancer and cancer of the stomach. Figure 6.3 shows that the overall contribution of chemotherapy to cure is low and that the proportion of all cancer patients who need, or will benefit from, current drug treatments is relatively small.

Classes of cytotoxic drugs, mode of action and toxicity

ALKYLATING AGENTS AND NITROSOUREAS

These very reactive compounds produce their effect by covalently linking an alkyl group ($R-CH_2{}^+$) to chemical moieties in proteins and nucleic acids. Nitrogen mustard, for example,

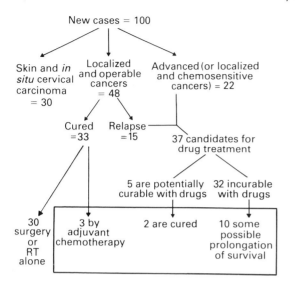

Fig. 6.3 The impact of cancer chemotherapy. The flow diagram gives the proportion of new cancer cases which might be expected to benefit from drug treatment.

has two chloroethyl side-chains (Fig. 6.4A) and one of these forms a cyclical, highly reactive immonium ion which binds to the 7-nitrogen group of guanine. After forming this bond, if there is another side-chain (as there is with nitrogen mustard), another link can be formed which may result in DNA strands being cross-linked, either within a strand or between strands. The commonly used alkylating drugs bind in the major groove of DNA. There is selectivity in the nucleotide sequence in which the drug forms the guanine N_7 bond. The cross-link is also dependent on the chemical structure of the drug — the length of DNA over which it can span and the nature of the chemical reaction on the opposite strand. Alkylating agent damage is therefore highly selective and this may account for some of the observed differences in response of different tumour types since some genes may contain regulatory sequences more vulnerable to alkylation than others or can repair these lesions more efficiently.

Many other molecules may be alkylated including cytoplasmic proteins and RNA. At therapeutic doses, however, it seems that impairment of DNA replication is the major mechanism of the cytotoxicity. Alkylating agents which are bifunctional (with two alkylation products) are more cytotoxic than monofunctional compounds by virtue of the cross-linking they produce. The cell can repair itself against

A

Fig. 6.4 The alkylating action of (A) nitrogen mustard and (B) chloroethylnitrosourea.

this kind of damage of excision of the damaged segment of DNA with formation of a new segment of DNA which is then linked to the strand. Although DNA alkylation occurs at any stage in the cell cycle, it seems to have more lethal consequences if it occurs during S phase, possibly because there is less time for DNA repair before cell division begins. For this reason, alkylating agents usually have greater effect on proliferating cells but are not cycle phase specific.

Nitrosoureas seem to act in part as alkylating agents linking an alkyl (Fig. 6.4B) or carbamoyl group to cell proteins. The compounds are unstable and decompose in water to liberate alkylating and carbamoylating groups. It seems probable that damage to cell proteins occurs with both types of reaction but alkylation is probably the main mechanism of damage to DNA.

Other alkylating agents have different structures. Busulphan is a methane–sulphonate ester which also binds to guanine in DNA and cross-links DNA strands. Dacarbazine (DTIC) is an analogue of an intermediary in purine metabolism but acts by alkylation, after enzymatic cleavage, to form a carbonium ion which binds to guanine and other bases. Thiotepa, and related compounds, are ethyleneimines which probably act by virtue of the aziridine ring structure with attachment to guanine N7 which is the initial step in alkylation. Both nitrosoureas and other alkylating agents are associated with leukaemia in long-term administration, and nitrosoureas cause brain and other tumours in animals.

Mechlorethamine (mustine, HN₂)

Mechlorethamine (mustine, HN$_2$)

Mustine is now seldom used except, in some centres, as part of the chemotherapy regimen in Hodgkin's disease. It is given by intravenous injection and undergoes rapid transformation so that within minutes it is no longer in active form. It must be given within a few minutes after it has been made up into a fast flowing intravenous drip and is an intense irritant outside a vein. The usual dose is $6\,mg/m^2$. The toxic effects are nausea and vomiting, leucopenia, thrombocytopenia, thrombophlebitis and tissue necrosis if extravasated.

Cyclophosphamide (Endoxana, Cytoxan) (Fig. 6.5)

Cyclophosphamide (Endoxana, Cytoxan) (Fig. 6.5)

This is a stable inactive compound which is well absorbed when given orally. It is activated in the liver by the cytochrome P450 system to 4-hydroxy-cyclophosphamide and thence to phosphoramide mustard and acrolein (Fig. 6.5). The latter is responsible for the haemorrhagic cystitis which is a complication of prolonged or high-dose administration. 2-Mercaptoethane sulphonate (mesna), which binds acrolein in the urine, prevents this complication. After oral administration maximal plasma concentrations are reached in 1 hour, and the plasma half-life of the drug is 5–6 hours. Little unchanged drug is excreted. The dosage, route and schedules of administration are very variable. In solid tumours such as small cell lung cancer, a single

Fig. 6.5 The metabolism of cyclophosphamide. The boxed compounds are alkylating agents. Acrolein is the major cause of haemorrhagic cystitis.

intravenous dose of the order of $1 g/m^2$ is often used, but in breast or ovarian cancer and some lymphomas it is often given orally in lower dose (e.g. $100 mg/m^2$ daily). There are numerous tumours in which the drug has been found to be useful, and it is the most versatile alkylating agent in terms of activity and method of administration.

Very high dose cyclophosphamide ($10 g/m^2$) has been used in solid tumour chemotherapy and in allogeneic marrow transplantation for leukaemia and aplastic anaemia. Because the drug must be converted to an active form in the liver, it is not suitable for local use.

Haematological toxicity is common, but thrombocytopenia is less marked than with other alkylating agents. Nausea and vomiting accompany intravenous administration, and nausea may also occur when it is given orally. The drug is not vesicant if extravasation occurs. Haemorrhagic cystitis and bladder fibrosis commonly occur and alopecia is frequent with higher doses. Pulmonary fibrosis occurs, as it does with other alkylating agents. High doses may be complicated by inappropriate secretion of ADH leading to hyponatraemia. As with most alkylating agents male infertility is usual. Haemorrhagic carditis has been reported with very high doses.

Ifosfamide

This compound is structurally closely related to a cyclophosphamide but the two chloroethyl groups are sited on the nitrogen atom and the other on the oxazophosphorine ring nitrogen. Like cyclophosphamide it is activated by hepatic P450 oxidases. Acrolein, liberated during its metabolism, causes haemorrhagic cystitis but this is prevented by mesna. Toxicity also includes a neurological syndrome with somnolence, confusion and fits. It is more frequent when given in high dose and if there is impaired liver function. The half-life is about 6 hours. It is given by short or long infusion and schedules vary greatly. Hydration is necessary. Renal tubular and glomerular dysfunction may occur.

The drug is moderately myelosuppressive. It may be more active than cyclophosphamide in squamous carcinomas and sarcomas.

Melphalan (Alkeran) (Fig. 6.6)

This is a stable alkylating agent in which the two chloroethyl groups are linked to phenylalanine. It was originally hoped that this would result in selective activity against melanoma, but in conventional doses this has not proved to be the case. It is usually given orally (for example, 10 mg daily to an adult for 7 days every 4−6 weeks). It is well absorbed, not vesicant and has a half-life of 90 minutes. Delayed leucopenia and thrombocytopenia occur but nausea, vomiting and alopecia are infrequent. The drug is often used in myeloma, ovarian and breast cancer and has a similar activity to cyclophosphamide in these tumours. With prolonged continuous use there is an appreciable risk of the development of myeloid dysplastic states leading to acute leukaemia. As with cyclophosphamide there is interest in its use at very high dose as treatment for neuroblastoma, melanoma and myeloma [7].

Fig. 6.6 The structures of other commonly used alkylating agents.

Chlorambucil (Leukeran) (Fig. 6.6)

In this compound the two chloroethyl groups are linked to a phenyl group. It is a stable compound, well absorbed orally with a plasma half-life of 90 minutes. The drug is usually given in low continuous dose (e.g. 4 mg daily) or as a higher intermittent dose (e.g. 10 mg daily for 2 weeks). It produces its antitumour effects slowly and its myelosuppressive effect is gradual in onset but persistent. Thrombocytopenia is frequent but haemorrhagic cystitis rarely occurs. It is generally well tolerated and is widely used in the treatment of ovarian cancer and low-grade lymphomas particularly in the elderly.

Busulphan (Myleran) (Fig. 6.6)

This compound differs in structure from other alkylating agents, being an alkyl sulfonate. It is exceptional in that it has very little action apart from bone marrow depression. Thrombocytopenia is frequent and pancytopenia develops which may be irreversible. Pulmonary fibrosis is a complication of long-term administration, which occurs with other alkylating agents but is especially frequent with this drug. Other side-effects include skin pigmentation, glossitis, gynaecomastia and anhidrosis. It is particularly used in the treatment of chronic granulocytic leukaemia and in some very high dose regimens.

BCNU (Carmustine) (Fig. 6.7)

BCNU (bis-chloroethylnitrosourea) was the first nitrosourea to be used clinically. It has a wide spectrum of activity similar to the alkylating agents. It is lipid soluble and penetrates the blood—brain barrier which is assumed to exist for primary brain tumours. However, the response rates are low in primary tumours and the effect usually transient. It has also been used in the treatment of small cell lung cancer and lymphoma, but does not have major activity in these disorders.

Fig. 6.7 The structure of nitrosoureas.

It is usually given intravenously and the half-life is very short, i.e. less than 5 minutes. The major toxic effect is bone marrow depression which is characteristically delayed for 5–6 weeks. Nausea and vomiting are frequent, renal and hepatic drainage may occur as does oesophagitis and flushing. It is not vesicant.

Long-term follow-up of children treated for brain tumours reveals a high incidence of asymptomatic pulmonary fibrosis which may become symptomatic at any time [8]. BCNU and CCNU (see below) bind to the O_6 position of guanine and the cross link is formed with the opposite cytosine.

Adducts formed by BCNU and CCNU with the O_6 position of guanine are repaired by the enzyme O_6 alkyl transferase. High levels of this enzyme are associated with resistance to nitrosoureas. The enzyme removes the adduct and is itself then inactivated. Prior treatment by drugs such as streptozotocin, which deplete the enzyme, increases susceptibility to nitrosoureas administered subsequently.

CCNU (Lomustine) (Fig. 6.7)

CCNU (cis-chloroethylnitrosourea) is rapidly absorbed and metabolized, and is usually given by mouth. The products of metabolism have a plasma half-life of 1–2 days, and the metabolites can be detected in the CSF. As with BCNU the major toxic effects are nausea, vomiting and delayed bone marrow depression. For this reason the drug is given at 6-week intervals. Nausea and vomiting can be reduced by spreading the dose over 2 or 3 days. Its spectrum of activity is similar to alkylating agents. It has been widely used in the treatment of primary and secondary brain tumours as well as in lymphomas and small cell bronchogenic cancer.

Dimethyltriazenoimidazole carboxamide (DTIC)

This drug probably produces its cytotoxic effect by functioning as an alkylating agent. It is administered intravenously and is vesicant if extravasated. There is an initial rapid clearance followed by slower clearance ($t_\frac{1}{2}$ 5 hours). Much of the drug is excreted unaltered in the urine. It was initially introduced as a treatment for melanoma but the results have proved disappointing. It is sometimes used in combination chemotherapy for soft tissue sarcoma but evidence for its value is meagre. It is also included in some regimens for Hodgkin's disease. It causes severe nausea and vomiting, and myelosuppression is frequent. Damage to liver and peripheral nerves occurs as does flushing and myalgia.

ANTIMETABOLITES: FOLIC ACID ANTAGONISTS

Several folic acid antagonists have been developed since the introduction of aminopterin in 1947, but only one, methotrexate, is now widely used. The antifolate action is complex and includes inhibition of the enzyme dihydrofolate reductase. This enzyme is essential for reducing dihydrofolate (FH_2) to tetrahydrofolate (FH_4),

which in turn is converted to a variety of coenzymes that are essential in reactions where one carbon atom is transferred in the synthesis of thymidylate, purines, methionine and glycine. Methotrexate, and other antifolates, are polyglutamated inside the cell. This process increases the efficiency of binding to dihydrofolate reductase. The critical effect in preventing cell replication appears to be the blocking of synthesis of thymidine monophosphate as shown in Fig. 6.8. The block of thymidine monophosphate synthesis results in inhibition of DNA and RNA synthesis and the drug is therefore S phase specific. The block in activity of dihydrofolate reductase can be bypassed by supplying an alternative intermediary metabolite. This is N_5-formyl-FH_4, variously termed leucovorin, citrovorum factor or, more commonly, folinic acid. It is converted to the FH_4 coenzymes, needed for thymidylate synthetase to function.

The most important mechanism of methotrexate resistance appears to be by production of large amounts of dihydrofolate reductase. In methotrexate-resistant cells there may be an increase in the number of copies of the gene coding for dihydrofolate reductase. An increase in gene copy number is shown by dense homogeneous staining regions on chromosomes or in small chromosome fragments called double minute chromosomes. The homogeneous

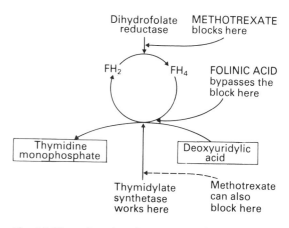

Fig. 6.8 The action of methotrexate and folinic acid.

staining regions appear stable and may be responsible for the continuation of methotrexate resistance in subsequent cell divisions.

Other described mechanisms are the production of variants of the enzyme with decreased affinity for methotrexate, and impaired transport into cells.

Methotrexate (amethopterin) (Fig. 6.9)

This drug is readily absorbed from the gut at low dosages, but higher doses are incompletely absorbed. After intravenous injection there is an initial rapid distribution phase ($t_{\frac{1}{2}}$ 45 minutes), then a slower phase of renal excretion ($t_{\frac{1}{2}}$ 2–3 hours) followed by a very slow phase when the drug concentration is low. It is this latter prolonged phase of clearance that is responsible for toxicity to marrow, gut and mucous membranes. If there is ascites or a pleural effusion the drug may accumulate in these sites and then be slowly released from the 'reservoir' (or third space) causing unexpected toxicity even from a low dose. The drug is 50% bound to albumin from which it can be displaced by drugs such as salicylates, sulphonamides, tetracycline and phenytoin. It is not metabolized significantly but is mainly excreted unchanged in the urine especially in the first 8 hours both by glomerular filtration and tubular secretion. Drugs which compete for tubular secretion, or the presence of renal failure, may greatly delay the excretion of the drug and thereby increase toxicity. The drug may remain bound to dihydrofolate reductase in kidney and liver cells for several weeks, only being released when these cells die. When given in very high dose renal excretion must be promoted by intravenous fluids and by alkalinization of the urine (see below).

In conventional doses the drug does not penetrate significantly into the CSF, but when given at high doses the CSF concentrations can achieve cytotoxic levels of up to 10% of the plasma concentration. The drug can also be administered intrathecally, usually at a dose of $10 \, mg/m^2$, and high CSF levels are thereby achieved, especially in the spinal CSF.

The toxicity is mainly haematological and to epithelial surfaces. Pancytopenia develops rapidly after a large dose. After 4–6 days there is oral ulceration, diarrhoea which may be bloody, and erythematous skin rashes. Other toxic effects include alopecia; renal failure with high doses; hepatic toxicity (occasionally leading to cirrhosis); pneumonitis; and osteoporosis after long-term therapy. The drug has a wide spectrum of activity and is part of the established treatment of acute lymphoblastic leukaemia. It is also widely used in non-Hodgkin's lymphomas, breast and ovarian cancer, soft tissue sarcomas and osteogenic sarcoma. It is an effective single agent for choriocarcinoma. Attempts have been made to overcome methotrexate resistance by using very high doses followed by folinic acid rescue. Doses of methotrexate can be increased over 100-fold provided the effect of the drug is reversed at 24 hours. Meticulous attention to hydration is essential. Urinary alkalinization is needed to prevent methotrexate deposition in the renal tubule. This is accomplished by sodium bicarbonate or acetazolamide. Plasma levels of methotrexate must be measured at 24 and 48 hours. Correctly monitored there is little toxicity, but the approach is potentially very dangerous. The cost is prohibitive and the value of the procedure uncertain although improved response rates have been claimed in osteosarcoma (see Chapter 23). Newer antifolates include edatrexate and trimetrexate. Their

Folic acid	R_1 = OH	R_2 = H
Methotrexate	$R_1 = NH_2$	$R_2 = CH_3$
Aminopterin	$R_1 = NH_2$	R_2 = H

Fig. 6.9 Folic acid analogues.

advantage over methotrexate is uncertain. Thymidylate synthase inhibitors are currently in Phase 2 evaluation. The pattern of toxicity appears similar to methotrexate.

ANTIMETABOLITES: PYRIMIDINE ANTAGONISTS

Drugs in this category either antagonize or mimic natural pyrimidine metabolites and thereby interfere with nucleic acid synthesis. The most important members of this group are 5-FU and cytosine arabinoside.

5-Fluorouracil (5-FU) (Fig. 6.10)

The fluorine atom which is substituted for hydrogen on the uracil molecule is similar in size to the hydrogen atom so that the 5-FU molecule can enter into many reactions where uracil would be the normal participant. 5-FU has first to be activated to 5-fluoro-2 deoxy-uridine monophosphate (FdUMP). This is the active form of the drug. The conversion of 5-FU to FdUMP can proceed through a variety of pathways, and resistance to the drug is associated with decreased activity of the enzymes necessary for this conversion. FdUMP interferes with DNA synthesis by binding to the enzyme

thymidylate synthetase and inactivating it (Fig. 6.8). The effect of the block can to some extent be overcome if thymidine is given (similar to the effect of folinic acid rescue for methotrexate). Folinic acid, on the other hand, enhances 5-FU activity by stabilizing the binding of FdUMP to thymidylate synthetase. Folinic acid is used as a means of increasing the effectiveness of 5-FU, although the degree to which this is selective for the tumours is not clear and the therapeutic ratio may not change greatly. Nevertheless, response rates of colorectal cancer metastases do appear to be increased with the combination. 5-Fluorouracil is also incorporated into RNA but the importance of this for its antineoplastic effect is not certain. 5-Fluorouracil is more toxic to proliferating cells, that is, it is cycle specific, but it does not seem to have an effect at a particular phase of the cycle. Recovery from 5-FU involves the synthesis of both thymidylate synthetase and the normal substrate deoxy-uridine monophosphate.

The intestinal absorption of 5-FU is erratic so the drug is normally given intravenously. Plasma clearance is rapid ($t_{\frac{1}{2}}$ 15 minutes). Much higher plasma concentrations are achieved by rapid intravenous injection than by continuous infusion, and the toxicity of the drug is greater when given by bolus injection. The drug penetrates the CSF well. The usual schedule of administration is 12 mg/kg daily for 4 days, then every 2–3 days at a dose of 6 mg/kg unless the patient develops diarrhoea or stomatitis. Myelosuppression is commonest between 10 and 15 days. Full doses are usually necessary to get a tumour response. Care is necessary in the presence of hepatic dysfunction. Intra-arterial infusion of 5-FU sometimes produces good results in hepatic metastases from gut cancer. The drug has activity against adenocarcinoma of the gut, breast and ovary, but responses are infrequent and tend to be transient. There is increasing evidence of the value of 5-FU as adjuvant therapy in colorectal cancer. In this situation, it has been given alone, or with folinic acid or with levamisole. The additional value of levamisole is uncertain (see p. 313).

Fig. 6.10 The structure of the pyrimidine analogues.

The drug is generally well tolerated but toxic effects include nausea, diarrhoea, stomatitis, alopecia, myelosuppression, cardiac disturbances and a cerebellar syndrome.

Cytosine arabinoside (Cytarabine, ara-C) (Fig. 6.10)

In this analogue of cytidine the pyrimidine base is unchanged but the sugar moiety differs by an alteration in the position of a hydroxyl group. This leads to impaired mobility of the pyrimidine base so that it cannot be effectively incorporated into DNA. The drug is converted by a series of enzymic steps to its active form known as ara-CTP. This is an inhibitor of DNA polymerase but it is not clear if this is the mechanism of its cytotoxic action. It would explain why the drug is markedly cell cycle, S phase, specific. Resistance to the effect of the drug could either be due to low levels of one of the converting enzymes (deoxycytidine kinase) or to increased rates of deamination. The former seems to be the major mechanism.

The drug is very poorly absorbed from the intestine. After intravenous injection there is a fast phase of clearance ($t_{\frac{1}{2}}$ 20 minutes) followed by a slower phase ($t_{\frac{1}{2}}$ 2 hours) and the clearance is largely determined by the speed of deamination in the liver and other tissues. The drug penetrates well into the CSF and deamination occurs slowly at this site. Because it is S phase specific it is usually given as multiple intravenous injections or as a continuous intravenous or subcutaneous infusion.

The agent is mainly of use against acute myeloblastic leukaemia (AML) but has been used in acute lymphoblastic leukaemia (ALL) and poor prognosis lymphomas as well. It is of little use in solid tumours which usually have a low growth fraction.

The toxic effects include marrow suppression, oral ulceration, diarrhoea, nausea and vomiting and, uncommonly, CNS toxicity. It is particularly toxic in the presence of hepatic dysfunction since the liver is the chief site of deamination.

ANTIMETABOLITES: PURINE ANTAGONISTS

There are several cytotoxic agents which are analogues of the natural purine bases and nucleotides. They are in wide use as cytotoxic and immunosuppressive agents. 6-Mercaptopurine and thioguanine are derivatives of hypoxanthine and guanine respectively but with the keto group on carbon-6 replaced by a sulphur atom. In many cases, the drugs of this class must undergo enzymatic conversion to the active form.

6-Mercaptopurine (6MP) (Fig. 6.11)

6-Mercaptopurine must be converted to the nucleotide to become active. This is done by the enzyme hypoxanthine-guanine phosphoribosyltransferase (HGPRT). The resultant nucleotide is 6-mercaptopurine ribose phosphate (6MPRP). 6-Mercaptopurine ribose phosphate accumulates in the cell and inhibits several important metabolic reactions in the formation of normal

Fig. 6.11 The structures of commonly used purine analogues.

nucleotides. The cytotoxicity of the drug cannot be ascribed to disruption of a single metabolic pathway and cell death probably results from multiple biochemical abnormalities. However, inhibition of purine nucleotide biosynthesis is a major action of the drug. 6-Mercaptopurine is also incorporated into DNA as 6-thioguanine but the contribution of this reaction to cyto-toxicity is not clear.

Resistance to the action of 6MP is often due to low levels of the converting enzyme HGPRT, and such cells also show resistance to 6-thio-guanine and azaguanine. There is evidence, however, that in leukaemia cells, deficiency of HGPRT is not the main mechanism of resistance, and that increased rates of drug breakdown are more important. Intracellular alkaline phospha-tase levels rise in treated patients, and dephos-phorylation may be a mechanism of resistance to 6-thiopurines generally.

6-Mercaptopurine is readily absorbed from the gut, and about half of an oral dose is excreted as antimetabolites in 24 hours. After intra-venous injection the drug is rapidly cleared from the plasma ($t_\frac{1}{2}$ 90 minutes) due to dis-tribution and metabolism. A major site of met-abolism is the liver where xanthine-oxidase rapidly converts the drug to an inactive form. The xanthine-oxidase inhibitor allopurinol blocks this conversion but this increases toxicity as well as effectiveness and the therapeutic ratio is unchanged. Allopurinol is sometimes used in the early stages of treatment of ALL and non-Hodgkin's lymphoma, to prevent hyper-uricaemia occurring during the rapid destruc-tion of the tumour. If 6MP is used as part of the initial treatment, allopurinol will increase its toxicity. 6-Mercaptopurine is widely used in remission maintenance in ALL and has been used in the treatment of chronic granulocytic leukaemia. Its use as an immunosuppressive agent has largely been superceded by azathio-prine although there is evidence that 6MP is a more powerful immunosuppressive agent. The frequent occurrence of cholestatic jaundice with 6MP has, however, made it less satisfactory for long-term administration. Its other toxicities

are nausea and vomiting with gradual and reversible bone marrow suppression. The usual maintenance dose in ALL is 50–100 mg/day.

Azathioprine (Imuran) (Fig. 6.11)

This drug was developed in an attempt to decrease the rate of inactivation of 6MP. The drug acts as a 'prodrug' whereby 6MP is slowly formed in the tissues. It is degraded in the liver by xanthine-oxidase, and allopurinol increases its toxicity. The drug is well absorbed orally and is partly excreted by the kidneys so that its toxicity is greater if renal failure is present. Reversible bone marrow depression is the major toxicity. It is most widely used as an 'immuno-suppressive' agent in connective tissue diseases and renal allograft recipients. The usual dose is 1–2 mg/kg/day.

6-Thioguanine (6TG) (Fig. 6.11)

This purine analogue has a mode of action similar to that of 6MP. It is well absorbed orally and peak concentrations are achieved in 6–8 hours. About half the dose is excreted in the urine as metabolites within 24 hours. Degra-dation by xanthine-oxidase does not appear to be an important aspect of detoxification and the drug can be used safely with allopurinol. The drug is widely used as part of remission induc-tion and maintenance in AML. It has also been used as an immunosuppressive. The average oral daily dose is 2 mg/kg. Reversible bone marrow depression is the major toxicity, but nausea and diarrhoea may also occur.

2-Deoxycoformycin (Pentostatin)

This increasingly used drug is closely related to adenosine and is a potent inhibitor of adenosine deaminase. Deficiency of adenosine deaminase is a rare, inherited cause of immune deficiency in which lymphocyte function is defective but other cells are relatively normal. The drug may prove to be valuable both as an immunosup-pressive and in treatment of lymphomas.

VINCA ALKALOIDS AND PODOPHYLLOTOXINS

Vinca alkaloids are extracted from the periwinkle, *Catharanthus roseus*, and were observed to cause granulocytopenia in animals. Subsequently they have been shown to be mitotic spindle poisons, and their mode of action is related to other agents such as colchicine.

In the *prophase* of normal mitosis the centrioles divide and move to opposite ends of the cell, the chromosomes appear as double strands and the nuclear membrane disappears. In the *metaphase* the chromosomes line up at the equator and the spindle of microtubules appears. In *anaphase* the chromosomes divide, are pulled to opposite ends of the cell and the cleavage furrow appears. In *telophase* the cells separate and the nuclear membrane forms. The vinca alkaloids and other mitotic inhibitors act by binding to tubulin which is the constituent protein of the microtubules. The assembly and function of the microtubules during metaphase is shown in Fig. 6.12. Colchicine and epipodophyllotoxin both bind to the same site on tubulin but vinca alkaloids bind differently. Exposure of the cell to vinca alkaloids leads to rapid disappearance of the microtubules because no further assembly can take place (Fig. 6.12).

Microtubules are involved in other cell functions such as secretion of hormones, axonal transport and cell mobility. It is generally assumed, however, that the cytotoxic activity of these agents is related to the effect on mitosis.

Little is known about the mechanisms of resistance to these drugs. In some cell lines vinca resistance is associated both with the appearance of the 180 kDa membrane glycoprotein and resistance to many other agents (MDR, p. 91). There is often cross-resistance from one vinca alkaloid to another and between vinca alkaloids and podophyllotoxins.

Vincristine (Oncovin)

The drug is administered intravenously usually in a dose of 1.5 mg/m^2 (maximum 2 mg) and can

Fig. 6.12 The assembly and function of microtubules during metaphase. (A) The chromosome pair (1) is attached to a microtubule (2) which is assembled at the equatorial region (3) and disassembled at the centriole (4). (B) In metaphase the chromosome pair is divided and pulled to opposite ends of the cell. (C) A microtubule is a polymer of the protein tubulin which is made up of α and β subunits. Vinca alkaloids bind to tubulin, blocking further assembly, but disassembly continues.

be repeated weekly when used in the young. The drug is poorly and unpredictably absorbed from the gut. It is vesicant if it escapes from the vein into the tissues. The pharmacokinetics are similar to those of vinblastine (see below).

The drug is useful in treatment of lymphatic malignancies such as Hodgkin's disease, non-Hodgkin's lymphoma and ALL. In these diseases it is usually used in combination with other drugs such as steroids and alkylating agents. It also has a place in treatment of other cancers such as breast cancers, small cell carcinoma of the bronchus and brain tumours.

The toxicity of the drug is mainly neurological and peripheral neuropathy is an almost invariable sequel to long-term administration. It is especially likely to occur in the elderly and those with liver disease, and may be severe and incapacitating. Loss of reflexes and paraesthesia occur early and are not usually regarded as indications for cessation of treatment, but severe myalgic and neuritic pain and motor weakness and/or peripheral sensory loss are signs that treatment should be stopped. Nerve conduction is usually preserved even with severe neuropathy, but electromyography shows a pattern of denervation. Cranial nerve palsies are occasionally encountered. Neurones are rich in tubulin, which appears to be important for axonal transport. It is postulated that vincristine blocks the passage of tubulin from proximal to distal axonal sites. Autonomic neuropathy often occurs, with constipation and ileus; symptoms can be partially alleviated with bulk laxatives. Myelosuppression is mild, increasing the usefulness of the drug when used in combination. Alopecia occurs in 20% of patients and a syndrome of inappropriate release of ADH occurs. The drug sometimes causes thrombocytosis.

Vinblastine (Velbe)

After intravenous injection the drug disappears from the plasma in three phases with half-lives of 4 minutes, 1 hour and 16 hours. Much of the drug remains tissue-bound for many days. In the blood it binds to platelets, red cells and plasma proteins. All vinca alkaloids behave in a similar manner and clinical differences cannot be explained on pharmacokinetic grounds.

Indications for the use of vinblastine are similar to those for vincristine. In addition, vinblastine is often used in high dose for the treatment of testicular teratoma in combination with cisplatin and bleomycin (see Chapter 19). In these high doses neutropenia and ileus are common. Vinblastine causes more myelosuppression but less neurotoxicity than vincristine. The usual intravenous dose is 6 mg/m² weekly. Extravasation leads to cellulitis. Alopecia and mucositis are infrequent side-effects.

Vindesine (Eldisine and Vinorelbine)

These new semi-synthetic additions to the vinca alkaloids have a similar spectrum of activity but appears to have additional activity in non-small cell lung cancer making them useful agents in diseases where response to chemotherapy is generally disappointing. The toxicity of the drugs is intermediate between that of vinblastine and vincristine. Myelosuppression and neurotoxicity both occur.

Paclitaxel (Taxol)

This new drug is an extract from the bark of the Pacific yew *Taxus brevifolia*. It promotes assembly of microtubules and inhibits their disassembly. It is poorly water soluble and is formulated in cremophor oil. When infused the dose-limiting toxicity is neutropenia. Other side-effects are neuropathy, alopecia and myalgia. It is active in advanced ovarian cancer with a response rate of 30%, and is also effective for breast cancer; responses have been reported in non-small cell lung cancer and melanoma. When combined with anthracyclines mucositis has been dose-limiting. It is currently given as a 3-hour infusion. A recent development is docetaxel (Taxotere), a novel semi-synthetic taxoid. It has demonstrated significant activity against breast cancer and non small cell lung cancer, and has also shown some activity in a number of other tumours, including cancers of the head and neck, ovary and pancreas. The dose-limiting toxicity is neutropenia, but other side-effects are hypersensitivity, skin reactions, fluid retention, neuropathy and alopecia. The current treatment schedule is usually a 1-hour infusion every 3 weeks.

Epipodophyllotoxin derivatives — VP16−213 and VM26 (vepesid)

These substances are semi-synthetic derivatives of extracts of *Podophyllum peltatum* — the American mandrake. Etoposide stabilizes the complex formed by the enzyme topoisomerase II with DNA. This enzyme is involved in reversibly cleaving DNA so that it unwinds during cell division. The drug stabilizes the enzyme–DNA 'cleavable complex' and results in DNA strand breaks. The drugs have an early rapid phase of clearance followed by a slower phase ($t_{\frac{1}{2}}$ 11–39 hours for vepesid and 2–13 hours for etoposide). They enter the CSF in low concentration. Etoposide is the drug most widely used at present. It is absorbed erratically from the gut with a plasma availability of about 50% of the intravenous dose which must be adjusted accordingly. The drug can be infused at high dose. However, mucositis then becomes dose limiting. At conventional doses bone marrow suppression is the major toxicity. Etoposide is highly protein bound and about half the drug is excreted in the urine in 72 hours. After dilution it is stable for about 24 hours depending on the concentration. The activity of etoposide has been shown to be highly schedule dependent. In small cell lung cancer the response rate is greatly increased by multiple daily administration compared with the same total dose as a single infusion. The drug is active orally but erratic absorption makes dosage difficult and toxicity unpredictable.

The drugs are useful in treatment of lymphomas, acute leukaemias, small cell lung cancer, testicular and brain tumours. The toxic effects are alopecia, leucopenia, nausea and vomiting, febrile reactions and peripheral neuropathy.

ANTITUMOUR ANTIBIOTICS

A wide variety of antitumour antibiotics has now been produced from bacterial and fungal cultures. They produce their effect by binding to DNA intercalating between base pairs.

Actinomycin D (dactinomycin)

This antibiotic was first isolated from *Streptomyces* in 1940. At low concentrations it blocks DNA-directed RNA synthesis and at higher concentration also blocks DNA synthesis. The drug does not react directly with RNA. The molecule intercalates between guanine–cytosine base pairs and the transcription of DNA is blocked. The drug inhibits the division of all rapidly dividing cells. Resistance appears to be associated both with impaired drug entry and increased drug efflux.

It is given intravenously and is cleared within a few minutes. The usual daily dose is 15 µg/kg and this can be repeated daily for 4–5 days. A further course of injections can be given 3–4 weeks later. It is, however, more usual to give the drug as a single injection of 15 µg/kg in combination with other agents (such as vincristine and cyclophosphamide).

Its main use has been in the treatment of childhood cancers, such as rhabdomyosarcoma, Wilms' tumour and Ewing's sarcoma. It is of less value in adult tumours. The toxicities are nausea and vomiting, myelosuppression, mucositis and diarrhoea. It sensitizes tissue to radiation.

Doxorubicin (Adriamycin) and daunorubicin (Cerubidin) [9]

These are anthracycline antibiotics produced from a species of *Streptomyces* fungus. Doxorubicin is a useful agent with a wide spectrum of activity against many tumours and differs from daunorubicin only in the substitution of an –OH group for a hydrogen atom.

Both drugs bind tightly to DNA, deforming the helical structure. The drugs intercalate between base pairs but there appears to be no base specificity in the binding. Breaks in DNA strands have also been shown to occur. The drugs also produce highly active intracellular free radicals and these may be important in producing some of the toxic effects, for example cardiac toxicity. Drug resistance is mediated, at least in part, through the MDR drug-efflux protein (p. 91). There appears to be complete cross-resistance between these two drugs as well as some degree of cross-resistance with vinca alkaloids and actinomycin, probably due to the MDR mechanism. The drugs are effective mainly against cells in S phase.

Both drugs are injected intravenously into a fast running drip, and are highly vesicant. They are cleared rapidly from the plasma, but there is a slow terminal clearance of doxorubicin. There is rapid uptake into spleen, kidney, lungs, liver and heart, but not into the brain. The drugs are metabolized in the liver and severe toxicity may result if they are given to patients with impaired liver function. With doxorubicin, 40% is excreted in the bile as free drug, adriamycinol and other metabolites. With both drugs the major and acute side-effects are bone marrow depression, nausea and vomiting, mucositis, alopecia and gastro-intestinal disturbance. Alopecia can perhaps be lessened by cooling the scalp with ice packs for 25 minutes before and after drug administration. The most important chronic and dose limiting side-effect is cardiotoxicity causing arrhythmias and heart failure. It is related to the total dose administered and is a major risk above a total dose of $500\,\text{mg}/\text{m}^2$. In addition to total dose the drug schedule may also be important. High peak plasma concentrations may be associated with more toxicity. In recent years it has become apparent that subclinical cardiac toxicity may be more frequent than suspected previously — which may be of great importance in the treatment of childhood tumours. Cardioprotective agents are currently under evaluation.

Daunorubicin is of value in the treatment of acute lymphoblastic and myeloblastic leukaemia. Dosage schedules vary but $50\,\text{mg}/\text{m}^2$ once weekly is often given. Doxorubicin has a wide spectrum of activity in childhood and adult tumours including lymphomas, small cell bronchogenic carcinoma, adenocarcinomas of ovary, breast and stomach, bone and soft tissue sarcomas, liver and bladder cancer.

Mitoxantrone

This is an anthraquinone related to doxorubicin which binds to DNA. When injected intravenously it has a terminal half-life of 36 hours. It is vesicant and has a spectrum of activity similar to doxorubicin with useful effects in metastatic breast cancer, lymphoma and leukaemia. The main toxicity is myelosuppression. It causes less alopecia than doxorubicin and possibly less cardiotoxicity. The usual single dose schedule is $12-15\,\text{mg}/\text{m}^2$ repeated every 3 weeks.

Mithramycin

This antibiotic is derived from *Streptomyces plicatus*. It had some clinical use in the treatment of hypercalcaemia, but also has activity against embryonal carcinoma of the testis. It inhibits RNA synthesis, possibly in a manner similar to actinomycin D. It crosses the blood–brain barrier and penetrates into brain tumours. It is locally irritant, is inactive orally, and is therefore given intravenously.

The hypocalcaemic effect of mithramycin appears to result from interference with bone resorption by osteoclasts. In full doses ($25\,\mu\text{g}/\text{kg}$) it causes nausea, stomatitis, thrombocytopenia, a haemorrhagic tendency and impaired renal and liver function.

Weekly doses of $15\,\mu\text{g}/\text{kg}$ can be given safely without serious toxicity and will often control hypercalcaemia refractory to steroids. Its use has been largely supplanted by biphosphonates.

Bleomycin

This antibiotic is a mixture of glycopeptides isolated from *Streptomyces verticillus* but has now been chemically synthesized. The commercial bleomycin consists mainly of bleomycin A_2. The drug inhibits DNA synthesis and causes breaks in the DNA chain. It arrests cells in G_2, and this has led to attempts to use it to synchronize cells for subsequent chemotherapeutic attack, although little therapeutic advance has come from this approach.

The drug can be given parenterally by any route. It disappears from the plasma with an initial $t_{\frac{1}{2}}$ of 1 hour and then more slowly ($t_{\frac{1}{2}}$ 9 hours). It is excreted in the urine and caution is needed with impaired renal function. The drug concentration is very low in the brain and CSF and it appears to be concentrated mainly in skin and lung. Many tissues contain an inactivating enzyme which hydrolyses the drug, and the levels of this enzyme appear to correlate with resistance. It is active in squamous carcinomas of the head and neck, skin and cervix and against lymphomas and testicular tumours.

The drug is valuable in combination with other agents because it causes little bone marrow toxicity. Skin toxicity is characterized by pigmentation, erythema and vesiculation. It also causes mucosal ulceration, pulmonary infiltrates and fibrosis. These toxic effects are serious, sometimes disabling and are related to total dose, with a high risk when the dose exceeds $300 \, \text{mg/m}^2$. Acute pyrexial reactions commonly occur, and can be relieved or prevented by hydrocortisone. Rarely, cardiorespiratory collapse occurs. A small subcutaneous test dose at the start of treatment is a wise precaution.

The dosage schedule varies considerably but is usually of the order of $15 \, \text{mg/m}^2$ as a single dose which can be repeated weekly.

MISCELLANEOUS AGENTS

Cis-diammine dichloroplatinum (cisplatin, DDP)

Following the observation by Rosenberg that certain platinum complexes inhibited bacterial replication, cisplatin was synthesized and shown to be active in experimental tumours. The drug is only active in the *cis* form. It diffuses into cells and the chloride ions are then lost from the molecule. The compound then binds to DNA producing inter- and intra-strand cross links. The binding appears to be mainly to guanine groups. The drug is administered intravenously; the early $t_\frac{1}{2}$ is about 40 minutes and the later phase of clearance is slow ($t_\frac{1}{2}$ 60 hours). It is 90% bound to plasma protein, and is taken up in the kidney, gut, liver, ovary and testis but not in the CNS.

The drug is highly nephrotoxic, and when administered in high dose a high urine flow is essential with intravenous fluids being administered before the drug and for 24 hours after. Renal function may worsen during repeated cycles and the plasma creatinine level and clearance should be checked regularly. With some high-dose regimens mannitol is used to maintain urine flow. Loss of K^+ and Mg^{2+}/Ca^{2+} in the urine may require electrolyte supplementation both in the short and long term. Nausea and vomiting are severe with higher doses, and ototoxicity may be irreversible so that pretreatment audiometry should be carried out. Myelosuppression is not severe, but peripheral neuropathy is frequent and often subclinical.

The drug is highly effective in the treatment of testicular tumours, and, in combination with vinblastine and bleomycin has revolutionized the outlook in advanced disease (see Chapter 19). It is also effective in cancer of the ovary and bladder as well as in lymphomas and small cell carcinoma of the bronchus. It is active in osteosarcoma and squamous cancer of the head and neck.

Carboplatin (Paraplatin)

This analogue of cisplatin has a different spectrum of toxicity from cisplatin but is active in the same tumours. It is given intravenously and the area under the concentration−time curve (AUC) is given by the formula (GFR (ml/min) + 25) $\times n$ where n is the desired multiple. Thus dose required for AUC 5 in a patient with a GFR of 120 is $(120 + 25) \times 5 = 725 \, \text{mg}$. Some drug regimens are given according to this formula, others on a conventional dose/m^2 basis. The main toxicity is myelosuppression which may be profound. Typically its onset is at 14−21 days and for this reason intervals between treatments may need to be 28 days. It causes less nausea and vomiting than cisplatin and is not as nephrotoxic or neurotoxic. The drug is given by intravenous injection in saline or dextrose/saline. Prehydration and posthydration are not necessary unless there is vomiting. In testicular cancer the drug is less effective than cisplatin since dose reduction is necessary due to myelosuppression. It is active in small cell lung cancer and ovarian cancer. In the latter its ease of administration makes it valuable for palliative treatment.

L-Asparaginase (Crasnitine, Elspar)

When L-asparaginase was first shown to have antitumour effects, it was hoped that this might prove to be an agent acting exclusively on malignant cells. The enzyme is produced by *Escherichia coli* and *Erwinia carotovora* and its action is based on the observation that while most normal tissues synthesize asparagine, some tumour cells need an exogenous source which the enzyme removes. Resistance may be related to the appearance of asparagine synthetase in the tumour cells.

The drug is initially eliminated rapidly from the circulation but the later $t_{\frac{1}{2}}$ is 6—30 hours. It does not penetrate into the CSF. There is no marrow, gut, or hair follicle toxicity but anaphylaxis, pancreatitis, hyperglycaemia, raised liver enzymes with fatty change in the liver, confusion, somnolence, coma, and hypofibrinogenaemia all occur and the drug is extremely nauseating.

The main use of the drug is in remission induction in acute lymphoblastic leukaemia. The dosage schedules vary considerably with different combinations of drugs.

Procarbazine (Natulan)

This drug is the most useful of the hydrazine derivatives which were originally synthesized as monoamine oxidase inhibitors and found to have antitumour activity. It causes inhibition of action in DNA and RNA, and protein synthesis is depressed. The mode of action is, however, unclear. Metabolic activation is needed and the active product may be a methyldiazonium ion which acts as an alkylating agent. The drug oxidizes at 37°C and hydrogen peroxide is formed but does not appear to be responsible for the cytotoxic effect. Interphase is prolonged and mitosis is suppressed with breakage of chromatin strands.

The drug is very well absorbed from the gut, and rapidly equilibrates with blood and CSF. After intravenous injection the $t_{\frac{1}{2}}$ is 7 minutes and the drug is rapidly metabolized. The toxic

effects are nausea and vomiting, leucopenia, CNS disturbances especially psychological upsets, flushing with alcohol, and hypertensive reactions to foods rich in tyramine.

The drug is usually given in a dose of $100 \, mg/m^2$ daily for 1—2 weeks. It is especially useful in Hodgkin's disease and brain tumours.

Hydroxyurea (Hydrea)

This drug was synthesized over 100 years ago, but was only found to have antineoplastic activity much later. It blocks the action of ribonucleoside diphosphate reductase and thereby interferes with DNA synthesis. It causes leucopenia and megaloblastic changes in the bone marrow. It is S phase specific, and has been used in attempts to produce cell synchronization.

The drug is well absorbed orally and enters the CSF. It is excreted in the urine. The usual dose is 20—30 mg/kg/day, or 80 mg/kg every 3 days. Toxic effects are mainly marrow suppression and gut disturbances. Its main use is in chronic granulocytic leukaemia resistant to other forms of therapy.

Hexamethylmelamine (Hexalon)

Although this drug has a similar structure to the alkylating agent triethylene melamine, it does not act as an alkylating agent itself. Indeed its mechanism of action remains largely unknown. It is well absorbed orally and is rapidly metabolized.

The drug is administered in 2—3-week cycles of 12 mg/kg/day and is active in ovarian and cervical cancer. Nausea, vomiting and neurotoxicity are major problems with its use. Abdominal cramps and diarrhoea occur and leucopenia may develop. Central nervous system toxicity includes altered mental state, extrapyramidal effects and convulsions.

The administration of cytotoxic agents

There is much to be said against the occasional chemotherapist. Most surgeons, gynaecologists

and physicians are quite unfamiliar with cytotoxic agents and when they attempt to use
them, often run into difficulty because of lack of
experience and also because of the lack of an
appropriate organization to give drugs, check
on blood counts and inquire into side-effects.
Just as hospitals concentrate expertise in other
activities — diabetic clinics, endoscopy clinics,
coronary care units — so, for best results, they
should bring chemotherapy into the hands of
those expert in its administration.

It is our practice to separate patients needing
chemotherapy into three groups:

Patients on out-patient regimens. The majority
of patients can receive their drugs in this way
especially if the person giving them is the same
each time and gets to know the best anti-emetic
or sedative regimen *for that patient.* Some
patients are not sick at all, others vomit several
hours later and prefer to get home quickly and
take a $5HT_3$ antagonist, others vomit at the
sight of the needle and require premedication
with diazepam or prochlorperazine. There is
little doubt that trained nurses are the best
people to give the drugs. They become very
expert in putting up intravenous infusions and
noting side-effects from previous drug treatment, and there are seldom difficulties with
extravasation. Newly qualified house staff are
not nearly so capable or as accessible to the
patient during the day.

Patients undergoing cytotoxic chemotherapy
should be aware of the nature of the treatment
and its possible hazards. It is easier to make
sure that patients receive adequate information
if the treatment is the responsibility of a single
department. The patient should be told of the
nature of the drugs, what the possible side-
effects might be and which of these effects
should lead him/her to contact the hospital.
This can be done in a way which is not frightening. For example, he or she should be told to
report fever or sore throat so that a blood count
can be taken. It is often worthwhile supplying
explanatory leaflets about chemotherapy, and
drug cards giving the names, dosage and purposes of the drugs are very useful.

Patients staying overnight. Some regimens
such as those containing high-dose platinum,
or a methotrexate infusion, require an overnight
stay. It is convenient and efficient to have
designated overnight-stay beds for this kind of
chemotherapy where the admission is planned
in advance and is relatively informal. It is our
practice to have the ward chemotherapy nurse
give the drugs after the patient has been seen
by a doctor, and to book the next admission.

Patients on lengthy regimens. These patients,
many of whom are on treatments where there is
a serious possibility of prolonged myelosuppression, are admitted in the usual way. They
are under the care of a single team, experienced
in the use of intensive cytotoxic regimens,
familiar with the supportive techniques
required (see Chapter 7) and in mitigating the
side-effects of the drugs.

This organization should be the responsibility of a senior member of staff whose particular interest is the medical treatment of
cancer. In most hospitals this will be a medical
oncologist and in others a radiotherapist or a
haematologist.

Chemotherapy-induced vomiting

The mechanisms by which chemotherapy induces vomiting are not well understood. Both
peripheral (gastric and intestinal) and antral
stimuli may be important. A schematic representation is shown in Fig. 6.13. Receptors for
serotonin (5HT) have been described in the rat
brain ($5HT_3$ receptors) and in peripheral nerve.
Studies on high-dose metoclopramide (see
below) have shown that blockage of $5HT_3$
receptors is part of its action and have led to the
introduction of $5HT_3$ antagonists as a new class
of anti-emetic.

Intravenous alkylating agents, doxorubicin
and cisplatin typically produce nausea and
vomiting 2–8 hours after injection and the
symptoms persist for 8–36 hours. Other drugs
do not cause vomiting so frequently. After one
or two cycles of chemotherapy some patients
suffer from anticipatory nausea and vomiting

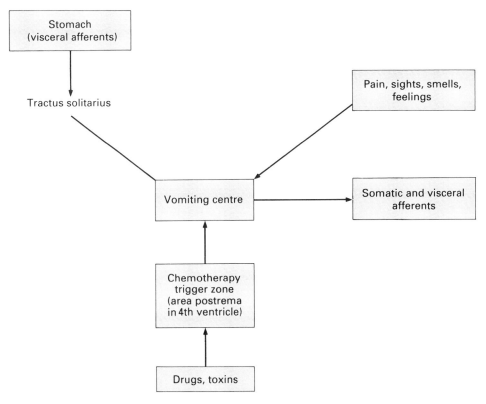

Fig. 6.13 A simplified scheme of events in chemotherapy-induced vomiting. The site of action of anti-emetics is not shown since the details are not clearly established. $5HT_3$ receptors are assumed to play a role in the central and peripheral mechanisms. Chemotherapy may damage cells of the intestinal lumen, liberating 5HT from enterochromaffin cells.

at the sight of the nurse, doctor, intravenous infusion or hospital or even on setting out on the journey to hospital. In these patients prophylactic anti-emetic therapy must be given a considerable time before chemotherapy.

There are several different types of drugs which can be used to prevent or treat vomiting (Table 6.4). None is satisfactory in all patients and most are only partially effective. Anti-emetic therapy should be started prophylactically and often a satisfactory regimen can be established in each individual patient by trial and error.

5HT₃ ANTAGONISTS

This new class of compound represents a major step forward in the control of vomiting. Control of cisplatin-induced emesis is achieved in 60% of patients — similar to optimum results obtained with combinations of metoclopramide, maxolon and dexamethasone. Ondansetron, tropisetron and granisteron are selective $5HT_3$ antagonists. The main site of action (central or peripheral) is still unclear. Ondansetron has good oral bioavailability. Both are safe and well tolerated. The terminal plasma half-life of ondansetron is approximately 3 hours. Side-effects include headache, flushing and constipation. Hepatic dysfunction decreases metabolism. The usual dose of ondansetron is 8 mg by slow intravenous infusion, then 2 further doses four hours apart followed, if necessary, by 8 mg twice daily to prevent delayed emesis, for 3 days.

Table 6.4 Anti-emetic agents

Drug	Dose	Action	Toxicity
Ondansetron	0.15 mg/kg 4-hourly	$5HT_3$ antagonist	Constipation, headache
Granisetron	3 mg i.v. over 5−10 mins	$5HT_3$ antagonist	Constipation, headache
Metoclopramide	10 mg p.o. or i.v. or 1−2 mg/kg i.v. repeated 3-hourly	Dopamine and $5HT_3$ antagonist (central and peripheral)	Extrapyramidal symptoms, diarrhoea
Dexamethasone	8−16 mg i.v. before treatment	Unclear	Restlessness, mood changes
Benzodiazepines, e.g. lorazepam	1−2 mg p.o. or i.v. every 4−6 hours	Cerebral cortex, ? histamine receptor blocking agent	Sedation, hypotension, hallucinations, dysphoria, dizziness, ataxia
Phenothiazines, e.g. prochlorperazine	12.5 mg i.m. or 25 mg suppository	Dopamine antagonist	Extrapyramidal symptoms, drowsiness
Butyrophenones, e.g. haloperidol	0.5−1 mg p.o. or i.v. repeated 4−8 hours	? Dopamine antagonist	Extrapyramidal symptoms, akasthesia

Piperazine phenothiazines

These include prochlorperazine and perphenazine. They are effective anti-emetics in some patients but need to be used near the maximum dose, at which point extrapyramidal reactions are common particularly with intravenous administration.

Aliphatic phenothiazines

The most commonly used agents are chlorpromazine and promazine. They have more sedative and less anti-emetic properties and are more liable to produce hypotension.

Metoclopramide

This drug appears to act on the trigger area, possibly through blocking dopamine receptors. It increases gastric emptying. The drug can be given intramuscularly or intravenously and may cause extrapyramidal side-effects, restlessness and diarrhoea. In low dose (10 mg orally or intravenously) it has little activity.

Metoclopramide is often used in high dose in the prevention of vomiting. It is probable that it is more effective at high dose and some studies have shown it to be more effective than phenothiazines and may act as a $5HT_3$ receptor antagonist. The incidence of extrapyramidal side-effects does not appear to be greater in high dose. Randomized trials have shown high-dose metoclopramide to be superior to phenothiazines.

Benzodiazepines

Although these drugs have no anti-emetic properties they may make the vomiting more tolerable by inducing a somnolent state in which the patient cannot remember the period of nausea clearly. Intravenous lorazepam is useful for this purpose.

Butyrophenone derivatives

These drugs are dopamine receptor blocking agents which work centrally. Haloperidol is the most widely used and is partially effective against cisplatin-induced vomiting.

Long-term complications
of cancer chemotherapy [1]

More children and young adults are now surviving diseases such as acute leukaemia, lymphoma and testicular cancer which were formerly incurable. Survival has been achieved by intensive combination chemotherapy. It has become apparent that chemotherapy of this type is associated with long-term complications in some patients. The recognition of these sequelae has emphasized that treatment of great intensity must be justified by a clear benefit in survival and that such drug and radiation therapies must be restricted to those categories of patients in which they are essential for survival. Long-term follow-up of patients is essential since some of the complications may develop many years after treatment is discontinued.

IMPAIRED GONADAL FUNCTION

Suppression of spermatogenesis occurs in the majority of men being treated with combination chemotherapy [10]. Procarbazine and alkylating agents seem to have the greatest adverse effect, methotrexate and doxorubicin less so. The degree of infertility and its permanence vary with different regimens. With MOPP therapy for Hodgkin's disease (Chapter 25) 95% of men will have long-lasting infertility. With the ABVD regimen this is less, and with the PVB regimen for teratoma there is frequent recovery of fertility. Damage to the germinal epithelium is associated with a rise in serum FSH (which normally stimulates spermatogenesis). While prepubertal boys do not appear to experience long-lasting endocrine changes from chemotherapy, intensive chemotherapy during puberty damages Leydig cells and is accompanied by a rise in both FSH and LH, low testosterone levels and gynaecomastia.

Pre-treatment storage of sperm is usually advised but in untreated Hodgkin's disease there may be pre-existing oligospermia. The number of successful pregnancies from stored sperm is disappointingly small.

Ovarian failure is often produced by combination chemotherapy and is more frequent the nearer the patient is to her natural menopause. Even if menstruation does not cease, subfertility is common and the duration of the reproductive years of life is shortened with earlier menopause. As with testicular failure, alkylating agents and procarbazine appear to be more likely to cause ovarian failure than antimetabolites.

PULMONARY FIBROSIS

Pulmonary damage is produced by many cytotoxic drugs (Table 6.5). Most alkylating agents will produce pulmonary fibrosis with long-term impairment of diffusing capacity. Busulphan is, however, more likely to do so than other drugs. Bleomycin causes pulmonary infiltrates, a total-dose related phenomenon which is very common over $300 \, mg/m^2$. These infiltrates may disappear when the drug is stopped but permanent fibrosis often follows.

LIVER DISEASE

Many drugs cause a transient rise in plasma enzymes (nitrosoureas, methotrexate, cytosine

Table 6.5 Pulmonary and hepatic toxicity of cytotoxic drugs

Drug	Effect
Pulmonary	
Busulphan and nitrosoureas (and other alkylating agents)	Fibrosis
Bleomycin Mitomycin C	Pulmonary infiltrates and fibrosis
Hepatic	
Methotrexate	Fibrosis
6MP and azathioprine	Cholestatic jaundice and necrosis
Asparaginase	Fatty infiltration

arabinoside) but permanent hepatic dysfunction is rare. Permanent liver damage can occasionally occur with antimetabolites (Table 6.5).

SECOND CANCERS

Second malignancies have been noted after long-term administration of alkylating agents particularly melphalan and chlorambucil, typically given to patients with ovarian cancer and myeloma. In both cases there is an increased risk of acute myeloid leukaemia. Almost all alkylating agents are leukaemogenic, and there is increasing evidence that second cancers are also induced by anthracyclines and epipodophyllotoxins.

In patients treated intensively for Hodgkin's disease there is also an increased risk of acute myeloid leukaemia. A recent case–control study [12] has clearly demonstrated the increased risk of leukaemia in Hodgkin's disease and ovarian cancer. In Hodgkin's disease the relative risk was higher in young patients and is greatly outweighed by the survival advantage of treatment. In ovarian cancer the survival benefit of chemotherapy is less marked. Chemotherapy-induced leukaemia is associated with non-random chromosomal deletions (e.g. on chromosomes 5 and 7), and the leukaemia tends to be refractory to treatment. Bladder cancer is a reported complication of cyclophosphamide therapy but the risk appears to be very small.

Long-term immunosuppressive therapy in renal allograft recipients (and the immune suppression in AIDS) also predisposes to the development of cancer [13]. Lymphomas are the commonest malignancy, particularly large cell lymphoma of the brain. The average time of onset is 2 years but the risk persists indefinitely.

The mechanisms whereby chemotherapy induces cancer are not known. Hodgkin's disease is associated with a slight increase in acute leukaemia even in patients who have not been treated with chemotherapy.

Postulated mechanisms are a direct carcinogenic effect of the drugs, diminished 'immune surveillance' and activation of oncogenic viruses in immune suppressed individuals.

PRINCIPLES OF HORMONE THERAPY

The demonstration by Beatson in 1896 that inoperable breast cancer sometimes regressed after oophorectomy was one of the most remarkable discoveries in the history of cancer treatment. Many years later Huggins demonstrated that metastatic prostatic cancer would regress with orchidectomy or the administration of oestrogens. A rational basis for the use of hormone manipulation in cancer treatment has, however, been hampered by lack of knowledge of how hormones act on cancer cells and of which cancer cells are likely to be affected. In recent years, there has been a transformation in our understanding and in at least one tumour — breast cancer — knowledge of the hormone receptor status of the tumour has become clinically important.

Steroid hormone receptors

It is now clear that there are receptor proteins for steroid hormones both in the cytoplasm and the nucleus and that interaction between the hormone and its receptor modifies DNA activity and hence cell growth and replication. These events are depicted diagrammatically in Fig. 6.14.

The steroid hormone, unbound to plasma protein, crosses the cell membrane by a mechanism which is not well understood. The hormone then links to the cytoplasmic receptor protein and the complex undergoes a conformational change either in the cytoplasm or in the nucleus. This hormone–receptor complex binds to a nuclear protein which in turn exerts a controlling activity on DNA. There then follows an increase in RNA polymerase activity which results in the synthesis, first of messenger RNA (mRNA), and then cytoplasmic protein. After 24 hours DNA synthesis occurs, followed by cell division.

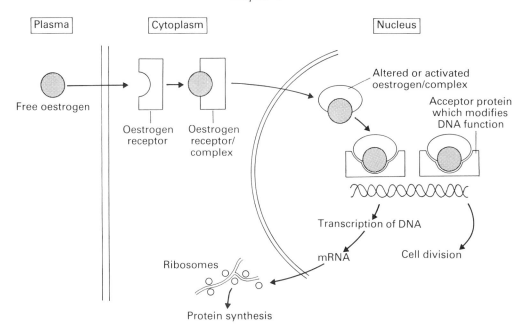

Fig. 6.14 A simplified scheme of the interaction between oestrogen and its receptor.

This model appears to be generally applicable to a variety of steroid hormones. There is evidence that the synthesis of the receptor proteins is promoted by the hormone to which they bind and that other hormones can reduce the synthesis of receptor proteins; for example, progesterone inhibits the synthesis of oestrogen receptor.

Using these concepts of hormone action, several strategies for modifying tumour growth can be developed: the plasma concentration of the stimulating hormone might be lowered by ablative therapy, either surgical, radiotherapeutic or chemical. Once the hormone has entered the cell it may be prevented from binding to the receptor either by competitive inhibitors or by reduction of receptor synthesis. It might also be possible to block the binding of the complex to the nuclear 'acceptor' protein.

In practice it is often difficult to determine the site of action of agents used in hormone therapy. Tamoxifen, for example, appears to bind to the oestrogen receptor but may also affect its synthesis, and the tamoxifen–receptor complex may also block the acceptor site in the nucleus.

The situation may become clearer when it is possible to measure the concentration of receptor molecules independently of their hormone binding properties. It may then be possible to say whether lack of oestrogen binding, for example, is due to lack of receptor protein or to lack of free binding sites.

Hormone receptor assays

Attempts to use the presence of a hormone receptor to predict the responsiveness of an individual tumour to hormone manipulation have been only partially successful. The usual assay is a measure of uptake of isotopically labelled hormone by homogenized tumour cells. The degree of binding varies and an arbitrary cut-off point has to be made in what is in fact a gradation from negative to positive. In studies on tissue sections it can be shown that in breast cancer some cells are oestrogen receptor (ER) positive and others negative. The overall expression of ER status is thus an over-simplification of the position. Furthermore, the presence of hormone receptors does not prove that they are functionally active. Oestrogen promotes the synthesis of progesterone receptor (PR) in breast cancer cells, and measurement of PR may thus provide a better measure of functionally active oestrogen receptor than measurement of ER itself. At present it is clear that in, for example, breast cancer, the absence (or very low values) of an oestrogen receptor strongly predicts a lack of response to hormone manipulation, and that high levels of receptor are indicative of probable response. Intermediate values are associated with a variable response rate.

The role of hormone therapy in individual tumours is discussed in detail in the appropriate chapters.

Approaches to hormone therapy

1 *Lowering the plasma hormone concentration.* This may be done by surgical or medical means:

Surgical. Oophorectomy (surgical or radiotherapeutic) will abolish oestrogen secretion by the ovary in premenopausal women and was widely used as a first step in hormone treatment of advanced breast cancer. Knowledge of the oestrogen receptor status is useful because the likelihood of response in ER +ve tumours is 50% compared with only 5% of ER −ve tumours in whom the procedure may not be worthwhile.

Adrenalectomy sometimes produces further responses in premenopausal patients with advanced breast cancer responding to oophorectomy. This is probably due to residual sex hormone synthesis by the adrenal. The tumour response occurs despite adequate glucocorticoid replacement. Hypophysectomy produces a similar effect. Both of these operations are less commonly performed since the advent of aromatase inhibitors (see below). Orchidectomy is effective in reducing plasma testosterone levels and has been widely used as treatment for metastatic prostatic carcinoma.

Medical. In premenopausal women the main source of oestrogens is the ovary, but some oestrogens are formed as a result of the peripheral conversion of androgens, formed in the adrenal. This conversion takes place in muscle, liver, and fat and is mediated by aromatase enzymes. After the menopause the adrenal becomes the main source of oestrogens by production of androgen (δ-4-androstenedione) which is converted in the peripheral tissues. However, the adrenal is not the only source of oestrogen precursors, and breast tissue itself can synthesize oestrogens. Aminoglutethimide and other more specific aromatase inhibitors block the action of aromatase enzymes and also depresses synthesis of androgens and cortisol in the adrenal itself. Premenopausal women (whose major source of oestrogen synthesis is the ovary which is not dependent on aromatase enzymes) do not respond to aminoglutethimide.

Approximately 30% of postmenopausal women will respond and the response rate of bone metastases is particularly striking (55%) while liver metastases are less responsive (20%). Toxicity includes somnolence, transient skin rash, and muscle cramps. Aminoglutethimide has been shown to be as effective as adrenalectomy in advanced breast cancer.

Luteinizing hormone releasing hormone (LHRH) is a decapeptide released from the hypothalamus to act on the pituitary (Fig. 6.15). Analogues of LHRH such as goserelin and leuprorelin cause an initial pituitary stimulation followed by an inhibition of gonadotrophin release which causes a profound fall in plasma testosterone. Goserelin is given by subcutaneous injection once a month. If combined with an anti-androgen such as flutamide (see below) more profound suppression of androgen effect is achieved, which may have some extra benefit in prostate cancer.

2 *Blocking the action of circulating hormones.* Anti-oestrogens, of which the most notable example is tamoxifen, have been a major advance in the treatment of metastatic breast cancer. The mode of action of tamoxifen is ill understood. The drug appears to exert its effect by binding with the cytoplasmic oestrogen receptor but its affinity for the ER is much less

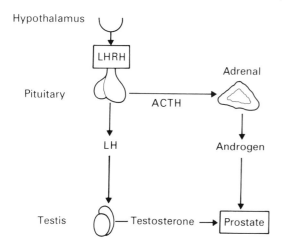

Fig. 6.15 LHRH analogues at first stimulate and then suppress LH release resulting in a fall in testosterone release from the testis. This results in regression in hormone-dependent prostate cancer.

than that of oestrogen itself. Possibly the drug–receptor complex undergoes a conformational change which blocks its entry to nuclear sites of activity. Other receptor sites which bind tamoxifen but not oestrogen have also been described, however the balance of evidence at present suggests that tamoxifen exerts its effect by competitively binding with ER thus displacing oestradiol. Tamoxifen does not increase plasma oestradiol levels in postmenopausal women but does do so in premenopausal women. Tamoxifen has a prolonged terminal half-life in plasma and after 1 month of treatment the plasma concentration exceeds that of oestradiol by up to a thousand fold. It is for this reason that a dose–response effect is not usually observed clinically. Toxic effects are uncommon the most frequent being mild nausea and hot flushes. Occasionally a flare-up of the breast cancer may be seen which is then sometimes followed by a response. The long-term use of tamoxifen is associated with a small increase in uterine cancer, and a possibly beneficial alteration in plasma lipid concentrations.

The mechanism of acquired resistance to tamoxifen is unclear since the cancer cells still contain ER. It is possible that the cell's dependence on oestrogen is bypassed by other mechanisms such as growth factor stimulation [14]. Megestrol acetate is a synthetic anti-androgen. It blocks the synthesis of testosterone, reducing plasma testosterone levels. Adrenal androgens (androstenedione) are also reduced. The drug also blocks the action of testosterone on prostatic carcinoma cells and this is a further mechanism for its action in the disease. Cyproterone acetate and flutamide have an anti-androgen effect which may be valuable in prostatic cancer. Flutamide does not inhibit pituitary LH release and blocks the negative feedback which testosterone produces resulting in a rise in serum testosterone. Flutamide has no progestogen activity.

3 *Additive hormone therapies.* In breast cancer these include oestrogens, androgens, glucocorticoids and progestogens. ER +ve breast cancers will sometimes regress with exogenous oestrogen which indicates that we still have gaps in our knowledge of the mechanism of action of hormone therapies. Medroxyprogesterone acetate and megestrol acetate produce responses in about 20% of patients. They possibly do this by lowering the cytoplasmic ER content and responses are usually only seen in ER +ve tumours, but appear independent of progesterone receptor status. Progesterone derivatives produce responses in about 30% of uterine carcinomas usually in cases which are ER +ve or PR +ve.

CYTOKINES IN CANCER TREATMENT

Cytokines are a group of proteins some of which regulate the growth of cells and others modulate the immune response and inflammation. They are usually glycosyslated and of low molecular weight. They are produced by cells of various types and usually act over short distances (as autocrine or paracrine stimuli) (Table 6.6). In cancer therapy they may regulate tumour cell growth, be directly cytotoxic, excite an inflam-

Table 6.6 Properties of interferons, tumour necrosis factor and interleukins

Cytokine	MW (kDa)	Chromosome location	Cell of origin
Interferons			
α	17–23	9	White cells
β	20	9	Fibroblasts
γ	20	12	T and NK cells
Tumour necrosis factor			
α	17	6	Monocytes
β	25	6	T cells
Interleukins			
1	17	2	Numerous cells
2	17	4	T cells
4	20	5	Numerous cells
5	18	5q	Numerous cells
6	26	7	Numerous cells

Table 6.7 Clinical activity of cytokines

INTERFERONS
α

Hairy cell leukaemia	90% response. Improved prognosis
Chronic myeloid leukaemia	70% response often with Ph' −ve marrow in chronic phase
Follicular lymphoma	60% response
Myeloma	Decreased relapse rate
Essential thrombocythaemia	50% response
Melanoma	20% response
Renal cell carcinoma	20% response
Kaposi's sarcoma	30% response

β and γ
Little activity in solid tumours. Some activity against chronic lymphatic leukaemia (γ)

TUMOUR NECROSIS FACTOR
Useful clinical activity not yet confirmed

INTERLEUKINS
IL-2

Renal cell carcinoma	15–30% response
Melanoma	15–30% response

IL-4
No clinical data to show antitumour activity in patients

IL-6
Possible effect in mitigating thrombocytopenia induced by cytotoxic drugs. ?Growth regulatory role in myeloma

matory or immune response in the tumour, or speed normal tissue recovery from the effect of cytotoxic drugs. Cytokine treatment has an established role in only one or two, rather uncommon, tumours.

Interferons (IFs)

Three classes of interferon have been defined: α, β and γ. At first they were of interest because of their antiviral properties but it is now clear they have a wide spectrum of activity (Table 6.6). Their antitumour activity is complex. They may have a direct antiproliferative effect on normal and neoplastic cells, they induce differentiation in some leukaemic cell lines, and enhance the cytotoxicity of T, NK, and LAK cells (see below). Expression of MHC class I and II is increased on tumour cells.

The clinical activity of interferons is summarized in Table 6.7. Side-effects include a 'flu-like illness with rigors, headache, muscle pains and fever; leucopenia may occur. These symptoms are dose related. Most patients can tolerate 3×10^6 units of α daily for many weeks. Neutralizing antibodies may develop.

Interleukins (ILs)

Interleukins are a family of peptides which act as modulators of immune and inflammatory responses. Interleukin 2 has received most clinical attention.

INTERLEUKIN 2 (IL-2)

This is a glycoprotein (molecular weight 15 kDa) produced by activated T cells. It was first called T cell growth factor because its main effect is to cause antigen-activated T cells to proliferate. It binds to a cell surface receptor on T cells. This receptor has 2 subunits each of which can bind IL-2 with low affinity but together bind with

Chapter 6

high affinity. IL-2 stimulates production of IFNγ, and TNF (see below) and activates killer lymphocytes which are then called lymphokine activated killer cells or LAK cells. These kill cells without the need for antigen recognition or histocompatibility specificity.

As a single agent IL-2 produces responses in 15–30% of patients with metastatic renal carcinoma and melanoma. Some of these responses are very durable. Continuous infusion may have some advantages over bolus injection (continuous activation, fewer side-effects). The combination of LAK cells (where the patient's own lymphocytes are activated and expanded *in vitro* and then returned to the patient) and IL-2 may produce more complete responses but overall response rates are similar. Expansion of a population of lymphocytes infiltrating the tumour (which might be thought of as 'committed') has not shown any clinical advantage over other LAK cell therapy or IL-2 alone. Nothing is known of the impact of these treatments on survival. Controlled comparisons are overdue. Side-effects of IL-2 are considerable: fever, lethargy, hypotension, adult respiratory distress syndrome, nausea, vomiting, anaemia, neutropenia, disorientation and somnolence. These effects are dose-related.

INTERLEUKIN 4 (IL-4)

This is a potent stimulator of cytotoxic T cells but there are, as yet, no clinical data to suggest it has activity in human cancer.

INTERLEUKIN 6 (IL-6)

This cytokine is produced in the bone marrow and by human osteoblasts. It appears to act as a paracrine growth factor in myeloma and is overproduced in this disease. The reason for the overproduction is unclear. Its production is dependent on IL-1. Interleukin 6 stimulates osteoclast activity and appears to stimulate platelet production.

Tumour necrosis factor (TNF) [15]

This group of cytokines obtained their name from experiments in which a serum protein component caused tumour necrosis in mice. *Cachectin* was a name given to a protein found to cause weight loss in animals and now shown to be TNFα. Two molecules have been described. TNFα is derived from macrophages and lymphoid cells and is a non-glycosylated protein of MW 17000 Da. It may assume dimeric or trimeric forms. TNFβ (MW 25000) is also called lymphotoxin and is produced by activated T lymphocytes. Both TNFs bind to specific cell-surface receptors (the same or closely related). The cytotoxic effect may be via free-radical generation inside the cell. TNF has been shown to be cytotoxic for leukaemic cells (including hairy cells) and B lymphoid malignancies. TNFs act on the vascular endothelium to release chemostatic factors, increase HLA class I expression and the production of procoagulants. These effects are essentially those of a mediator of acute inflammation. TNFs are produced in a wide range of bacterial infections and in chronic inflammatory and malignant diseases.

So far, Phase 1 studies have indicated some activity in lymphoma. More work needs to be done to reduce the considerable toxicity and to explore its use in conjunction with other therapies.

Monoclonal antibodies in cancer therapy

Monoclonal antibodies (mAbs) are secreted by antibody producing hybridoma cells, which are made by fusing immunocompetent cells (taken from an animal which has been immunized with tumour cells or extract) with an immortal myeloma cell line. The mouse is the animal most widely used. The immunocompetent cells provide the genetic programme for specificity of antibody response, and the myeloma line provides the permanent production of mAb. The immune response is directed to cell surface and cytoplasmic constituents and a wide variety of antibodies result. Screening of the hybrid-omas yields the mAb of interest.

The resulting mAbs are not tumour specific. Among the structures recognized are:

1 human histocompatibility antigens;
2 growth factor receptors;
3 cell surface glycoproteins associated with function and differentiation;
4 glycolipids (e.g. blood group antigens); and
5 cell matrix proteins.

The mAbs may be used for localization of tumours and metastases (but the sensitivity does not generally exceed other methods of imaging). They may also be used for attempted therapy by attaching a cytotoxic component. This may be ionizing radiation such as ^{131}I, ^{211}As, ^{111}Ind; drugs such as alkylating agents; or toxins such as ricin or abrin [16].

There are many difficulties with this approach to therapy.

1 Tumour heterogeneity means that not all cells will express the antigen. This may not matter greatly if ionizing radiation is used since associated antigen-negative cells may be killed if adjacent to antigen-positive cells.
2 Normal tissues express the antigen. This may or may not lead to toxicity depending on the cells concerned (e.g. marrow is more important than skin).
3 There is considerable non-specific uptake in the liver spleen and marrow. There may be technical ways of overcoming this limitation by using sophisticated methods of coupling to the antibody.
4 Anti-mouse antibody is often produced by the patient (this can be minimized by cyclosporin).
5 There is relatively low uptake (as a percentage of injected dose) by the tumour.
6 Free antigen in the plasma may bind to the mAb and result in clearance in the reticulo-endothelial system.

For these reasons more work has yet to be undertaken before mAb therapy becomes established in the treatment of cancer.

REFERENCES

1 McVie J.G., Bast R.C. jnr. Therapeutic modalities. *Current Opinion in Oncology* 1989; **1**: 171–73.
2 Nowell P.C. The clonal evolution of tumour cell populations. *Science* 1976; **194**: 23–8.
3 Brown R., Kaye S.B. Drug resistance and the problem of treatment failure. In Ponder B.A.J. & Waring M.J., eds. *The Science of Cancer Treatment*. Kluwer Academic Publishers, 1990.
4 Simon S.M., Schindler M. Cell biological mechanisms of multidrug resistance in tumors. *Proceedings of the National Academy of Sciences* 1994; **91**: 3497–504.
5 Moscow J.A., Cowan K.H. Multidrug resistance. *Journal of the National Cancer Institute* 1988; **80**: 14–20.
6 Salmon S.E. Chemosensitivity testing: Another chapter. *Journal of the National Cancer Institute* 1990; **82**: 82–83.
7 Prichard J., McElwain T.J., Graham-Pole J. High-dose melphalan with autologous marrow for treatment of advanced neuroblastoma. *British Journal of Cancer* 1982; **45**: 86–94.
8 O'Driscoll B.R., Hasleton P.S., Taylor P.M. *et al*. Active lung fibrosis up to 17 years after chemotherapy with carmustine (BCNU) in childhood. *New England Journal of Medicine* 1990; **323**: 378–82.
9 Young R.C., Ozols R.F., Myers C.E. The anthracycline antineoplastic drugs. *New England Journal of Medicine* 1981; **305**: 139–53.
10 Chapman R.M., Sutcliffe S.B., Malpas J.S. Male gonadal dysfunction in Hodgkin's disease. *Journal of the American Medical Association*. 1981; **245**: 1323–28.
11 Weiss R.B., Muggia F.M. Cytotoxic drug-induced pulmonary disease. *American Journal of Medicine* 1980; **68**: 259–66.
12 Kaldor J.M., Day N.E., Clarke E.A. *et al*. Leukaemia following Hodgkin's disease. *New England Journal of Medicine* 1990; **322**: 7–13 (pp. 1–6 for study of ovarian cancer).
13 Sheil A.G.R. Cancer in organ transplant recipients: part of an induced immune deficiency syndrome. *British Medical Journal* 1985; **288**: 659–60.
14 Johnston S.R.D., Dowsett M., Smith I.E. Towards a molecular basis for tamoxifen resistance in breast cancer. *Annals of Oncology* 1993; **3**: 503–11.
15 Semenzato G. Tumour necrosis factor: a cytokine with multiple biological activities. *British Journal of Cancer* 1990; **61**: 354–61.
16 Wawrzynczak E.J. Systemic immunotoxin therapy of cancer: advances and prospects. *British Journal of Cancer* 1991; **64**: 624–50.

Chapter 7
Supportive Care and Symptom Relief

PSYCHOLOGICAL ASPECTS OF CANCER MANAGEMENT

Talking about the diagnosis and treatment

Major disease brings anxiety and worry, but few diseases are associated with such dread as cancer, with its imagined inevitable sequel of certain death, pain, lingering and suffering. One of the most difficult, and most rewarding tasks for the physician is to set the disease in its right context, to explain the treatment, to give enough information at the correct rate and time, to sustain hope, and to be accessible, competent, open minded and, above all, kind.

It is easy to forget that the patient has a life outside the consulting room and that he or she will interpret what is said in the light of his or her own experience and apprehensions. Cancer is commonest in the elderly. In the course of a long life many patients will have had friends or relatives who have died of the disease or may perhaps have cared for a member of the family with cancer. These experiences will have an important influence on a patient's outlook and expectations. In recent years cancer and its treatment has been widely discussed in the media of mass communication. Although patients are better informed now than 20 years ago, their knowledge is often fragmentary and disorganized. Some patients may have recognized the seriousness of a symptom — haemoptysis, unexplained weight loss, a lump, or backache, but be too anxious (or too afraid of surgery) to voice their suspicions. Other patients may have no idea of the possible diagnosis.

As with patients, the attitude of physicians is influenced by their experience and training. Frequently the diagnosis of cancer is made by a specialist in another area such as general surgery, gynaecology or chest medicine. Some of these doctors may themselves have a very pessimistic view of cancer and what can be achieved by treatment. Furthermore, in hospital medicine the specialist has often had little opportunity to get to know the patient before the diagnosis has been made. A lack of familiarity both with what can be achieved by treatment and also with the patient, combined sometimes with the fear of the disease, may lead the physician or surgeon into euphemisms and half-truths. Words may be used such as 'growth' or 'ulcer' to soften or obscure the diagnosis, while the doctor often betrays his real meaning by appearing evasive or unclear.

This attitude means that, unless the patient is bold and asks for a more frank statement of the diagnosis, the doctor may be unable to assess what impact his words have had. Because the meaning of the diagnosis is being avoided it becomes difficult to allow the patient to express his or her fears or ask the appropriate questions. The patient may in fact be under the impression that the diagnosis is worse than it actually is, that he has only a short time to live, or that treatment will be to no avail. The doctor's evasions may then strengthen this opinion. Another failing is that there will be many clues to the patient as to where the truth lies. He may learn the diagnosis from a pathology request form, from a hospital porter, a well meaning friend or an overhead remark. If the diagnosis is discovered accidentally the patient may realize that the intention behind concealment was to spare him anxiety, but may sometimes feel let down by the doctor and be cautious in accepting any further reassurance.

In recent years the attitude of cancer specialists has moved decisively towards a fuller discussion of the diagnosis and treatment. What is said to the patient must, however, be well-judged and carefully delivered. Every physician makes errors of judgement which shake his confidence with the next patient he sees, but it is important not to retreat from these discussions when difficulties have occurred. It is important to learn from one's mistakes.

If possible it is useful to assess the attitude of the patient before the diagnosis is made. Questions such as 'what do you feel is wrong with you' or 'have you any particular anxieties about what might be wrong' are often very revealing since the patient will sometimes admit to a fear of malignancy and, if so, it allows the physician to ask the patient whether, if this proves to be the diagnosis, he would want to know the details of what is found.

It is sometimes possible to make the diagnosis before major surgery is undertaken; by bronchoscopy for lung cancer, needle biopsy in breast cancer, or endoscopy for gastro-intestinal disease. When the diagnosis has been established pre-operatively and treatment by surgery is necessary, it is hardly possible, still less desirable, that the diagnosis is not discussed and the probable operative procedure described. Often the diagnosis only becomes apparent after an operation and the patient will be waiting to hear the result. In either case when talking to the patient about the diagnosis, the doctor needs to have a clear idea of what he is going to say and the words he will use, although he must be prepared to modify the approach if the situation demands it.

In explaining the diagnosis the word 'cancer' is the only word which unequivocally conveys the nature of the complaint. Many physicians use the words 'malignancy', 'tumour' or 'growth' with the best of intentions, but this carries the risk that the patient will fail to realize the true nature of the disease (indeed this is often what

is intended). It is true that in the elderly or very anxious, the word cancer may occasionally be very frightening and there are some patients for whom other terms may be necessary. Many patients have only a vague idea of what cancer means and are surprised that the disease is nearly always treatable and sometimes curable. The explanation of the diagnosis must be combined with a realistic but hopeful account of what can be done. Few patients can exist without hope of any kind. It is nearly always necessary to hold out the hope of cure if this is possible, or of a period of healthy normal life even when the prognosis is poor. This does not mean that a cure is promised but that the patient can feel confident that every attempt will be made to cure him and that there is a possibility of success. Of course, if it is likely that the patient will be cured this must be stressed and a much more optimistic account of the disease can be given.

The manner in which the explanation is given is critical. The doctor should be unhurried, speak clearly and not technically, look at the patient's face while speaking, and show that he is not frightened or discomfited by the diagnosis and indicate by look and gesture that he is competent and prepared to discuss the problem calmly. There is a limit to the number of facts which a patient can assimilate during one conversation, particularly under stressful circumstances. Too much information may progressively extinguish the understanding which a short account would achieve. Not infrequently the patient may seem to understand, but in fact be too anxious to take in anything of what is being said. This failure of understanding is not 'denial' but is due to confusion and anxiety. It is a good policy to stop frequently and enquire if what is being said is clear or if there are questions which the patient wants to ask. When the patient is able to ask questions it implies that he or she has understood at least part of the explanation. The doctor should make it quite clear that he or she or a member of the team will always be pleased to answer questions and that there will be an opportunity to talk again in a day or two. One discussion is seldom enough. It may take a few days for the patient to start to understand and to take a realistic view of the situation and at that stage want to know more. It is usually advisable therefore to impart the details of the diagnosis and treatment over a period of time. The facts of the diagnosis are given first with a brief outline of treatment, gradually giving more information as the patient begins to come to terms with his or her position.

Some physicians ask relatives for advice on how much to tell the patient, particularly when they are in doubt about the correct approach. This can be helpful but there is a risk that the relatives may misjudge the patient and, out of love and sympathy, suggest that the truth be withheld when the patient would have wished otherwise. It is of course essential that relatives have a clear understanding of what has been said and why, and that the medical team do not give contradictory accounts. For this reason, after talking to the patient, the doctor should explain to the rest of the medical and nursing team exactly what has been said, with an idea of the words that have been used and what the reaction has been. The same information should be conveyed to the relatives but the discussion about prognosis may have to be more pessimistic with relatives. We think it almost always wrong to give patients a prognosis measured in a finite time because they tend to remember the stated number of months or years however many qualifications are made, and such predictions are often incorrect.

The patient's reaction may be a mixture of acceptance, anxiety, anger and grief. Some of this emotion may be directed at the doctor and this is one of the challenges of the job. It is essential to be understanding and not to be irritated by unjustified hostility if it occurs. This demands a lot from the doctor who must have enough self-confidence and maturity to realize that, in the end, the patient will come to trust his honesty and rely on his support.

At a later stage the physician, while discussing the details of investigation and treatment, may wish to explain that an illness such as cancer will alter the patient's perception of herself. That is, she will tend for a while to view herself as 'ill' and minor aches and pains which would previously have been ignored, may be magnified in her mind and be interpreted as symptoms of relapse. In explaining that this is an understandable but usually temporary phase, the physician should make it clear that he will be seeing the patient regularly and, if symptoms occur which cause anxiety, the patient should get in touch. The best cancer departments operate an 'open-door' policy of this type, eliminating a lot of bureaucratic difficulty for the patient who may otherwise be given an appointment weeks ahead for a problem which is immediate. The ideal arrangement is where the hospital specialist works in close collaboration with the family doctor in providing support and reassurance. The family practitioner may have long and invaluable experience of the patient and his or her family.

Whenever a patient visits, either for a regular review or because of a symptom, the physician should give equal priority to discussion as to the technical aspects of examination and investigation. It is greatly to be regretted that some doctors, and most health administrators, regard heavily booked clinics as a sign of efficiency. A 5-minute consultation with a cancer patient is nearly always bad medicine. These are conditions which may be forced upon doctors but should never be accepted by them.

Many cancer treatments have a bad reputation. Before the era of megavoltage equipment, high-dose radiotherapy required multiple fields if severe skin reactions were to be avoided (see Chapter 5). Fear of being burnt or scarred by radiotherapy is very common and a careful explanation of modern advances is sometimes needed. Alopecia, nausea and vomiting are unpleasant side-effects of chemotherapy and increasing numbers of patients have heard of these and, understandably, fear them. If chemotherapy is judged necessary, then the reasons should be explained. Patients will easily grasp the idea that cancer may not be localized and that a systemic treatment is being given to prevent or treat any recurrence from cancer cells which may have spread to other sites. Indeed they often find the idea of a systemic as well as a local treatment, reassuring. The ways in which the side-effects can be mitigated should be clearly explained.

Although patients will usually accept the need for radiotherapy or chemotherapy they may find the reality worse than they had imagined. This is particularly true for chemotherapy which often goes on for many months. There can be few things more miserable than repeated, predictable episodes of severe nausea and vomiting. Many patients begin to feel that they cannot go through with treatment and then find themselves in a frightening dilemma. On the one hand they are fearful of jeopardizing their chance of cure and of disappointing the doctor, but on the other the side-effects may produce progressive demoralization. In the case of a potentially curative treatment, for example for Hodgkin's disease, testicular tumours or acute lymphoblastic leukaemia, the doctor must try to sustain the patient through the treatment and do all he can to see it completed. For many cancers of adult life the benefits of chemotherapy are, however, much less clear. In these cases the worst outcome is that a patient is made to feel wretched by the treatment and guilty at stopping, and is then frightened of the prospect that he or she has jeopardized the chance of survival. If relapse occurs there may be self-blame and depression. The responsibility for this situation is as much the doctor's as the patient's. When chemotherapy is being given without a reasonable prospect of cure and the patient cannot continue, the physician should be sympathetic and reassuring and explain that he does not feel let down by the patient or that the prognosis has been materially worsened.

There are few other branches of medicine which demand simultaneously such technical expertise and kindly understanding as does cancer medicine. The strains on the doctor are considerable, especially if he takes the human aspect of his work seriously. It is a great failing in a doctor if he talks to his patients only about the physical and technical aspects of the illness, relies heavily on investigation in making treatment decisions and finds it difficult to give up intensive measures and accept that the patient cannot be cured. Technical prowess has then replaced a thoughtful analysis of the patient's feelings and what is in his or her best interests.

Treating patients with cancer demands great resources of emotional energy on the part of the doctor. In some units, part of the work of talking to patients is taken over by psychiatrists, psychologists, social workers or other counsellors. Invaluable though help from these persons may be, we do not think it desirable that doctors should see themselves as technical experts and that when human feelings intrude into the medical situation, the patient should be sent to talk to someone else about their problems. Sustaining and counselling a patient and his relatives is a matter of teamwork, but the doctor in charge of the case must make it clear that he or she regards the psychological aspects of the disease as being as important as the physical. The special problems of dealing with children with cancer are discussed in Chapter 24.

SUPPORT, COUNSELLING AND REHABILITATION

With any disease it is important to put oneself in the patient's position and try to anticipate the problems which are likely to arise. For example, it may seem obvious that mastectomy is a mutilating operation and that some psychological support pre- and postoperatively will be necessary. Nevertheless, many women do not receive adequate advice from their doctors. What may be less obvious (until one thinks of it) is that partners of women with mastectomy may be in need of explanation too. Indeed the reaction of a partner to the operation may be of fundamental importance in helping the patient to recover from her illness. Such advice is seldom offered.

In addition many patients with cancer face specific problems of rehabilitation as a result of surgical and other treatments. Rehabilitation and counselling are an essential part of the general care of cancer patients. In recent years specialized support services have developed to help patients overcome the effects of the illness and its treatment, and to return as far as possible to a normal life.

Stoma care

Successful treatment of cancer of the bowel or bladder will sometimes require permanent colostomy or ileostomy. Similarly in the treatment of gynaecological cancers, there will be a few patients in whom a permanent colostomy, resulting from radiation damage to the large bowel, is the price of a radiotherapy cure (see Chapter 17). Although some patients manage their stoma without difficulty, others require a great deal of education and help, and the role of the stoma therapist has now become established. Patients must learn not only how to keep the stoma clean and healthy, but also how to recognize the complications that might demand further surgical review, such as prolapse or stricture. Although a left-sided colostomy is relatively easy to manage, there are considerable difficulties with an ileostomy because of the fluid loss of 400−500 ml/day which can lead to electrolyte disturbance, dehydration (especially if gastro-intestinal infection occurs) and greater aesthetic difficulties. Surgery advances may yet lead to continent ileostomies, but at present most patients need to wear an appliance. The British Colostomy Association and Ileostomy Association offer support and practical help.

Breast prostheses

Most large hospitals should now have some form of mastectomy counselling service, to provide not only psychological support for patients who have undergone mastectomy, but also to offer expert advice regarding external prostheses. Almost all patients, including those with very radical operations, can now, when clothed, disguise their defects since a wide variety of prostheses, brassières and swimsuits are available. A nurse/counsellor specializing in the problems of mastectomy is of great help and many patients will benefit from the advice available from the Mastectomy Association. None the less, an increasing number of women are unhappy with any form of external prosthesis and request prosthetic implantation surgery which they hope will give them a more normal contour and the opportunity for more adventurous dress. Part of the mastectomy counsellor's job is to advise such patients that, contrary to their expectation, following surgery they cannot expect to look completely normal.

Laryngectomy rehabilitation

Following total laryngectomy, the patient has to be taught how to create an oesophageal voice, using techniques of air swallowing and careful phonation which can only be acquired with the help of an experienced speech therapist. Although some patients find this straightforward, the majority require careful tuition, and some never achieve a satisfactory voice. From these patients, a vibrating device or 'artificial larynx' should be available. The vibrating device is held against the neck, and permits a vibrating column of air to be produced which, with careful phonation by the patient, gives monotonous, barely acceptable but comprehensible speech. In a few centres, permanent valves are now being implanted which increase the power and durability of speech. Although these experimental techniques may well have a place in the future rehabilitation of laryngectomy patients, it should be stressed that well taught oesophageal speech can be very acceptable indeed. The National Association of Laryngectomee Clubs may provide further helpful advice.

Limb prostheses

The regional limb-fitting centres are responsible for providing both temporary and permanent external prostheses for those who have lost limbs whether through trauma or surgery. Traditionally, amputation has been the mainstay of treatment for bone and soft tissue sarcoma. Most patients, including children, adapt remarkably well to the loss of a limb, and many are able to drive a car, participate in sport, and lead a full and active life. In children, the limb must be replaced as the child grows and care must be taken with the details of weight, length, construction and fitting in order to avoid unequal pressure on the spine which might lead to scoliosis.

Other prostheses

Other sophisticated prostheses may also be necessary, particularly for patients with facial defects following radical surgery of the head and neck region. In particular, radical surgery for tumours of the maxillary antrum, orbit and nasal fossa, though curative, may result in substantial disfigurement which can only be covered by external prostheses. Remarkable results can be obtained but the work is highly specialized.

Home support

Learning how to use a colostomy bag or walk with an artificial limb is the start of a much more complex process of rehabilitation, in which the development of self reliance and self esteem needs encouragement. Whilst many patients achieve this with the help of their family, some are more isolated and require more professional help. The importance of, for example, a modified bathroom with supporting rails and wheelchair access may well be underestimated compared with the surgical and oncological challenge that the patient represented, but may help to make independent existence at home possible. District nursing help may allow patients to leave hospital relatively early after major operations, improving morale and reducing both the cost of the operation and also its morbidity from postoperative complications.

National counselling organizations

In a general hospital the work of counselling patients and their families is made easier if much of the in-patient treatment is in a specialized unit. In such a unit the nursing staff become very skilled in anticipating the problems of the disease and its treatment. When frequent admissions are necessary, for example for chemotherapy, it is of great help to the patient to see familiar faces. There is also a considerable benefit to be gained by having medical social workers who are especially skilled and interested in the problems of cancer. Not only do they provide another source of advice and reassurance but they will be knowledgeable about the local availability of counselling groups, nursing support, bereavement organizations and facilities for the care of the dying.

Self-help groups have arisen in many counties, organizing themselves nationally. Such groups have an enormous amount to offer, provided that they take care to give well-balanced and sensible advice. Many patients find it very helpful to talk about their problems with fellow sufferers and much detailed practical advice may be given which few doctors are in a position to match.

A fairly comprehensive list of support organizations in Britain and Ireland is provided in Appendix 7.1 (p. 136).

CANCER TREATMENT AND THE QUALITY OF LIFE

Most cancer treatments are unpleasant, producing short and long-term side-effects which interfere with the patient's quality of life. Assessment of the quality of life in cancer patients is not straightforward. Obvious criteria include length of time spent in hospital, the ability to get back to work, or at least to an independent life after treatment, and the degree of relief from troublesome symptoms, particularly pain. These parameters give an incomplete description of morbidity, and fail to draw attention to important symptoms such as nausea, fatigue, depression and anorexia.

Wherever possible, the distinction between *radical* and *palliative* treatment intent should be clear in the doctor's mind. For example, patients with widely metastatic breast cancer are often treated with combination chemotherapy, and remissions, often lasting several months, are frequently seen. However, since cure is never achieved, such treatment must be viewed as palliative and offered to patients with symptomatic deposits which are likely to respond. It is surprising how frequently this approach is not followed and patients with widely disseminated cancers (including far less sensitive tumours than carcinoma of the breast) are treated routinely with combination chemotherapy.

Where two types of treatment appear to give similar results, one should undoubtedly choose the less toxic. For example, chemotherapy for Hodgkin's disease has been made much more acceptable by the substitution of chlorambucil and vinblastine for mustine and vincristine (see Chapter 25). In certain situations, where there is a slight possible advantage to a more toxic treatment, the greater toxicity might outweigh the slight improvement in results. For example, in infiltrating carcinoma of the urinary bladder, there may be a slight survival advantage in a combination of irradiation and radical cystectomy, compared with treatment by radiotherapy alone (see p. 362). However, the extra few months of median survival are obtained at the cost of both a permanent ileostomy and a high risk of impotence. Given a choice, many of us might opt for radiotherapy alone, despite the slightly greater risk, particularly since surgery is still possible if there is local recurrence.

The use of surgery when there is radiation failure at the primary site (salvage surgery) is now widely accepted as it has become apparent that the treatment of solid tumours by radiotherapy can give local control rates which are the equal of surgery. This is clearly shown by the increasing use of radiotherapy for carcinoma of the cervix, of the head and neck, bladder, prostate and breast. In each of these sites, there are important physiological and psychological advantages to treatment with radiotherapy. Radical surgery can usually be performed if relapse occurs. Finally one should remember that there are some patients with malignant disease in whom treatment may not be immediately necessary. Many patients with follicular lymphoma harbour a disease whose course is so indolent that treatment is unnecessary, often for several years. In patients with asymptomatic but inoperable squamous carcinoma of the bronchus, there is generally no advantage to early treatment with radiotherapy or chemotherapy since such treatment does not prolong life and may cause side-effects (see Chapter 12). Treatment is better withheld until a troublesome symptom such as haemoptysis, dyspnoea or pain from a secondary deposit becomes apparent.

For these reasons, when trials of cancer treatments are undertaken it may be important to include some assessment of quality of life, especially if there is unlikely to be a substantial difference in cure rate. In this way, any advantage in terms of survival or local control can be set against the morbidity which the treatment has induced.

THE CARE OF THE DYING

In England and Wales alone, 135 000 people die each year of cancer, some 20% of all deaths. Of these about 60% die in district general hospitals, 30% at home and the remainder in hospices, nursing homes and non-NHS hospitals. About half of all cancer patients present with incurable conditions at the time of diagnosis, and in the more fortunate half with potentially curable cancers, the majority develop recurrent disease and require palliative symptomatic care. The WHO have estimated that about 3.5 million people are suffering worldwide from cancer pains each day — a sad reflection on the quality of care available to the majority of cancer patients.

It has become increasingly apparent that patients dying from cancer have particular needs which are often poorly served by traditional means of support. Even the most well meaning doctors frequently find themselves out of their depth either through inadequate training in the use of the appropriate drugs (particularly analgesics) or because of the difficulties of exploring the patient's needs. It is against this background that interest and expertise in the management of terminally ill patients has developed, and as so often happens, it has been the determined work of a few individuals which has identified the problem and developed principles which are now widely adopted.

First and foremost, it is always wrong for a doctor to say, or feel, 'there is nothing more that I can do'. The enthusiastic oncologist may feel that his or her work is over when the specific anticancer treatment is at an end. The patient will in general make a much less clear distinction between *active* and *supportive* treatment so that from the patient's point of view, careful treatment with analgesics, concern about appetite, constipation, mobility and so on, may be equally important. Second, it is largely through the work of hospice staff that we are beginning to learn the critical importance of adequate symptom control. The symptoms most commonly causing distress are pain, anorexia, nausea and vomiting, constipation, weakness and lassitude.

PAIN RELIEF WITH ANALGESICS

Relief of pain is a particularly important aspect of the care of the dying. There is no single ideal analgesic and most patients will require drugs of different strength and dosage during the course of their illness. It is convenient to group analgesics into the three classes according to their strength as shown in Table 7.1.

1 *Mild analgesics.* This group includes aspirin, paracetamol, dextropropoxyphene and non-steroidal anti-inflammatory agents. These can be valuable for considerable periods of time. Aspirin and the non-steroidal anti-inflammatory agents (indomethacin, ibuprofen, etc.) are particularly helpful in bone pain. Side-effects include dyspepsia and gastro-intestinal bleeding. They can be combined with agents from a more powerful class (e.g. aspirin and papaveretum tablets). Dextropropoxyphene is sometimes combined with paracetamol and many patients prefer this to paracetamol alone. The combination has been criticized because of the possibility of habituation but this is not important in the present context.

2 *Moderate analgesics.* This group includes codeine derivatives, oxycodone, pentazocine and dipipanone. These agents are more effective than those in the mild analgesic group but at the cost of greater side-effects, particularly constipation. Oxycodone is particularly valuable as it is available in the form of suppositories. Pentazocine should be avoided because it commonly produces hallucinations. It has a partial antagonist action to morphine and should not be used in combination with opiates.

3 *Powerful analgesics.* These drugs, which include morphine and related compounds (synthetic and semi-synthetic derivatives), are powerful in their pain-relieving effects and are the mainstay of analgesic therapy for patients with unremitting pain. Almost all patients with terminal cancer pain require regular medication with analgesics of this type. Useful agents include morphine, diamorphine, methadone, pethidine, dextromoramide, papaveretum (often combined with aspirin as effervescent compound tablets) and buprenorphine. Ordinary morphine and diamorphine have activity only for 4 hours and should be given 4-hourly, but long-acting oral tablets of morphine sulphate are now available, as described below.

The choice of opiate analgesic and dosages should be determined by the patient's need. For example, many patients are comfortable and pain-free with small regular dosage (10–20 mg every 4 hours) of morphine or diamorphine where others require 20 times this dose. There are few other drugs with a dose-range as wide. In most patients, oral medication is appropriate and effective though in those with, for example, complete obstruction from pharyngeal or oesophageal cancer, an alternative

Table 7.1 Analgesics for pain relief in cancer

Drug	Duration of action	Toxicity
Mild analgesics		
Aspirin	4–6 hours	Gastro-intestinal bleeding and abdominal pain.
Paracetamol	2–4 hours	Skin rash. Hepatic damage with overdose.
Propionic acid derivatives (e.g. ibuprofen)	2–6 hours	As aspirin
Indole derivatives (e.g. indomethacin)	8 hours	As aspirin
Moderate analgesics		
Codeine and dihydrocodeine	4–6 hours	Constipation, excitement
Oxycodone	8–10 hours	Constipation, hypotension, nausea, dysphasia
Pentazocine	3–4 hours	Nausea, dizziness, palpitations, hypertension, dysphasia
Dipipanone	6 hours	Constipation, mental confusion, respiratory depression
Powerful analgesics		
Morphine sulphate	4–6 hours (longer with sustained-release preparations)	Constipation, hypotension, nausea, dysphasia
Diamorphine	4–6 hours	As morphine sulphate
Methadone	15–30 hours	As morphine sulphate, more nausea, cumulative
Dextromoramide	6 hours	Dizziness, sweating, constipation, respiratory depression
Pethidine	3 hours	Nausea, dry mouth, respiratory depression

route will have to be found. Sublingual buprenorphine can be a useful alternative but it antagonizes the effect of morphine and should therefore not be abruptly substituted for morphine nor given with it concurrently. Treatment by rectal suppositories of oxycodone or morphine can be extremely effective. In very occasional cases, where both the oral and rectal routes are unavailable, suppositories can be given vaginally.

Regular intramuscular or intravenous treatment with opiates is almost never required though subcutaneous or intravenous infusions of diamorphine can be valuable if treatment by other routes proves unsatisfactory. Diamorphine is preferable because of its very high solubility, allowing volumes for injection to be small. Very rarely, regular administration of subdural or intrathecal morphine may be necessary for pain relief, but this should never be considered as a long-term solution unless other methods of regular opiate administration have been tried.

An important addition to the family of useful opiates is the long-acting morphine now available in oral tablets of 10, 30, 60, 100 and 200 mg strength; sachets are also available. The tablets are formulated in a long-acting base and give sustained pain relief for 12 hours. Since both morphine and diamorphine must be given frequently throughout the day, the availability of long-acting morphine is of real value, particularly to the active patient who is disinclined to carry bottles of diamorphine elixir with him. It is important to remember, when changing the treatment from diamorphine elixir to long-acting morphine that the dose ratio of diamorphine to morphine is 2:3 so that a patient on, say, diamorphine 20 mg 4-hourly (i.e. total daily dosage 120 mg), will require 180 mg of morphine daily, or long-acting morphine 90 mg twice daily, given orally at a 12-hour interval. In a small proportion of patients, treatment with slow-release morphine appears more effective if given three times per day (8-hourly) than the usual twice daily recommendation.

All patients taking regular opiate medication will require advice regarding constipation. Regular laxatives are usually (but not always) necessary, and may need to be given in above normal doses. We usually recommend regular danthron–poloxamer mixture (Codalax) but the standard daily dose of 10–12 ml in divided daily doses may be required for patients on large doses of morphine or diamorphine elixir

or tablets. Nausea, vomiting and sedation are the other important side-effects of opiate analgesics but are less consistent and often disappear rapidly. We do not find it necessary to offer routine anti-emetics with diamorphine elixir.

GUIDELINES FOR PAIN CONTROL IN TERMINAL CANCER PATIENTS (Fig. 7.1)

1 *Use enough analgesia to be effective.* Regular aspirin, or compound paracetamol/dextropropoxyphene tablets can be effective for many weeks. A change to dihydrocodeine will then usually give further pain relief. Use of morphine or related agents should be considered when drugs of lesser effect are inadequate for the patient's pain. At this stage less powerful agents

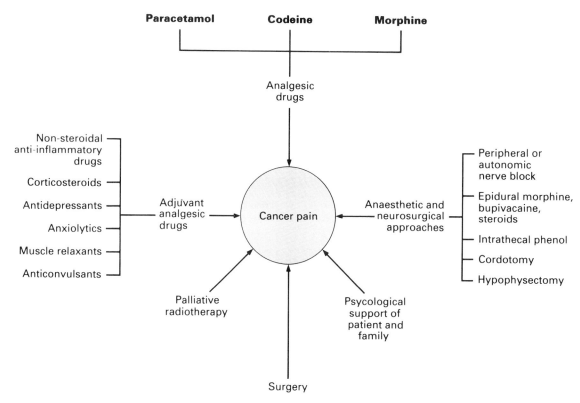

Fig. 7.1 Treatment of cancer pain. Reproduced from Baines M. *British Medical Journal* 1989; **298**: 36–38 with permission.

such as dipipanone, aspirin or non-steroidal anti-inflammatory agents may be useful to supplement the regular morphine dose. A common useful starting dose of diamorphine elixir is 10 or 20 mg every 4 hours, but some patients need more than 1 g of diamorphine daily for adequate pain relief. Addiction is not a problem and opiates should not be withheld for fear of producing it. Dysphoria and loss of lucidity may occur and can be distressing. In such cases a lower dose may have to be accepted, even if pain relief is incomplete, and additional analgesia attempted by other means (see below).

2 *Give analgesics regularly rather than on a 'when required' basis.* This is one of the commonest of prescribing errors. Patients should not have to 'earn' their analgesia. Morphine and diamorphine need to be given every 4 hours to be effective but most patients can be managed very comfortably on slow-release morphine tablets (see above).

3 *Warn patients about side-effects.* This particularly applies to constipation. High-fibre diet and regular laxatives are sufficient to deal with this important and painful problem in most cases. Metoclopramide, prochlorperazine or cyclizine can be useful if nausea is a persistent problem.

4 *Keep drug prescriptions as simple as possible.* Some opiates antagonize each other and should never be given together (e.g. sublingual buprenorphine and oral diamorphine).

5 *Consider alternative methods of pain control.*

(a) Alternative routes of analgesic administration. Oral, sublingual, rectal, vaginal or even (rarely) via colostomy; subcutaneous, intramuscular, intravenous, intrathecal using fentanyl. Transdermal patches are just becoming available. The past 5 years have seen a welcome increase in familiarity with subcutaneously administered morphine infusions, using a simple, constant rate syringe-driver which the patient can usually manage very effectively at home, with a boost facility for additional flexibility.

(b) Alternative approaches. Consider radiotherapy for painful bone metastases, surgical internal fixation for pathological fractures and other procedures such as nerve block and neurosurgical approaches.

NERVE BLOCKS, SURGICAL PROCEDURES AND OTHER APPROACHES

Some patients with cancer have intractable pain at a particular site, which responds poorly even to high doses of opiates. In such cases, a nerve block which destroys pain and other sensations in the affected part of the body can be extremely valuable. The technique requires great skill and is usually performed by an anaesthetist with special training. Local dorsal root block using fine-needle insertions of phenol or absolute alcohol is the commonest method. Careful positioning of the patient is important and advantage can be made of the fact that phenol is heavier, and absolute alcohol lighter than CSF, so choice of agent and patient position can result in effective blockage of pain at different sites (Fig. 7.2). A similar technique can be used to produce coeliac or brachial plexus block.

Surgical destructive procedures may have to be considered if all else fails. Spinothalamic tractotomy is an operation performed on the spinal cord in which the fibres carrying pain are divided. Anatomical specificity is often possible since the pain fibres are arranged in the lateral spinothalamic tract in an orderly fashion (Fig. 7.3). Pain relief may, however, not be complete since other spinal pathways may also subserve pain sensation. Operations can also be considered at higher levels (e.g. thalamotomy) if tractotomy is ineffective.

EPIDURAL INFUSIONS

Epidural infusions of local anaesthetic or opiates can sometimes be used to control pain. The infusions are intermittent or continuous and use an infusion pump (such as that used for subcutaneous infusion) which is connected to a catheter in the epidural space. Tolerance to local anaesthetics occurs quickly so that effect only lasts a few weeks. Infection may occur.

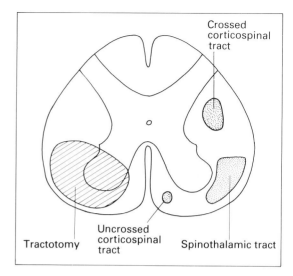

Fig. 7.3 Spinal tractotomy. Often carried out at T_1 or T_2. Included in the operation are vestibulospinal, rubrospinal, ventral corticospinal and ascending ventral spinocerebellar tracts. It is increasingly performed percutaneously.

Fig. 7.2 Coeliac plexus and dorsal root blocks to relieve pain. (A) Anatomical relations of coeliac plexus. The plexus is comprised of a number of ganglia situated in front of T_{12} and L_1. The injection is made in front of the anterior border of the body of L_1. The needle is inserted below the 12th rib. (B) Dorsal root block and section. 1. Block of root inside dura. 2. Block of dorsal root outside dura. 3. Excision of dorsal root ganglion. 4. Coagulation of nerve trunk. 5. Coagulation of medial branch of primary ramus.

Pain relief may be obtained without paralysis or autonomic disturbance.

Continuous opiate infusion results in higher drug concentrations in the CSF. Systemic absorption occurs rapidly. Localized analgesia may be achieved without motor or sensory loss or the drowsiness induced by systemic opiates. There is, however, cross-tolerance with systemically administered opiates so the value is limited in patients already on high doses of these drugs.

Alternative procedures include transcutaneous nerve stimulation and acupuncture analgesia, both of which can be valuable even in patients taking large doses of opiates. The mechanisms of these methods may involve a stimulation of endogenous endorphins at a central level.

ANOREXIA AND NAUSEA

Anorexia is a very common accompaniment of terminal cancer and there is of course no long-lasting remedy. There is, however, much that can be done to relieve the anxiety which the patient feels about the continued wasting. Small meals should be offered, particularly the patient's favourite dishes, and a glass of wine or sherry may stimulate appetite. One of the great ironies of faddish 'alternative' diets is the denial of the simple pleasure of eating and drinking in the final weeks of a patient's life. Steroids may be extremely valuable and are underused in this situation. Steroid side-effects will not be a problem if the prognosis is a matter of weeks. Dexamethasone is probably the drug of choice (2 mg given three or four times a day) though lower doses may be adequate.

Treatment of nausea (and vomiting) may be difficult. If there is a mechanical cause, such as intestinal obstruction from intra-abdominal cancer, a fine-bore nasogastric tube may have to be passed for aspiration of stomach contents. In most cases symptomatic treatment with prochlorperazine, chlorpromazine or meto-clopramide given regularly before meals may help. Rectal administration may be necessary.

DEPRESSION AND ANXIETY

Most patients will have episodes of depression and anxiety, and sympathetic conversation with family, friends, doctors and nurses will usually help the patient over bad days. Persistent, disturbing or suicidal depression (fortunately very uncommon) may require additional treatment with tri- or tetracyclic antidepressants and occasionally skilled psychiatric help is needed. Some authorities find amphetamines are helpful in special circumstances. Benzodiazepines are useful for acute or persistent anxiety.

Terminal care: home, hospice and support teams

Many patients like to remain at home for as long as they can and to die there if possible. Familiar surroundings and family life offer great comfort. The care of a dying patient is, however, extremely demanding and a great deal of support is always required if home care is to be achieved successfully. Women generally look after dying men much better than men care for their wives. There are many factors which determine the feasibility of home care. These include whether the patient lives alone; the continued presence of family or friends to provide support (the spouse or partner may have to go to work); whether there are young children at home to be cared for; the availability of adequate local support services such as nursing, laundry, home helps and meals-on-wheels; and the degree and nature of the patient's disability and symptoms. It may be necessary to provide specialized aids to nursing and mobility, such as hand rails in the bathroom, commodes, a ripple or water bed, a hoist or a wheelchair.

A flexible approach is essential. Even if the intention is to care for the patient at home, the circumstances may change and the situation become more difficult, making hospital or hospice care necessary. This may lead to feelings of guilt or of defeat in the family and the doctor should realize this and explain that continuous care of the dying patient is a highly skilled task and that professional help is often needed and the change in plan is not a sign of failure.

The first UK hospice, St. Christopher's, was opened as recently as 1967. Since then we have seen a dramatic growth, not just in the United Kingdom, of palliative care teams and in-patient hospices such that palliative care has now emerged as a new medical specialty. By December 1989 there were 145 in-patient hospice units in the UK, with over 2600 beds. There are also nearly 300 home-care teams caring for cancer patients at home and reducing the need for long-stay cancer in-patient beds in acute hospitals.

Hospices for terminally ill cancer patients have taught us the importance of careful pain control, attention to the patient's physical and spiritual needs, and the important ways in which medical, nursing and other staff can make enormous contributions by spending a little more time with patients, often just by listening or simply by being there. None the less, the hospice movement is itself aware of the disadvantages of hospice care. Hospices are expensive to set up and maintain, and demand a high staff–patient ratio. Some patients find the concept of moving to a 'terminal home' difficult to accept, even though the majority are content once they arrive. Psychologically, many patients find it difficult to accept that the doctor who had been treating them, in whom they had trust and confidence, no longer has any treatment to offer. Doctors with a genuine interest in the management of terminally ill cancer patients often find it upsetting if they are made to feel that they have no further role, as sometimes happens where hospice support teams take the view that they should be entirely responsible for the patient. For the general practitioner who will have to look after the family after the death of the patient with cancer, this sudden role change can create real difficulty.

The traditional alternative, and the place where many cancer patients die, has been the general hospital ward. Undoubtedly there are advantages, in particular the continuity of care afforded by familiar staff and surroundings. Some patients might gain comfort from the fact that many of the patients on the ward will be suffering from non-malignant conditions, and that the general atmosphere is likely to be brisk and active. However, most of us would agree that for patients in the final stages of their illness, the ideal environment would be more tranquil and the staff rather less busy so that there is more time for reflective discussion. It is well known that on many general medical or surgical wards, the cancer patient is all too often hurriedly passed by, particularly by the medical staff, who perhaps feel pressured and unable to help, and embarrassed or discomfited by this inadequacy.

A solution which is rapidly becoming more popular is the setting up of community or hospital-based supportive care teams, which consist of medical and nursing staff, usually with a social worker. This team exists to help both hospital specialists and also the local general practitioners, by providing expertise, assistance and time for terminally ill cancer patients, maintaining continuity of support whether the patient has been admitted to a hospital bed or is at home under the care of the local practitioner. From our own experience of working with such a team it is apparent that there are benefits both for the patient and also for his family. Supportive care teams can assist by providing an expert service regarding, for example, choice of analgesic or anti-emetic, as well as arranging for essential facilities such as commodes, home oxygen, rapid installation of telephone services and so on. Although all of these roles could be undertaken by general practitioners, district nurses or social workers, there is no doubt that the presence of a team entirely committed to the improvement of standards in terminal care enormously improves the efficiency of the service. Many teams also take on a bereavement counselling role, and remain closely in touch with bereaved relatives particularly if problems have been perceived before the death of the patient. Although there is no ideal time to refer patients to such a team, we feel that early referral is to be encouraged so that possible problems can be rapidly identified, and a close relationship quickly established.

CANCER QUACKERY

Quackery: the pretensions or practice of a quack.
Quack: shortened form of quacksalver — a charlatan.
Quacksalver: one who quacks about his salves (derived from Dutch).

Patients with cancer may decide to abandon medical treatment and opt for false or unproven remedies such as dietary manipulation, 'natural' or herbal medicines, homoeopathy, faith healing, visualization therapy, immunizations, multivitamin supplements and enemas. They may be urged to do so by relatives or other cancer patients and they sometimes try these treatments in addition to conventional methods.

Patients who do this are usually frightened and anxious; some may see doctors as members of a conspiratorial establishment who have closed minds to any alternative approach. They may have strong ideas about the way their body works or what causes cancer, believing for example that the disease is the result of lifestyle, diet, psychological stress or pollution. However, even if dietary factors are important in aetiology it is illogical to expect that the cancer can therefore be cured by alterations in diet, emotional attitude, or by taking natural products such as herbal remedies. Sadly, giving up smoking does not cure lung cancer. Many august personages are prepared to lend their support to these notions, their names often being more impressive than their intellectual credentials.

There is also no shortage of doctors, naturopaths or homoeopaths to support the public in these beliefs, as well as some more tough-minded charlatans out to make money. There are many damaging aspects to their activities.

First, there is no evidence that any of these remedies work. No evidence for antitumour activity is presented, no evaluation of results and no independent or critical assessment of data. Instead cases are quoted, anecdotes offered and spurious facts and figures are produced. In one of the few controlled studies of alternative cancer treatments, Laetrile (amygdalin), a 'harmless yet effective' remedy approved by most alternative cancer 'authorities' was found to be entirely without benefit and yet with significant side-effects when assessed in over 500 cancer patients treated at the Mayo Clinic [3]. Randomized trials of the 'holistic' approach against conventional treatment have not been undertaken partly due to reluctance by the practitioners of alternative medicine to put their beliefs to the test, and partly due to the ethical difficulties. Two case−control studies have been carried out in advanced cancer neither of which have shown any benefit for survival in the 'alternative' approach, and one of which showed no improvement in quality of life either [4]. The widely-promoted vitamin C remedy was shown in a randomized trial to be of no value in advanced cancer. Objective but uncontrolled studies of macrobiotic diets and immuno-

augmentative therapy have found no evidence of efficacy.

Second, the proponents may say that they do not pretend to offer a cure-all, but it is clear that patients believe that they *will* be cured or the disease arrested. The process of mental adjustment to the diagnosis may be badly shaken by false optimism followed by despair at failure. The term *alternative medicine* is in itself a lie when it is used to imply that a proven method of treatment is being offered. Third, the patient may delay conventional treatment occasionally with tragic consequences in the case of a potentially curable tumour. Fourth, the treatment is often expensive and the patient may waste a lot of money. Finally, these 'remedies' may create a great deal of conflict within the family. Patients with advanced cancer can be cajoled or even bullied by their well-meaning relatives into taking an entirely 'natural' diet; then find it intolerable and lose what remaining interest they may have in nutrition. They may even feel that they have to continue in order not to let their children down.

It must be admitted, however, that one reason that patients seek these remedies is a dissatisfaction with conventional medicine or with their doctor which may in part be well-founded [5,6]. Patients will often say that they tried these treatments because they were given no hope or emotional support, because they found the prospect of radiotherapy or chemotherapy unnatural, because there was inadequate explanation and reassurance or because treatment was being unreasonably and thoughtlessly prolonged or aggressive without any hint of benefit. The first question a doctor should ask himself when faced with a patient who has decided to undergo a quack treatment is 'Have I given enough explanation and reassurance?'

If a patient or relative decides to discontinue treatment it is of course essential to say what the consequences might be, but cruel to overstate the case in order to browbeat the patient into continuing. Much cancer treatment is palliative and no great harm may be done by stopping it. It is kind to make it clear that, although the proposed alternative is bogus, the patient will be welcome to come back at a later date.

REFERENCES

1 Twycross R.G. Pain relief in cancer. *Clinics in Oncology* 1984; **3**: (1).
2 Saunders C.M., Sykes N. *The Management of Terminal Malignant Disease.* London: Edward Arnold, 1993.
3 Moertel C.G., Fleming T.R., Rubin J. *et al.* A clinical trial of amygdalin (Laetrile) in the treatment of human cancer. *New England Journal of Medicine* 1991; **306**: 201–06.
4 Cassileth B.R., Lusk E.J., Guerry P. *et al.* Survival and quality of life among patients receiving unproven as compared with conventional cancer therapy. *New England Journal of Medicine* 1991; **324**: 1180–85.
5 Cassileth B., Lush E.J., Strouse T.B. *et al.* Contemporary unorthodox treatment in cancer medicine: a study of patients, treatments and practitioners. *Annals of Internal Medicine* 1984; **101**: 105–12.
6 Downer S.M., Cody M.M., McCluskey P. *et al.* Pursuit and practice of complementary therapies by cancer patients receiving conventional treatment. *British Medical Journal* 1994; **309**: 86–9.

Appendix 7.1 Cancer support organizations in Britain and Ireland

Organization	Address	Organization	Address
England BACUP	3 Bath Place, Rivington Street, London EC2A 3JR (Helpline: 0800 181199)	Hodgkin's Disease Association	PO Box 275, Haddenham, Aylesbury, Bucks HP17 8JJ (Tel: 0844 291500)
Breast Cancer Care	15–19 Britten Street, London SW3 3TZ (Helplines: 071 867 1103; 0500 245 345)	Hospice Information Service	St Christopher's Hospice, 51–59 Lawrie Park Road, Sydenham, London SE26 6DZ (Tel: 081 778 9252)
British Association for Counselling	1 Regent Place, Rugby CV21 2PJ (Tel: 0788 578328)	Hysterectomy Support Network	3 Lynne Close, Green Street Green, Orpington, Kent BR6 6BS
British Colostomy Association	15 Station Road, Reading, Berkshire RG1 1LG (Tel: 0734 391537)	Leukaemia Care Society	14 Kingfisher Court, Venny Bridge, Pinhoe, Exeter, Devon EX4 8JN (Tel: 0392 464848)
Cancer Care Society	21 Zetland Road, Redland, Bristol BS6 7AH (Tel: 0272 427419)	Marie Curie Cancer Care	28 Belgrave Square, London SW1X 8QG (Tel: 071 235 3325)
Cancerlink	17 Brittania Street, London WC1X 9JN (Tel: 071 833 2451)	National Association of Laryngectomee Clubs	Ground Floor, 6 Rickett Street, Fulham, London SW6 1RU (Tel: 071 381 9993)
Cancer Relief Macmillan Fund	Anchor House, 15–19 Britten Street, London SW3 3TZ (Tel: 071 351 7811)	National Cancer Alliance	PO Box 579, Oxford OX4 1LP (Tel: 0865 793566)
Carers National Association	20–25 Glasshouse Yard, London EC1A 4JS (Tel: 071 490 8898)	Neuroblastoma Society	Mrs A Ward, 41 Towncourt Crescent, Petts Wood, Kent BR5 1PH (Tel: 0689 873338)
CRUSE (Bereavement care)	126 Sheen Road, Richmond TW9 1UR (Tel: 081 940 4818; Helpline: 081 332 7227)		

continued

Appendix 7.1 *contd*

Organization	Address	Organization	Address
Retinoblastoma Society	c/o Academic Department of Paediatric Oncology, St Bartholomew's Hospital, West Smithfield, London EC1A 7BE (Tel: 071 600 3309)	Cancerlink	9 Castle Terrace, Edinburgh EH1 2DP (Tel: 031 228 5557)
		Cancer Relief Macmillan Fund	9 Castle Terrace, Edinburgh EH1 2DP (Tel: 031 229 3276)
Sue Ryder Foundation	Cavendish, Sudbury, Suffolk CO10 8AY (Tel: 0787 280252)	*Wales* Tenovus Cancer Information Centre	142 Whitchurch Road, Cardiff CF4 3NA (Tel: 0222 619846; Helpline: 0800 526527)
Urostomy Association	Buckland, Beaumont Park, Danbury, Essex CM3 4DE (Tel: 0245 224294)	*Northern Ireland*	
Women's Nationwide Cancer Control Campaign	Suna House, 128–130 Curtain Road, London EC2A 3AR (Tel: 071 729 4688; Helpline: 071 729 2229)	Ulster Cancer Foundation	40–42 Eglantine Avenue, Belfast BT96 DX (Tel: 0232 663281; Helpline: 0232 663439)
Scotland Breast Cancer Care	9 Castle Terrace, Edinburgh EH1 2DP (Tel: 031 221 0407) and Suite 2–8 65 Bath Street, Glasgow G2 2BX (Tel: 041 353 1050)	*Republic of Ireland* Irish Cancer Society	5 Northumberland Road, Dublin 4 (Tel: (01) 6681855; Helpline: 1 800 200 700)

Chapter 8
Medical Problems and Radiotherapy Emergencies

Acute and often life-threatening medical problems may arise as a result of the cancer and its treatment. Iatrogenic deaths are not infrequent because many treatments, particularly intensive chemotherapy, are inherently very dangerous. Nevertheless the majority of deaths are avoidable and many oncologists prefer to look after their patients in specialized cancer units with staff skilled in anticipating, avoiding and managing these problems.

BONE MARROW FAILURE AND ITS CONSEQUENCES

Cytotoxic drugs damage the reproductive integrity of cells. Bone marrow haemopoietic cells are among the most rapidly dividing cells in the body and are extremely sensitive to the action of most antineoplastic agents. Some drugs, for example vincristine and bleomycin, produce only slight bone marrow depression while the majority impair haemopoiesis. With drugs such as doxorubicin, myelosuppression is one of the major toxicities. There is some evidence that cytotoxic agents affect different proliferative compartments within the marrow. This leads to non-uniform patterns of toxicity even within the same class of cytotoxic agent. For example cyclophosphamide, administered as a single intravenous injection, causes predictable granulocytopenia 4–7 days later with a less marked effect on platelet count. In contrast, melphalan and busulphan produce a slower marrow suppression with onset at 7–8 days and maximum depression of white count at about 2–3 weeks. Nitrosoureas such as CCNU

characteristically exert a delayed effect on the blood count occurring at about 4–5 weeks.

The speed of onset and the severity with which the marrow is affected also depend on dose and timing of drug administration. Although the platelet count does not fall significantly with cyclophosphamide given in conventional doses, it will do so at much higher doses. Similarly although neutropenia and thrombocytopenia usually occur at 4–5 weeks after CCNU administration in conventional doses, at very high doses such as those which have been used experimentally in the treatment of brain tumours, an earlier onset of neutropenia and thrombocytopenia may be seen, occasionally as early as 4–5 days after the drug has been given.

Although some agents (melphalan, busulphan, CCNU) may cause prolonged marrow suppression even when given on the first occasion, in a patient receiving intermittent cytotoxic chemotherapy for the first time the marrow depression is usually transient and the blood count normal in 2–3 weeks when the next cycle can be given. With increasing duration of chemotherapy, however, the proliferative compartments in the marrow may become progressively more depleted and the nadir of the white count then becomes lower and recovery less rapid, so that chemotherapy cycles may have to be delayed or the dose reduced. In order to avoid life-threatening marrow suppression a familiarity with the cytotoxic regimen is essential and the physician must be aware of the likelihood of increasing marrow depression with time.

However experienced the clinician, marrow depression does occur unexpectedly. With some treatment regimens, for example during the induction of remission in acute myeloblastic leukaemia, or with the use of very high dose chemotherapy in some solid tumours, pancytopenia is an inevitable consequence of treatment.

Granulocytopenia is symptomatic only when infection supervenes. Then there may be fever, malaise, shaking and chills sometimes accompanied by oral ulceration and perineal inflammation. If the platelet count is depressed the patient may develop epistaxis or purpura. It is unusual for symptoms of anaemia to occur acutely even if erythropoiesis ceases altogether as a result of cytotoxic agents, since the half-life of red cells (25 days) is such that the haemoglobin does not usually fall appreciably.

The management of marrow suppression by blood component therapy

BLOOD TRANSFUSION [1,2]

Many patients undergoing combination intermittent chemotherapy for solid tumours develop moderate anaemia with a haemoglobin of 10–12 g/dl. The blood count will recover when treatment is discontinued and transfusion is not usually required unless the haemoglobin falls below 9 g/dl. In deciding whether to transfuse a patient, the symptoms of anaemia (i.e. fatigue, malaise and breathlessness) must be balanced against the risks of transfusion, in particular volume overload in elderly patients. If a patient is at risk of cardiac failure because of ischaemic heart disease, volume overload can be minimized by the use of packed cells and diuretics. There is some evidence that, in the presence of thrombocytopenia, a transfusion can precipitate episodes of bleeding, in particular intracerebral haemorrhage. For this reason, many physicians prefer to use a platelet transfusion before giving blood or packed cells in severely thrombocytopenic patients.

Many patients with advanced malignant disease become anaemic due to an effect of the tumour itself or to marrow infiltration (e.g. in myeloma, leukaemia or widespread bone secondaries). This occurs even when patients are not having treatment with chemotherapy or radiotherapy. Even if no active treatment for the tumour is planned, a patient may gain symptomatic relief from blood transfusion. Since the symptoms of anaemia will be similar to those of the tumour, it is often difficult to anticipate whether blood transfusion will help a patient. Precise guidelines cannot be drawn, but in general transfusion should be considered only if the haemoglobin falls below 9 g/dl.

PLATELET TRANSFUSION

The risk of bleeding is related to the platelet count and rises sharply below $20 \times 10^9/l$. Ecchymosis and purpura are characteristically found in pressure areas and on the shins. Major bleeding is life-threatening and intracerebral haemorrhage is often fatal.

The lifespan of platelets is approximately 10 days, but transfused platelets have a half-life of only a few days. Platelets have a variety of antigens on their surface including HLA antigens. Repeated transfusion may be accompanied by immunization against these antigens with the result that further platelet transfusions lead to rapid platelet destruction and a failure to elevate the platelet count. Nevertheless, platelet transfusion has been a major factor in decreasing the morbidity of intensive chemotherapy regimens and most patients can be protected during periods of hypoplasia without serious haemorrhage [3]. A unit of platelets is derived from one fresh unit of whole blood and yields about 0.5×10^{11} platelets. Although theoretically a unit of platelets should raise the platelet count by $10 \times 10^9/l$ this seldom happens, particularly if patients have had many previous transfusions or if there is fever, infection or bleeding.

There is no single level of platelet count at which transfusion should be given. Platelet transfusion is rarely required at counts above $30 \times 10^9/l$. Indications for platelet transfusion are:

1 A rapidly falling platelet count following the start of intensive chemotherapy in which it can be predicted that the circulating platelets will fall below $20 \times 10^9/l$ within a 24-hour period. This is particularly important when making arrangements for the care of patients at weekends. The trend of the platelet count will help in deciding if a further transfusion will soon be necessary.

2 If there is evidence of bleeding (such as widespread ecchymoses, epistaxis or gastrointestinal bleeding), platelet transfusion is essential, even at levels higher than $30 \times 10^9/l$.

3 Platelet transfusions are sometimes necessary at higher levels of platelet count (above $30 \times 10^9/l$), if there are other complicating factors such as anaemia, peptic ulceration or infection which predispose to bleeding.

Occasionally, patients will become refractory to platelet transfusions, with little or no rise in platelet count. Fever, infection and splenomegaly may all contribute to this, but the usual cause is immunization to platelet antigens. This can be avoided by using HLA-matched donors, generally obtained from the patient's family. In immunized patients a rise in platelet count can sometimes be produced by the use of corticosteroids.

GRANULOCYTE TRANSFUSION

A great deal of controversy has surrounded the use of granulocyte transfusion in the aplastic patient. Granulocytes can be collected using blood cell separators, and function after injection into the recipient. However, with the advent of modern broad-spectrum bactericidal antibiotics, particularly of the aminoglycoside group, the frequency of granulocyte transfusion has diminished, particularly in patients where the aplasia is expected to be transient. From $5-25 \times 10^9$ cells are transfused which is less than one-tenth of the normal daily granulocyte production. Early studies showed that granulocyte transfusion was of value in patients whose granulocyte count was less than $0.5 \times 10^9/l$. There is, however, little evidence that they are useful

prophylactically in patients who do not have evidence of infection or fever. The use of granulocyte transfusion has diminished greatly since the introduction of haemopoietic growth factors.

HAEMOPOIETIC GROWTH FACTORS [4]

Short-term cultures of human bone marrow cells has allowed identification of progenitor cells which form colonies and whose growth is dependent on colony stimulating factors (CSFs). The progenitor cells may form cells of several lineages but they are not the self-renewing stem cells (detected in the mouse spleen colony-forming assays). Cloning of the genes of these CSFs has led to the characterization of many of these molecules. Some of these are interleukins (see p. 117). CSFs are glycoproteins, active at extremely low concentrations (which usually interact between cells at short range) and which may stimulate a variety of functions in marrow precursor and mature cells. The chromosomal location and source of the factors are shown in Table 8.1.

The factors bind to specific, high-affinity receptors on the target cell. Granulocyte CSF (G-CSF) and macrophage-CSF (M-CSF) stimulate the late stages of division and the differentiation of the granulocyte and macrophage lineage respectively, and affect the function of mature cells. Other CSFs such as granulocyte–macrophage GM-CSF stimulate several cell lineages earlier in differentiation. GM-CSF also increases neutrophil phagocytosis of bacteria and yeasts. IL-1 and IL-6 act on early progenitor cells stimulating cell division and making cells more sensitive to GM-CSF, G-CSF and M-CSF by increasing the number of surface receptors. The earlier return of the white count may allow increased intensity of chemotherapy and possibly improve results of treatment. This has not yet been shown to occur in any chemo-curable cancer.

Table 8.1 Haemopoietic growth factors: chromosomal location and cellular source

Factor	Molecular weight (kDa)	Chromosome	Source
G-CSF	18	17q 11.2–21	Monocytes Endothelium
M-CSF	40–50	5q 23–31	Monocytes, T cells Endothelium
GM-CSF	14–35	5q 23–31	Monocytes, T cells Endothelium
EPO	36	7q 11–22	Renal peritubular cells Macrophages
IL-3	14–28	5q 23–31	T cells

Clinical use of haemopoietic growth factors

GRANULOCYTE CSF (G-CSF)

In normal individuals G-CSF causes a temporary fall in neutrophil count (possibly due to sequestration of cells). It has been shown to hasten the return of the neutrophil count with conventional myelosuppressive chemotherapy [5] and after autologous bone marrow transplantation (ABMT). The platelet count is unaffected. G-CSF has become widely and rather uncritically used in cancer therapy. Before using G-CSF the physician should decide whether it is wise or necessary to use chemotherapy at a dose which will dangerously depress the WBC. This is clearly not the case for palliative treatment. Using drugs intensively can only be justified if the cure rate is thereby increased. G-CSF may then have a role in improving treatment. There is no place for its routine use, the more so since it is very expensive and inconvenient.

MACROPHAGE CSF (M-CSF)

M-CSF derived from human urine is said to hasten the return of neutrophil count after chemotherapy. No studies with the recombinant product have yet been reported.

GRANULOCYTE–MACROPHAGE CSF (GM-CSF)

GM-CSF causes a rise in granulocyte and platelet count in patients not receiving chemotherapy. Immediately after injection it causes a fall in neutrophil count due to margination especially in the lungs. It accelerates recovery following conventional chemotherapy and after ABMT. Fever and thrombophlebitis are side-effects. In spite of the more rapid recovery of the blood count, length of hospital stay and mortality do not appear to be reduced during ABMT.

ERYTHROPOIETIN (EPO)

Patients with anaemia due to malignant disease have lower plasma erythropoietin levels than non-deficient patients with comparable haemoglobin values. It is not known yet whether EPO will diminish transfusion requirements in anaemic cancer patients.

INFECTIONS IN THE IMMUNE-COMPROMISED PATIENT

Infections are a major cause of death in cancer. Not only do they occur frequently, they are often more severe than in other patients, less responsive to therapy and are sometimes produced by organisms which are not pathogens in healthy people. This susceptibility results from depression of host defence mechanisms produced by the tumour and its treatment.

Host defence mechanisms in cancer

PHAGOCYTE FUNCTION

Advanced cancer is sometimes associated with reduced function of both neutrophils and monocytes. Depression of chemotactic, phagocytic and bactericidal activity have all been described. There is some evidence that chemotherapy can cause a deterioration in function as well as granulocytopenia.

CELL-MEDIATED IMMUNITY (CMI) AND HUMORAL IMMUNITY

Anergy to delayed hypersensitivity antigens is common in advanced untreated Hodgkin's disease but less common in other malignancies. Lymphopenia is an invariable accompaniment of treatment with alkylating agents and radiotherapy — the effect of the latter lasting for many months. CMI is particularly important in host defence against fungi, viruses, tuberculosis and protozoa. Cytotoxic T cells and natural killer cells are especially important in the control of herpes virus infections. Several studies have shown that intensive cytotoxic chemotherapy leads to impaired production of antibody to bacterial and viral antigens [6].

RETICULOENDOTHELIAL (RE) FUNCTION

Circulating bacteria are cleared by the phagocytic cells lining the sinuses of the RE system especially in the liver and spleen. Antibody and complement are important for this clearance. Splenectomy increases the risk of severe bacterial infection, especially pneumococcal septicaemia in young children and to a lesser extent in adults [7].

THE MUCOSAL BARRIER

The skin and mucosal surfaces are a barrier to infection. Tumour infiltration and local radiotherapy may lead to damage to lymphatic or venous drainage, with resulting susceptibility to local infection. The turnover of gastro-intestinal epithelial cells is normally very rapid and this is depressed by chemotherapy leading to mucosal damage and ulceration which allows gut organisms to escape into the portal system. The skin is breached by intravenous needles and cannulae, especially tunnelled, subcutaneous lines, and nasogastric tubes act as a focus for infection with *Candida albicans*.

Bacteraemia and septicaemia [8]

Bloodstream infections are particularly frequent in granulocytopenic patients. Gram-negative bacteria (*Escherichia coli*, *Pseudomonas aeruginosa*), staphylococci and streptococci are frequent pathogens. Fever in a neutropenic cancer patient is an indication for blood cultures, but an organism is often not isolated. Treatment should not be delayed in the neutropenic patient. An aminoglycoside (gentamicin) is usually given with penicillin and metronidazole or with a semi-synthetic penicillin such as ticarcillin. Cephalosporins and β-lactamase resistant penicillins are valuable for gram-positive septicaemia. The prognosis depends mainly on the time it takes for the bone marrow to recover. In patients who are undergoing intensive chemotherapy or a bone marrow allograft, prophylactic gut sterilization is attempted with oral antibiotics. If there is an obvious source of the infection such as infected infusion sites, cultures should be taken and the cannula removed. The widespread use of subcutaneous intravenous infusion lines has led to a large number of *Staphylococcus epidermidis* infections. In such patients the cultures should be taken from blood and the line. If the line is removed the fever may subside but the line should be cultured. Vancomycin is an effective antibiotic against this organism.

Respiratory infection

Fever with pulmonary infiltration is a common

occurrence in the severely immunocompromised patient. The major causes are given in Table 8.2. The difficulties in making a diagnosis can be considerable because sputum and blood cultures may be negative, and more invasive procedures such as transbronchial biopsy may be impossible because of thrombocytopenia or the general condition of the patient.

There are some clinical features which are helpful in diagnosis. Cavitation is more common with anaerobic bacteria, staphylococci, and mycobacteria. Pneumocystis infection causes marked dyspnoea, and the chest X-ray shows bilateral infiltrates typically radiating from the hilum. The disease may, however, be indolent, and can cause lobar consolidation. Cytomegalovirus infection mainly occurs in severely immune-depressed patients, particularly during allogeneic bone-marrow transplantation. The disease may also cause myocarditis, neuropathy and ophthalmitis. The pulmonary infiltrate is usually bilateral. Candida infection can cause a wide variety of X-ray changes. There is often candida infection elsewhere. Panophthalmitis may occur and the organism can sometimes be isolated from the blood. Aspergillus infection is usually rapidly progressive in these patients. Blood cultures are usually negative and the infiltrate can be in one or both lungs.

Table 8.2 Causes of fever and pulmonary infiltration in immunocompromised patients

Bacteria	*Streptococcus pneumoniae*
	Gram-negative organisms
	Mycobacteria
	Legionella
Fungi	Aspergillus
	Candida
	Cryptococcus
Viruses	Cytomegalovirus
	Herpes simplex
	Measles
Protozoa	Pneumocystis
Treatment	Cytotoxic drugs
	Radiation pneumonitis

Faced with this diagnostic uncertainty the following scheme can be adopted.

In the patient without neutropenia or thrombocytopenia. Investigate with blood cultures, sputum culture, bronchoscopic washings, transbronchial biopsy, where possible.

If blood and sputum cultures are negative, treat with broad-spectrum bactericidal antibiotics (usually with an aminoglycoside, penicillin and metronidazole or equivalent combination). If pneumocystis is a possible cause, high-dose co-trimoxazole should be given. If there is no response consider acyclovir for herpes simplex infection and antifungal therapy with amphotericin or ketoconazole. Acyclovir is not effective against cytomegalovirus.

If blood or sputum cultures are positive treat as appropriate but if there is no response consider a mixed infection.

In the patient with neutropenia or thrombocytopenia. Bronchoscopy can be carried out, but biopsy may not be possible and treatment may have to proceed along the lines indicated above without further diagnostic investigation. Before and after bronchoscopy, antibiotics and platelet transfusion may be necessary.

Urinary tract infections

Infection is common in patients with obstruction to outflow, particularly from the bladder. Obstruction may be by tumour or due to an atonic bladder in a patient with cord compression. Diagnosis is made by urine culture and treatment is with antibiotics and relief of obstruction if possible.

Gastro-intestinal infections

Oral thrush (infection with *Candida albicans*) is a frequent complication of chemotherapy. It is particularly likely to occur in immunosuppressed patients, in patients on steroids and in those treated with broad-spectrum antibiotics. The mouth and pharynx become very sore and white plaques of fungus are visible on an erythematous base. The infection may penetrate more deeply in some malnourished patients and extend down into the oesophagus, stomach and bowel. Oral nystatin, amphotericin or miconazole are usually effective. Herpes simplex cold sores are often troublesome in leucopenic patients and the lesions may become very widespread. Treatment is with acyclovir given topically for minor infections in immunosuppressed patients, and systemically for more serious infections.

Candida infection in the oesophagus requires treatment with oral nystatin suspension, but if this is ineffective treat with ketoconazole or a short course of amphotericin. Candida infections of the bowel should be treated with amphotericin.

Perianal infections are common in neutropenic patients. Preventative measures should always be employed, with scrupulous perineal hygiene and stool softeners to prevent constipation and anal tears. Spreading perineal infection can be a life-threatening event, and urgent treatment with intravenous antibiotics active against gram-negative and anaerobic bacilli is required.

Meninges

CNS infections are rare, but patients with lymphoma or leukaemia occasionally develop meningitis due to *Cryptococcus neoformans*. The onset is insidious with headache. The organism can be detected by India ink staining of the CSF. Detection of cryptococcus antigen in blood and CSF is possible in most patients. Many patients will improve with amphotericin and some will be cured.

Skin

Apart from infection introduced at infusion sites the most common skin infection is shingles (varicella zoster). This infection, which is due to a reactivation of varicella zoster virus in dorsal root ganglia, is a dermatomal vesicular eruption which is particularly severe in immune-compromised hosts and which may disseminate as chickenpox and cause a fatal pneumonia. Severely compromised patients, those with a progressive local eruption and widespread dissemination should be treated with acyclovir.

Prevention of infection in the leucopenic patient

When a patient is leucopenic reverse barrier nursing procedures are often used. How rigorous these need to be is a matter which has provoked much discussion. Many of the infections are from the patient's own bacteria rather than from staff or relatives. For most episodes of granulocytopenia, disposable aprons, face masks and careful washing of hands is probably satisfactory. For more persistent leucopenia (e.g. with allogeneic bone marrow transplantation) a protected environment has much to commend it. Here the air is filtered free of bacteria and a laminar air flow is established from one end of the room to the other. The patients are 'decontaminated' before entry with oral antibiotics to kill intestinal bacteria, and cutaneous antiseptic cleansing. Protected environments can lower the infection rate but their contribution to overall reduction in mortality is small since the hazards of the disease and other effects of treatment are greater. The psychological stress and cost of isolation are other major disadvantages.

Other important preventative measures are scrupulous hygiene in the placing of intravenous drugs, perineal hygiene, and high standards of staff training. It has recently been shown that prophylactic oral acyclovir is effective in preventing varicella zoster, and ketoconazole appears to lower the incidence of fungal infections.

CANCER CACHEXIA AND THE NUTRITIONAL SUPPORT OF THE CANCER PATIENT [9,10]

Weight loss is a common symptom of cancer but profound and rapid weight loss usually indicates disseminated tumour. When cancer recurs and is widespread, loss of weight is an almost invariable accompaniment. This leads finally to the cachectic state in which the patient becomes wasted, weak and lethargic.

Occasionally, rapid weight loss and weakness may occur with a small tumour which, when removed, leads to restoration of normal health. It is more usual to find that profound cachexia is an indication of advanced malignancy and attempts to reverse it are inappropriate.

Pathogenesis of malnutrition in cancer

Anorexia is a major factor in causing weight loss in patients with cancer. The mechanism of the anorexia is poorly understood. It frequently accompanies widespread disease, in particular the presence of hepatic metastases. In the case of tumours of the gastro-intestinal tract, anorexia may be profound even when the tumour is small. Typically the patient loses all interest in food and has an altered perception of taste and smell such that the thought of eating can become repugnant.

There have been many studies on the metabolism of patients with cancer cachexia. A variety of abnormalities has been found (Table 8.3) but the findings are not consistent from patient to patient and there is no uniform abnormality which is always present in cachectic individuals. The abnormalities which have been demonstrated are:

1 An increased metabolic rate which has been demonstrated in some patients but by no means all. The mechanism is unknown.

2 An abnormality of glucose metabolism has been suggested. It is proposed that the metabolism of glucose is altered with a production of excess lactate by the tumour, which is then reutilized to form glucose — a process wasteful of energy.

3 An overall increase in protein metabolism associated with a negative nitrogen balance has been demonstrated in some patients.

It has frequently been proposed that the tumour might itself contribute towards cachexia

Table 8.3 Factors contributing to weight loss and cachexia

Factor	Cause
Anorexia, nausea and vomiting	Tumour
	Treatment
	Psychological factors (pain and depression)
Loss of protein, blood and minerals	Diarrhoea
	Ulceration
	Bleeding
Malabsorbtion and intestinal obstruction	Carcinoma of pancreas and ovary
Metabolic abnormalities induced by the tumour	Increased protein breakdown, metabolic rate or fat breakdown
	Altered glucose metabolism due to increased lactate recycling or insulin resistance
	Tumour metabolism of protein and carbohydrate
Iatrogenic factors	Chemotherapy (nausea, vomiting, mucositis)
	Radiotherapy (nausea, vomiting, diarrhoea)

by metabolizing essential nutrients, and that tumours continue to utilize proteins and amino-acids while other body tissues have diminished uptake. More recently inflammatory mediators (produced by the tumour) have been implicated in the anorexia–cachexia syndrome. TNFα (p. 118) has been shown to be a cause of cachexia in animals and may be part of the pathogenesis in humans.

Similarly the consumption of glucose by the tumour, at a time when there is decreased carbohydrate intake, might contribute towards the wasting seen in these patients. It has been calculated that a 1 kg tumour might consume as much as 100 g of glucose daily. The remote metabolic effects on the host might also be due to so-far unidentified products released from the tumour.

On the face of it, it seems sensible to try and reverse the cachectic process in patients with cancer. In considering nutritional support for an individual cancer patient, the objectives of treatment must be clear. First the question must be answered as to whether the cancer is curable or not. If a potentially curative treatment is being considered either with surgery, chemotherapy, or radiotherapy then there is some evidence (see later) that effective nutritional support may improve the result. Well-nourished cancer patients frequently lose weight as a result of cancer treatment, whether with surgery, chemotherapy or radiotherapy. If the effects of radical treatment are likely to persist over a week or more, and considerable weight loss can be anticipated, it is probable that nutritional supplements will decrease morbidity. If, on the other hand, there is no prospect of cure and treatment is to be palliative, then nutritional support should also be seen as a palliative procedure. Aggressive and uncomfortable means of maintaining nutrition are in this case completely inappropriate. There is no evidence at present that the malnutrition and wasting which accompany advanced and incurable cancer can be reversed by any form of feeding. If nutritional support is thought to be necessary it must be given in a form which will be effective in reversing the malnourished state, and a decision made as to whether this should be enteral or parenteral.

Nutritional support available for the cancer patient

ENTERAL FEEDING

If the patient can be fed by mouth then this is clearly the best method. At the simplest level, careful attention to diet and to the foods available to the patient is of great importance. This involves discussions with the patient about which food he fancies, careful dietary advice by a skilled dietitian and the support of members of the family in providing favourite foods which might encourage the patient to eat. A variety of nutritional supplements can be added to the patient's diet, including high calorie liquids such as Hycal and more complete protein and carbohydrate mixtures (e.g. Complan or Clinifeed). Protein hydrolysates, providing small peptides and amino acid fragments, are also available (Vivonex). These dietary supplements can be taken by mouth. Their main advantage is the delivery of calories in liquid form at a time when the patient finds it difficult to eat solid food. The disadvantage is that they can cause osmotic disturbances and for many patients they are quite unpalatable.

Occasionally a patient may find it difficult to swallow or eat at all. Enteral support with liquid dietary supplements can be given by using a fine bore flexible nasogastric feeding tube. The aim is to provide about 2000–3000 kcal/24 hours. These supplements have a high osmolality. They can cause nausea and diarrhoea and provide a large solute load for renal excretion. Large amounts of fluid are required to excrete this solute load, even in the presence of normal renal function. If fluid is not provided, osmotic diuresis may occur leading to salt and water depletion and pre-renal uraemia.

TOTAL PARENTERAL NUTRITION

It is now possible to provide adequate calories intravenously for patients who cannot take food by mouth or by nasogastric tube. Access must be through a catheter placed in a deep vein, since parenteral nutritional solutions cause irritation and venous thrombosis will quickly occur in small peripheral veins. The incidence of venous thrombosis when catheters are inserted into the subclavian vein is small. With all subcutaneous catheters there is a risk of infection which is particularly likely to occur in the immune-compromised individual. A variety of synthetic total parenteral nutrition solutions are available commercially, usually consisting of amino acid solutions with dextrose, vitamins, electrolytes and trace elements.

Several of the metabolic defects present in the malnourished patient can be reversed by total parenteral nutrition. Although it is difficult to demonstrate benefit, it is reasonable to support a patient with parenteral nutrition during intensive but potentially curative treatment. This includes patients undergoing major gastro-intestinal surgery, or chemotherapy with marrow ablation. Total parenteral nutrition is complex, expensive and potentially hazardous, and is of no proven value as a routine measure in patients undergoing cancer therapies, or in the vast majority of patients with malnutrition from cancer who have disseminated disease in whom curative treatment is out of the question.

ACUTE METABOLIC DISTURBANCES

Hypercalcaemia

A raised plasma calcium is a frequent accompaniment of cancer. In a hospital population, carcinomas of the bronchus, breast and kidney are, together with multiple myeloma, the commonest malignant causes of hypercalcaemia. Life-threatening hypercalcaemia is usually due to cancer. Minor elevations of plasma calcium (up to 2.8 mmol/l) are not usually associated with any symptoms. As the plasma calcium rises, patients experience anorexia, nausea, abdominal pain, constipation and fatigue. There may be proximal muscle weakness, polyuria and polydypsia. With increasing hypercalcaemia, severe dehydration, confusion and finally coma may supervene.

Bone metastases are much the commonest cause of hypercalcaemia in cancer. Most patients with severe hypercalcaemia have demonstrable metastases on X-ray or on bone scanning. Bone marrow aspiration may show infiltration with tumour. Even if metastases are not detectable at presentation, they usually quickly become apparent. Metastases in bone may liberate factors which are responsible for bone dissolution. Amongst the factors which have been incriminated are transforming growth factor TGFα, TGFβ, epidermal growth factor, interleukin 1 (α and β forms) [11]. These factors may act locally to cause bone dissolution.

In addition to direct bone lysis by metastases, cancers may produce hypercalcaemia by re-mote, humoral mechanisms — the syndrome of humoral hypercalcaemia of malignancy (HHM). The mechanism of HHM has been partly elucidated with the discovery of a parathyroid hormone-related protein (PTHrP) [12]. PTH itself was not found in plasma or tumour extracts in many patients, yet the metabolic features were remarkably similar to hyperparathyroidism. PTHrP was isolated from cell lines. The protein has striking homology to PTH in the first 13 amino acids but differs in the remainder. It seems that alternatively spliced forms of messenger (RNA) may yield two or more different proteins. The normal function of this protein (it is found in the normal hair follicle and in human milk) is not known, but it may be important in fetal calcium metabolism. Most squamous carcinomas express the protein (whether the patient is hypercalcaemic or not). Its metabolic effect is similar to PTH with increased bone reabsorption of calcium.

The treatment of hypercalcaemia in cancer may be a medical emergency and this is particularly true in the elderly and in patients with myeloma. The raised plasma calcium may be accompanied by uraemia which is due to salt and water loss as a result of the effect of calcium on the distal tubule making it unresponsive to ADH. In addition to this element of pre-renal uraemia, the high calcium appears to reduce glomerular filtration rate directly, by ill-understood mechanisms. Hypokalaemia may also accompany hypercalcaemia, and may in part be due to a renal loss of potassium. Elderly patients, and those with impaired renal function, are unable to withstand the effects of the raised plasma calcium, and life-threatening renal failure may quickly develop. In myeloma it is particularly likely to occur since other causes of renal failure are present (see Chapter 27).

In severe hypercalcaemia, the first line of treatment is therefore with salt and water replacement using isotonic saline. In the first 24 hours, 4−8 litres may be required. This may be sufficient to lower the plasma calcium to normal. In the elderly, care must be taken not to overload the patient with fluids. If the plasma calcium does not begin to fall within 24 hours, prednisolone given orally (30–60 mg/day) or hydrocortisone intravenously (50–100 mg 6-hourly) is often helpful in reducing the calcium but not all patients will respond. Frusemide promotes calciuresis but care must be taken with volume replacement, to avoid further salt and water depletion.

Biphosphonates reduce serum calcium by inhibiting bone resorption (Fig. 8.1) and are effective in hypercalcaemia due to metastases or PTHrP. Pamidronate is effective in 80% of patients. A dose of 30 mg is probably as effective as 60 mg and a single infusion is usually adequate. It can be repeated every 2–3 weeks. Mild fever and skin irritation can occur and it is preferable to use biphosphonates after rehydration since temporary renal impairment can occur. Etidronate seems rather less effective — it is usually given as three infusions of 7.5 mg/ kg. Clodronate in a dose of five daily infusions of 300 mg restores normo calcaemia in 90% of cases. Oral clodronate can be given (1600 mg/ daily) but causes gastro-intestinal upset.

Mithramycin has been largely replaced by the biphosphonates. The usual dose is 15–25 mg/kg and a single injection usually causes a fall in plasma calcium after 24–48 hours. Occasionally it may be necessary to use mithramycin on 2 or 3 successive days. This carries a risk of thrombocytopenia. Doses of 15 μg/kg can be repeated every 4 or 5 days without serious risk of thrombocytopenia, but regular blood counts are essential especially in the presence of renal failure.

Intravenous or oral *phosphate* therapy is seldom necessary to control the plasma calcium, but phosphate infusions (usually with serum calcium of 4 mmol/l or more) may be helpful in patients who are gravely ill.

Calcitonin may produce a fall in the plasma calcium but its effect is variable and its usefulness is limited. It may be more effective combined with steroids. The usual dose is 100–200 units of salmon calcitonin subcutaneously 12-hourly.

Although it is not usually difficult to diagnose the cause of malignant hypercalcaemia, diagnostic problems can occur when hyperparathyroidism is an alternative diagnosis in cancer patients who do not have evidence of disseminated disease. The steroid suppression test will not reduce the plasma calcium in hyperparathyroidism, but 75% of patients with cancer show a fall after 10 days of hydrocortisone administration. If serious doubt remains, elevation of plasma parathormone is found in 80% of patients with primary hyperparathyroidism, but not in patients with cancer.

Tumour lysis syndrome

An acute metabolic disturbance may occur as a result of the rapid dissolution of tumour following chemotherapy. This is particularly likely to occur in children in Burkitt's lymphoma or acute lymphoblastic leukaemia, and in non-Hodgkin's lymphomas in children, adolescents and young adults. The syndrome occurs when there is extreme sensitivity of the tumour to treatment, and is uncommon in adults with non-lymphoid neoplasms. When it occurs, tumour masses may disappear very rapidly and as the cells are killed they release products of nitrogen metabolism especially urea, urate and large amounts of phosphate.

The rapid reduction in tumour mass causes hyperuricaemia, hyperphosphataemia, hyperkalaemia and uraemia. The hyperuricaemia may result in acute urate deposition in the renal tubules (urate nephropathy) leading to acute renal failure or, less dramatically, to a reduction in glomerular filtration rate which exacerbates the hyperuricaemia. Occasionally, the syndrome can be sufficiently severe to cause an acute and prolonged uraemia. The hyperphosphataemia results in a reciprocal lowering of the plasma calcium and can result in tetany.

The syndrome is more likely to occur in children with Burkitt's lymphoma who have extensive disease, particularly if there are intra-abdominal masses, impaired renal function from tumour infiltration of the kidney, or post-renal obstruction due to lymph node enlargement. The syndrome is rare in adults since the tumours are generally less sensitive to chemotherapy, and their dissolution less rapid. It may, however, occur if there is coincidental renal failure due to some other cause, ureteric obstruction, or infiltration of the kidney with tumour.

The tumour lysis syndrome is usually preventable. Before beginning chemotherapy in a high-risk patient, allopurinol should be given (usually by mouth) in full dose (50–100 mg 8-hourly in children, twice this dose in adults) for 24 hours. This xanthine-oxidase inhibitor partly prevents the formation of urate. Allopurinol should be continued for the first few days of treatment and discontinued when the plasma urate is in the normal range. If 6-mercaptopurine is being given the dose should be reduced to 25% since allopurinol inhibits its metabolism. At the same time the patient should be given adequate fluids usually in the form of intravenous saline to establish a good diuresis. These measures should prevent both hyperuricaemia and hyperphosphataemia. In Burkitt's lymphoma, the induction chemotherapy is sometimes given at reduced dose until there has been considerable tumour shrinkage and then the full dose is administered. In adults with high-grade lymphoma starting treatment with intensive chemotherapy, allopurinol should be given and its use should be considered in other cases if there is any possibility of renal impairment.

If hyperuricaemia and acute renal failure develops this can usually be treated by cessation of chemotherapy, cautious administration of intravenous fluids with alkalinization of the urine to promote urate excretion, and allopurinol. If the blood urea and plasma urate continue to rise, peritoneal dialysis may be needed to tide the patient over the acute renal failure. If preventative measures are taken this should rarely be necessary.

EFFUSIONS AND ASCITES

Many patients with cancer develop a pleural or pericardial effusion or ascites during the course of their illness. These can be difficult to treat and can be a major cause of discomfort and breathlessness.

Pleural effusion

Pleural fluid must reach a volume of about 500 ml before it can be detected clinically, though lesser degrees can be radiologically apparent.

The commonest malignancy to cause pleural effusion is a primary lung cancer with involvement of pleura. This may be the first evidence of the tumour but more commonly it occurs later in the disease. Typically the effusion is substantial in volume (1–4 litres), accumulates rapidly, and may be blood-stained. It often causes dyspnoea with dry cough probably due to irritation of central mediastinal structures particularly the phrenic nerve. Although cytological demonstration of cells confirms the nature of the effusion, it is common for a malignant effusion to be repeatedly cytologically negative, in which case pleural biopsy will often be indicated if there is clinical doubt as to the diagnosis. Other important tumours causing pleural effusion include pleural metastases (sometimes from an unknown primary site), lymphoma and mesothelioma. Pleural metastases are common in cancer of the breast, bronchus and ovary.

Occasionally, patients with cancer develop a pleural effusion from a non-malignant cause and alternative explanations should always be considered if a patient with apparently controlled cancer unexpectedly develops a pleural effusion. Diagnosis is by clinical examination and chest X-ray supported by cytological examination and microscopy of the pleural fluid.

Management is rarely straightforward. Most patients require therapeutic aspiration (thoracocentesis) to improve symptoms of cough and dyspnoea, and large volumes (1–5 litres) may have to be removed for worthwhile benefit. Since aspiration of volumes above 1.5 litres can sometimes cause re-expansion of pulmonary oedema, the aspirations may have to be performed slowly over several days, or on several occasions over a week. In some patients, particularly those with secondary pleural deposits and disseminated disease elsewhere, chemotherapy or endocrine therapy will be given as well. In these patients, this systemic treatment may prove effective in preventing re-accumulation of pleural fluid. In others, where effective systemic therapy is unavailable the question of whether to instil an intrapleural sclerosant, to prevent or reduce fluid accumulation, will arise.

Treatment with simple physical or antibiotic sclerosants (talc, tetracycline or quinacrine), cytotoxic drugs (mustine, thiotepa, doxorubicin, bleomycin and others) or radioactive colloids are all commonly used. Each has its disadvantages and is effective only in a proportion of cases. Tetracycline can cause severe local pain, mustine and doxorubicin are painful and may be nauseating and bleomycin can cause fever and chills. There are few direct comparisons of one treatment with another and many clinicians feel that there is little to choose between them.

However, in a controlled study comparing bleomycin, doxorubicin and tetracycline, the cytoxic agents were more effective (the response to bleomycin is approximately 60%). Although intrapleural bleomycin can be effective and may at present be the treatment of choice, it requires careful preliminary drainage so that the pleural space is as dry as possible, and a subcutaneous test dose (5 mg) is advisable. The intrapleural dose is 30–60 mg. Colloidal ^{32}P or ^{198}Au have been used with success rates of the order of 50% but they are expensive, and require particular care over administration and patient position to produce maximal effect with minimal staff exposure. External beam irradiation has also been used but its value is restricted because of the wide field of irradiation which limits the total dose to the hemithorax to approximately 20 Gy (2000 rad) in 3 weeks.

If simple measures fail, thoracoscopy and tube drainage with talc insufflation and pleurodesis is often more successful than simple intrapleural drug instillation. Occasionally, pleurectomy will be required for adequate control of an effusion due to pleural secondary deposits and should be considered if the patient's general condition warrants [13].

Pericardial effusion

This is an infrequent clinical problem and in contrast to pleural effusion, pericardial effusions are less commonly due to malignancy than other causes such as infections, myxoedema, collagen disorders and rheumatoid arthritis. Although the diagnosis is often a radiological one, with 'globular' enlargement of the heart shadow, clinical signs include faintness of the heart sounds, pericardial friction rub and loss of apex beat. Tamponade may occur, with raised venous pressure, hypotension and paradoxical pulse.

The commonest causes of malignant pericardial effusions are carcinomas of breast and bronchus, and lymphoma including Hodgkin's disease. Post-mortem studies have shown that pericardial effusion is substantially underdiagnosed during life. In patients with widespread metastases, it may occur concurrently with a malignant pleural effusion. The diagnosis can be simply confirmed by echocardiography, which also gives useful quantitative information regarding the volume of the effusion. Because pericardial aspiration is both more hazardous and technically more difficult than pleural aspiration, it should not be undertaken in asymptomatic patients where the diagnosis is almost certain.

Treatment is by means of the same agents that are used for pleural effusion including cytotoxic drugs, tetracycline, radioactive gold and external beam irradiation. There may in addition be a useful response to systemic chemotherapy or endocrine therapy in which case intrapericardial instillation should be withheld. Pericardectomy has no place in the management, but creation of a surgical 'pericardial window' into the mediastinum may be beneficial if the condition is persistent and the patient relatively fit.

Ascites

Ascites is a common clinical problem in cancer. The usual cause is widespread peritoneal seedlings which cause exudation of fluid and lymphatic metastases block lymphatic drainage. Liver metastases are often present and hypoalbuminaemia contributes to the accumulation of fluid by lowering plasma osmotic pressure. Common cancers causing ascites include carcinomas of ovary, breast, bronchus (especially small cell), large bowel, stomach, pancreas and melanoma.

Patients usually present with abdominal distension, bulging of the flanks and with peripheral oedema if there is associated hypoalbuminaemia and/or IVC obstruction. The umbilicus may be everted and some patients have a fluid thrill. Some patients with moderate ascites are unaware of the distension, taking more note of the ankle oedema. It is important not to assume a malignant diagnosis, particularly when the tumour was previously thought to be localized or controlled by treatment. Important non-malignant causes include: portal hypertension (usually from cirrhosis or portal vein thrombosis), hepatic vein thrombosis (Budd–Chiari syndrome), raised systemic venous pressure as in long-standing cardiac failure and hypoalbuminaemia from other causes.

Diagnosis is by clinical examination, abdominal X-ray, ultrasound and aspiration cytology. Plain X-ray of the abdomen often shows a 'ground-glass' appearance due to a general blurring of the bowel and other intra-abdominal images by the fluid. There may be dilatation of the bowel and fluid levels indicating partial or subacute obstruction if the ascites is accompanied by an intra-abdominal tumour such as carcinoma of the ovary or bowel. Ultrasound examination is a sensitive technique for demonstrating ascites. Malignant ascites is usually turbid and straw-coloured with a protein concentration above 25 g/l. Malignant cells may be detected cytologically though this examination is frequently negative even in cases confirmed by other means.

Treatment includes both therapeutic aspiration (paracentesis) and general measures designed to prevent recurrence. Slow drainage over several days, via a peritoneal dialysis catheter, may be necessary to give relief of symptoms. Instillation of cytotoxic agents is less frequently practised and less frequently successful than in malignant pleural effusion, but intraperitoneal thiotepa, mustine, bleomycin and other agents have all been used. Systemic chemotherapy (or endocrine therapy in breast cancer) may occasionally help to control ascites and should be considered if the patient's general condition warrants it. Intraperitoneal radioactive colloids can be given via peritoneal dialysis catheter, and are reportedly effective in about half of all cases [14]. External irradiation is of little value except in some cases of ovarian cancer.

In the presence of hypoalbuminaemia, treatment with diuretics can be helpful in preventing recurrence. Combination treatment with frusemide and spironolactone is often used. Surgical procedures such as peritoneo-venous shunts have been attempted if the patient is fit and suffering from repeated episodes of ascites, with a reported success rate of over 70%. The prognosis for patients with malignant ascites is poor, the majority dying within 6 months of diagnosis.

CARCINOMATOUS MENINGITIS

Malignant meningitis is increasingly recognized as a complication of cancer. It is common in acute leukaemia. The most frequently associated solid tumours are non-Hodgkin's lymphoma, breast cancer and melanoma. Management is discussed further in Chapter 11.

MANAGEMENT OF HEPATIC METASTASES

Many patients with cancer will develop hepatic metastases and when these are widespread the expectation of life is only 2–3 months. In many cases there will be widespread dissemination and the liver involvement will not be a separate medical problem. In some tumours such as small cell carcinoma of the bronchus, breast cancer or lymphoma there is a reasonable likelihood of a response to chemotherapy with symptomatic and biochemical improvement. There are, however, many occasions when the liver is involved with metastatic cancer for which chemotherapy is inappropriate due to primary or acquired drug resistance.

The usual symptoms are fatigue, weight loss, anorexia and right upper quadrant pain. There may be abdominal distension from ascites. Episodes of sudden severe pain may occur when there is haemorrhage into a metastasis. Later, jaundice develops with advancing cachexia. Survival is usually a few months depending on the extent of involvement and rate of progression. Metastatic carcinoid tumours may be very slow growing and in this disease hepatic metastases are compatible with survival of 3–5 years.

Almost all treatment of hepatic metastasis is palliative and the value of each approach depends on the circumstances of each patient. The main symptoms are anorexia, nausea, pain, fever and malaise. Jaundice is a late feature unless there is obstruction to the porta hepatis by a tumour or lymph node mass. Itching and steatorrhoea may then be major symptoms. The following approaches can be taken to relieve symptoms.

Pharmacological

Anorexia, fever and malaise may all be relieved for a time by corticosteroids. Prednisolone 20–30 mg/day is usually adequate but the symptoms often recur after a few weeks and muscle wasting becomes profound if this dose is continued for long. Phenothiazines or metoclopramide before meals may help a little with the nausea, and aspirin or indomethacin may also relieve fever. Pain is treated with analgesics as described in Chapter 7.

Radiotherapy

Although the liver does not tolerate large doses (above 35 Gy), radiotherapy has a useful role in palliation of pain and may also improve nausea and vomiting. With a dose of 20–35 Gy to the whole liver, over 70% of patients will experience some improvement, particularly relief of pain. In chemoresistant tumours the addition of chemotherapy or hypoxic cell sensitizers does not improve these results. Often a particularly painful metastasis can be treated with a local field using a few large fractions, producing quick relief of pain without adverse effects.

Chemotherapy

In the case of responsive tumours such as small cell lung cancer or breast cancer, chemotherapy may be very effective, with responses in 50–60% of patients. If the primary tumour is of a type not usually amenable to chemotherapy, it is unlikely that cytotoxic agents will be of much value. For metastatic adenocarcinoma of the bowel, 5-fluorouracil (5-FU) has been most widely used but the objective response rate is only 10–20%. Subjectively, particularly with respect to pain, the response rate is higher. Modern regimens use 5-FU in conjunction with folinic acid (p. 100), and prolonged infusion regimens have been advocated.

Surgical

Hepatic artery ligation or embolization can produce pain relief and shrinkage of metastases but they recur rapidly with regeneration of the blood supply. Occasionally a slowly growing solitary metastasis is worth resecting in a fit patient with, for example, a carcinoid tumour.

RADIOTHERAPEUTIC EMERGENCIES

There are two common clinical situations which require urgent consideration by the radiotherapist. These are acute spinal cord compression, and superior vena caval obstruction.

Acute spinal cord or cauda equina compression

This syndrome results from pressure on the cord, usually as a result of tumour extending from a vertebral body to compress the cord from the epidural space. Compression may also occur as a result of direct extension from a mediastinal tumour or the cauda equina from a retroperitoneal tumour. If the vertebra is weakened a crush fracture may precipitate cord compression. Extradural compression may develop in the absence of deposits in the spine. Very occasionally, intramedullary metastases will cause acute cord compression from within. Cord compression most commonly occurs in diseases where bony metastases (particularly spinal metastases) are frequent. Carcinomas of the breast, prostate and lung (particularly small cell carcinomas), lymphoma and myeloma are the commonest causes followed by carcinomas of the thyroid, kidney, bladder, bowel and melanoma. Lymphomas may produce cord compression by extension from paraspinal lymph nodes through the intervertebral foramina.

Characteristically, the patient complains of back pain often with a root distribution, weakness of the legs, dribbling, hesitancy and incontinence of urine and sluggish bowel action. In most cases, only one or two of these symptoms will be present, and limb weakness and bladder dysfunction are late signs. Higher cord lesions will also be accompanied by symptoms and signs in the upper limb.

The cauda equina syndrome, where the compression occurs below the lower level of the spinal cord L_1 or L_2, is often difficult to diagnose (see p. 220). The features include leg weakness, sacral anaesthesia, retention of urine and erectile failure. Clinical diagnosis is particularly important since in this syndrome radiological studies, including myelography, often fail to demonstrate any definite abnormality. Careful neurological examination may reveal loss of sacral sensation (saddle anaesthesia) which will only be detected if perianal sensation is tested with a pin, and anal sphincter tone is assessed on rectal examination.

Spinal cord compression may occasionally occur at more than one site, giving rise to neurological signs (for example a mixture of upper and lower motor neurone weakness) which would otherwise be difficult to explain on the basis of a single lesion.

Investigation should include plain X-ray of the spine and myelography. Plain X-ray may show evidence of multiple bone metastases, a crush fracture at the site of pain, or less obvious changes such as erosion of a pedicle (Fig. 8.1). Myelography will delineate the site of block if it is above $L_{1/2}$. Increasingly MR imaging is used as an alternative. It demonstrates the site of block with great accuracy and often gives a clear view of its extent and whether multiple lesions are present (Fig. 8.2).

Cord compression is a medical emergency

Fig. 8.1 X-ray of lumbar vertebrae showing destruction of the left pedicle L_3.

Fig. 8.2 MRI scan showing acute spinal cord compression.

where treatment must begin within hours not days. Any patient with cancer who develops severe back pain with a root distribution is at very high risk and must be investigated at once.

Treatment of cord compression is either by surgery, radiation therapy, or a combination of both [15,16]. With acute cord compression in a patient in good general health and with no other evidence of metastatic disease, decompressive laminectomy is the treatment of choice. Most neurosurgeons feel that laborious attempts to remove all of the tumour are generally fruitless, so that in the majority of cases neurosurgical treatment will be followed by radiotherapy in an attempt to control the residual local disease. In patients with multiple metastases and with a short life expectation, radiotherapy may be used without surgery. This will of course be particularly beneficial in

patients with radioresponsive tumours. In small cell carcinoma of the bronchus, it has been shown that treatment with radiotherapy alone is as beneficial as treatment by surgery and radiotherapy in combination, as judged both by recovery of power, mobility and also survival. Where radiotherapy is employed as the sole method, dexamethasone is often used routinely as a means of reducing local oedema, particularly where acute radiation hyperaemia of the cord might pose additional problems. In multiple myeloma, radiotherapy is often preferred to surgery since there may be multiple sites, and patients with cord compression from myeloma are often unfit for surgery. Myeloma deposits are very sensitive to irradiation.

The prognosis for patients with cord compression relates to the degree of neurological damage before treatment and the underlying cancer. Delayed diagnosis results in a bad outcome. Speedy and efficient treatment are essential. If the patient has progressed to paraplegia before treatment, the chance that he will walk after treatment is less than 5%. Early diagnosis is essential since with less severe damage, 50% will be ambulatory. Widespread radioresistant tumour (e.g. melanoma) has a bad prognosis. Chemotherapy plays no part in the initial management of cord compression.

Superior vena caval obstruction (SVCO)

This most commonly results from a right-sided carcinoma of the bronchus (particularly small cell carcinoma). It also occurs in lymphoma (particularly Hodgkin's disease, in which mediastinal involvement occurs in about one-quarter of all patients), as well as carcinoma of the breast, kidney and other tumours which may metastasize to mediastinal nodes. Occasionally, it may be a presenting feature of a primary mediastinal tumour such as a thymoma, or a germ cell tumour. It is characterized by swelling of the face, neck and arms, sometimes with a typical plethoric cyanotic facies. There is non-pulsatile engorgement of veins and large collateral veins may be visible over the surface of the shoulders, scapulae and upper chest. Retinal veins may also be engorged and there is often conjunctival oedema. The most constant physical sign is that of leashes of tiny bluish venules which occur over the chest wall, particularly in the precordial, subcostal and infrascapular regions. Patients are almost always dyspnoeic and hypoxic, and the chest X-ray usually shows a substantial right-sided mass (Fig. 8.3).

Urgent treatment with radiotherapy is the mainstay of management and is undoubtedly the treatment of choice for non-small cell carcinomas of bronchus and other tumours not amenable to chemotherapy, and where treatment must be started before the diagnosis is known. However, with the advent of effective chemotherapy for lymphoma and small cell carcinoma of the bronchus, combination chemotherapy should be considered in SVCO due to these conditions and has a number of advantages. In the first place, patients may be several miles (and an uncomfortable journey) from a radiotherapy centre, whereas chemotherapy can be given without moving the patient; secondly, many of them will have extensive disease which would be left untreated by local irradiation; thirdly, chemotherapy is given as a single intravenous injection whereas radiotherapy has to be given daily for several days or weeks. Finally, the response to chemotherapy is often at least as quick as with radiotherapy, which can still be given if chemotherapy fails.

Radiation dosage in treatment of SVC obstruction should depend on the primary diagnosis. In small cell carcinoma of the bronchus, a total of 40 Gy (4000 rad) midline dose is given in 20 daily fractions over 4 weeks (or the equivalent over a shorter time). However, in non-small cell lung cancer, this dose is generally inadequate and treatment with radical intent will demand that at least 56 Gy (5600 rad) be given over 5–6 weeks, using a planned multifield arrangement in order to avoid overtreatment of spinal cord. As with spinal cord compression, dexamethasone is a useful addition to treatment. Although in lung cancer SVC obstruction has long been considered a serious prognostic sign, in small cell carcinoma of the bronchus, which is the commonest cause, this does not appear to be the case.

Other radiotherapy emergencies

Orbital or intra-ocular metastases most commonly occur in carcinoma of the breast and in malignant melanoma. They present with proptosis, oculomotor palsy or visual loss which may be acute if there is bleeding into the eye from a choroidal deposit. These metastases may be bilateral. Early treatment with radiotherapy is important since permanent visual loss or ocular palsy may occur in a patient whose lifespan may be several years. Careful radiation planning is required in order to avoid treatment to the anterior half of the eyes and to the contralateral lens. A single lateral radiation field with a dose of 30 Gy (3000 rad) in 10 daily fractions over 2 weeks of treatment is usually adequate. Chemotherapy plays no part in the management of these complications.

Primary or secondary cancers at other critical sites may also lead to a necessity for urgent

Fig. 8.3 Typical radiological findings in superior vena caval obstruction. The tumour is usually right-sided. In this case the diaphragm is raised because of involvement of the phrenic nerve.

treatment. Impending collapse of a lung from severe bronchial narrowing may be the cause of an urgent referral from a chest physician who has been following an asymptomatic patient with known carcinoma of the bronchus for months or even years. The development of a unilateral monophonic wheeze, usually heard at its loudest over the main or lobar bronchus, is the most reliable physical sign. The sequence of chest X-rays often shows increasing shadowing and obstruction of part of the lung. Radiotherapy may well reverse this picture and relieve the patient's dyspnoea. The role of radiotherapy in carcinoma of the bronchus is more fully discussed in Chapter 12.

For the severe, localized and unremitting pain of bony metastases, radiotherapy is preeminently the treatment of choice. Palliative radiotherapy is often given as a matter of urgency in patients with severe bone pain who have not previously been treated maximally with radiotherapy to the painful site especially if a single metastatic site is evident on clinical examination, X-ray or isotope bone scan. Analgesics (usually opiates) will need to be given during the course of treatment and often afterwards as well (see p. 128 for discussion of pain control). If an area of spinal cord is included in the field, the treatment is often fractionated over 2 weeks (30 Gy (3000 rad) in 10 daily treatments) though shorter treatment periods are certainly acceptable for patients with a short lifespan, and may be perfectly safe. Common regimens for the relief of bone pain include 5 fractions of 5 Gy (500 rad) calculated at depth, or 4 fractions of 6 Gy (600 rad). Single fraction treatments of 8–14 Gy (800–1400 rad) are becoming more popular and are certainly more convenient. It is becoming increasingly clear that such treatments are probably as effective as more conventional regimens [17].

CANCER DURING PREGNANCY [18]

Cancer is not uncommon in women during the childbearing years of life. Breast and cervical are the commonest tumours, but leukaemia, lymphoma, melanoma and colorectal cancers frequently affect this age group especially as more women start families later. The approach to management will depend on the curability of the tumour, the stage of pregnancy and the wishes of the patient with respect to continuation of the pregnancy.

Treatment with cytotoxic drugs is especially hazardous during the first trimester. Pooled data suggest that the risk of fetal malformation if alkylating agents are used at this period is about 15%. For antimetabolites the figure is the same. Methotrexate is particularly likely to cause malformation. There are few data on other drugs. Large doses early in pregnancy will often cause abortion. The deformities are in skeletal and limb formation. There is no evidence of increased risk of malformation if treatment is in the second or third trimester, but it is not known if long-term consequences of drug treatment such as leukaemia will occur.

If the patient refuses termination and the cancer is curable with drug treatment then this must be given in full dosage (there is no evidence that drug combinations or full dosage carries a greater risk of fetal injury). Where possible this treatment should be delayed to the second trimester. Local treatment, for example surgery for breast cancer, or involved field radiation for lymphoma can be given safely. Abdominal radiation must be avoided throughout pregnancy, and if given will be very likely to lead to abortion. Radiation causes fetal growth retardation, CNS damage (microcephaly) and malformation of the eyes. The degree of microcephaly is related to radiation dose. The malformations can occur with irradiation at any stage in the pregnancy but are more severe earlier. Abdominal surgery for cancer can be performed but clearly presents major difficulties if the pregnancy is advanced. Safe delivery of the fetus can now usually be attained at 30 weeks gestation. This has made cancer management easier during the third trimester.

REFERENCES

1 Petz L.D. Red blood cell transfusion. *Clinics in Oncology* 1983; **2**(3): 505−27.

2 Kelton J.B., Ali A.M. Platelet transfusions — A critical appraisal. *Clinics in Oncology* 1983; **2**(3): 549−85.

3 Groopman J.E., Molina J.-M., Scadden D.T. Haemopoietic growth factors: Biology and clinical applications. *New England Journal of Medicine* 1989; **321**: 1449−59.

4 Devereux S., Linch D. Haemopoietic growth factors. *Quarterly Journal of Medicine* 1990; **75**: 537−50.

5 Gabrilove J.L., Kubowski A., Scher H. *et al.* Effect of granulocyte colony stimulating factor on neutropenia and associated morbidity due to chemotherapy for transitional cell carcinoma of the urothelium. *New England Journal of Medicine* 1988; **318**: 1414−22.

6 Siber G.R., Weitzmann S.A., Aisenberg A.C., Weinstein H.J., Schiffmang. Impaired antibody response to pneumonococca vaccine after treatment for Hodgkin's disease. *New England Journal of Medicine* 1978; **299**: 442−48.

7 Weitzman S., Aisenberg A.C. Fulminant sepsis after the successful treatment of Hodgkin's disease. *American Journal of Medicine* 1977; **62**: 47−50.

8 Joshi J.H., Schimoff S.C. Therapy of infection in granulocytopenia patients with cancer. *Clinics in Oncology* 1983; **2**(3): 611.

9 De Wys W. Management of Cachexia. *Seminars in Oncology* 1985; **12**: 452−60.

10 Theologides A. Anorexins, asthenins and cachectins in cancer. *American Journal of Medicine* 1986; **81**: 696−98.

11 Linkhart T.A., Mohan S., Jennings J.C. *et al.* Copurification of osteolytic and transforming growth factor β activities produced by human lung tumour cells associated with humoral hypercalcaemia of malignancy. *Cancer Research* 1989; **49**: 271−78.

12 Martin T.J. Properties of parathyroid hormone-related protein and its role in malignant hypercalcaemia. *Quarterly Journal of Medicine* 1990; **76**: 771−86.

13 Anderson C.B., Philpott G.W., Fergison T.B. The treatment of malignant pleural effusions. *Cancer* 1974; **33**: 916−22.

14 Dybiki J., Balchum D.J., Meneely G.R. Treatment of pleural and peritoneal effusion with intracavitary colloidal radio-gold (^{198}Au). *Archives of International Medicine* 1959; **104**: 802−15.

15 Bruckman J.E., Bloomer W.D. Management of spinal cord compression. *Seminars in Oncology* 1978; **5**: 135−40.

16 Gilbert R.W., Kim J.H., Posner J.B. Epidural spinal cord compression from metastatic tumour. Diagnosis and management. *Annals of Neurology* 1978; **3**: 40−51.

17 Hoskin P. Changing trends in palliative radiotherapy. In Tobias J.S., Thomas P.R.M. (eds) *Current Radiation Oncology*, Vol. 1. London: Edward Arnold, 1994, pp. 342−364.

18 Doll D.C. (Ed.) Cancer and pregnancy. *Seminars in Oncology* 1989; **16**(5) (see reviews by Doll *et al.* (p. 337) for effects of cytotoxic drugs, and Brent (p. 347) for effects of radiation).

Chapter 9
Hormonal and Paraneoplastic Syndromes

Cancers are frequently associated with constitutional disturbances which are not due to the local effect of the tumour. For example, although cancer of the head of the pancreas will frequently cause obstructive jaundice leading to steatorrhoea and weight loss, these metabolic upsets are due to the physical presence of the tumour obstructing the common bile and pancreatic ducts. However, the tumour may occasionally give rise to remote effects such as fever, thrombophlebitis or mood change, and the mechanisms whereby these symptoms are caused are poorly understood. Such systemic metabolic effects of cancer are common and often add to the patient's symptoms. Sometimes these paraneoplastic syndromes may be the presenting feature of cancer and lead to other diagnoses being made in error, before a cancer is suspected. An awareness of these complications of cancer is therefore essential for proper management because the symptoms can often be controlled and the patient made more comfortable even when the primary tumour cannot be removed. Furthermore, the symptoms may be wrongly interpreted as being due to metastases and an opportunity for effective treatment.

In recent years the pathogenesis of these syndromes has become clearer. The syndromes of ectopic hormone production have been further elucidated, antibody-mediated syndromes have been defined, and syndromes due to secretion of colony-stimulating and growth factors have been described.

Table 9.1 illustrates metabolic and paraneoplastic syndromes in non-endocrine neoplasms. The pathogenesis and management of weight loss, cachexia, and hypercalcaemia are discussed in Chapter 8.

FEVER DUE TO MALIGNANT DISEASE [1]

Most patients with cancer who develop a fever do so because of infection. Fever is, however, a symptom of cancer itself and may be the presenting feature. The pathogenesis is obscure. Lymphomas, especially Hodgkin's disease, are often accompanied by fever and in these diseases the pyrexia usually indicates an aggressive and advanced tumour. The typical relapsing Pel−Ebstein fever is only present in a minority of patients with Hodgkin's disease. Non-specific intermittent or remittent fever is much more common.

Hypernephroma is notorious for its tendency to cause fever and to present in this way. It may be associated with leucocytosis (often extreme) and thus mimic a pyogenic infection. Other carcinomas may present similarly especially if they are metastatic to the liver and bone marrow. Sarcomas and primary liver cancer are also frequently associated with pyrexia.

When cancer is the cause of the presenting pyrexia it can usually be diagnosed fairly easily. Isotope or ultrasound scans of the liver are often abnormal, the liver enzymes are elevated, especially alkaline phosphatase, and there are usually symptoms and signs of the primary tumour. If nothing can be done to treat the cancer itself, symptomatic relief can sometimes be obtained by aspirin, non-steroidal anti-inflammatory agents and by steroids. The

Table 9.1 Metabolic paraneoplastic syndromes in non-endocrine neoplasms

Syndrome	Tumour	Syndrome	Tumour
Endocrine and metabolic		*Haematological*	
Cushing's syndrome	Small cell bronchogenic cancer, thymoma, bronchial carcinoid, neuroblastoma, phaeochromocytoma, medullary carcinoma of the thyroid	Multiple thromboses	Pancreatic cancer, other adenocarcinomas
		Erythrocytosis	Renal carcinoma, hepatoma, uterine cancer, cerebellar haemangioblastoma
Inappropriate ADH secretion	Small cell bronchogenic cancer, thymoma, lymphoma, duodenal carcinoma, pancreatic carcinoma	Red cell aplasia	Thymomas
		Disseminated intravascular coagulation	Mucinous adenocarcinomas
		Neurological	
Gynaecomastia	Teratoma, large cell lung cancer, adenocarcinomas (breast, pancreas and gut), tumours of liver and adrenal	Peripheral neuropathy	Small cell bronchogenic carcinoma, breast, ovary, lymphoma
		Cerebellar degeneration	Small cell lung cancer
		Eaton–Lambert syndrome	Small cell lung cancer
Hypoglycaemia	Retroperitoneal sarcoma and lymphoma, hepatoma	*Muscle and joint*	
		Polyarthritis	Adenocarcinomas (gut, breast, ovary)
Hypercalcaemia (see Chapter 8)	All cancers with widespread bone metastases, squamous cancers, renal and ovarian carcinoma	Dermatomyositis	Lung cancer, oesophageal cancer, adenocarcinomas
		Skin See Table 9.2	
Hyperpigmentation	Small cell bronchogenic cancer	*Renal*	
Cachexia, anorexia, altered taste	All tumours	Nephrotic syndrome	Adenocarcinomas

control of symptoms usually lasts a few weeks or months.

ECTOPIC HORMONE PRODUCTION IN CANCER

Many cancers (perhaps the majority) produce hormone precursors and peptides, some of which have biological activity [2]. In the formation of a hormone in an endocrine gland the precursor hormone (pro-hormone) is often the major storage form and is biologically inactive but is cleaved to the active hormone at the time of secretion. In the blood and tissues the hormone is degraded to the inactive carboxyl fragment and the amino fragment which may retain activity. Tumours may produce inactive pro-hormones or the active principle. They may also produce biologically active peptides such as HCG or variants of HCG which have a reduced carbohydrate content and which have lost activity. Similarly a biologically active glycopeptide hormone may have two chains both of which are necessary for biological activity. If only one chain is made by the tumour it will be inactive.

The mechanism of ectopic synthesis is not clear but may be due to abnormal gene activation as a result of malignant transformation. In this section, 'ectopic' hormone is taken to mean production of a hormone by a non-endocrine tumour. Clearly cancers of the adrenal, pancreas or endocrine cells in the gut may cause hormonal disturbances. These are discussed in the appropriate chapters.

Syndrome of inappropriate ADH secretion (SIADH)

The syndrome is due to ectopic production of arginine vasopressin by the tumour — usually small cell lung cancer (SCLC). An elevated level of ADH and impaired water handling is present in 30% of SCLC patients. The syndrome is characterized biochemically by a plasma sodium below 130 mmol/l with a low plasma and high urine osmolality. Clinically it usually becomes apparent only when the plasma sodium reaches 120 mmol/l or below, when the patient becomes tired, then drowsy and confused. The commonest underlying tumour is SCLC which is usually apparent on chest X-ray. A CT brain scan may be necessary to exclude cerebral metastases as a cause of the neurological picture, since they are common in SCLC. Cyclophosphamide, vincristine and morphine can also cause hyponatraemia due to either pituitary ADH release or a direct effect on the renal tubule. Although 30% of patients have impaired water handling, only 10–20% have a plasma sodium below 130 mmol/l [3]. The ADH is identical with that produced by the neurohypophysis. A low plasma sodium may be found in very ill patients regardless of cause. This is probably due to inappropriate ADH release from the posterior pituitary. This syndrome is occasionally difficult to distinguish from ectopic ADH production. In SCLC, marked hyponatraemia (assumed to be a reflection of ectopic ADH) is associated with a worse prognosis.

Treatment of the tumour with drugs and radiotherapy may improve the metabolic abnormality. While this is being done, demeclocycline (300 mg by mouth 6–8-hourly at first then 8–12-hourly) is effective in correcting the plasma sodium. It does this by rendering the distal tubule unresponsive to the ectopic ADH.

This drug can impair renal function and the blood urea should be measured regularly. In severe cases water restriction may be temporarily required but this is difficult to sustain and is sometimes ineffective. In an acutely ill patient with life-threatening hyponatraemia, a 3% saline infusion combined with intravenous frusemide (to increase free water clearance) is effective emergency treatment.

Ectopic adrenocorticotrophic hormone (ACTH) production

Excess production of ACTH is an uncommon metabolic complication of cancers which are normally neuroectodermal in origin. The commonest tumour to produce the syndrome is small cell carcinoma of the bronchus. Small carcinoid tumours in the lung, thymus and pancreas may also cause the syndrome. Raised ACTH levels have been found in half of all patients with SCLC and immunoreactive ACTH can be extracted from the majority of these tumours [4]. In SCLC clinical manifestations of ectopic ACTH production are very unusual, and when they occur the clinical picture is usually different from classical Cushing's syndrome. There is generally hyperkalaemia, glucose intolerance, hypertension and muscle weakness, but without the long-term weight gain of typical Cushing's syndrome. These patients usually have extensive disease with a poor prognosis. Estimates of the frequency of this syndrome vary depending on the criteria used to define it. In indolent or benign tumours such as bronchial carcinoid, typical Cushing's syndrome occurs. The syndrome also occurs rarely in squamous lung cancer, adenocarcinomas of the lung, gut or kidney and medullary carcinoma of the thyroid. It also occurs in thymoma and ganglioneuroblastoma in childhood. Some of these tumours contain molecules of a pro-hormone with a higher molecular weight than normal ACTH which may not be biologically active. Other tumours can produce a corticotrophin releasing factor which acts on the pituitary.

Clinically, the syndrome caused by SCLC is

rarely confused with other forms of Cushing's syndrome. The diagnosis is more difficult when the tumour is a bronchial carcinoid. The urinary free cortisol is increased and plasma cortisol is greatly raised. In lung cancer with ectopic ACTH, high-dose dexamethasone does not suppress the plasma cortisol level, in contrast to pituitary-dependent Cushing's syndrome. Some patients with ACTH from carcinoid tumours will show suppression with dexamethasone. The plasma ACTH will be very low with an autonomous adrenal adenoma or carcinoma. In the latter, the plasma cortisol may also fail to suppress with dexamethasone.

Treatment is to the primary tumour. If this is ineffective then aminoglutethimide will block steroid synthesis. Metyrapone will also block 11-hydroxylation of corticosteroids causing a fall in plasma cortisol. This drug can be useful in seriously ill patients before definitive treatment of the tumour begins, but neither drug will produce lasting benefit in the absence of treatment of the disease.

Hypoglycaemia

Hypoglycaemia is a very uncommon complication of some cancers. It occurs with large thoracic and abdominal sarcomas, especially those situated retroperitoneally, and with hepatomas, mesotheliomas, adrenal carcinomas and lymphomas [5]. It does not seem to be produced by insulin which cannot be found in plasma or tumour extracts. Elevated plasma levels of somatomedin-like peptides have been found. These are peptides normally made in the liver as a result of stimulation by growth hormones and which have an action like insulin. These peptides have occasionally been extracted from the tumour itself. Other substances may be produced which have insulin-like activity or which bind to insulin receptors.

The hypoglycaemic attacks may be spontaneous or associated with fasting and can be very severe. Emergency treatment requires glucose infusion. Clinically the episodes are indistinguishable from those produced by islet-

cell tumours, but the plasma insulin is not raised. If the tumour cannot be completely removed the hypoglycaemia may be partially controlled by frequent feeding, diazoxide, glucagon or corticosteroids.

Gynaecomastia and gonadotrophin production

Gynaecomastia is an increase in the glandular and stromal tissue of the male breast. In most instances when it complicates a non-endocrine malignancy, it is probably caused by tumour-related HCG production. In women oligomenorrhoea may occur. In children precocious puberty may occur with hepatoblastoma or hepatoma. Teratoma and seminoma may both be associated with HCG production and so may carcinoma of the bronchus of all histological types. Other HCG-producing tumours include pancreas (both exocrine and islet-cell tumours), liver, adrenal and breast. In most cases of non-germ cell neoplasms, HCG is produced in amounts too small to be clinically significant although it may occasionally be useful as a tumour marker [6]. In other cases the hormone may not be glycosylated by the tumour and this results in its rapid removal from the blood. Some tumours secrete free subunits which are not associated with biological activity. The increased oestrogen production which is the cause of the gynaecomastia is probably due to the action of the ectopic HCG on the testis. The correct treatment is removal of the tumour, but if this is not possible, or is incomplete, the HCG inhibitor danazol may be useful if the gynaecomastia is painful. Painful gynaecomastia can also sometimes be relieved by local irradiation of the breasts. Further details on HCG are given in Chapters 4 and 19.

Other ectopic hormones

Bronchial carcinoids may rarely produce growth hormone releasing substances over sufficient length of time to cause acromegaly. Galactorrhoea has been reported with cancer, due to hyperprolactinaemia [7]. Hyperthyroidism may occur in trophoblastic tumours producing HCG. This does not appear to be due to thyroid-stimulating hormone (TSH) production, but the HCG may have TSH-like activity. Hypercalcaemia is discussed in Chapter 8.

HAEMATOLOGICAL SYNDROMES

Anaemia

Anaemia is an almost universal accompaniment of advanced cancer. Many factors contribute including gastro-intestinal bleeding leading to iron deficiency, and poor appetite with resulting iron and folate deficiency. Even if there are no secondary deficiency states, anaemia can still develop and can be regarded as a 'paraneoplastic' syndrome. Characteristically it is similar to the anaemia of other chronic diseases. It takes a few months to develop and the haemoglobin does not usually fall below 8 or 9 grams. The anaemia is normocytic and normochromic or slightly hypochromic. The serum iron is low but so is the total iron binding capacity (TIBC), in contrast to the anaemia of iron deficiency where the TIBC is high. The marrow shows stainable iron in macrophages. The red cell survival is often shortened to some degree without an increase in erythropoiesis sufficient to compensate for this. There also appears to be a block in release of iron from macrophages into the plasma. Serum erythropoietin levels are low.

Treatment of the anaemia depends on the successful treatment of the cancer. If this is impossible, and there are no secondary deficiencies of iron or folate, the anaemia can only be corrected, albeit temporarily, by blood transfusion. This can be of value when the anaemia may be contributing to fatigue and the transfusion may allow the patient a little more useful and active life. Response to erythropoietin occurs but is temporary.

An autoimmune haemolytic anaemia (AIHA) which usually responds to treatment with steroids may complicate B cell neoplasms and Hodgkin's disease. It is much less common to find AIHA associated with non-lymphoid neoplasms but it has been reported as an association with cancers of many types.

Erythrocytosis

The commonest cancer to produce this syndrome is renal carcinoma. Rarer causes include cerebellar haemangioblastoma, hepatoma, uterine leiomyosarcoma and fibroids [8]. The probable explanation is the production of an erythropoietin-like substance in renal cancer although this may not be the cause with cancers from other sites. Only 2–5% of cases of renal cancer are associated with polycythaemia though excess production of erythropoietin occurs in over half of all patients. However, if the investigation of a high haematocrit confirms a true polycythaemia, an IVU should be performed to exclude renal carcinoma. The white blood count and platelet count are often raised in polycythaemia rubra vera but unless these values are greatly elevated it is not wise to rely on this alone in making the distinction from renal carcinoma.

The erythrocytosis usually responds to removal of the primary tumour whether or not it is due to erythropoietin production by the tumour.

Migratory thrombophlebitis

Carcinoma of the pancreas, especially of the body or tail, is occasionally associated with multiple thromboses often in superficial veins and migratory in nature. Other adenocarcinomas may give rise to the same syndrome. The tumours tend to be inoperable. The venous thromboses are sometimes in an unusual site such as the arm, and this may arouse the suspicion of the underlying diagnosis. Pulmonary embolism seldom occurs. These tumours probably liberate thromboplastins which promote clotting in veins.

Disseminated intravascular coagulation (DIC) [9]

This is a complication of malignancy which has been described in many different types of cancer of which the commonest are adeno-carcinomas (prostate, breast, pancreas, ovary) and other tumours such as metastatic carcinoid, neuroblastoma and rhabdomyosarcoma. It is probably due to the liberation of thromboplastin-like material from cancer cells, but some cancers secrete thrombin-like enzymes. Many patients with cancer have increased levels of fibrin degradation products in the blood but the degree of intravascular coagulation is usually mild. Problems with haemorrhage are very unusual except in acute promyelocytic leukaemia where DIC can be severe when treatment has been started. In solid tumours, where the DIC is chronic and low-grade, treatment is by removal of the cancer where possible. Occasionally the DIC can be associated with red cell fragmentation (microangiopathic haemolytic anaemia) especially in stomach cancer [10]. This syndrome may also be accompanied by acute renal failure (the haemolytic-uraemic syndrome).

Red cell aplasia

Acquired suppression of erythropoiesis has been described in adults as an accompaniment of tumours, particularly thymomas, although in many of these cases the thymoma is benign. It occurs rarely in association with a variety of other cancers such as carcinoma of the bronchus. The anaemia, which is often severe, is normocytic and erythropoiesis is selectively absent from the marrow. An immune suppression of erythropoiesis provoked by the tumour is the postulated cause.

NEUROLOGICAL SYNDROMES

Cancers can be associated with neurological syndromes unrelated to direct compression or infiltration. While interesting and import-ant, these syndromes are uncommon, their frequency often being over-estimated by neurologists who, because of their specialty, see these complications not infrequently. From the point of view of the cancer specialist the non-metastatic neurological complications of malignancy are infrequently encountered, at least in a clinically significant form. Most neurological complications of cancer are due to metastases or compression and it is a grave error to fail to treat a cancer causing, for example, fits or spinal cord compression, because of a mistaken diagnosis of a non-metastatic manifestation of the tumour. The major clinical syndromes are discussed briefly below.

Peripheral neuropathy

The commonest variety of neuropathy seen in association with cancer is a *distal sensory and motor neuropathy* [11]. Pathologically there is segmental demyelination of nerves, usually distally, and axonal degeneration. It is possible that the neurones themselves may also be the site of the initial damage. The neuropathy varies in its severity. There is a mild form developing late in the course of the disease, and a more severe form occurring earlier, sometimes before the tumour is manifest and occasionally following an intermittent course. The CSF shows a modest increase in protein (1–2 g/l), without excess cells.

The second form of neuropathy is carcinomatous *sensory neuropathy*. This is a slowly progressive sensory neuropathy, associated with pains and paraesthesiae in the limbs, which may spread to the trunk and face. There is degeneration of dorsal root ganglia sometimes associated with a mononuclear cell infiltrate. Later, there is loss of the posterior columns leading to ataxia. The patient may become chair or bed-bound before the primary tumour has declared itself. Cancer of the lung (especially small cell cancer) is the commonest tumour [12] but lymphoma and many other cancers can be associated. Removal of the tumour usually does not produce improvement and the neuropathy is progressive. Steroids may sometimes help.

An *acute ascending paralysis* of the Guillain–Barré type may also occur, and has been noted in Hodgkin's disease especially.

The diagnosis of carcinomatous neuropathy is often very difficult. Infiltration of the meninges with carcinoma and lymphoma may occasionally cause peripheral sensory and motor damage. The CSF should therefore always be examined for malignant cells. In young patients with lymphoma, where the risk of CNS involvement is high, it is usually best to treat the patient for CNS relapse if there is doubt about the diagnosis.

Carcinomatous myelopathy

This rare syndrome can present as a flaccid paraplegia of acute onset with loss of sphincter control [13]. The primary tumour is usually lung cancer. There is necrosis of the cord with little inflammation. The mechanism is unknown and the damage irreversible. A less acute myelopathy can also occur, associated with loss of anterior horn cells and a slowly progressive lower motor neurone weakness. It is usually associated with lymphoma and lung cancer.

The diagnosis of carcinomatous myelopathy is difficult to make. Cord compression must be excluded and the CSF examined for malignant cells. Other diseases such as amyotrophic lateral sclerosis may cause a similar picture. The association with carcinoma may become apparent only late in the evolution of the disease.

Cerebellar degeneration

This rare syndrome is most commonly associated with carcinoma of the bronchus and Hodgkin's disease. It differs from the chronic idiopathic cerebellar degenerations of adult life by being more rapid in evolution, sometimes progressing to severe disability in a few months, even before the primary tumour is apparent. Unsteadiness of gait, truncal ataxia, vertigo and diplopia (sometimes with oscil-

lopsia and opsoclonus) occur. Long tract signs due to spinal cord degeneration may develop. Unlike idiopathic cerebellar degeneration, the CSF may be abnormal with a raised protein and a few lymphocytes. Pathologically there is global cell loss in the cerebellar cortex and some perivascular inflammatory infiltrate. Degenerative changes may be found in the cord. Treatment of the primary tumour, although necessary, does not usually help. A CT scan is essential to exclude a cerebellar metastasis as far as possible. The syndrome is associated with the presence of antibodies to Purkinje cells. In Hodgkin's disease the response to treatment of the tumour is very unpredictable.

Limbic encephalitis

In this exceedingly rare syndrome an underlying small cell carcinoma is likely to be responsible [14]. It is characterized by the fairly rapid onset of confusion, memory disturbance and agitation. It may be associated with a cerebellar disturbance due to degeneration. There is temporal lobe degeneration with some perivascular infiltrate. A viral aetiology has been suspected but not proven. As with cerebellar degeneration, the main differential diagnosis is from intracranial metastasis.

Progressive multifocal leucoencephalopathy (PML)

This rare syndrome is not always associated with cancer, but lymphoma is by far the commonest associated disorder. The clinical features are aphasia and dementia leading to coma, visual field loss which may progress to blindness, fits and focal paralyses. The differential diagnosis includes metastases, lymphomatous meningitis, herpes encephalitis and cerebrovascular disease. The CSF is usually normal.

The brain shows patchy demyelination throughout the white matter with abnormal oligodendroglia, the nuclei of which contain viral inclusions. Papova viruses (JC and SV40) have been isolated from these brains [15]. Antibodies to these viruses may be present in blood or CSF and may help in diagnosis. Response to intrathecal and intravenous cytosine arabinoside have been reported.

Lambert—Eaton myasthenic syndrome [16]

In this rare syndrome, which is found almost exclusively with SCLC, the patient complains of weakness, aching and fatique in the shoulder and pelvic girdle muscles, and sometimes impotence. It resembles myasthenia except that the relationship of fatigue to repeated muscular activity is less clear-cut and the electromyogram (EMG) shows an increase in muscle action potentials at higher rates of nerve stimulation. The ocular and bulbar muscles are usually spared. The syndrome may appear before the tumour. Unfortunately there is little response to oral anticholinesterases. The syndrome is produced by an IgG antibody which impairs calcium influx and acetylcholine release. Treatment of the tumour may help. Guanidine hydrochloride, which enhances acetylcholine release, may be used but it is nephrotoxic and myelosuppressive. 3—4 Diaminopyridine, which prolongs calcium channel activation, may be a useful new agent.

MUSCLE AND JOINT SYNDROMES

Many patients with cancer complain of fatigue and sometimes of aching in the muscles which is occasionally out of proportion to the amount of weight loss. It has often been postulated that some of these patients have a more specific muscle disturbance. On the other hand, unequivocal myopathic syndromes are unusual. Arthritic complications of cancer are also uncommon.

Polymyositis and dermatomyositis [17]

A syndrome which is typical of polymyositis, and which may be associated with skin changes indistinguishable from dermatomyositis, can,

rarely, accompany cancer. All types of tumours have been reported in association. It is often stated that polymyositis in a middle-aged patient should lead to an extensive search for a cancer, which may at that stage be clinically inapparent. On the other hand, the likelihood of an occult, localized and remediable tumour being discovered is small, only 10—15% of cases being associated with a neoplasm, and by no means all curable. One therefore has to judge the extent to which investigation should be undertaken in each patient. A cancer is much more likely to be present in men over the age of 50 and when the syndrome is dermatomyositis. In this group bronchial carcinoma is by far the commonest associated malignancy. A reasonable policy is to carry out a minimum of investigations in middle-aged patients presenting with dermatomyositis. These would include chest X-ray, acid phosphatase and abdominal ultrasound in a man and pelvic ultrasound and mammograms additionally in a woman. Clinical pointers such as rectal or vaginal bleeding or persistent cough should of course be further investigated.

The syndromes are characterized by symmetrical proximal muscle weakness which is slowly progressive. The skin changes consist of facial erythema and oedema especially over the nose and around the eyes. The chronic contractures and calcification typical of the childhood disease do not usually have time to occur. Steroids produce temporary improvement. Where possible, the underlying cancer should be treated.

Hypertrophic pulmonary osteoarthropathy

Nowadays, bronchogenic carcinoma is almost exclusively the cause of this uncommon syndrome although it can occur with lung metastases. The periosteum at the ends of the long bones (tibia, fibula, radius and ulna especially) is raised, thickened and inflamed and periosteal new bone formation is shown by a typical layer of calcification parallel to, and 2—3 mm above, the periosteal surface of the bone. The neighbouring joints may be hot and swollen and clubbing is usually present. The pathogenesis of the syndrome is unknown, but it may regress on treatment or removal of the cancer. A rare form of the syndrome may be associated with features of acromegaly, with raised growth hormone levels in the plasma.

Polyarthritis [18]

An asymmetrical polyarthritis is a rare complication of many types of cancer. The differential diagnosis is from rheumatoid arthritis, but tests for rheumatoid factor are negative and the arthritis is less erosive. The syndrome may subside with removal of the tumour. An SLE-like syndrome has also been reported in association with lymphoma.

DERMATOLOGICAL SYNDROMES

The skin manifestations of malignancy are extremely varied (Table 9.2). First, the skin may be infiltrated by primary or secondary cancer. Second, it may be indirectly affected by general

Table 9.2a Non-metastatic dermatological manifestations of malignancy

Tumour	Syndrome
Metabolic	
Hyperpigmentation	MSH-producing carcinoma (usually bronchial)
Erythema	Carcinoid, glucagonoma
Fat necrosis	Pancreatic carcinoma
Eruptions associated with cancer	
Acanthosis nigricans	Adenocarcinomas, lymphomas
Dermatomyositis	Most cancers
Hypertrichosis	Adenocarcinomas
Thrombophlebitis	Adenocarcinomas
Thrombophlebitis migrans	Adenocarcinomas especially pancreas and ovary
Erythroderma	Lymphomas
Pyoderma gangrenosum	Myeloproliferative syndromes, leukaemia, myeloma
Bullous eruptions	Many neoplasms
Generalized pruritus	
	Lymphoma, leukaemia, polycythaemia

Table 9.2b Inherited disease (associated with cancer and with non-malignant skin lesions)

Gardner's syndrome: epidermal cysts and dermoids with multiple colonic polyps leading to carcinoma

Neurofibromatosis: neurofibromas, café au lait patches and other skin lesions, with sarcomatous change, medullary carcinoma of thyroid and phaeochromocytoma

Tylosis palmaris: hyperkeratosis of palms and soles with oesophageal cancer

Peutz—Jeghers syndrome: buccal, oral and digital pigmentation with multiple intestinal polyps leading uncommonly to gut carcinomas, ovarian tumours

Ataxia-telangiectasia: Telangiectases on neck, face, behind elbows and knees with cerebellar ataxia, IgA deficiency and increased incidence of lymphoma and leukaemia

Chediak—Higashi syndrome: defective skin and hair colour, recurrent infections, high incidence of lymphoma and leukaemia

Wiskott—Aldrich syndrome: eczema, purpura, pyoderma, thrombocytopenia, low IgM, leukaemia and lymphoma

Tuberose sclerosis: adenoma sebaceum on cheeks, mental retardation and epilepsy. Hamartomas and astrocytoma

Bloom's syndrome: photosensitive light eruptions, facial erythema, dwarfism, leukaemia, squamous cell carcinoma of the skin

Adult progeria (Werner's syndrome): thickened tight skin, soft tissue calcification, growth retardation; soft tissue sarcomas

Fanconi's anaemia: patchy hyperpigmentation, skeletal abnormalities, anaemia leading to acute myelomonocytic leukaemia metabolic consequences of cancer at other sites (e.g. due to obstructive jaundice or steatorrhoea). Third, some inherited disorders are associated with skin manifestations and an increased likelihood of developing cancer. Finally, some skin eruptions are non-specific manifestations of internal malignancy. Some of these (such as dermatomyositis and thrombophlebitis) have previously been described in this chapter. The following is a brief account of some dermatological syndromes not discussed elsewhere.

Acanthosis nigricans

This is a brown/black eruption in the armpits, groins and on the trunk which has a velvety surface and multiple papillary outgrowths. A familial form occurs which is not associated with cancer, and the syndrome can develop without any underlying malignancy in middle age. However, when it occurs in adult life, a cancer is often present, usually an adenocarcinoma and often a gastric neoplasm. Lymphomas are also associated. The skin lesion may antedate the cancer, and when it recurs after treatment, may herald a recurrence.

Hypertrichosis (lanuginosa acquisita)

Very rarely an adenocarcinoma of the lung, breast, or gut, or a bladder carcinoma, may be associated with lanugo, which is fine downy hair on the face, trunk or limbs. The syndrome may be associated with acanthosis nigricans or ichthyosis. The hair growth does not usually regress after treatment of the primary tumour.

Erythroderma

A generalized, red, maculo-papular rash may complicate cancer and the underlying disease is nearly always a lymphoma. The condition may progress to exfoliative dermatitis. Control of the underlying lymphoma is essential in treatment. As the rash fades it becomes slightly scaly and bran-coloured. Relapses of the lymphoma may result in further skin rash.

Pyoderma gangrenosum

This is an infrequent complication of malignancy and can occur with other diseases such as ulcerative colitis. The lesions start as red nodules and then expand rapidly, breaking down in the centre to form necrotic, painful, infected ulcers with a rolled, erythematous edge. Although the condition responds to steroids, the dose needed is usually very high. An underlying lymphoma or myeloproliferative syndrome is the most commonly associated malignancy and the skin lesion may regress with successful treatment of the tumour.

Bullous eruptions

Very uncommonly, typical bullous pemphigoid and dermatitis herpetiformis are associated with underlying cancers.

Ichthyosis

Hodgkin's disease and other lymphomas are occasionally associated with thickened and flaking skin with hyperkeratosis of the palms and soles. Histologically there may be epidermal atrophy or hyperkeratosis. Tylosis palmaris is an inherited hyperkeratosis of the palms associated with oesophageal cancer.

Alopecia

Patchy alopecia occasionally accompanies lymphoma (usually Hodgkin's disease). There may be follicular mucinosis. The disorder may be self-limiting.

Generalized pruritus

Occasionally patients present with a generalized itching without any rash. Although cancer is not a frequent cause of this problem, it is an important one and the itching may precede the clinical appearance of the tumour, sometimes by a few years.

Hodgkin's disease is one of the commonest cancers to be associated and the itching can, in this disease, become intolerable. Pruritus is usually worse at night, and in the case of polycythaemia, worse after a hot bath. Lung, colon, breast, stomach and prostate are other sites to bear in mind. Effective treatment of the cancer will often alleviate the condition and will certainly do so in Hodgkin's disease.

NEPHROTIC SYNDROME

The kidney may be involved by cancer in many ways but non-metastatic manifestations are unusual, apart from amyloidosis complicating myeloma (see Chapter 27). Massive proteinuria leading to nephrotic syndrome may occur as a direct result of glomerular damage [19]. In the elderly especially, a small proportion of patients with membranous glomerulonephritis have an underlying cancer, removal of which results in remission of the renal lesion. The cancer is usually an adenocarcinoma (breast, colon, stomach). Hodgkin's disease is also associated although here there is usually minimal-change glomerulonephritis. In membranous lesions it is thought that complexes of tumour products and antibody are deposited in the glomeruli.

REFERENCES

1 Bodel P. Tumours and fever. *Annals of the New York Academy of Science* 1974; **230**: 6—13.
2 Blackman M.R., Rosen S.W., Weintraub B.D. Ectopic hormones. *Advances in Internal Medicine* 1978; **23**: 85—113.
3 Richardson R.L., Greco F.A., Oldham R.K., Liddle G.W. Tumour products and potential markers in small cell lung cancer. *Seminars in Oncology* 1978; **5**: 253—62.
4 Hansen M., Hansen H.H., Hirsch F.R. *et al.* Hormonal polypeptides and amine metabolites in small cell carcinoma of the lung with special reference to stage and subtypes. *Cancer* 1980; **45**: 1432—37.
5 Chandalia H.B., Boshell B.R. Hypoglycaemia associated with extra-pancreatic tumors. *Archives of International Medicine* 1972; **129**: 447—56.
6 Muggia F.M., Rosen S.W., Weintraub B.D., Hansen H.H. Ectopic placental proteins in nontrophoblastic tumors. Serial measurements following chemotherapy. *Cancer* 1975; **36**: 1327—37.
7 Odell W.D., Wolfsen A.R. Humoral syndromes associated with cancer. *Annual Review of Medicine* 1978; **29**: 379—406.
8 Hammond D., Winnick S. Paraneoplastic erythrocytosis and ectopic erythropoiesis. *Annals of the New York Academy of Sciences* 1974; **230**: 219—27.
9 Colman R.W., Robboy S.J., Minna J.D. Disseminated intravascular coagulation: a reappraisal. *Annual Review of Medicine* 1979; **30**: 359—74.
10 Antman K.H., Skarin A.T., Mayer R.J. *et al.* Microangiopathic haemolytic anaemia and cancer. A review. *Medicine* 1979; **58**: 377—84.
11 Croft P.B., Urich H., Wilkinson M. Peripheral neuropathy of sensorimotor type associated with malignant disease. *Brain* 1967; **90**: 31—66.
12 Grans F., Eklon K.B., Cordon-Cardoc, Posner J.B. Sensory neuropathy and small cell lung cancer: antineurone antibody that also reacts with the tumour. *American Journal of Medicine* 1985; **80**: 45—52.
13 Handforth A., Nag S., Sharp D., Robertson D.M. Paraneoplastic sub-acute necrotic myelopathy. *Canadian Journal of Neurological Science* 1983; **10**: 204—7.
14 Brennan L.V., Craddock P.R. Limbic encephalopathy as a non metastatic complication of small cell lung cancer. *American Journal of Medicine* 1983; **75**: 518—20.
15 Weiner L.P., Hernden R.M., Nareayan O. *et al.* Virus related to SV40 in patients with progressive multifocal leucoencephalopathy. *New England Journal of Medicine* 1972; **286**: 385—90.
16 O'Neill J.H., Murray N.M.F., Newsom Davis J. The Lambert—Eaton myasthenic syndrome: a review of 50 cases. *Brain* 1988; **III**: 577—96.
17 Barnes B.E. Dermatomyositis and malignancy. A review of the literature. *Annals of Internal Medicine* 1976; **84**: 68—76.
18 Calabro J. Cancer and arthritis. *Arthritis and Rheumatism* 1967; **10**: 553—67.
19 Gagliano R.G., Costanzi J.J., Beathard G.A., Sarles H.E., Bell J.D. The nephrotic syndrome associated with neoplasia: An unusual paraneoplastic syndrome. *American Journal of Medicine* 1976; **60**: 1026—31.

Chapter 10
Cancer of the Head and Neck

INTRODUCTION, AETIOLOGY AND EPIDEMIOLOGY

Carcinomas of the upper air and food passages are a varied and important group of tumours with particular epidemiological features. They pose exceptionally difficult management problems, and together account for approximately 4% of all carcinomas in Britain. Table 10.1 shows mortality from cancers of the commonest sites and Fig. 10.1 shows age-specific incidence rates.

Important aetiological factors include excessive intake of tobacco either by smoking or chewing (a common practice in many parts of Asia and India where, as a result, oral cancer is among the commonest of all tumours). Alcohol, particularly spirit, ingestion is also an important contributing agent. In the past, syphilitic leucoplakia was an important predisposing factor in carcinoma of the tongue. Dental or mechanical trauma have also been incriminated, but with improvements in oral and dental hy-

giene these factors are perhaps less important today [1]. The Paterson–Kelly (Plummer–Vinson) syndrome of chronic anaemia, glossitis and oesophageal web appears to predispose to postcricoid carcinoma, particularly in women. More recently, adenocarcinoma of the nasal cavity has been described in hardwood workers in the furniture industry. Several clusters have now been reported.

Important racial differences have also emerged, particularly in relation to carcinoma of the nasopharynx, commonly seen in the Chinese and in particular those of the Mongolian race. It is especially common in Hong Kong and south China, and in male Formosans it is much the most common cause of death, three times the rate of any other neoplasm. It is also common in the Philippines, Malaysia, Greenland, Malta, North Africa and Saudi Arabia. Curiously, it may develop in far younger patients than typically occurs with other head and neck cancers. There appears to be a bimodal age distribution with 20% of all cases (in high-prevalence areas) recognized in patients (usually male) under the age of 30 years. Environmental agents have been suggested, including dietary factors such as salted fish and vegetables which are popular amongst many Chinese, Eskimos and North Africans. Case–control studies in Chinese patients have suggested a link between salt fish consumption and incidence of nasopharyngeal carcinoma [2].

Apart from possible dietary causes of nasopharyngeal carcinoma, it is also known that patients with this condition generally have evidence of Epstein–Barr virus genome in the

Table 10.1 Annual mortality (England and Wales) from major sites of cancer of the head and neck

Site	Males	Females
Lip	42	9
Tongue	206	141
Oral cavity	188	106
Pharynx	422	293
Nose, middle ear and sinuses	143	113
Larynx	608	149

Modified from data supplied for years 1971–78, from OPCS Monitor, DH1 80/3, 11.11.1980.

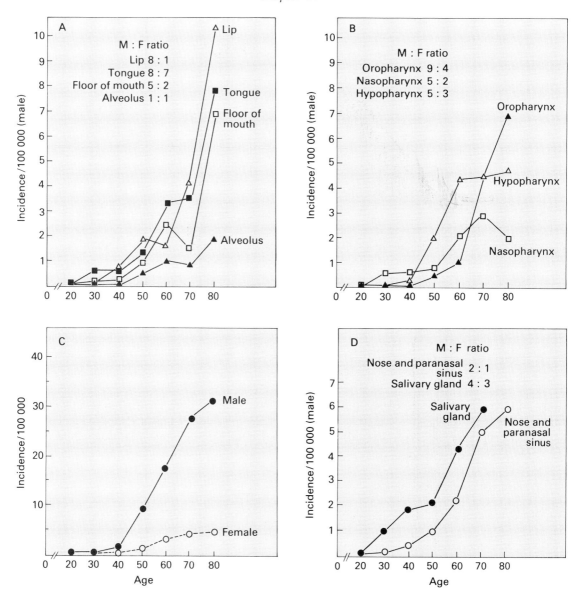

Fig. 10.1 Age-specific incidence for cancers of the head and neck. (A) Oral cavity (male); (B) pharynx (male); (C) larynx (male and female); (D) nose and paranasal sinuses, and salivary gland (male).

epithelial tumour cells [3] and a characteristic EBV antibody pattern. There is generally a rise in IgA and IgG anti viral capsid antigen (VCA) and EBV-associated nuclear antigens (EBVNA).

In head and neck cancers generally, there is a male predisposition (except possibly for postcricoid carcinomas), with a common male : female ratio of 3 : 1. For some sites, notably carcinoma of the larynx, the male : female ratio has been reportedly as high as 10 : 1. Data from the Thames Cancer Registry of London indicate that if the heavily sex-determined laryngeal cancers are excluded, the true male : female ratio for other sites is approximately 2 : 1.

Improvements in dental and oral hygiene, coupled with reductions in intake of spirits and cigarette consumption have led to a falling incidence of cancers of the head and neck. In 1987, the number of new cases in the United States was 42 000 with an age-adjusted incidence rate of 17.2 per 100 000 for white males and 5.6 per 100 000 for white females. Approximately 40% of these tumours prove fatal. In Britain, Scandinavia, Germany, Japan and Israel the figure is somewhat lower, but elsewhere in North-West Europe (France, Switzerland, Italy and Scotland) the death rate is slightly higher. These survival figures may correlate with alcohol intake.

PATHOLOGY

The overwhelming majority of these tumours are squamous cell carcinomas, though the frequency of other histological types and the degree of differentiation varies markedly with site. Nasopharyngeal carcinoma is clearly an exception and indeed differs from other head and neck cancers in a number of ways. For example, in one large series the commonest tumours were anaplastic and squamous cell carcinomas, though lymphoepitheliomas (undifferentiated squamous cell carcinomas), malignant lymphomas, adenoid cystic carcinomas (cylindromas) and plasmacytomas were also seen, as well as rarer tumours such as melanoma or undifferentiated sarcoma. Together these constituted a significant group of carcinomas of non-squamous origin amounting to almost 30% of all cases [4]. By contrast, in a series of over 2000 cases of carcinoma of the larynx, 95% were squamous showing varying degrees of differentiation and including 97 patients with carcinoma *in situ*. Interestingly, some 20% or more of patients with head and neck carcinomas develop multiple primary lesions, most notably within the oral cavity.

Malignant lymphomas can arise anywhere within the head and neck but particularly from Waldeyer's ring. In such cases special care should be taken to establish the correct histo-logical diagnosis since prognosis and management of lymphomas is very different from epithelial carcinoma.

CLINICAL STAGING

Although no staging system is entirely satisfactory, careful staging is essential, both as a reminder to carry out full clinical and radiological assessment in each case, and also in order to develop logical treatment strategies and to attempt worthwhile documentation for comparison of cases. In Europe, the UICC proposals for standard TNM staging have gained wide acceptance [5]. This has been facilitated by the adoption of the same staging notation for lymph node spread regardless of the primary head and neck site. New guidelines for staging of neck nodes were issued in 1987 (Table 10.2). Unfortunately this uniformity of notation has not been possible for T staging, where some primary sites are still staged according to their spread (see Table 10.3 and Table 10.4 for examples).

In all cases, routine assessment and staging should include careful inspection of the primary site with measurement of its dimensions and examination for direct extension into adjacent tissues and local lymph node areas. Although a reasonable attempt at clinical examination and staging can be made in the out-patient clinic, often using indirect laryngoscopy and nasopharyngoscopy with mirror techniques, most patients require an examination under anaesthetic with direct endoscopic evaluation of the upper food and air passages, before firm conclusions can be drawn. This is particularly true of nasopharyngeal carcinoma, since mirror examination of the postnasal space can be demanding for the patient, and unreliable even in the hands of an expert. Out-patient nasendoscopy has also become standard practice in the past 5 years and has proven extremely valuable. Histological confirmation must ideally be obtained in every case of head and neck cancer and can usually be performed at endoscopy under general anaesthesia, though more accessible lesions, such as those in the oral cavity, can

Table 10.2 Current UICC staging system in nasopharyngeal carcinoma

T stage	N stage	M stage
T_x not assessed	N_x not assessed	M_x not assessed
T_0 no primary found in nasopharynx	N_0 no palpable lymph nodes	M_0 no distant metastases
T_1 one site within nasopharynx, or positive biopsy	N_1 N < 3 cm ipsilateral	M_1 distant metastases present
T_2 two sites within nasopharynx	N_2 N 3–6 cm ipsi- or bilateral	
T_3 extension to nasal cavity or oropharynx	N_3 N > 6 cm	
T_4 invasion of skull, or cranial nerve involvement		

Table 10.3 Histological classification of pharyngeal cancer

	Nasopharynx (%)	Oropharynx (%)	Laryngopharynx (%)
Squamous cell carcinoma:			
well-differentiated	21	60	75
anaplastic	42	12	13
Lymphoma	20	15	0
Others (including unbiopsied cases)	17	13	12

From Lederman and Mould [4]. With permission.

occasionally be diagnosed and staged without undertaking this procedure.

Investigation

Plain, tomographic and computed tomographic (CT) radiography are of great value. In carcinomas of the larynx and hypopharynx, for example, the soft tissue lateral X-ray of the neck often gives a useful indication of the anatomical extent of the lesion, particularly when coupled with coronal or sagittal tomography, which may show more extensive spread than is obvious clinically. This is particularly valuable in subglottic tumours of the larynx, where extension or origin of the lesion may be difficult to assess even with direct inspection under anaesthetic. The advent of CT scanning has made a dramatic impact on the accuracy with which deep-seated lesions can now be visualized, particularly those of the nasopharynx, parotid gland, retro-orbital area and paranasal sinuses, and where there is involvement of the skull base or other evidence of bony erosion (Fig. 10.2).

Haematogenous spread is uncommon at presentation, but when it does occur the lungs are the most common site of spread. The risk is highest with advanced tumours, and in particular, in cases of nasopharyngeal carcinoma. A chest X-ray should always be performed and will also disclose the occasional simultaneous carcinoma of the bronchus. A routine blood count and liver function tests should also be performed.

Epithelial carcinomas of the head and neck region are best managed jointly by a surgeon and a radiotherapist with particular interest in this area, since they present technical problems

Table 10.4 Staging of nodes and metastases in head and neck cancers

Regional lymph nodes

The definitions of the N categories for all head and neck sites except thyroid gland are:

N — Regional lymph nodes

N_X Regional lymph nodes cannot be assessed
N_0 No regional lymph node metastasis
N_1 Metastasis in a single ipsilateral lymph node, 3 cm or less in greatest dimension
N_2 Metastasis in a single ipsilateral lymph node, more than 3 cm but not more than 6 cm in greatest dimension, or in multiple ipsilateral lymph nodes, none more than 6 cm in greatest dimension, or in bilateral or contralateral lymph nodes, none more than 6 cm in greatest dimension
   N_{2a} Metastasis in a single ipsilateral lymph node, more than 3 cm but not more than 6 cm in greatest dimension
   N_{2b} Metastasis in multiple ipsilateral lymph nodes, not more than 6 cm in greatest dimension
   N_{2c} Metastasis in bilateral or contralateral lymph nodes, none more than 6 cm in greatest dimension
N_3 Metastasis in a lymph node more than 6 cm in greatest dimension

Distant metastasis

The definitions of the M categories for all head and neck sites are:

M — Distant metastasis

M_X Presence of distant metastasis cannot be assessed
M_0 No distant metastasis
M_1 Distant metastasis

of management unequalled by those at any other site. Because of the extreme variation in presentation, natural history, and response to treatment, this chapter only gives a brief outline of general principles of management; for those with a particular interest specialist texts can be recommended [6].

CARCINOMA OF THE LARYNX

Carcinomas of the larynx form the largest single group and there has been a fascinating and rapid evolution of ideas in management over the past century [7]. Although the first laryngectomy for carcinoma is generally credited to Billroth in 1873, laryngofissure for tumour excision was performed 3 years before the invention and development of the laryngeal mirror.

The human larynx is an unusually complex organ (Fig. 10.3) combining the role of a protective sphincter largely responsible for keeping the lower respiratory tract free from foreign bodies, with the highly sophisticated function of speech production. This demands extraordinary precision in the tone of the laryngeal musculature and in the approximation of the vocal cords themselves.

Laryngeal cancer accounts for about 2–3% of all malignant disease, but the distress it causes is disproportionately high because of the severe social consequences of loss of speech. Indeed, the quality of voice and speech production is an important factor in choice of treatment [8]. The larynx is sufficiently accessible to be viewed directly with ease, using mirror techniques (indirect laryngoscopy), nasendoscopy or by direct vision under anaesthesia. It contains epithelial and mesodermal tissue components which lend themselves well to the study of radiation effects on both normal and abnormal tissues. For these reasons, the larynx has always been of particular interest to the radiotherapist.

Of the aetiological factors previously mentioned, cigarette smoking is undoubtedly the most important. It almost certainly accounts for the male predominance of this disease, and there is a known correlation between precancerous laryngeal mucosal changes and the number of cigarettes smoked. The rise in incidence of laryngeal carcinoma has been shown to parallel the rising incidence of carcinoma of the bronchus, and in patients cured of early laryngeal carcinoma but continuing to smoke, carcinoma of the bronchus has become the commonest cause of death.

Hoarseness is the principal and often the only symptom, and any patient with hoarseness of more than 3 weeks duration should be

Fig. 10.2 CT scanning in head and neck tumours. (A) CT scan through nose and paranasal sinuses showing a large tumour of left maxilla with extensive local invasion and bone destruction (see also Fig. 4.5); (B) CT scan through orbits showing large left-sided tumour (arrowed) displacing the globe forwards and downwards.

referred for immediate laryngoscopy since early (T_{1-2} N_0) carcinomas can almost always be cured by radiotherapy (see below). *Dysphagia* is much less common, though important in patients with supraglottic carcinoma, particularly when there is extension to the oropharynx.

Dyspnoea, sometimes with stridor, is a feature of subglottic carcinomas where early obstruction is the rule and immediate tracheostomy frequently required before definitive management can be undertaken.

Carcinomas can arise from any of the three

Fig. 10.3 Anatomy of the larynx. (A) From above; (B) coronal plane; (C) median sagittal plane. 1. True vocal cord; 2. false vocal cord; 3. thyroid cartilage; 4. laryngeal ventricle; 5. cricoid cartilage; 6. arytenoid; 7. epiglottis; 8. subglottic area; 9. base of tongue.

anatomical regions of the larynx, though not with equal frequency (Fig. 10.4). Lesions of the glottis are much the commonest, followed by supraglottic and finally subglottic cancers. Though early supraglottic cancer is uncommon in Britain these tumours are commoner than cancer of the glottis in some parts of Europe including Spain, Italy and Finland. In glottic lesions, the commonest site is the anterior third of the cord, often with extension to anterior or (more rarely) the posterior commissure. The whole cord can, however, be involved. Direct spread can take place upwards via the laryngeal ventricle to the false cord and then to the remainder of the supraglottic region; or downwards directly to the subglottic area. Lymph node metastases are uncommon in early glottic carcinoma since the lymphatic drainage of the true cord is so sparse, but prognosis is highly dependent on the T stage. Most patients with T_1 and T_2 tumours are curable, whereas the majority of T_3 and T_4 lesions are not. Tumours of the epiglottis are usually advanced at presentation because there is little anatomical hindrance to direct tumour extension, particu-

larly into the pre-epiglottic space. They do not cause hoarseness initially, and may elude diagnosis at laryngoscopy particularly if the tumour arises on the inferior surface.

Management and prognosis

CARCINOMA OF THE GLOTTIS

Radiotherapy cures at least 75% of patients where the vocal cord remains mobile (T_1, over 90% and T_2, 65%). Where failure occurs with radiotherapy treatment, salvage surgery is curative in over half of all cases. Total laryngectomy is usually necessary but some cases can be treated successfully by partial laryngectomy with preservation of the voice, particularly if the initial tumour was well localized. Although conservative surgery (usually by partial vertical laryngectomy) can deal effectively with most early glottic carcinomas, the resulting voice is inferior to what can be achieved with radiotherapy. In these early cases, there are few drawbacks to radiotherapy, particularly since the field of treatment is small (often only 5 × 5 cm) with no need — at least in T_1 tumours — to irradiate local lymph node areas because of the rarity of nodal involvement.

Treatment of the *advanced* case is more difficult, and always requires full discussion between surgeon and radiotherapist. Surgery may sometimes be required as an emergency procedure, particularly with subglottic extension. Many centres still employ a policy of planned radiotherapy and surgery in combination for the majority of these advanced lesions, especially if there is evidence of cartilage invasion, perichondritis, extralaryngeal spread, or nodal metastases where the ultimate prospect for cure is so poor. In many centres, a pre-operative radiation dose of 40 Gy (4000 rad) in daily fractions over a 4-week period is followed by an attempt at surgical removal of all gross tumour about 4 weeks later. However, in other clinics, radiotherapy in combination with multi-agent chemotherapy has replaced this approach (see below), reserving 'salvage'

Sites

Supraglottis 35%

Glottis 57%

Subglottis 8%

TNM Staging

T_{is} Carcinoma *in situ*
T_1 Confined to site of origin
T_2 Involves adjacent site: mobile
T_3 Spread within larynx, with fixation
T_4 Beyond larynx

See Table 10.4 for N-staging

Fig. 10.4 Relative frequency and TNM staging system in laryngeal cancer.

surgery for cases in which non-surgical treatment had been unsuccessful. This approach has become more widely practised in recent years, and has led to a higher proportion of patients cured of the carcinoma yet with retention of the larynx and satisfactory speech production [9]. As with many tumours, adverse prognostic factors such as fixation of the primary tumour, early local invasion, extrinsic spread and lymph node metastasis are interrelated and often occur together. For the majority of these patients, even the most intensive combinations of surgery, radiotherapy and chemotherapy will fail to cure, and the ultimate 5-year survival rate for T_3 lesions is about 25%.

CARCINOMA OF THE SUPRAGLOTTIS

These tumours are more difficult to treat. They often present late because early symptoms are few. Dysphagia may not develop until ulceration and local extension takes place. Both local invasion and lymph node involvement are more common than with glottic carcinomas, and almost a quarter of supraglottic lesions extend down to the glottis. By locally invading in other directions, these tumours frequently involve the oropharynx (particularly the posterior third of the tongue) and the hypopharynx (particularly the pyriform fossa). For early lesions, a policy of radical irradiation with salvage surgery (total laryngectomy) where required (as for glottic tumours) is currently adopted in most centres, though surgery may be preferable for accessible lesions, such as those at the tip of the epiglottis. Conservative surgery is not normally undertaken for supraglottic carcinoma. An important difference in radiotherapy technique between treatment of this region and the true glottis is that the radiation fields should routinely include the local lymph node areas, since clinical and occult lymph node metastases are common [10]. For more advanced supraglottic lesions, the combination of total laryngectomy with pre-operative radiotherapy has traditionally been employed. Although this policy can be successful when wide field laryn-

gectomy and a full dose of radiotherapy are routinely used, the morbidity is considerable. In expert hands, a 5-year survival rate of 60% has been achieved but at the cost of performing a number of laryngectomies only to find that on histological examination the pre-operative radiation has already produced a probable cure. For this reason it may be preferable to withhold surgery until there is evidence of recurrence or residual disease after radiation.

CARCINOMA OF THE SUBGLOTTIS

The outlook is much less satisfactory with these difficult tumours. In many cases there will be vocal cord fixation at the time of diagnosis, and invasion of the cricoid cartilage is common. Involvement of the thyroid gland or paratracheal lymph nodes is frequent, possibly in as many as 65% of cases, and surgical excision, if undertaken, must be radical. Such operations, which may have to include removal of the manubrium, dissection of paratracheal lymph nodes and total thyroidectomy, are performed less often nowadays, in favour of a planned combination of radiotherapy and chemotherapy, with surgery reserved for residual or recurrent disease.

CONSERVATIVE SURGERY IN LARYNGEAL CANCER

Although long-term survival in patients with laryngeal cancer has remained unchanged for the past 20 years, the quality of life of survivors has improved considerably. Where surgery proves necessary in radiotherapy failures, there has been increasing interest in conservation techniques where the purpose is to ensure control of the primary lesion whilst at the same time offering the patient some chance of reasonable speech production. With *horizontal* supraglottic laryngectomy (Fig. 10.5), the upper part of the larynx is removed but the cords preserved. At *vertical* partial laryngectomy, the surgeon removes one vocal cord, the false cord and the vocal process of the arytenoid with part of

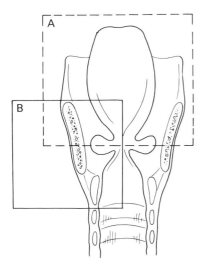

Fig. 10.5 Conservative laryngectomy operations in laryngeal cancer. (A) Horizontal supraglottic laryngectomy; (B) vertical partial laryngectomy.

the adjacent thyroid cartilage, and if necessary up to one-third of the contralateral vocal cord. Success in these procedures lies in accurate evaluation of tumour extent even though pre-operative assessment can never be completely reliable. None the less the case for conservative surgery, particularly in supraglottic lesions, has been argued more strongly over the past few years.

REHABILITATION

Following any type of laryngectomy, and particularly after total laryngectomy, social rehabilitation is of great importance (see Chapter 7, p. 125), and all surgeons and radio-therapists working with these patients are aware of the immense contribution made by the speech therapist. With the appropriate training of oesophageal voice technique and stoma care, most patients who have undergone total laryngectomy can look forward to a full and enjoyable life, usually with an adequate voice. Although this is difficult to define, the ability to speak on the telephone is often used as an important criterion.

Permanent vocal rehabilitation prostheses are now used more frequently in patients who find it difficult to develop adequate oesophageal speech. These devices contain valves which, for some patients, offer a striking improvement in voice quality. An example is the Blom–Singer valve, which requires a permanent pharyngeal puncture with placement of a small tube which is brought forward to the skin of the anterior neck. By occluding the opening with a finger, many patients can produce adequate speech, although care of the valve can be difficult and high standards of personal hygiene must be observed.

CARCINOMA OF THE PHARYNX

Anatomy and patterns of metastasis

The pharynx is best considered as a passage with two distal sphincters serving the function of channelling both food and air in the right directions, namely to the digestive and respiratory passages. It is only by laryngeal constriction that the respiratory tract is effectively closed during deglutition, protecting the trachea and bronchi from inhalation of food or foreign bodies. The pharynx has three concentric coats: an internal mucous membrane, a supporting fibrous tunica and a muscular coat with a series of deficiencies for entry of vessels and nerves. These defects are important because they are the principal sites through which malignant tumours of the pharynx spread to adjacent tissues, particularly lymph nodes, in the neck.

Anatomically, the pharynx is usually described in three contiguous parts (Fig. 10.6). The *naso-pharynx* is situated behind the nasal cavity and extends from the base of the skull above to the superior aspect of the soft palate below. It is bounded posteriorly by prevertebral fascia, and extends anteriorly to the junction of the hard and soft palate. The *oropharynx* is situated behind the oral cavity, extends inferiorly to the floor of the vallecula sulcus and includes the posterior third of tongue, vallecula, soft palate, uvula, faucial pillars and tonsils. The

Fig. 10.6 Anatomical divisions of the pharynx.

Fig. 10.7 Lymphatic drainage of the head and neck. 1. Jugulo-digastric; 2. jugulo-omohyoid; 3. deep cervical; 4. submental; 5. submandibular; 6. pre-auricular; 7. parotid; 8. postauricular; 9. occipital; 10. posterior triangle; 11. supraclavicular.

laryngopharynx or *hypopharynx* is situated behind the larynx, extending from the floor of the vallecula sulcus above to the level of the lower border of the cricoid cartilage below, where it joins the oesophagus. It includes the pyriform fossae, posterior pharyngeal wall and postcricoid area. The whole pharynx has a rich lymphatic drainage and early nodal involvement is common, with a predictable clinical pattern (Fig. 10.7). The important but inaccessible node of Rouvière is situated in the lateral retropharyngeal area, closely related to the jugular foramen and situated over the lateral masses of the atlas. Its importance lies in its critical position, making it an early site of invasion, particularly by nasopharyngeal tumours.

The relative frequency and the histological variation of neoplasms in the three pharyngeal sites, is shown in Table 10.3. Lymphomas most commonly arise in the oropharynx (particularly the tonsil) and nasopharynx. Nasopharyngeal carcinomas are more frequently anaplastic than

well-differentiated, which is the reverse of the position with oropharyngeal and hypopharyngeal carcinomas. There are also important differences in the probability of lymph node involvement at presentation. Three-quarters of all nasopharyngeal lesions present with obvious lymphadenopathy, whereas in hypopharyngeal cancer, almost half of all cases are clinically free of nodes.

CARCINOMA OF THE NASOPHARYNX

Although relatively uncommon in the Western world, these tumours are the commonest of all malignant tumours in many parts of China, accounting in some areas for half or more of all cancers (see p. 8). Clinical staging is more difficult than in any other of the head and neck sites, because of the inaccessibility of the lesion and its drainage routes. The TNM staging system is now widely used.

Cancers of the nasopharynx often have an insidious onset and tend to present late, often with nodal disease in the neck. Nasal obstruction, usually unilateral, and secretory otitis media are also common presenting features. Because of the close proximity of the nasopharynx to the base of the skull, many patients present with cranial nerve involvement, particularly nerves III−VI, since these pass through the cavernous sinus which the tumour frequently invades. The IX−XII nerves may also be involved by direct tumour extension where they pass through the parapharyngeal space in proximity to the lateral nasopharyngeal wall. Cranial nerve involvement usually implies bony destruction of part of the base of the skull. Other extrapharyngeal sites include the paranasal sinuses, nasal cavity, orbit and middle ear. Involvement of these regions causes pain, nasal stuffiness or discharge, unilateral deafness and ophthalmoplegia.

Treatment is by radical radiotherapy. In order to encompass the likely local extension of disease, particularly when lymph node involvement is known to be present (i.e. in the majority of cases), the irradiation volume must be large. This must be achieved without any concession in total dosage, which should be at least 60 Gy (6000 rad) delivered within 6−6½ weeks. Higher doses may be delivered to the primary site but the many challenging technical difficulties include avoidance of the upper part of the spinal cord and temporal lobe of the brain (both of which have limited radiation tolerance yet are unavoidably included in the treatment portals), as well as the minimization of mucosal reaction as far as possible. The classical approach of Lederman (Fig. 10.8) is still widely employed and aims at non-uniform high-dose irradiation to the primary and bilateral cervical nodes. Lateral and anterior fields are employed, with appropriate shielding and field changes to avoid dangerous overtreatment of the upper cervical spinal cord without compromising the dosage to the lymph nodes. Even with this technique, a small portion (usually about 4 cm) of the spinal cord is treated to a dose of 50 Gy

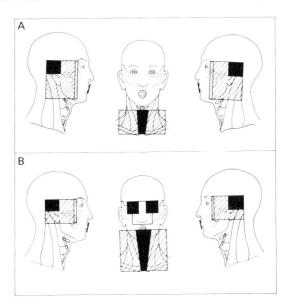

Fig. 10.8 Radiation field arrangement for radical treatment of carcinoma of the nasopharynx. (A) First phase of treatment (40 Gy in 4 weeks); (B) second phase of treatment (to 60 Gy total dose in 6 weeks). (From Lederman and Mould [4]. With permission.)

(5000 rad), and treatment complications will be inevitable in some cases. Other complications of treatment such as perichondritis or radionecrosis are uncommon with careful fractionation and avoidance of over-dosage. A sensible dental policy is required, and it is important to avoid removal of teeth during or shortly after treatment. Local shielding to sensitive areas such as the cornea and buccal cavity can often be safely achieved, and penumbra trimming is also important when using equipment with poorly defined beam margins (see Chapter 5). It is generally accepted that surgery has no place other than biopsy of the primary lesion, and occasionally in removal of residual lymph node disease by block dissection if the primary appears controlled.

Results of treatment are closely related to stage (Table 10.2); median disease-free 5-year survival, even in patients with early disease, is less than 50%. The largest single group ($T_2N_{0−1}$), with an intermediate prognosis, have a 5-year disease-free survival of about 30%. A significant number of patients alive at 5 years will ultimately die of recurrence, and prolonged control followed by late relapse is common in this tumour. With $T_{3-4}N_{2-3}$ disease very few patients survive 5 years. Overall 5-year survival is better in younger people and in women. Recent attempts to improve results have included the use of intracavitary caesium implants to increase the dose to the primary site.

CARCINOMA OF THE OROPHARYNX

These are more accessible, and in many ways simpler to treat. The important sites in this area include the soft palate, faucial pillars, tonsil, posterior third of tongue, and pharyngeal wall. The relative incidence of tumours of these sites is shown in Fig. 10.9. TNM staging is now standard for oropharyngeal tumours and is shown in Table 10.5. The presenting symptoms include dysphagia with pain as well as aspiration of liquids. There may also be dysarthria with large tumours of the posterior tongue. The tumour is usually easily visible providing the anterior portion of the tongue is carefully retracted. There may be enlarged cervical lymph nodes. Radiological assessment can be very useful. Plain lateral views of the neck, tomography, barium contrast studies and CT scanning may all help to delineate the tumour.

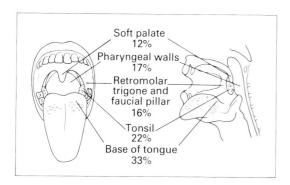

Fig. 10.9 Carcinoma of the oropharynx: relative frequency at different sites.

Table 10.5 TNM staging for oropharyngeal and oral cavity carcinoma

T — Primary tumour

T_{is}	Pre-invasive carcinoma (carcinoma *in situ*)
T_0	No evidence of primary tumour
T_1	Tumour 2 cm or less in its greatest dimension
T_2	Tumour more than 2 cm but not more than 4 cm in its greatest dimension
T_3	Tumour more than 4 cm in its greatest dimension
T_4	Tumour with extension to bone, muscle, skin, antrum, neck, etc.
T_X	The minimum requirements to assess the primary tumour cannot be met

N — Regional lymph nodes
See Table 10.4 for N staging notation

M — Distant metastases

M_0	No evidence of distant metastases
M_1	Evidence of distant metastases
M_X	The minimum requirements to assess the presence of distant metastases cannot be met

Stage grouping

Stage I	T_1	N_0	M_0
Stage II	T_2	N_0	M_0
Stage III	T_3	N_0	M_0
	T_1, T_2, T_3	N_1	M_0
Stage IV	T_4	$N_0.N_1$	M_0
	Any T	$N_2.N_3$	M_0
	Any T	Any N	M_1

There are important differences in the presenting stage of tumours at different sites within the oropharynx; lesions of the tonsillar fossa are more often T_3 and T_4 at presentation than tumours of the retromolar trigone or anterior faucial pillar. Lymph node involvement is common, and again varies with the site. Half of all patients with soft palate, retromolar trigone and anterior faucial pillar tumours have lymph node involvement at presentation, whilst with carcinomas of the tonsil three-quarters of patients have palpable lymph nodes. About 20% of patients with positive nodes have bilateral involvement, and it is common for lymph node enlargement to be the presenting sign, sometimes preceding the primary site by more than a year.

In most centres, combinations of surgery and radiotherapy are routinely used in managing these lesions though increasingly the emphasis has been on radical radiotherapy (sometimes in combination with chemotherapy) with surgery reserved for radiotherapy failures. The radiotherapeutic technique is much simpler than with carcinoma of the nasopharynx since direct extension of tumour can usually be dealt with simply by extension of the field in the appropriate direction. The direct route of spread is via the parapharyngeal space lying between the mandible and the pharynx. More difficult problems arise when there is extension into the hard palate, mandible, tongue or larynx, and these are usually best dealt with by high-dose radiation (with or without chemotherapy), or by surgery if treatment by irradiation and chemotherapy is unable to control the primary tumour. This is also true of lymphatic metastases. *En bloc* radical neck dissection may be required and can even be performed bilaterally if necessary. Despite this, most of the representative series continue to show that a more aggressive surgical attack on the primary does not lead to better control or to a worthwhile improvement in recurrence-free survival [11]. However, a recent large randomized study from Europe [12] has suggested a real advantage in tumour control following hyperfractionated radiotherapy using two fractions of treatment per day (see also Chapter 5).

Surgery and radiation are probably equally effective in controlling both the primary and the node metastases though with a far better functional result in patients treated by radiotherapy. Combined surgery and radiation may be valuable in more advanced tumours, particularly those arising in the anterior faucial pillar. For tonsillar tumours, excision biopsy of the whole tonsil is usually advisable for reliable histology and may be sufficient if the resection margins are clear.

For patients with oropharyngeal cancers who relapse after radical irradiation to the primary site, surgical removal offers the only prospect of cure. These operations are complex and require careful consideration, usually demanding close co-operation between the head and neck surgeon who will undertake the radical excision and the plastic surgeon who is responsible for the reconstruction. Modern repair techniques, for example using jejunal replacement of the pharynx, are beginning to improve the functional results. Rehabilitation of oropharyngeal function, especially deglutition, can be exceptionally difficult after successful treatment. Patients may need many months of skilled support and may suffer from long-term problems with oral lubrication since the radiation fields are likely to cover the parotid glands.

LYMPHOMAS OF THE PHARYNX

A significant proportion of nasopharyngeal and tonsillar tumours will prove histologically to be lymphomas rather than epithelial tumours. Invariably these are non-Hodgkin's lymphomas, usually lymphocytic B-cell neoplasms. It is wise to undertake full investigation as for non-Hodgkin's lymphomas at other sites, because distant spread occurs. The stomach is involved in 20% of cases at some stage but spread to the marrow and other extranodal sites is unusual at presentation. Nasopharyngeal lymphomas also have a tendency to spread directly to the paranasal sinuses and nasal fossae. Routine treatment of these contiguous areas is often recommended whenever a primary nasopharyngeal lymphoma is encountered. Although this represents an unusually large treatment volume, local control can usually be achieved with a more modest dose than for epithelial tumours. Generally 40 Gy (4000 rad) in 4 weeks is adequate.

CARCINOMA OF THE LARYNGOPHARYNX (HYPOPHARYNX)

These are at least as common as those of the oropharynx, and accounted for 960 cases in Lederman's comprehensive review of 2400 carcinomas of the pharynx seen in his 30 years experience at the Royal Marsden Hospital,

London [4]. As with other sites, excessive cigarette and spirit consumption are the chief aetiological factors, and common symptoms include dyspnoea, dysphagia, anorexia, inanition and sometimes stridor. Most are well-differentiated squamous carcinomas. Palpable lymph nodes are present in about half the cases at diagnosis and a quarter of these have bilateral lymphadenopathy. The majority of patients have advanced lesions at presentation.

Although the prognosis in general is poor, some sites are prognostically more favourable than others. Carcinomas of the upper part of the laryngopharynx, including the aryepiglottic fold and exophytic lesions of the pharyngolaryngeal fold have a better prognosis than those of the more infiltrating or ulcerative variety, which usually arise from the pyriform fossa, cervical oesophagus and posterior pharyngeal wall. In general, these tumours have a very poor prognosis despite intensive treatment with radiotherapy, surgery and chemotherapy in patients whose general condition warrants it. Five-year survival rates remain no better than 10–15% overall, regardless of the specific hypopharyngeal sub-site or method of treatment. A small group of tumours without direct extension or node involvement has a better prognosis, including a remarkable 5-year survival rate of 50% for early ($T_1 N_0$) lesions of the pyriform fossa. Although good results with radiotherapy alone have occasionally been claimed for individual patients with advanced disease, it is clear that the chief use of radiotherapy lies in palliation, and the avoidance of mutilating surgery which would in all probability fail to cure. Radical surgery is, however, occasionally indicated in patients with operable lesions and in good general health; these individual decisions are best made by a surgeon and radiotherapist working jointly in a combined clinic. Most patients ultimately die of local or regional recurrence (rarely because of lymph node disease alone) although an increasing proportion have evidence of more widespread dissemination at the time of death.

Radiation technique in these tumours is complicated by the large volume which is frequently required, especially since delineation of the lower extent of spread in laryngopharyngeal tumours is often very difficult. When the disease is localized to the neck, the technique usually consists of lateral opposed field treatment with either open (direct) or wedged fields (see Chapter 5). A major technical problem arises when the tumour has extended below the thoracic inlet since easy access by lateral fields is limited by the shoulders. In this situation, a more complicated radiation field arrangement is required, and these tumours pose some of the greatest technical challenges in clinical radiotherapy. This particularly applies to postcricoid tumours. For treatment to be curative, a radical dose of 60 Gy (6000 rad) in 6 weeks, or equivalent, is always necessary.

TUMOURS OF THE ORAL CAVITY

Tumours of the oral cavity include those arising from the lip, the mobile portion of the tongue (anterior to the circumvallate papillae), buccal musosa, alveolae (gingiva), floor of mouth, hard palate and retromolar trigone. Age-specific incidence is shown in Fig. 10.1. Although these tumours became less common in the early part of this century due to better dental and oral hygiene, possibly coupled with more moderate consumption of tobacco, they are still among the commonest tumours seen in any combined head and neck oncology clinic, and are often surprisingly advanced at presentation. There is evidence that the incidence is again rising, particularly among younger men [13]. These tumours also appear to be commoner in rural than urban populations, and in black people rather than white. TNM staging is now widely used (Table 10.5), and clinical photographs are particularly valuable as a permanent and routine part of clinical staging since most of these tumours are easily visible. There is increasing evidence that use of retinoids in high-risk populations may prevent the development of dysplastic premalignant intra-oral lesions into frankly invasive tumours [14].

Cancers of the oral cavity usually present as non-healing ulcers on the lip, tongue, cheek or floor of the mouth. Pain, though usually present, is not invariable. Cancers of the lip can arise on the upper or lower vermillion borders, or an adjacent area such as the philtrum, with direct involvement of the lip itself. The primary lesion can be raised, ulcerated, excavated, pigmented, well or poorly demarcated, painful or painless. Many oral cavity lesions are first diagnosed by a dentist and are sometimes hidden by dentures. Leucoplakia is a predisposing cause. On examination the usual findings are of a raised erythematous ulcerated lesion, often with an area of necrosis. Large tumours of the tongue may reduce mobility and interfere with speech.

Clinical examination should include careful bimanual palpation and the lesion should always be measured. Examination of the neck may reveal enlarged lymph nodes.

Investigation should include chest X-ray, full blood count and liver function tests. In patients with tumours of the floor of mouth or lower alveolus, investigation should always include radiological examination (orthopantomogram) of the lower jaw since asymptomatic involvement can occur, even when the lesion is not tender on digital palpation. Fine-needle aspiration cytology of neck nodes is easily performed and may confirm a clinical suspicion of lymph node metastasis.

The clinical behaviour and probability of metastases varies with the site. For example, carcinomas at the tip of the tongue are far easier to control than tumours of its lateral margins, although cancers of the dorsum are most difficult (Fig. 10.10). In general, tumours of the floor of mouth, buccal mucosa, hard palate and alveolus show similar and relatively low metastatic rates whereas tumours of the oral portion of the tongue have a higher propensity for nodal spread.

Metastases are more frequent with poorly differentiated tumours. Large oral cavity

Fig. 10.10 Relative frequency (in parentheses) and control rates in carcinoma of the tongue.

tumours (more than 4 cm in diameter) are both more difficult to control at the primary site, and more likely to be accompanied by cervical node metastases. Bilateral node involvement is common in patients with lesions of the floor of the mouth and faucial arch. The anatomical position of the abnormal nodes varies with the primary site. For carcinomas of the oral tongue and floor of mouth, the commonest sites are the jugulodigastric and submaxillary nodes, whereas palatine and retromolar trigone lesions are more frequently accompanied by lymphadenopathy at the angle of the jaw.

Management

Optimum management is best achieved in joint consultative clinics staffed by a surgeon, radiotherapist and medical oncologist. Principles of management are similar for the major sites within the oral cavity and will be considered together, except for carcinomas of the lip (see p. 187).

SMALL ACCESSIBLE TUMOURS (T_1) OF THE ORAL CAVITY

These have an excellent cure rate with radical radiotherapy, with very good preservation of function. Most radiotherapists employ interstitial implantation techniques for intra-oral tumours (i.e. excluding those of the lip), since the treatment volume can be kept sufficiently small for a high dose to be given with safety. Implants of radium, caesium, gold, tantalum and iridium are all satisfactory. Intra-oral sites often treated by interstitial irradiation include tongue, buccal mucosa, floor of mouth, palate and lower alveolus. Very small lesions (less than 1 cm) can be treated with an interstitial implant alone, without external beam irradiation, though most radiotherapists use a combination of interstitial and external irradiation in larger tumours which are still small enough to implant (T_1 and small T_2 cancers). With an interstitial implant, a tumour dose of 60 Gy is usually given over 4−7 days. Where interstitial and external radiation are used together, many authorities recommend that the volume implant is taken to 50 Gy in 5−7 days, followed by external beam irradiation to 30 Gy in 3 weeks. In some clinics, excisional surgery is preferred for small tumours of the anterior tip of the tongue.

LARGER TUMOURS OF THE ORAL CAVITY ($T_2 - T_4$)

In these tumours, external beam irradiation has traditionally been the mainstay of treatment, though a dual modality approach using combined radiation and chemotherapy is increasingly being employed (see below). With external irradiation, doses of 60 Gy (6000 rad) over 6 weeks are usually considered essential for adequate control and it is known that tolerance is related to the volume irradiated. Radiation technique usually involves treatment by lateral open (direct) or wedged fields, to include both the primary tumour and the initial drainage node group since these are so commonly involved. For cancers of the tongue, floor of mouth and lower jaw, the palate can safely be excluded from treatment by means of a mouth gag which depresses the tongue.

The proper management of metastases in neck nodes remains contentious. Many clinics recommend routine radical neck dissection in patients with mobile nodes, and prophylactic node dissection in clinically node-negative patients has revealed a significant incidence of micrometastatic tumour. In patients without evidence of neck node involvement (N_0), most radiotherapists give prophylactic treatment to the neck, to a slightly lower dose (50 Gy (5000 rad) in 5 weeks or equivalent) than radical dosage, on the grounds that occult nodal spread is common and that nodal recurrence is reduced by such treatment. Most centres employ external beam irradiation, sometimes in combination with surgery, to control metastatic neck nodes, though ultimate survival rates in patients with N_2 and N_3 nodes is poor whatever the approach.

Patterns of recurrence and overall survival are clearly dependent on the size and stage of the tumour. Although some intra-oral sites (particularly floor of mouth) have a notorious reputation, there is little evidence that, stage for stage, this is borne out in survival figures. In one study the cumulative 3-year survival in mobile tongue/floor of mouth lesions without lymphadenopathy was 57% whereas for patients with palpable lymphadenopathy, the survival rate fell to 42% [15]. Where lymph node involvement is obvious at presentation, failure at the primary site is common despite intensive radiotherapy.

Occasionally it is possible to control a limited relapse (usually the primary site) with an interstitial radioactive implant though radical surgery is usually required later since durable control is rarely achieved.

In the United Kingdom, surgery is usually undertaken if local relapse occurs after primary radiation therapy, though increasingly some centres are recommending primary surgical excision instead of radical irradiation because of the long-term problems of radiation damage to the oral cavity. A wide resection is invariably required, preferably with sophisticated reconstructive surgery. The advent of free flap grafting with microvascular anastomosis has dramatically improved the cosmetic results. The difficulty is that in general, complete surgical extirpation of the initial area at risk has to be undertaken, and may result in substantial local damage with loss of function despite recent improvements in reconstructive surgery. A typical operation for a recurrent lesion of the floor of the mouth might include a hemiglossectomy, excision of the floor of the mouth, hemimandibulectomy, and neck dissection (commando procedure) with pedicle and/or microvascular free flap grafting in order to achieve adequate healing — a major undertaking in patients who are often debilitated enough to require hyperalimentation before surgery. Intensive rehabilitation and speech therapy are also critically important. Chapter 7, pp. 126–7, and pp. 145–8, provides a fuller discussion of rehabilitation of patients following this type of extensive surgery.

Chemotherapy may also be valuable in the primary or secondary management of these tumours and is further discussed in the final section of this chapter.

CARCINOMA OF THE LIP

Carcinomas of the lip constitute about one-fifth of all oral cavity lesions. These are almost always squamous cell carcinomas, often well-differentiated and presenting relatively early since the tumour is usually visible. The incidence has fallen rapidly during the past 25 years, and less than 300 new cases are now seen annually in Britain. Cancers of the lower lip are much commoner than the upper lip (20 : 1) but upper lip cancers are relatively commoner in women.

Metastasis is relatively uncommon, and is to local lymph nodes. About 7% of patients have involvement of local nodes at diagnosis, and the same proportion will develop metastases in local lymph node groups after primary treatment. Nodal invasion is usually directly to the submaxillary or submental nodes. Metastases to other node groups or organs is extremely unusual.

Treatment

Treatment is by surgery or radiotherapy. Most carcinomas of the lip are curable by radiation therapy, particularly where the tumour is small (T_1). External beam therapy with photons or electrons, and brachytherapy with radium moulds or interstitial iridium implants have all been used, and local recurrence is very rarely seen. Surgery also offers excellent local control, though the cosmetic result may be slightly less satisfactory, particularly where excision of a substantial portion of the lip needs to be undertaken. In larger tumours (T_2), which might require reconstructive surgery, radiotherapy is generally accepted to be the better method of treatment, both cosmetically and functionally, since excision of large portions of the lip leads to poor closure of the mouth and may interfere with phonation. With large destructive cancers of the lip (T_3, T_4) it is difficult to achieve an adequate cosmetic and functional result by either method of treatment, and the incidence of local recurrence is higher. Fortunately, very few cancers of the lip now fall into this category. Healing may be excellent even following large doses of radiation therapy, but surgical reconstruction will often be necessary.

External beam irradiation is most commonly employed though formerly the lip was one of the classic sites for brachytherapy with a radium mould. Superficial X-ray therapy (100–150 kV) has the advantage of adequate penetration with simple and effective protection of gums, teeth and mandible by intra-oral lead shielding which can be positioned by the radiographer for each fraction of treatment. As with treatment of skin cancer, an individually designed lead cut-out can be used to allow for treatment of any size and shape of field. Tumours larger than 3 cm are usually treated with higher energy

(200–250 kV). Electron therapy has also been used and possibly offers superior cosmetic results. Treatment schedules are varied, though the best cosmetic schedules include 40 Gy (4000 rad) applied dose in 10 fractions daily over 2 weeks, 50 Gy (5000 rad) applied dose in 20 fractions over 4 weeks, 45 Gy (4500 rad) in 10 fractions given on alternate weekdays over 3½ weeks, or, in centres preferring lengthy radical dosage, 60 Gy (6000 rad) in 30 consecutive daily fractions over 6 weeks. This latter regimen is probably the most suitable for large volumes.

In the rare patient with nodal metastases, radical neck dissection is the treatment of choice though radiotherapy can also be effective. With radical radiation therapy, surgery or a combination of both techniques, the results in carcinoma of the lip are excellent, and virtually all patients without lymph node involvement should be considered curable. Even with lymph node metastases, the overall survival is 60–70% at 5 years.

NASAL CAVITY AND PARANASAL SINUSES

These uncommon tumours, where presentation is often late and accompanied by early invasion of critical structures, are amongst the most difficult of all tumours of the head and neck region. The exposed nature of these facial cancers adds to the patient's burden, and demands great skill not only in eradicating the tumour, but also in offering acceptable reconstruction. They tend to be slow-growing tumours, usually well-differentiated squamous carcinomas, in which local recurrence is the major problem. Other tumour types are occasionally encountered, with differing patterns of clinical behaviour and natural history. Melanoma of the nasal cavity is well recognized, accounting for almost 10% of nasal cavity cancer. Tumours of the nasal cavity and paranasal sinuses spread to other paranasal structures and to the nasopharynx (Fig. 10.11). Although late presentation is the rule in tumours of the paranasal sinuses,

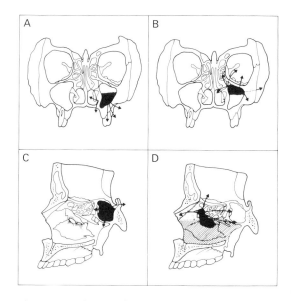

Fig. 10.11 Pathways of local spread of tumours of the nasal cavity and paranasal sinuses. (A) and (B) lower and upper maxillary tumours spreading to orbit, nasal fossa, palate, upper alveolus and soft tissues; (C) sphenoid sinus tumours (lateral view) into nasopharynx, base of brain, ethmoid and nasal cavity; (D) nasal fossa tumours (lateral view) into orbit, base of skull, sphenoid and posterior choana. (From Boone *et al.* *American Journal of Roentgenology* 1986; **102**: 627–636. With permission.)

those originating in the nasal cavity tend as a group to present earlier, usually with nasal obstruction, stuffiness or offensive discharge. Anatomically, the commonest tumours are those of the maxillary antrum, followed by tumours of the nasal cavity (Table 10.6).

Localized tumours of the maxillary antrum are usually asymptomatic; symptoms such as swelling and erythema of the cheek should raise a suspicion that the disease has extended beyond the confines of the primary site. Upward extension results in erosion of the floor of the orbit and displacement of the globe, leading to diplopia and ophthalmoplegia. Spread may also occur downwards into the oral cavity or posteriorly into the pterygoid region. Adjacent sites such as the nasal cavity, the ethmoid and sphenoidal sinuses are often involved (Fig. 10.11).

Table 10.6 Distribution of tumours of nasal cavity and paranasal sinuses

	Frequency (%)
Site of primary	
Maxillary antrum	60
Nasal cavity	20
Ethmoid sinus	15
Nasal vestibule	4
Frontal and sphenoid	1
Histological type	
Squamous carcinoma	54
Anaplastic carcinoma	17
Transitional cell carcinoma	7
Adenocarcinoma	6
Melanoma	5
Lymphoma	6
Other	5

From Robin *et al.* [16]

Aetiologically, little is known of the predisposing factors, though excessive alcohol intake, cigarette smoking and oral hygiene are held to be important. Adenocarcinoma of the nasal cavity is known to be commoner in hardwood furniture makers, and is presumably due to the inhalation of an occupational carcinogen. Because of difficulties in accurate assessment of the size and local extension of these tumours, staging by TNM or other conventional criteria has on the whole been disappointing. CT scanning gives far more information (Fig. 10.2) and this investigation should now be routinely performed, although simpler radiographic examinations are also of value.

Although some groups recommend either radical surgery or radical radiotherapy alone, the concept of combined modality treatment is well established. In 1933, Ohngren advocated treatment by a combination of surgery and irradiation on the grounds that this combination gave better results than either treatment alone. In general, this approach has been validated and remains the standard policy in many large centres, particularly for treatment of the maxillary antrum. Fortunately, surgical healing after radical doses of radiotherapy is not usually a problem at this site, and conversely there seems little prospect of reducing the extent of surgery for tumours which have usually spread beyond their primary confines at the time of the diagnosis. Although no worthwhile comparative trials have been reported, many large series have demonstrated a 5-year survival of up to 40% with combined treatment. More localized cases are occasionally treated by surgery alone, but even in patients too frail to undergo an operation a 20% 5-year survival has been achieved with the use of radiotherapy alone. Modern prosthetics have allowed many of these patients to face the world with a reasonably normal appearance despite substantial anatomical deficiencies.

TUMOURS OF THE MIDDLE EAR

Cancer of the middle ear is extremely unusual, and tends to occur in middle-aged men with a history of chronic otitis media, often making diagnosis difficult since the symptoms may well be little more than an accentuation of the discharge which the patient has suffered for many years, with the addition of bleeding and pain. Direct local spread to mastoid air cells or external auditory canal is the rule, sometimes producing severe pain particularly when bony erosion (usually of the temporal bone) has occurred. The tumours are usually squamous carcinomas, presumably arising as a result of squamous metaplasia of the columnar epithelial cells normally present. Adenocarcinoma is very rarely encountered. Both radical surgical removal and radical irradiation have been advocated, but complete surgical removal is often impossible, and local control difficult to achieve. Extension beyond the temporal bone makes the prognosis very poor. Local extension to the brain may occur. Since survival rates are similar (about 25% at 5 years) whichever local method of treatment is employed, radical irradiation is usually preferred. Other rare tumours include soft tissue sarcomas and primary tumours of bone. In these cases, radical surgery is seldom possible and the mainstay of treatment is radiotherapy.

Glomus jugulare tumours arise from neuro-endocrine chemoreceptors of the jugular bulb, and should be considered with similar tumours (chemodectoma, paraganglioma) arising at other sites such as the bifurcation of the carotid artery (carotid body tumour) or posterior mediastinum. They are three times commoner in women, and may occasionally be bilateral. Although histologically benign, these tumours invade locally. Surgery is hazardous, since they are highly vascular and usually involve the middle ear and petrous temporal bone. Presentation is with a classical cluster of symptoms including deafness, cranial nerve palsies, local pain and tinnitus. Radiotherapy is the treatment of choice and modest doses (40−50 Gy, 4000−5000 rad in 4−5 weeks) are adequate though regression may be slow.

CARCINOMA OF THE PINNA AND EXTERNAL AUDITORY CANAL

In this group of tumours, the pinna is the commonest primary site, followed by the external auditory canal. Tumours of the external auditory canal are usually squamous cell carcinomas. On the pinna, the commonest cell type in Britain is the basal cell carcinoma though squamous carcinomas are commoner in the United States. Malignant melanoma of the pinna is occasionally encountered. These tumours present either with a visible lesion of the pinna, or, in the case of tumours of the external canal, with discharge (sometimes bloodstained), crusting, or unilateral deafness. Pain is unusual. Local extension of tumours of the external canal may occur to pre-auricular structures, tympanic membrane, middle ear or mastoid and can be difficult to detect even with isotope bone scanning or CT scanning.

Although removal by radical surgery can be curative, it is widely accepted that treatment by radical radiotherapy is equally effective and offers a better functional result even though mucosal oedema, sterile fluid collections in the middle ear and perforation of the eardrum may occur with high radiation dose.

CHEMOTHERAPY IN SQUAMOUS CARCINOMAS OF THE HEAD AND NECK

Although both surgery and radiotherapy can be curative for localized squamous cancers of the head and neck (and even in some cases with lymph node involvement), the prognosis of patients with recurrent or disseminated disease is very poor. The first attempts at using cytotoxic chemotherapy in these patients were made at least 30 years ago, often using intra-arterial perfusion. More recently, interest has shifted from the use of single agents to combination chemotherapy, and from treatment of recurrent disease to the use of adjuvant chemotherapy in the initial management. Both of these approaches remain controversial [17].

Methotrexate was the first drug shown to be capable of producing responses, though it rapidly became apparent that with conventional doses the response duration was short, often a matter of a few months or less. The ill health of many of these patients, coupled with the wide variety of clinical presentations and primary sites, has made it difficult to assess this drug. Treatment by the intravenous or intra-arterial route gives an overall response rate of about 50%, with no obvious advantage in favour of either method [17]. Although attempts have been made to increase the response rate by the use of high doses of methotrexate with folinic acid rescue, the evidence in favour of this approach is limited; recent studies have demonstrated slightly higher response rates can be expected, but the duration of response and overall survival are not significantly improved. Where methotrexate has been employed concomitantly with surgery and radiotherapy, mucosal reactions have often been dose limiting. In addition, these patients are usually poorly nourished, cachectic and elderly, making aggressive treatment hazardous.

Other well studied agents include bleomycin,

cisplatin, 5-fluorouracil and mitomycin C. All of these show some degree of activity and in the past few years there has been a tendency towards combination chemotherapy for recurrent disease, increasingly employing combinations of cisplatin—5-fluorouracil or methotrexate—bleomycin (Table 10.7), although the duration of response tends to be short. There is at present no definite evidence that multi-drug regimens are superior in survival to single agents [18].

A major area of controversy surrounds the use of adjuvant combination chemotherapy immediately following (or in some cases preceding) local treatment with surgery or radiotherapy [19]. Both American and European groups have reported better local control and survival by comparison with historical controls. Indeed, randomized studies have been reported, using chemo-radiotherapy compared with conventional radical irradiation [20,21] and increasingly suggesting a possible benefit for the combined modality group, especially

in terms of freedom from local recurrence. In a large study from the Christie Hospital, Manchester, the addition of two pulses of single-agent methotrexate proved clearly beneficial in a series of over 300 patients with advanced disease. A smaller study from Yale University employed mitomycin C as the chemotherapeutic agent [22] and also showed a clear improvement. Several uncontrolled series have investigated cisplatin—5-fluorouracil combinations and found them both active and feasible in combination with radical irradiation. Other active agents include carboplatin and ifosfamide. Despite encouraging data from a number of studies it remains difficult to evaluate the role of chemotherapy in primary treatment until larger scale randomized trials have been completed. Chemotherapy for advanced disease should probably not be used outside controlled clinical trials [23].

Patients with nasopharyngeal carcinoma appear to have a higher response rate to chemo-

Table 10.7 Chemotherapy in squamous carcinoma of the head and neck

Regimen	Total response* (%)
Single-agent response rates	
Methotrexate**	
Low-dose	30—40
High-dose	40—50
Bleomycin	30
Cisplatin	30
Vinblastine	25
5-FU	15
Cyclophosphamide	35
Doxorubicin	20
Hydroxyurea	30
Typical combination chemotherapy regimens	
Cisplatin and 5-FU	80
Cisplatin and bleomycin	50
Cisplatin, bleomycin and methotrexate	60
Bleomycin, methotrexate, cyclophosphamide and 5-FU	55
Vincristine, bleomycin, methotrexate, 5-FU, doxorubicin and hydrocortisone	67
Methotrexate, bleomycin and vinblastine	75

* These are approximate response rates from several studies. ** Low dose: below $80\,mg/m^2$. Considerable variability in reported response rates.

therapy [24]. One large series reported a response rate as high as 80% for patients with metastatic disease, using a combination of bleomycin, cisplatin and epirubicin, with some long-term successes.

TUMOURS OF SALIVARY GLANDS

Although uncommon, accounting for about 2% of all neoplasms, salivary tumours are of great interest to pathologists and clinicians since they are of varied histology and present technical problems in management. The most common primary site is the parotid, accounting for almost 80% of all cases though the other major (submandibular and sublingual) and minor salivary glands can be affected. Occasionally, tumours of minor salivary glands can grow to a large size, mimicking cancers of the nasopharynx or palate.

Anatomy

The parotid gland is an accessible organ, overlying the styloid process and situated between mastoid and mandible, for the most part lying anterior to the pinna. Its deep aspect is in close relation to the parapharyngeal space and lateral pharyngeal wall. Superiorly, it rarely extends beyond the zygomatic arch. The gland is divided by the facial nerve and its branches into a superficial and deep lobe, and surgical excision of parotid tumour is often limited for fear of surgical damage to this nerve. The submandibular gland lies beneath the horizontal portion of the mandible, and the sublingual gland (the smallest of the three major salivary glands) lies in the floor of the mouth, in contact with the inner surface of the mandible, often extending to the midline where it meets the contralateral gland.

Pathology

The wide variety of histological types of salivary tumour encompasses both benign and malignant disorders (Table 10.8). About three-quarters are benign, mostly pleomorphic adenomas or 'mixed salivary tumours', which is much the commonest tumour in the parotid gland and less frequently found in other sites (only 40% of tumours in minor salivary glands). About 65% of these tumours occur in women, mostly in the age group 50–65, though pleomorphic adenomas of the parotid have been reported in children and adolescents. Histologically, the tumours are very varied, with epithelial cells showing either acinar formation or arranged in clumps or sheets of cells, and

Table 10.8 Histological types and prognosis in salivary gland tumours

	% Frequency	5-year survival	10-year survival*
Pleomorphic adenoma	75	96	93
Adenocarcinoma	8	50	—
Mucoepidermoid			
low-grade	3	90	80
high-grade	3	20	10
Adenoid cystic	4	60	38
Malignant mixed	2	55	30
Acinic cell	1	80	65
Squamous	3	25	—
All types — men			60
— women			75

* Where available

situated within a stroma which is often myxoid in consistency. Several populations of cells may be present, but in general the overall pattern, though bizarre, pleomorphic and disorganized, is not one of malignancy.

Twenty-five per cent of parotid tumours are malignant. *Malignant mixed tumours*, or pleomorphic adenocarcinomas, often resemble pleomorphic adenomas histologically though foci of malignant change are typically scattered throughout the specimen. These patients usually give a history of slow-growing and painless parotid swelling, often for several years, followed by a sudden change, with increased swelling and pain. This well recognized development represents one of the best examples of malignant change within an area of benign neoplasia — a most unusual phenomenon at other sites. The *adenoid cystic carcinomas* or cylindromas are rather more common (about 15% of malignant salivary tumours) and arise not only in major salivary glands but also quite typically in the minor glands, for example in the palate. Characteristically, these tumours spread by direct extension along perineural spaces, a feature which may lead to unusual presentations of this tumour. Pain and perineural extension have been well correlated in clinicopathological studies. *Mucoepidermoid carcinomas* are now well recognized, and consist histologically of two distinct populations of cells, with both mucus secretion and typical epidermoid features. These often tend to be less malignant tumours and the lowest grade ones are clinically benign, though at the other end of the spectrum is a high-grade mucoepidermoid carcinoma which can be difficult to control and may be rapidly fatal. *Acinic cell tumours* are rare, more common in females, with a slow clinical evolution and an unusual histological picture suggesting an origin in acinic epithelial cells. Squamous cell carcinomas and *anaplastic carcinomas* of the salivary glands must be diagnosed with caution since there is a problem in distinguishing these from secondary deposits arising from a head and neck tumour site of more typical squamous origin.

Histologically, the squamous or anaplastic element may be one component of a mixed malignant or other type of salivary tumour. True anaplastic or squamous tumours of the salivary gland are amongst the most malignant of tumours, with a very poor prognosis. *Lymphoma* of the parotid is occasionally seen, but it is difficult to be sure if its site of origin is the parotid itself or an adjacent lymph node. *Adenolymphoma* (Warthin's tumour) is an unusual lesion, sometimes misdiagnosed as an abscess, and of doubtful origin. It is never malignant, may even be degenerative, and is characterized by large pink-staining cells surrounded by a lymphoid 'follicle'. The 'oncocytic epithelium' may enclose a centrally cystic area.

Clinical features

Benign salivary tumours usually present with a slowly growing painless mass. The onset of pain or a facial palsy is a sinister development suggestive of malignancy in a parotid tumour. The most rapidly growing tumours are anaplastic and squamous carcinomas, when the history of swelling will be shorter. Most of the other malignant salivary tumours tend to present with a more insidious onset. With adenoid cystic carcinomas, pain is a common feature due to the perineural spread which characterizes these tumours. Lymph node involvement is unusual in salivary tumours though reportedly higher in high-grade mucoepidermoid carcinoma. Haematogenous spread is well recognized, particularly with anaplastic, mixed malignant tumours and cylindromas.

Management of salivary gland tumours

Surgical excision is undoubtedly the most important method of treatment for both benign and malignant salivary tumours. For benign parotid tumours, which occur most commonly in the superficial portion of the gland, superficial parotidectomy with preservation of the facial nerve is the operation of choice, giving excellent results provided that complete excision is possible. When excision is incomplete, postoperative radiotherapy is indicated since recurrence rates following this combined treatment are as low as those following complete excision. Although some surgeons recommend follow-up observation after incomplete excision, this policy carries the disadvantage that a second operation may then be required, with the consequent risk of damage to the facial nerve. It would seem safer to offer routine postoperative radiotherapy to patients with incompletely excised parotid tumours. At other sites such as the submandibular and sublingual glands, experienced surgeons are often able to achieve wider excision than with parotid lesions since they are freed from the fear of facial nerve trunk damage.

The indications for routine radiotherapy in malignant tumours are: inadequate surgical excision margins; tumours of high grade (particularly squamous, anaplastic and mixed malignant lesions); when surgery has been performed for recurrent disease; and for malignant lymphoma of the parotid, where surgery plays no part in the management, other than for biopsy. Lymphomas and adenocarcinomas are generally the most radiosensitive types of salivary tumour. Occasionally, surgery is contraindicated, for example in unfit or elderly patients, or those with malignant tumours of the minor salivary glands in nasopharynx or palate. In these circumstances, long-term control can sometimes be achieved with radiotherapy alone.

In summary, the usual policy for malignant parotid and other salivary tumours is one of excisional surgery followed routinely by postoperative radiotherapy. Exceptions might include low-grade malignant lesions with complete surgical excision, particularly where a capsule or pseudocapsule can be demonstrated in the specimen. The radiotherapy technique may be technically demanding since large volumes of tissue need to be uniformly irradiated and care is required to avoid overtreatment to sensitive structures — the brain stem, eye and mucous membranes. The usual arrangement is a wedged pair of fields. Particular care must be taken to avoid irradiation of the contralateral eye from the exit beam. A dose of $50-55\,\text{Gy}$ $(5000-5500\,\text{rad})$ in $5-5\frac{1}{2}$ weeks is adequate treatment for residual benign tumours. Malignant parotid tumours need higher doses and $60-70\,\text{Gy}$ in $6-8$ weeks is often recommended if there is residual disease postoperatively. Because of the initially large treatment volume, a shrinking field technique may be necessary (see Chapter 5). Careful planning should allow treatment of the whole parotid bed as high as the zygomatic arch and inferiorly to the level of the hyoid, in order to include the jugulodigastric and upper cervical nodes. For submandibular and sublingual tumours, large treatment volumes are also required since in general the whole gland will need to be irradiated. With adenoid cystic lesions, it is particularly important to treat widely in view of the perineural invasion; with parotid cylindromas, the mastoid should always be treated.

Opinions vary as to whether the whole of the cervical node chain should be irradiated in patients with malignant parotid tumours. Since the frequency of lymph node involvement varies with the histology, routine cervical node irradiation is only necessary in patients with squamous or anaplastic tumours, adenocarcinomas or mucoepidermoid and malignant mixed tumours of high grade. In some clinics, particularly in the United States, these patients are treated by elective lymph node dissection.

Promising preliminary results have been reported for neutron therapy (Chapter 5) as primary treatment for malignant salivary gland tumours [25], but this treatment is not generally available. The role of neutron therapy in these diseases remains uncertain.

Prognosis

Prognosis in salivary gland tumours depends on the histological type [26] as well as its operability (Table 10.8). Routine use of postoperative radiotherapy has been shown to increase local control in all of the major types, but squamous, anaplastic and high-grade mucoepidermoid carcinomas carry a poor prognosis because of both local recurrence and metastatic spread [27]. Better results are seen with low-grade mucoepidermoid tumours and acinic cell tumours, with adenoid cystic and malignant mixed tumours carrying an intermediate prognosis. Overall, women have a better prognosis than men (10-year survival of 75% and 60% respectively).

Further surgical excision is sometimes possible for recurrent disease at the primary site, whilst for distant metastases palliative radiotherapy is sometimes useful, particularly with less aggressive slow-growing tumours. Pulmonary and other distant metastases are occasionally encountered, particularly with adenoid cystic carcinoma. Treatment with chemotherapy has no established place in management.

TUMOURS OF THE ORBIT AND EYE

Orbit

Both primary and secondary neoplasms occur in the orbit (Table 10.9). Lymphoma and rhabdomyosarcoma are the commonest primary tumours. Soft tissue sarcoma, nerve and nerve sheath tumours (including optic nerve gliomas) and meningiomas are all seen occasionally. Orbital secondary deposits are likely to be due to carcinomas of the breast, bronchus or thyroid.

Table 10.9 Tumours of the orbit (excluding globe)

Benign	Malignant
Haemangioma	Lymphoma
Lachrymal gland tumours	Rhabdomyosarcoma
Meningioma	Optic nerve glioma
Lymphangioma	Metastases
Neurofibroma	Angiosarcoma and other
Dermoid cysts	sarcomas
(Pseudotumour)	Myeloma

CLINICAL FEATURES

Because of its rigid bony structure, forward displacement of the globe (proptosis) is the cardinal physical sign. Ophthalmoplegia may also occur because of interference with the external ocular muscles or, less commonly, because of a III cranial nerve palsy, particularly with posteriorly placed tumours. Proptosis can be extreme and disfiguring, particularly in children. Chemosis and infection are common and may lead to a misdiagnosis of cellulitis. Panophthalmitis can lead to perforation of the globe and unilateral blindness is common with advanced tumours. The rapid onset of chemosis and lid oedema suggest that the tumour is malignant. Marked proptosis with normal ocular movement usually indicates a slow growing benign tumour. Tumours within the muscle cone produce less disturbance of ocular movement but more proptosis and greater visual loss; those outside the cone produce eccentric proptosis and affect vision later.

INVESTIGATION

Plain X-rays and tomography can be extremely helpful and give good views of the orbital margins and optic canals. Even greater detail is obtained with CT scanning which gives reliable information on the site, size and degree of intra- and extra-orbital spread as well as a clear indication of bony erosion and soft tissue tumour invasion (Fig. 10.2). This is now an essential investigation. Ultrasound examination is often helpful in providing a rapid demonstration that a tumour is present. Biopsy confirmation of the diagnosis should be obtained where possible, but there may be formidable difficulties in so doing with a risk of tumour spillage, haemorrhage and blindness. If the tumour is encapsulated it is usually best to excise it entirely.

Lymphoma

Malignant lymphomas of the orbit are almost

always of the non-Hodgkin's variety and may be isolated or seen as part of a more generalized lymphoma (see Chapter 26). Full investigation is usually required as for any other lymphoma, since evidence of systemic disease will be found in a proportion of patients. Biopsy of these lesions is usually easy since they tend to be anteriorly placed, and treatment with radiotherapy is usually successful in eradicating all signs of disease. Even where systemic lymphoma is discovered, radiotherapy is used as an addition to systemic treatment in order to prevent local recurrence, and modest doses of the order of 30 Gy (3000 rad) over 3 weeks are usually adequate.

Orbital pseudotumour

This condition usually presents as a painful ophthalmoplegia often accompanied by swelling of the eyelids. CT scanning shows a retro-orbital mass, often ill defined and surrounding the optic nerve. Histologically there is a pleomorphic inflammatory infiltrate but occasionally monotypic B cells can be demonstrated, indicating a low-grade lymphoma.

The disease responds rapidly to steroids which may prevent visual loss. Relapses occur and the 'tumour' may spread back through the orbital fissure to the base of the brain. Radiotherapy may help but, rarely, the disease can be relentlessly progressive.

Rhabdomyosarcoma

This is usually embryonal in type, occurring chiefly in infants, young children and adolescents, and slightly more commonly in males. Local spread may involve the maxilla, paranasal sinuses, frontal bone or even the brain, via the anterior or middle cranial fossa. Haematological spread may also occur, chiefly to lung or bone, but tends to be less common than with rhabdomyosarcomas presenting at other sites. Lymph node involvement, present in about one-quarter of cases, usually involves the upper deep cervical or pre-auricular nodes. Once

established, these tumours tend to advance rapidly, leading to particularly severe proptosis with chemosis and lid oedema. Wherever possible, full staging, including bone marrow aspiration, should be performed before treatment, in order to formulate a rational treatment plan. Although surgery was formerly used for control of the primary lesion, radiotherapy has become increasingly recognized as a satisfactory alternative, with low local recurrence rates. High doses of the order of 50 Gy (5000 rad) over 5–6 weeks are required and a high proportion of these patients will preserve useful vision in the affected eye provided that the lachrymal apparatus is shielded to ensure against xerophthalmia (see below).

Routine adjuvant chemotherapy is now an established part of treatment, and combinations of cyclophosphamide, vincristine and actinomycin D or doxorubicin are recommended. Generally at least one course of combination chemotherapy is given before the orbital radiation, because of the high probability of extraocular spread and also because rapid resolution occurs which will make the child more comfortable and the radiotherapy technically easier. The chemotherapy should normally be continued for about 1 year. Local irradiation is important as a means of ensuring local control even when metastases are present. Routine use of chemotherapy has improved prognosis from a survival rate of less than 40% using surgery and radiotherapy alone to about 75% at 5 years, with a particular improvement in tumours of younger children, which were previously notorious for their high probability of dissemination (see Chapter 24).

Lachrymal gland tumours

These are usually considered with orbital tumours, though they are extremely rare. Commonest in young adults, their histological spectrum is reminiscent of that of salivary gland tumours, with pleomorphic adenomas and adenoid cystic carcinomas the most frequently encountered types. There is usually a long history (longer than a year) of a slowly expanding, hard, painless mass. With more rapidly growing lesions, a biopsy is imperative and complete surgical removal of the tumour should be carried out if possible. Where total removal of the lachrymal gland cannot be performed (either for a patient with a pleomorphic adenoma or any of the malignant tumours) radiotherapy should also be given. Local recurrence is very common even after a high dose, so every effort should be made to remove these tumours. True carcinomas of the lachrymal gland are rare, and extra-orbital spread tends to occur early. Malignant lachrymal gland tumours are a miscellaneous group, difficult to treat and with a poor overall prognosis and a 5-year survival rate in the order of 20%.

Optic nerve glioma

This is discussed on p. 212.

RADIATION TECHNIQUES FOR
TUMOURS OF THE ORBIT

Although lead shielding of the cornea, lens and lachrymal sac is routinely recommended, it is impossible to arrange for homogeneous irradiation of the whole of the orbital content as well as adequate shielding of sensitive structures. A wedged pair of fields (see Chapter 5, Fig. 5.8) is the usual arrangement. Great care must be taken to avoid irradiation of the contralateral eye, even though useful vision is sometimes retained in the treated one. It is often useful to ask the patient to look directly into the beam during treatment both to fix the gaze and to avoid the inevitable build-up effect of the closed lid. With supervoltage beams, the maximal energy deposition is deep to the cornea and may even partly spare the lens. Partial or complete corneal shielding can usually be achieved with a simple cylindrical shield, and conjunctival damage is uncommon particularly as low doses of radiation are well tolerated by this part of the eye. Where shielding is impossible, painful keratitis, sometimes with

iridocyclitis or even corneal ulceration may occur. Failure to shield the lachrymal gland will usually pose a greater threat to the integrity of the eye since the lachrymal apparatus has a lower tolerance, and doses of greater than 30 Gy (3000 rad) over 3 weeks will cause significant reduction of tear production with consequent dryness of the eye, requiring regular instillation of lubricant drops.

The most radiosensitive structure in the eye is the lens itself (see Chapter 5, p. 75) and cataracts can develop after doses of a few Gy though clinically important lens opacity is rarely seen with doses below 15 Gy (1500 rad). With doses above 25 Gy (2500 rad), progressive cataract is almost invariable; fortunately, these cataracts can be removed. Other parts of the eye such as the retina and the sclera have a much higher radiation tolerance closely similar to that of the central nervous system, and clinically important changes are uncommon where doses of less than 60 Gy (6000 rad) are given by carefully fractionated external beam therapy.

Tumours of the eyelid and conjunctiva

Tumours of the eyelid are not uncommon and include basal cell and squamous cell carcinomas mostly occurring in elderly patients. The lower lid and inner canthus of the eye are the commonest sites. The management is discussed in Chapter 22. In the conjunctiva both melanoma and squamous cell carcinoma are occasionally encountered, and are important to diagnose early since small lesions can be effectively treated by radiation, with conservation of the eye and preservation of vision. In general, local surgical excision is advisable, followed by radiotherapy using an applicator carrying a radioactive source, often [90]Sr. It is important to distinguish true melanomas from precancerous ocular melanosis (a diffuse flat pigmented lesion) which can be clinically diagnosed with confidence, and should be observed without biopsy since malignant change may take years to develop. Overall prognosis of conjunctival melanoma is good (5-year survival about

75%), though patients with bulky lesions have a high risk of early fatal dissemination. Squamous carcinomas have an even better prognosis provided that adequate surgery and/or radiotherapy can be given.

Tumours of the globe

The two main tumours are retinoblastoma and uveal (choroidal) melanoma. Retinoblastoma is discussed in Chapter 24.

Malignant melanoma of the uveal tract is the commonest intra-ocular tumour of adults (6 per 1 000 000 per year). Blood-borne metastases are common, but may not become clinically apparent for many years. Only 15% arise in the ciliary body and iris. These present earlier and they are more easily visible. Choroidal melanomas (85% of the total) may cause no symptoms at first unless they are at the macula. At other sites a peripheral field defect may go unnoticed. Retinal detachment may occur.

The diagnosis is normally made on inspection. Primary choroidal melanomas must be distinguished from secondary deposits since the choroid is a known site of metastasis of cutaneous melanoma.

In the past immediate enucleation has been preferred to biopsy in the belief that biopsy was dangerous. A more conservative approach has been adopted in recent years especially in the elderly. Small melanomas can probably be watched and surgery only considered when the tumour enlarges. Treatment is then by photocoagulation, cryotherapy, local irradiation to a high dose, or surgery. In small lesions and tumours of the iris, enucleation can sometimes be avoided though it may be necessary for large lesions or where there is macular/optic nerve involvement or retinal detachment. Pain, local extension and secondary glaucoma are also indications for enucleation.

REFERENCES

1 Silverman S., Jr. *Oral Cancer*, 3rd edn. Atlanta: American Cancer Society, 1990.

2 Yu M.C., Ho J.H.C., Lai S. *et al.* Cantonese-style salted fish as a cause of nasopharyngeal carcinoma: a case control study in Hong Kong. *Cancer Research* 1986; **46**: 956–61.

3 Lyn T.C., Hsieh R.P., Chuang C.Y. *et al.* Epstein–Barr virus associated antibodies and serum biochemistry in nasopharyngeal carcinoma. *Laryngoscope* 1984; **94**: 485–88.

4 Lederman M., Mould R.F. Radiation treatment of cancer of the pharynx: with special reference to tele-cobalt therapy. *British Journal of Radiology* 1968; **41**: 251–74.

5 Union Internationale Contre le Cancer (UICC) *TNM Classification of Malignant Tumours*. Spiessl B., Beahrs O.H., Hermanek P. *et al.*, eds. Berlin: Springer Verlag, 1987.

6 Suen J.Y., Myers E.N. *Cancer of the Head and Neck*. Edinburgh: Churchill Livingstone, 1981.

7 Lederman M. Cancer of the larynx. Part 1: Natural history in relation to treatment. *British Journal of Radiology* 1971; **44**: 569–78.

8 McNeil B.J., Weichselbaum R., Parker S. Speech and survival. Trade-offs between quality and quantity of life in laryngeal cancer. *New England Journal of Medicine* 1981; **305**: 982–87.

9 Veteran Affairs Laryngeal Cancer Study Group. Induction chemotherapy plus radiation compared with surgery plus radiation in patients with advanced laryngeal cancer. *New England Journal of Medicine* 1991; **324**: 1685–90.

10 Harwood A.R., Beale F.A., Cummings B.J. *et al.* Supraglottic laryngeal carcinoma: an analysis of dose-time-volume factors in 410 patients. *International Journal of Radiation Oncology, Biology and Physics* 1983; **9**: 311–19.

11 Gelinas M., Fletcher G.H. Incidence and causes of local failure of irradiation in squamous carcinoma of the faucial arch, tonsillar fossa and base of tongue. *Radiology* 1973; **108**: 383–87.

12 Horiot J.C., Le Fur R., N'Guyen T. *et al.* Hyperfractionation versus conventional fractionation in oropharyngeal carcinoma: final analysis of a randomized trial of the EORTC cooperative group of radiotherapy. *Radiotherapy and Oncology* 1992; **25**: 229–32.

13 MacFarlane G.J., Boyle P., Scully C. Rising mortality from cancer of the tongue in young Scottish males. *Lancet* 1987; **ii**: 912.

14 Lippman S.M., Batsakis J.G., Toth B.B. *et al.* Comparison of low-dose isotretinoin with beta-carotene to prevent oral carcinogenesis. *New England Journal of Medicine* 1993; **328**: 15–20.

15 Montana F.S., Hellman S., von Essen C.F., Kligerman M.M. Carcinoma of the tongue and floor of the mouth: Results of radical radiotherapy. *Cancer* 1969; **23**: 1284–89.

16 Robin P.E., Powell D.J., Stansbie J.M. Carcinoma of

the nasal cavity and paranasal sinuses: incidence and presentation of different histological types. *Clinical Otolaryngology* 1979; **4**: 431−56.

17 Vokes E.E., Weichselbaum R.R., Lippman S.M. *et al.* Medical progress: head and neck. *New England Journal of Medicine* 1993; **328**: 184−94.

18 Tobias J.S. Current issues in cancer: cancer of the head and neck. *British Medical Journal* 1994; **308**: 961−66.

19 Stell P.M., Rawson N.S.B. Adjuvant chemotherapy in head and neck cancer. *British Journal of Cancer* 1990; **61**: 779−87.

20 Gupta N.L., Pointon R.C.S., Wilkinson P.M. A randomised clinical trial to contrast radiotherapy with radiotherapy and methotrexate given synchronously in head and neck cancer. *Clinical Radiology* 1987; **38**: 575−81.

21 Merlano M., Vitale V., Rosso R. *et al.* Treatment of advanced squamous-cell carcinoma of the head and neck with alternating chemotherapy and radiotherapy. *New England Journal of Medicine* 1992; **327**: 1115−21.

22 Weissberg J.B., Son Y.H., Papac R.J. *et al.* Randomised clinical trial of mitomycin C as an adjunct to radio-

therapy in head and neck cancer. *International Journal of Radiation Oncology, Biology and Physics* 1989; **17**: 3−9.

23 Tannock I.F., Browman F. Lack of evidence of the role of chemotherapy in the routine management of locally advanced head and neck cancer. *Journal of Clinical Oncology* 1986; **4**: 1121−26.

24 Gasmi J., Bachouchi M., Cvitkovic E. *et al.* Nasopharyngeal carcinoma: A medical oncology viewpoint. The Gustave Roussy Experience. *Annals of Oncology* 1990; **1**: 245−53.

25 Griffin T.W., Pajak T.F., Laramore G.E. *et al.* Neutron vs photon irradiation of inoperable salivary gland tumors: results of an RTOG : MRC cooperative randomised study. *International Journal of Radiation Oncology, Biology and Physics* 1988; **15**: 1085−90.

26 Hickman R., Cawson R.A., Duffy S.W. The prognosis of specific types of salivary gland tumours. *Cancer* 1984; **54**: 1620−24.

27 Armstrong J.G., Harrison L.B., Spiro R.H. *et al.* The role of postoperative radiation in malignant tumors of salivary gland origin: a matched pair analysis using historical controls. *International Journal of Radiation Oncology, Biology and Physics* 1988; **15**: 176.

Chapter 11
Tumours of the Nervous System

BRAIN TUMOURS

Brain tumours are amongst the most devastating of all malignant diseases, frequently producing profound and progressive disability leading to death. In addition they may be difficult to diagnose and are invariably challenging to treat. Their incidence appears to be rising steadily, at least in the United States; the peak incidence is in the first decade of life and at age 50–60 years. Brain tumours are one of the most important groups of childhood tumours, second only to the leukaemias and lymphomas in frequency. In Britain the incidence is approximately 6 per 100 000, with 2200 deaths each year.

Almost nothing is known of the aetiology. An increase in both benign and malignant brain tumours has been noted following radiation of the scalp for benign conditions in childhood. Epidemiological studies have confirmed that significant differences exist in the frequency of brain tumours throughout life, sufficient to suggest the possibility of different aetiological factors in their causation [1]. Clearly, childhood and adult central nervous system tumours have different biological behaviour; only haemangioblastomas have an equal incidence in both childhood and adult life. The hormonal influences on certain pituitary adenomas and meningiomas may explain the earlier peak age incidence of these tumours in females, and to some extent account for the apparent sex ratio differences.

The previously uncommon primary cerebral lymphoma has been diagnosed far more frequently with the advent of the AIDS pandemic over the past decade. The other important 'new' aetiological factor in cerebral lymphoma is the increase over the past 20 years of increasingly successful organ transplantation. Perhaps surprisingly, the increased incidence of primary cerebral lymphoma is not entirely attributable to these causes [2].

Over the past 25 years, refinements of both neurosurgical and radiotherapeutic techniques have resulted in changes in management and, in some instances, improvement in prognosis. More recently, medical oncologists have begun to demonstrate a possible role for cytotoxic drugs, although their contribution is not yet fully established.

Cellular biology of brain tumours

The growth kinetics of malignant brain tumours have been widely studied in recent years, mostly using incorporation of radiolabelled DNA precursors such as ^{3}H-thymidine or bromodeoxyuridine (BUdR) and then quantifying the result by immunological techniques with a specific anti-BUdR-DNA monoclonal antibody. Many studies have now shown that the higher grade tumours have much higher labelling indices, and possibly offer useful prognostic data as well [3]. Such techniques can also be used as the basis of flow cytometry studies, which have themselves demonstrated a strong correlation between aneuploidy and degree of malignancy in adult glioma.

Oncogene analysis of human brain tumours has also proven valuable in recent years. In over 50% of glioblastoma multiforme, amplification of N-*myc*, C-*myc*, N-*ras* or other oncogenes is present, often with simultaneous over-expression of more than one. In addition, the epidermal growth factor receptor (EGFR; see Chapter 3) is also usually highly expressed, and is encoded for by the *erb*-B encogene [4].

At least six specific and frequently occurring molecular genetic alterations have been identified in the pathogenesis of gliomas. In the amplification of EGFR, a specific gene appears responsible. In high-grade tumours, hemi- and homozygous deletion of interferon loci at chromosome 9p has frequently been demonstrated. In primitive neuroectodermal tumours including medulloblastoma, deletion of the short arm of chromosome 17 is a commonly observed karyotype abnormality.

Other specific aberrations are beginning to emerge, particularly involving chromosomes 1, 3, 7, 10 and 22 [5]. One particularly well studied brain tumour is the meningioma, which frequently displays monosomy 22.

Pathological classification of brain tumours

The majority of brain tumours are gliomas, thought to arise from malignant change of mature glial elements, usually with differen-

tiation towards one particular type of glial cell [6]. Although it now seems clear that tumour progression does occur, for example from astrocytoma to glioblastoma, no premalignant states have been recognized in human glioma — unlike many other human solid tumours.

Taken together, astrocytomas, ependymomas, oligodendrogliomas and medulloblastomas comprise over 90% of all primary brain and spinal cord tumours. In cases where the tumour is well differentiated, there is usually no difficulty in recognizing the type of cell from which the tumour has arisen.

These tumours are classified according to the cell of origin and a widely accepted working classification is given in Table 11.1. Other more detailed classifications have been proposed by the World Health Organization but the simpler system outlined in Table 11.1 is used in this chapter.

GLIOMAS

Astrocytomas

These are much the commonest variety and arise from astrocytes which are the supporting

Table 11.1 Classification of brain tumours

Primary tumours	Primary tumours	Secondary tumours
Gliomas	*Pineal tumours*	*Common sites of origin*
Astrocytoma	Pinealoblastoma	Lung
Glioblastoma multiforme	Pinealocytoma	Breast
Ependymoma	Germinoma	Melanoma
Oligodendroglioma	Teratoma	
Primitive neuroectodermal		*Less common sites of origin*
tumours (incl.	*Intracranial lymphoma*	Ovary
medulloblastoma)	'Histiocytic' lymphoma	Testis
	Microglioma	Gut
Pituitary tumours		Bladder
Pituitary adenoma	*Acoustic*	Kidney
Craniopharyngioma		Pancreas
Pituitary carcinoma	*Chordoma*	Liver
		Leukaemia and lymphoma
Meningioma	*Neuronal tumours*	
Benign	Ganglioneuroma	*Miscellaneous*
Malignant (meningiosarcoma)	Ganglioglioma	Histiocytosis X
	Colloid cyst	

cells of the brain. They are divided into four grades (according to Kernohan) on the basis of cytomorphological characteristics. Grade I is the least malignant. Grades II–IV show progressively more malignant characteristics. The degree of malignancy is assessed according to histological features such as invasion, tumour necrosis, cellularity and mitotic activity together with cytological features including nuclear abnormality and variation in cell size and morphology. Low-grade gliomas (Fig. 11.1A) occur most commonly in the frontal, parietal and temporal lobes and in the brain stem and cerebellum of children. Because of their relatively slow evolution, local destruction is not usually encountered, in contrast to the more high-grade gliomas, in which degeneration, necrosis, haemorrhage, infarction and local destruction are characteristically found.

As with tumours at other sites, biopsy specimens may not necessarily be representative of the whole tumour, and mixed varieties are common. Descriptive terms are sometimes used where a particular morphological feature predominates. Pathologists may use the terms fibrillary, protoplasmic, gemistocytic or pilocytic to describe relatively well differentiated types of astrocytoma. These subdivisions may have considerable prognostic significance (see below). In highly malignant gliomas it may be quite impossible to recognize the initial cell of origin, and these tumours are amongst the most bizarre and undifferentiated of all, often termed *glioblastoma multiforme* (Fig. 11.1B). They grow rapidly by direct extension, and are always much larger than suggested by pre-operative angiography, CT or MRI studies. They are rarely operable, do not as a rule respond to irradiation, and are usually fatal within a year. By contrast, grade I gliomas enlarge much more slowly and can usually be excised completely though local recurrence does sometimes occur.

True grade I gliomas are, however, extremely unusual — most low-grade gliomas are grade II. Gliomas at different sites may behave quite differently despite a similar histological appearance. For this reason, localized gliomas of the optic nerves are often left untreated and may regress spontaneously whilst gliomas of the pons or brain stem behave much more aggressively and demand urgent attention with wide field irradiation. In recent years it has become possible to grow cell lines of high-grade glioma in tissue-culture laboratories, a useful technique for determining cytotoxic drug sensitivity [7].

Ependymal tumours

These comprise about 5% of all primary brain tumours and are derived from the ciliated lining cells of the CNS cavities. The tumour cells form characteristic rosettes. (Fig. 11.1C). This tumour most commonly occurs in childhood and early adult life, and just over half arise from infratentorial sites. Tumour spread occurs by direct invasion and also by seeding throughout the CNS, particularly with high-grade ependymoma and where the primary tumour is infratentorial. Although tumour grading is perhaps less important than with astrocytomas there is general agreement that low-grade ependymomas have a far better prognosis than the higher grades. Most aggressive of all is the ependymoblastoma.

Oligodendrogliomas

These are derived from other supporting cells and are usually very indolent in their growth pattern with a long history, often calcifying. The cells have a typical appearance (Fig. 11.1D) with a clear zone around the nucleus, the cells appearing 'boxed-in'. Typical sites are the frontal, parietal and temporal lobes. The commonest age range is 40–60 years.

Medulloblastoma

The term 'primitive neuroectodermal tumour' (PNET) is now increasingly preferred to describe these, and certain other, embryonal tumours. Their cytogenetic characteristics are at least partly understood (see above), with loss of genetic information from chromosome 17, the most frequently observed abnormality.

Fig. 11.1 Histological appearance of the commoner brain tumours. (A) Low-grade glioma showing sparse cellularity with no vascular proliferation (original magnification × 200); (B) high-grade glioma showing cellular pleomorphism and necrosis (arrowed) (×200); (C) ependymoma: tumour forms typical rosettes (×400); (D) oligodendroglioma showing typical 'boxed-in' cell appearance (×400); (E) medulloblastoma showing small, darkly staining, closely packed cells (×400); (F) pituitary adenoma: appearance is characteristic of endocrine tumours (×250).

They comprise 3% of all brain tumours and are predominantly diagnosed in childhood and young adult life, with a few cases occurring after the age of 25 years. There is a peak age incidence of 4–10 years, and the male : female ratio is over 2 : 1. The tumour cells often form rosettes (Fig. 11.1E). Medulloblastoma chiefly arises in the posterior fossa, from the vermis, cerebellar hemispheres or the fourth ventricle. Patients usually present with raised intracranial pressure (see below). Because of close proximity to the CSF the tumour metastasizes via CSF, either to the spinal cord, or elsewhere in the brain. Occasionally, distant metastases are seen outside the central nervous system, and bone metastases (mostly osteosclerotic) and marrow involvement are occasionally encountered. Other sites include lung and lymph nodes.

PITUITARY TUMOURS

These account for about 10% of all primary intracranial neoplasms. They usually arise from the glandular epithelial cells, producing tumours which are histologically classified according to the staining characteristics of the cytoplasmic granules. In most of these, granular staining is absent (chromophobe tumours, Fig. 11.1F) but in a minority there is characteristic acidophilic or basophilic staining. Increasingly, these tumours are pathologically classified using functional and immunological criteria rather than simple staining. Non-epithelial pituitary tumours are thought to arise from cell rests from Rathke's pouch, producing tumours of the hypothalamus or true pituitary known as craniopharyngiomas. The pituitary and hypothalamus are not uncommon as sites of secondary cancer, chiefly from breast and small cell lung cancers.

Chromophobe adenomas comprise about three-quarters of all pituitary tumours, and are most frequently encountered in adult life. They tend to be non-functional (endocrine-inactive), though ACTH, growth hormone, prolactin and other hormones are sometimes produced. They frequently attain a large size, particularly if non-functioning, and may extend upwards out of the sella, to involve the optic chiasm leading to the characteristic visual disturbance of bitemporal hemianopia (Fig. 11.2). Of the chromophil tumours, the acidophil adenomas are chiefly associated with excessive production of growth hormone, leading either to acromegaly if the tumour arises in adult life, or very rarely to gigantism when the tumour is encountered in childhood. Basophilic tumours tend to be smaller, and usually secrete ACTH and/or MSH leading to Cushing's syndrome sometimes with hyperpigmentation. These tumours are usually small and rarely involve the suprasellar area, so visual signs are unusual.

Craniopharyngiomas

Craniopharyngiomas, unlike the other common pituitary tumours, are most frequently encountered in children. These tumours may be solid or cystic, and radiologically show characteristic calcification. They often involve suprasellar structures and can be particularly difficult to remove surgically, especially when there is heavy calcification.

MENINGIOMA

These tumours comprise about 10% of all brain

Fig. 11.2 Local effects of pituitary tumours. Extension commonly produces pressure on the optic chiasm, base of brain and anterior and posterior clinoid processes. Extension occurs inferiorly and laterally, to sphenoid and cavernous sinuses.

tumours and arise from the meninges. There is a predilection for certain sites, particularly the parasagittal region and sphenoid ridge. They tend to compress the brain from without, and frank invasion is very uncommon except for the rare malignant meningioma, sometimes referred to as meningiosarcoma. Pressure outwards may cause bony erosion of the inner table of the skull, whilst inward displacement of the brain may lead to epilepsy as an early feature. Meningiomas may be chiefly fibrous in nature (fibroblastic meningioma) or very vascular (angioblastic meningioma), the latter having a more rapid evolution and more frequent malignant transformation. A specific genetic abnormality, monosomy 22, is present in up to 70% of cases.

OTHERS

Tumours of the pineal and third ventricle

These are now increasingly recognized, and are a diverse group arising either from the pineal itself, the third ventricle, or less commonly from ectopic sites of pineal tissue, particularly in the hypothalamus. Common types include the pinealoblastoma which histologically resembles medulloblastoma; the pinealocytoma which is a tumour of mature pineal cells; and germ cell tumours, which can be either pure seminoma (pineal germinoma) or teratoma which often contains highly differentiated mesenchymal structures. These latter tumours may produce AFP and HCG which can be measured in CSF or in blood and which can be helpful in diagnosis and management (see Chapter 4). At the anterior end of the third ventricle, the histological types are even more varied and include pituitary tumours, germinomas, meningiomas, optic nerve glioma, histiocytosis X and non-malignant granulomas which can occasionally cause diagnostic difficulty, such as tuberculosis and sarcoidosis. In proven pineal and suprasellar germinomas there is a high risk of spinal seeding (20–30%), possibly aggravated by attempts at surgical excision.

Intracerebral lymphomas

These are unusual, but now far more common as one of the AIDS-related malignancies. The two chief types are the 'histiocytic' lymphoma which can occur at any site in the brain and appears more frequently in immunosuppressed patients such as renal transplant recipients; and the microglioma, a rare intracranial lymphoma not seen outside the central nervous system (Chapter 26).

Thalamic and brain stem tumours

These are usually gliomas, though surgical biopsy is generally thought inadvisable. Thalamic gliomas are seen both in children (usually well-differentiated tumours) and adults (usually glioblastoma multiforme). Brain stem tumours are also chiefly encountered in children and are usually astrocytomas of variable differentiation.

Tumours of cranial nerves and nerve sheaths

Acoustic neuroma is a tumour of adult life, rather more common in females, and arising from the VIII cranial nerve, usually in its vestibular part. These tend to be slow-growing tumours which present with unilateral deafness, vertigo, tinnitus, and involvement of other cranial nerves. Although strictly benign, they exert a local space-occupying mass effect. Other less common neuronal tumours include the ganglioneuroma and ganglioglioma which are also typically benign though dangerous because of local pressure effects.

Chordomas

Chordomas are uncommon malignant tumours, originating from the remnants of the embryonic notochord. Although occasionally encountered in children and young adults the peak age of incidence is 50–60 years and the characteristic sites are in the extremes of the spinal cord: a spheno-occipito-cervical group (40% of all cases) and a sacro-coccygeal group (equally frequent). The tumour consists of very characteristic solid cords of polygonal or mucin containing 'physalipherous' cells sometimes with a lobulated pattern. Local pressure symptoms are common, including bulbar, occipital or neck symptoms from tumours at the upper end of the spine, or constipation and low back pain from sacro-coccygeal tumours. Extensive bone destruction may occur.

Colloid cysts

Colloid cysts occur chiefly in the cerebellum and masquerade as malignant tumours because of their space-occupying nature. Although these tumours are rare they can usually be diagnosed with confidence on CT scanning.

Clinical features

Brain tumours can be difficult to diagnose. The onset of symptoms may be late, particularly in tumours situated in less critical areas of the brain. In these parts of the cerebral hemispheres, they may grow to a substantial size before diagnosis, and may only produce rather subtle changes in personality, muscular power or co-ordination. In more critically sited tumours, obvious symptoms such as convulsions, ataxia or sensorimotor loss will lead to much earlier diagnosis.

In general, the symptoms can be broadly divided into four main groups. First, brain tumours can exert a mass effect and lead to raised intracranial pressure, with headache, drowsiness, nausea and vomiting as the cardinal symptoms. The headache is often worse in the morning, typically clearing by lunchtime. Vomiting may be sudden, unexpected and not preceded by nausea. Tumours situated around the fourth ventricle, in the cerebellum and around the pons are particularly likely to lead to raised intracranial pressure while tumours situated in the cerebral hemispheres may reach a large size without producing such symptoms. Papilloedema is usually present though it may be unilateral. With the advent of CT scanning (Fig. 11.3) it is now recognized that ventricular enlargement, presumably caused by raised intracranial pressure, can be unaccompanied by papilloedema.

Secondly, there is a large group of focal symptoms caused by damage to local structures. These symptoms are determined by the site and size of the tumour. In a relatively small space, occupying lesions can cause devastating

Fig. 11.3 (A) CT scan showing a large mass (glioma) in the left hemisphere; (B) MRI scan from same case as (A); (C) CT brain scan showing large midline tumour of the posterior fossa. This was a medulloblastoma; (D) CT brain scan showing large parieto-occipital glioma. Note the obvious rim of contrast with oedema and ventricular dilatation.

symptoms if sited in the motor cortex, Broca's area or the base of the brain. Accurate siting of tumours is often possible as a result of these specific symptoms: myoclonic seizures, development of late-onset grand mal epilepsy or hemiparesis all point to lesions in the motor cortex, whereas lip smacking, hallucinations and other psychotic disturbances are typical of a temporal lobe lesion. For tumours situated more deeply, abnormalities of the visual pathways may give helpful diagnostic information since the optic nerves, chiasm, tract, radiations and visual cortex traverse the brain from front to back and interruption at a particular site will lead to recognizable abnormalities of the visual fields. At the base of the brain, the classical features are those of cranial nerve lesions, often multiple. In particular, tumours near the jugular foramen may cause a specific pattern of cranial nerve palsies since many of the lower cranial nerves exit at or near this point. Ataxia, nystagmus and diplopia are typical of cerebellar lesions, and are often coupled with nausea and headache due to raised intracranial pressure.

The third group of symptoms results from remote endocrine effects and occurs with tumours of the pituitary and hypothalamus. Damage to local structures is of great importance in pituitary tumours which can extend upwards to the suprasellar area and optic chiasm, inferiorly into the sphenoid sinus or laterally to the cavernous sinus or beyond, sometimes into the middle or posterior fossa (Fig. 11.2). Damage to the III, IV and VI cranial nerves may occur. Bleeding into a pituitary tumour (pituitary apoplexy) may result in sudden deterioration of vision, severe headache and hypopituitarism. Lesser degrees of panhypopituitarism are common in pituitary tumours though different endorgans may be variably affected. The florid syndrome includes hypothyroidism from reduction in TSH production, hypocorticism with hypotension from reduction in ACTH and hypogonadism with loss of secondary sexual characteristics, libido and amenorrhoea with infertility. In adults, lack of growth hormone results in hypoglycaemia. In children, reduction or cessation of growth is more characteristic. Sophisticated endocrinological investigations are often required to determine the full extent of the pituitary syndrome, but simple measurements of T_3, T_4, TSH, cortisol and gonadotrophins are usually sufficient for demonstration of the basic defects.

Finally, tumours of the central nervous system occasionally metastasize. Although this usually occurs late in the disease, patients may rarely present with symptoms caused by the metastases becoming apparent before the primary tumour itself. Although very unusual in adults, metastases are well recognized in children with medulloblastomas and poorly differentiated ependymomas. Secondary spread from these tumours is almost always through the CSF, usually presenting as spinal or meningeal deposits. Bone metastasis is also a well recognized complication of medulloblastoma.

Diagnosis

The accurate diagnosis of brain tumours has been revolutionized by the advent of CT and MRI scanning. Both carry the advantages of high definition and easy repeatability, invaluable for post-treatment assessment. The routine use of intravenous contrast material has increased their sensitivity still further (Fig. 11.3), as has the continual evolution of technological refinements and the ability to reconstruct the image in sagittal and other planes. CT brain scanning does, however, have its limitations particularly in tumours of the posterior fossa and brain stem. In these sites, MRI is clearly superior [8]. Pituitary tumours require high resolution since they are often small and close to bony structures. Most CT scanning machines can reliably detect lesions of greater than $1\,cm^3$ but low-grade gliomas are sometimes poorly visualized. Angiography is still indicated to exclude arteriovenous malformations and occasionally to visualize posterior fossa, deep-seated and thalamic lesions and other sites poorly visualized by CT or MRI scanning. In addition, pre-operative angiography may be helpful in defining the tumour's vascular supply. Digital subtraction techniques are generally felt to give the best image display in these situations.

Management of brain tumours

The approach to management depends on the histological nature of the tumour and its site. Surgical removal is desirable both for histological diagnosis and sometimes for definitive treatment. Radical excision can, however, be extremely hazardous and occasionally impossible. Stereotactic CT-guided biopsy can be useful for histological confirmation in inoperable cases. Where hydrocephalus is present surgical decompression by ventricular drainage results in dramatic improvement. Both ventriculoperitoneal and ventriculo-atrial shunts are employed and can be permanently implanted. For deep-seated tumours (e.g. thalamic, pineal and brainstem) even a biopsy may be out of the question. Urgent reversal of acute cerebral oedema may be necessary which may include the use of intravenous urea, mannitol, or high doses of dexamethasone (see p. 218 for management details). Radiotherapy is frequently employed as an adjunct to surgery and sometimes as the definitive treatment [9]. The role of chemotherapy is still debatable though cytotoxic drugs are increasingly used.

GLIOMAS

Low-grade (Kernohan Grades I and II). For low-grade astrocytomas, complete surgical excision is often undertaken since these lesions tend to be well localized and can often be removed from adjacent structures without causing too much damage. In many cases surgery is the sole method of treatment. However, late local recurrences may occur. Routine irradiation is now established as an important mode of treatment in incompletely resected tumours. Leibel and colleagues, in a series of over 100 patients with incompletely resected low-grade astrocytomas [10] showed that the 10-year survival rate was only 11% in patients where radiotherapy was not given, compared with 35% in patients who were irradiated. At 20 years, the survival difference was more striking still: 0% compared with 23%. These results lend support to the conclusions of Bouchard and Peirce who suggested over 30 years ago that irradiation was a useful adjunct to surgery for well-differentiated astrocytomas [11]. A more recent study from the Mayo Clinic supported these general conclusions [12]. Of 167 low-grade astrocytomas, the pilocytic group (41 cases) had a good prognosis regardless of postoperative treatment but in the remainder, radiotherapy clearly prolonged survival especially if the tumour dose was >53 Gy, in which the 5-year survival rate was 68% compared with 21% when radiotherapy was not given. Interestingly, complete surgical excision did not appear critically important so radiotherapy may become the dominant therapeutic modality in low-grade gliomas. Whereas previously a total surgical excision seemed adequate treatment, postoperative irradiation is now increasingly recommended in all cases. An alternative view, however, is provided by a series in which active treatment was limited to patients with progressive symptoms, large tumours or those in cerebellar sites [13]. Careful CT or MRI monitoring was offered in their cases, and the results of this policy seemed generally satisfactory. In general the radiation treatment volume can be limited since these tumours do not infiltrate widely.

High-grade (Kernohan Grades III and IV). For these tumours radiotherapy is almost always employed as an adjunct to surgery (Fig. 11.4), firstly because complete surgical removal is rarely possible, and secondly because the results of surgery alone are so poor. As long ago as 1962 Taveras *et al.* [14] asked the pertinent question: 'should we treat glioblastoma multiforme?' In a study of over 400 patients, these authors showed that where patients had undergone biopsy alone or partial resection postoperative irradiation was beneficial. Their

Fig. 11.4 External beam radiation for cortical glioma. Typical three-field plan treating whole hemisphere. The irradiated volume is shown by the broken line.

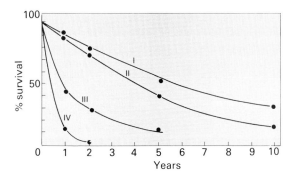

Fig. 11.5 Survival related to grade in malignant glioma. Note the small proportion of 10-year survivors even with low-grade tumours.

recommendations of adequate surgical decompression with partial or gross surgical removal where possible and radiation therapy shortly after operation, are still followed. More recent studies of postoperative irradiation for glioblastoma multiforme have demonstrated that, although at 1 year there are no survivors with surgery alone, almost one-fifth of patients receiving postoperative radiation are still alive. With these high-grade tumours, large radiation volumes are required and some radiotherapists routinely treat the whole of the brain. Doses of 40–50 Gy (4000–5000 rad) in 4½–6 weeks are often used (Fig. 11.4). However, the ultimate prognosis is very poor indeed, less than 6% of patients with Grade IV disease surviving for 5 years. For patients with Grade III tumours, the survival is better, and over half of the surviving patients achieve an independent life (Fig. 11.5).

Attempts to improve these dismal figures have led to the use of wide-field irradiation or treatment to higher dosage, since local recurrence at the initial tumour site is almost always the cause of death. A recent Medical Research Council (MRC) randomized study has shown that higher external beam doses (60 Gy) gave a small but significant survival advantage [15]. Autopsy findings on patients with glioblastoma dying shortly after diagnosis have confirmed that the tumour has almost always infiltrated

much more widely than is apparent even on surgical inspection. Nevertheless, even where the treatment field is increased to include the whole brain, with boosting of the primary site to a very high dose, later local recurrence is almost inevitable. If a means of increasing the dose could safely be found, better local control might yet be obtained. Unfortunately neither radiosensitizer studies nor novel high LET radiation techniques has yet proven to be of value. However, there is increasing interest in at least three novel radiation techniques: interstitial brachytherapy, stereotactic external beam irradiation and hyperfractionated radiotherapy. Interstitial brachytherapy, often using ^{125}Ir or ^{60}Co sources, permits the delivery of high doses of radiotherapy to the volume without unnecessary treatment of large areas of normal brain, and can be used in conjunction with stereotactic surgery. A large series from San Francisco suggested that this technique might be valuable both for primary treatment and also recurrent disease [16], particularly in Grade III lesions, though the excellent results from this group probably reflect careful selection of tumours which are limited by size and the performance status of the subject. Indeed, these features, together with age and clinical history, are known to be important prognostic factors [15].

There has been increasing interest in the use

of cytotoxic agents as an adjuvant to surgery and radiotherapy for high-grade gliomas. The nitrosoureas, BCNU and CCNU have received most attention, since they are known to be lipid soluble and cross the hypothetical blood–brain barrier (see Chapter 6). Assessment of response of brain tumours to chemotherapy is difficult, but there is no doubt that some patients with recurrent disease benefit with an objective response rate of about 40% (Table 11.2). Unfortunately, most of these responses are short-lived and are seen in patients with relatively well-differentiated gliomas. Patients with Grade IV tumours are very unlikely to respond. In a large prospective multicentre trial, Walker and colleagues showed that routine use of BCNU as an addition to surgery and radiotherapy prolonged the median survival by a few weeks [17]. The study also confirmed that treatment by surgery and chemotherapy (but no irradiation) was much less successful. Other data also suggest that nitrosoureas do offer a small survival advantage, with a possible superiority for CCNU over BCNU.

Other agents with known activity are vincristine and procarbazine (Table 11.2). These drugs have the added advantage of being relatively non-toxic. Cisplatin and vepeside (VM26) have recently been shown to have some activity.

One commonly used combination is PCV (procarbazine, CCNU and vincristine), a well tolerated regimen often used as adjuvant therapy and given on a 6-weekly out-patient basis. It is thought to be superior to single-agent nitrosourea treatment [18] and is currently

Table 11.2 Response to cytotoxic drugs in gliomas

Drug	Responders* (%)
BCNU	47
CCNU	44
Procarbazine	52
Vepeside (VM26)	25
Cisplatin	30
BCNU and vincristine	44

* Most of these are partial responses. Criteria of response vary considerably.

being tested in a prospective randomized study by the Medical Research Council. Previous work from the same group suggested that probability of chemotherapy responsiveness could to some extent be predicted by *in vitro* tissue-culture studies [7].

Unfortunately, intra-arterial chemotherapy (via the carotid artery) has proven unacceptably toxic. Of the newer agents recently tested, temozalamide has attracted particular interest, in view of a promisingly high preliminary response rate; these findings have yet to be verified.

Ependymoma. This tumour is far less common than astrocytoma and behaves rather differently. It arises from cells lining the ventricles and central canal of the spinal cord, and has a tendency to seed throughout the subarachnoid space giving rise to symptomatic spinal deposits in about 10% of patients. Spinal seeding is particularly likely in patients with high-grade lesions, especially those arising from the lining cells of the fourth ventricle. For this reason, routine craniospinal irradiation is usually recommended in all patients with high-grade ependymomas and for ependymomas of the posterior fossa regardless of grade (see pp. 213–14 for details of technique and toxicity). The primary site should receive a high dose (50 Gy or greater in 5–7 weeks) with full craniospinal treatment in patients with high-grade tumours. There is evidence that spinal cord primaries tend to be of lower grade than intracerebral tumours, with a better survival rate.

The overall survival of ependymomas is better than with astrocytomas. At least 50% of patients live for 5 years. Several series have, however, confirmed the importance of radiation dose. In a report by Phillips and colleagues [19] the 5-year survival of patients given *intensive* radiotherapy was almost 90%, twice the *overall* survival rate of 40% (which included those who died postoperatively without treatment as well as patients who received inadequate irradiation dosage). From this it is clear that the approach should be intensive with full treatment to the whole craniospinal axis at least in patients with high-grade or infratentorial tumours.

Oligodendrogliomas. These are uncommon tumours, often relatively well-differentiated, slow growing and amenable to complete surgical removal. In such cases there is no definite indication for postoperative irradiation although treatment is usually advised where there has been incomplete surgical excision, or where there are histologically aggressive features (sometimes termed oligodendro-blastoma). In a group of over 30 patients, reported by Sheline, the 5-year survival with surgery alone was 31% compared with an 85% survival rate in patients receiving postoperative irradiation [20]. From these and other data, the 10-year survival rate is of the order of 35%.

For recurrent oligodendroglioma there is increasing evidence of chemo-responsiveness, using either PCV or cisplatin [21].

Deep-seated gliomas. Gliomas situated deep to the cerebral cortex present particular problems of diagnosis and management. Important sites include the thalamus and hypothalamus, pons, brain stem, pineal region and optic nerves. The common difficulty with tumours in these areas is that histological confirmation is often not possible because any attempt at surgical inter-vention would be hazardous though gliomas of the pineal area are increasingly being con-sidered suitable for surgical removal.

Their clinical behaviour varies at each of the different sites. Optic nerve gliomas, which usually present with proptosis or blindness, are often thought to be benign and unresponsive to radiotherapy. However, in some cases the tumours are bilateral, involve the optic chiasm or extend backwards to the ventricles, some-times with hydrocephalus. These patients should be treated with radiotherapy. Although uncomplicated lesions may be self-limiting, radiotherapy may produce complete relief of distressing proptosis, and objective response verified on CT or MRI scanning. Pierce *et al.* [22] reported a series of 24 children with optic

nerve glioma with lengthy follow-up (median 6 years) and an overall 6-year survival rate of 100%. Over 90% of patients had improvement or 'stabilization' of vision.

For thalamic tumours, radiotherapy is almost invariably indicated. Surgical attempts at excision or even histological confirmation are particularly dangerous at this site.

The prognosis for these tumours appears to vary with age, though as expected, histological grade (usually obtained only at autopsy) is also important. The 5-year survival rate in young patients with Grade III lesions is about 25%. Tumours of the pons and brain stem carry a particularly poor prognosis and often present with florid symptoms including cranial nerve palsies, ataxia or involvement of the long tracts. These are usually high-grade astrocytomas and infiltrate widely, often attaining a large volume before diagnosis. They are a challenge to the radiotherapist since they are surgically untreat-able, but often present with urgent problems in management. Although the majority show some symptomatic response to radiotherapy, the ultimate survival rate (approximately 15%) is poor. A large review of patients with brain stem tumours showed an average survival of 4 years for irradiated patients compared with only 15 months if untreated [23]. In patients who showed a response to treatment, the average survival was over 5 years. In general, there seems to be no point in attempting to treat these lesions with highly localized radiation fields. Large lateral opposed fields are required since the tumour has usually spread throughout the whole of the pons, brain stem and medulla and often to the upper cervical spine. Doses of 40−55 Gy in 4−5 weeks daily treatment are usually recommended although some centres employ fewer fractions, for example a total dose of 45−48 Gy in 15 daily fractions.

Medulloblastoma (and other primitive neuroecto-dermal tumours). Surgical treatment alone is unsuccessful, and postoperative radiotherapy has been routinely employed since the 1920s, when the marked radiosensitivity of this tumour was first noted. With increasingly accurate treatment planning, the use of supervoltage equipment and prophylactic irradiation of the whole brain and spinal cord, the 10-year survival rate has improved and is now in the order of 40% [24].

Many surgeons limit their operation to biopsy and decompression, recognizing that an attempt at bulk removal is bound to increase the complication rate. The operative mortality is still in the region of 7%. However, although these tumours are radiosensitive, they do recur at the primary site, and it is possible that removal of tumour bulk might reduce the rate of local recurrence. Most neurosurgeons excise as much tumour as is safely possible, and survival following 'complete' removal of the tumour is better than when the tumour has been only partially removed. It is now routine practice to irradiate the whole of the craniospinal axis, as soon after surgery as possible. Treatment planning must be meticulous, taking particular care to treat the base of the brain, retro-orbital area and brain stem. (Fig. 11.6). These sites can be undertreated if adult surface anatomical boundaries are used without regard to the anatomy of the developing brain. The technique which we employ is carried out as follows.

1 Irradiation of the whole brain with large lateral opposing fields, including the midbrain and upper cervical vertebrae as far as the lower limit of C_2, to a midline dose of 30 Gy in 3 weeks.

2 Boosting of the posterior fossa and midbrain as far anteriorly as the anterior clinoid process, to 45 Gy at the same rate.

3 At the same time as the posterior fossa boost is commenced, spinal irradiation is begun, from the lower border of the cerebral fields to the lower border of vertebra S_2 so that the entire spinal cord including the conus medullaris and cauda equina are treated. A dose of not less than 30 Gy is given to the spine over 4−5 weeks.

4 For the final part of treatment, the posterior fossa is boosted to a still higher dose. The final

Fig. 11.6 Craniospinal irradiation. Schematic representation of the field arrangement for craniospinal irradiation in medulloblastoma and other tumours which seed through the CSF.

brain doses are as follows: posterior fossa 50−55 Gy in 6−7 weeks, midbrain 45 Gy in 5−6 weeks, cerebral hemispheres and anterior part of brain 35 Gy in 4 weeks, spinal cord 30 Gy minimum dose in 4−5 weeks.

5 Further boosting of limited areas of the spine if shown to be positive for tumour seeding, using myelographic or MRI imaging.

It is important to monitor the blood count during treatment of the spine, but with this technique and dose rate the treatment rarely has to be discontinued, although the white blood count frequently falls to about 2×10^9/l by the end of treatment.

Irradiation of the whole neuraxis carries a number of drawbacks. Fortunately, skull growth is usually almost complete by the time of treatment, so that permanent reduction in skull volume is very rarely seen. Nonetheless, some degree of shortness of stature (particularly sitting height) must be expected from irradiation of the whole spine coupled with pituitary irradiation (see Chapter 5). In addition, midline organs such as the thyroid, larynx, oesophagus, thymus and heart are directly in the path of the exit beam, and the kidneys and female gonads are also likely to receive a significant amount of scattered irradiation despite the most careful planning. The need for whole spine irradiation has therefore been questioned, especially as only 1 in 10 children will develop spinal cord metastases. However, current practice favours more extensive surgery even though there is a theoretical risk of spinal seeding because of shedding of tumour cells during the operation.

Despite these hazards and the possible added problem of cognitive and learning defects, over three-quarters of surviving children with medulloblastoma lead independent and active lives and at least one study has shown that intellectual achievement in these children is not impaired [25]. In the context of possible curative treatment for children with medulloblastoma, there seems little doubt that the possible hazards of treatment have to be accepted [26].

Chemotherapy has mainly been used for treatment of recurrent disease and as initial treatment in very young children (under 2 years). Lipid-soluble agents have been used both singly and in combination. The approximate response rates are shown in Table 11.3. The responses are usually short-lived and combination chemotherapy may be difficult if relapse follows soon after craniospinal irradiation because of the volume of bone marrow which has been irradiated. Methotrexate, which may be of some value, may be hazardous within 6 months of irradiation as it can cause a severe leucoencephalopathy.

Combination chemotherapy is increasingly preferred to single-agent treatment, and response rates up to 75% have been reported. It has recently been established that both cis- and carboplatin are active agents. Chemotherapy is

Table 11.3 Chemotherapy of recurrent medulloblastoma

Drug	Response rate
Single agent	
Vincristine	Probably 50%
CCNU	Probably 50%
High-dose methotrexate	Uncertain 0–60%
Cisplatin	Probably 50%
Combinations	
Procarbazine	
Vincristine	60%
CCNU	
Mustine	
Vincristine	
Procarbazine	Approximately 50%
Prednisolone	

also increasingly used for recurrent childhood malignant glioma, and at least one randomized study has produced encouraging results using CCNU, vincristine and prednisone [27]. The 5-year survival rates with and without adjuvant chemotherapy were 43% and 17% respectively, and the advantage was particularly striking in the very high-grade tumour subset.

Since there is modest responsiveness to drugs in patients with advanced disease and radiotherapy is often not curative, there has been considerable interest in using cytotoxic drugs as an adjuvant to surgery and radiotherapy. The International Society for Paediatric Oncology has undertaken a large trial to assess the role of adjuvant chemotherapy with vincristine and CCNU, given both during the radiotherapy treatment and as maintenance for 2 years afterwards [28]. In a series of over 330 cases, a number of points have now emerged. The main beneficiaries of adjuvant chemotherapy appear to be the groups where the tumour was incompletely removed, with brain stem spread and below 3 years.

It is often possible to obtain symptomatic improvement in patients with recurrence by further radiotherapy, particularly if the initial treatment was given at least 3 years beforehand.

PITUITARY TUMOURS

Pituitary tumours are usually treated surgically, both in order to make the diagnosis and in many cases to provide definitive therapy. For small tumours without suprasellar extension, many surgeons now favour the trans-sphenoidal route, which avoids the complications of craniotomy, although infection and CSF rhinorrhoea are occasionally encountered. In one large series, over 90% of patients with visual field defects had satisfactory postoperative reversal of the visual symptoms with only a few requiring craniotomy after trans-sphenoidal resection [29]. Many of these patients had large non-active macroadenomas with a suprasellar extension. However, for larger tumours and particularly for those with extension outside the pituitary fossa, a craniotomy is generally necessary. In children with craniopharyngioma, surgery can be particularly difficult because the chalky calcific material which is often encountered can be impossible to remove completely.

The routine addition of postoperative irradiation for patients with pituitary tumours decreases the likelihood of local recurrence. Chromophobe pituitary adenomas are probably more radiosensitive than chromophil tumours. In patients with acromegaly (almost always due to a chromophil tumour) arrest or reversal of the syndrome can be achieved with surgery and postoperative irradiation in 75% of cases. Craniopharyngioma requires a high local dose for eradication (50–60 Gy in 5–7 weeks).

Careful tumour localization, multifield planning and attention to detail are essential for successful radiation treatment. A three-field plan is normally employed, with particular care to avoid overtreatment of the eyes and optic chiasm. For most tumours the field size can be limited, although chromophobe pituitary adenomas can reach a very large size. In some centres a rotational plan is used. The radiation technique is the same regardless of whether the patient is treated postoperatively as an adjuvant to surgery, or later for recurrence — though in the latter instance, the treatment volume may have to be larger.

Alternatives to the use of conventional external beam irradiation include interstitial yttrium seeds or heavy particles (proton or α particle) irradiation. The use of bromocriptine has been advocated in recent years as an alternative to surgery and/or radiotherapy treatment for pituitary adenomas. This agent is particularly useful for small tumours producing prolactin only (prolactinomas). Although widely used, patients on bromocriptine do sometimes develop frank recurrence; it is also uncertain how long the drug needs to be continued. If bromocriptine fails, prolactinomas may have to be removed surgically.

MENINGIOMAS

Meningiomas should be surgically excised. If they arise at an inaccessible site they can be difficult to remove and in such cases postoperative irradiation should reduce the incidence of local recurrence. As these tumours are not very sensitive to radiation, high doses are usually required (50–60 Gy over 5–7 weeks). For patients with 'malignant' meningioma, radiotherapy is always required though the overall prognosis in these cases is very poor. Occasionally they metastasize to distant sites.

PINEAL TUMOURS

These present particular problems of management since they are often not biopsied by the surgeon for fear of causing irreparable damage. Many pineal tumours are curable by radiotherapy (particularly the 'pure' non-teratomatous pineal germinomas), and in patients without histological verification of the type of pineal tumour a brief trial of radiotherapy is generally justified unless there is strong evidence of a teratomatous tumour such as raised markers (AFP or βHCG, see below) or clear-cut radiological heterogeneity within the primary tumour. Pineal germinomas and pinealoblastomas are the most radiosensitive of pineal tumours, and repeat CT or MRI scanning after as little as 2 weeks treatment often shows dramatic reduction in the size of the primary. In these cases, it can reasonably be assumed that the diagnosis is either pineal germinoma or pinealoblastoma since other pineal tumours (generally glioma or pineal teratoma, pinealocytoma) are less radiosensitive. Although radiotherapy is often appropriate for pineal tumours in general, the technique varies with different types of tumour. With the radiosensitive group, there is a tendency for involvement by tumour seeding throughout the CNS, and full craniospinal irradiation should be employed. This is not required with other pineal tumours, though they require a high local dose to the primary itself. Neurosurgeons are increasingly prepared to attempt biopsy or even total removal of pineal tumours, so an accurate histological diagnosis is now more frequently available. For the less radiosensitive group, total surgical removal is likely to be of particular benefit. Pineal teratomas, like teratomas at other sites, can produce AFP and HCG which can be measured both in CSF and also in the blood. Chemotherapy clearly has a part to play in management and is certainly effective in recurrent disease, using conventional teratoma regimens (see Chapter 19).

Overall survival of pineal tumours (including unbiopsied cases) is close to 80% in young patients under the age of 30, reflecting the high incidence of radiocurable germinomas in this group. For older patients the prognosis is much worse, of the order of 25%, due no doubt to the higher incidence of gliomas and other less radiosensitive tumours.

INTRACRANIAL LYMPHOMA

Microgliomas and histiocytic lymphomas are also radiosensitive. The surgical approach depends on the site of the lesion and surgery is sometimes complete. None the less, radiotherapy should be offered in all cases and a remarkable degree of radiosensitivity is sometimes encountered although durability of response is often disappointing (see Chapter 26). In general, the best results have been obtained with high dosage, and full craniospinal irradiation is generally advocated since these tumours can spread throughout the nervous system.

CHORDOMA

Surgical removal is essential though often difficult because of the anatomy of the tumour. These tumours often have a 'dumbell' appearance with an intraspinal component, making total removal impossible. Postoperative radiotherapy is therefore usually necessary, although these lesions are rather insensitive. High radiation dose is particularly difficult to achieve in the cervical spine, though sacral chordomas can often be treated to a high dose since there is no danger of damage to the spinal cord. Despite the marginal radiosensitivity of chordomas, long survival has occasionally been documented in patients treated by subtotal surgical removal and radical postoperative radiotherapy.

OTHER TUMOURS

Acoustic neuromas, and other neuronal tumours, are best treated surgically and are only minimally radiosensitive. None the less, postoperative radiotherapy should be considered where surgery has been incomplete. The surgical approach depends both on the site of the tumour and also on the degree of hearing loss. The prospect for preservation of functional hearing is much better with tumours under 2 cm and where auditory brain stem responses and other audiological assessments are only minimally abnormal. With elderly patients or poor operative risk candidates, sequential MRI imaging may allow for a conservative non-intervention policy without significant danger.

Treatment on relapse

For recurrent brain tumours, the question of

retreatment radiotherapy often arises. When the disease-free interval has been short, as with high-grade gliomas, there is little value in retreatment since only a modest radiation dose can be safely achieved and is of doubtful benefit where more intensive radiotherapy has already failed. However, in patients with low-grade glioma of any type, or those with medulloblastoma, late recurrences are common. The feasibility of retreatment radiation therapy increases according to the time interval from first treatment, and if a sufficient time has elapsed (10 years or more), a complete retreatment dose can be contemplated. With medulloblastoma particularly, widespread late primary, cerebral and spinal metastases can develop, with continued responsiveness to repeated courses of radiotherapy. Dexamethasone often provides valuable symptomatic relief. Chemotherapy may produce transient responses and is discussed above.

Prognosis of brain tumours

For malignant gliomas, the prognosis is heavily dependent on tumour grade and on other well-established prognostic factors. Although there are four pathological (Kernohan) grades, patients with malignant glioma fall chiefly into two prognostic groups since those with Grades I and II tumours have a relatively good prognosis and 5 and 10-year survival rates of approximately 65% and 35%, whereas those with Grades III and IV tumours have a 5-year survival rate of under 10% (Fig. 11.5), with a much worse prognosis in the Grade IV category. In all grades incomplete removal is associated with a worse prognosis.

In medulloblastoma, a variety of factors are thought to contribute to prognosis. Patients undergoing total excision undoubtedly do better though this may be as much a result of tumour size as the contribution of surgery *per se*. Age at diagnosis is also important and children over 15 years of age have a better prognosis. Children with spinal metastases at presentation are not usually cured. The

adequacy of the irradiation, both in technique and dose, is crucial and 5-year survival rates of over 40% should now regularly be expected with modern techniques.

In ependymoma, overall prognosis depends on tumour grade and the median survival following surgery in low-grade ependymoma is approximately 10 years. When recurrences occur, they are frequently of a higher histological grade, and median overall survival in high-grade ependymoma is no better than 2–3 years.

Both pituitary tumours and meningiomas have an excellent prognosis following surgical removal and, where appropriate, postoperative radiotherapy. Few large series of pineal tumours have been reported. Survival is very variable (see above). In chordoma, the prognosis is poor since these tumours are not usually entirely resectable or fully radiosensitive.

SECONDARY DEPOSITS

Cerebral metastases are common and account for about a third of all brain tumours. The commonest primary sites include carcinoma of the breast and bronchus and melanoma. In each of these tumours, autopsy series confirm that the probability of dissemination to the brain is very much greater than the frequency of pre-mortem diagnosis. About 60% of all patients with small cell lung cancer have demonstrable brain metastases at autopsy, and in melanoma about three-quarters of patients who die from disseminated disease have brain metastases. Many other tumours can metastasize to the brain, though at a much lower frequency (Table 11.1).

Metastases may be either single or multiple and diagnostically may be difficult to distinguish from primary brain tumours, particularly when, as occasionally occurs, there is no known primary. Small cell lung cancer and melanoma are particularly likely to give rise to multiple intracerebral deposits.

About half of all brain metastases are found in the distribution of the middle cerebral artery and are characteristically cortical deposits.

Any other site may be involved and cerebellar, thalamic and pituitary deposits are all encountered. As with primary brain tumours, the characteristic symptoms are those of raised intracranial pressure, focal neurological damage or convulsions. The diagnosis is usually suggested by isotope or CT brain scanning which may show single or multiple abnormal areas of increased uptake of isotope or a typically spherical lesions often with obvious contrast enhancement on CT scanning. Although local oedema is often present, this is usually less than that seen with high-grade primary brain tumours. In patients with known cancer, particularly lung or breast cancer or malignant melanoma, further investigation is not usually indicated, especially where the primary diagnosis has been made within the previous 5 years, although alternative diagnoses should always be considered. With apparently solid metastases, the most important differential diagnosis is from benign brain tumour, particularly meningioma (especially of course if the tumour is anatomically located at a common meningioma site). In cases of multiple metastases, the presumed diagnosis is almost always correct, though occasional confusion with intracerebral abscesses may occur.

Occasionally patients with a known primary cancer develop headache, mental confusion or focal signs suggestive of cerebral metastases, yet the CT scan fails to show an abnormality. Such patients may well have cerebral secondaries and a trial of dexamethasone may be indicated. A good response usually implies that the diagnosis is correct and that radiotherapy to the brain should be considered.

TREATMENT OF SECONDARY DEPOSITS IN THE BRAIN

Reversal of oedema

Treatment with dexamethasone, often at high dosage (6 mg every 6 hours, initially by intramuscular or intravenous administration) is often valuable to provide rapid reduction of intracranial pressure and relief of cerebral oedema. Response to this powerful agent is a useful indicator that an intracerebral tumour is present, and is often thought to be a helpful determinant of the likelihood of response to radiotherapy. The important clinical point about dexamethasone treatment is that it exerts its effect rapidly, and can often be quickly reduced in dosage. It is a great mistake to allow patients to remain on dexamethasone for too long, because of the inevitability of steroid complications, particularly proximal myopathy and facial swelling. In general, we usually recommend gradual discontinuation of dexamethasone after 4–6 weeks, though this policy occasionally results in patients developing symptoms and signs of raised intracranial pressure because of too rapid reduction. In these cases, the dose can easily be increased again, and patients almost always respond quickly. There is considerable variation in the rapidity with which patients can be weaned off dexamethasone. In patients where dexamethasone is ill-advised or dangerous (e.g. where there is a history of bleeding peptic ulcer or severe hypertension or diabetes) it is sometimes possible to achieve the desired reduction in cerebral oedema by the use of intravenous urea (1 g/kg, in dextrose solution), mannitol (2 g/kg as a 20% solution) or oral glycerine which can be made palatable by making it up in a 50% mixture with lemonade. Most patients dislike this latter treatment because it rapidly induces diarrhoea, but it can be a highly effective means of improving symptoms of raised intracranial pressure.

Radiotherapy

Radiotherapy is indicated in a large proportion of patients with secondary brain deposits, though the decision to treat requires careful thought. Patients likely to benefit include those with known radiosensitive tumours (particularly small cell carcinoma of the bronchus and to a lesser extent carcinoma of the breast), those where there has been a good response to dexamethasone, where the patient's general condition is good (particularly if there is no other evidence of distant metastases) and in patients with multiple intracerebral deposits in whom there can be no question of surgery.

The choice of fractionation and dosage remains contentious. A recent large multicentre study has suggested that there is no advantage to prolonged fractionation and that a total dosage of 20 Gy (2000 rad) in 5 daily fractions, or 30 Gy (3000 rad) in 10 daily fractions over 2 weeks, are as effective as much more prolonged treatment regimens [30]. In patients with less radiosensitive tumours (adenocarcinomas, melanoma and others) higher doses may be required, particularly in the case of single metastatic deposits where the relatively limited volume can be treated to a higher dose.

Surgery

Neurosurgical removal of metastases is occasionally performed in the mistaken supposition that the surgeon is dealing with a primary brain tumour. In these cases, where there has been complete macroscopic removal, it is not clear whether treatment with postoperative radiotherapy is of benefit. Deliberate surgical removal of metastases is valuable in a small proportion of patients. Relative indications for surgery include: young fit patients with a solitary brain metastasis and with no evidence of disease elsewhere; where there has been a long treatment-free interval (this is often the case in patients with breast cancer); and where the single metastasis is unlikely to be radiosensitive (as for example in adenocarcinoma of the bronchus or thyroid). In this selected group of patients, surgical removal can be the treatment of choice.

Chemotherapy

Although this is not an established form of treatment it is clear that, in chemosensitive tumours such as small cell carcinoma of the bronchus or testicular teratoma, intravenous chemotherapy is effective in producing tumour response [31]. The role of chemotherapy requires further definition. The long held concept of a blood–brain barrier seems to be erroneous, possibly because the changes in vasculature following establishment of a secondary deposit result in a breach of the physiological barrier. Intrathecal chemotherapy is of no value for intracerebral metastases.

Patients with intracerebral metastases have a very poor survival, particularly where the primary diagnosis is a small cell lung cancer or melanoma. In other cases such as breast cancer and adenocarcinoma from other sites, survival may be more prolonged, particularly where neurosurgical removal of a solitary metastasis has been successfully accomplished, and in patients where the cranial involvement represents a late solitary site of recurrence.

Lymphomatous or carcinomatous meningitis is increasingly recognized in a variety of tumours, particularly acute leukaemia, non-Hodgkin's lymphoma, breast cancer, lung cancer, melanoma and ovarian cancer. It typically presents with the symptoms and signs of headache, clouding of consciousness, ataxia and focal cranial nerve palsies, particularly of the III, IV, VI and VII cranial nerves. Although an extremely grave site for metastasis, it may temporarily be responsive to treatment both with whole brain irradiation and also with intrathecal chemotherapy. In patients with breast cancer (much the commonest primary site in patients with carcinomatous meningitis), we employ whole brain irradiation to 30–40 Gy (3000–4000 rad) in daily fractions over 2–3 weeks, initially coupled with twice weekly intrathecal methotrexate 10–12.5 mg. If there has been a good response to treatment during the first 3 weeks, it is best to continue with regular, less frequent intrathecal chemotherapy for a prolonged period. Insertion of an Ommaya or Rickham intraventricular reservoir makes drug administration easy, avoiding repeated lumbar punctures, and should be considered in patients where obvious response to the initial treatment justifies continued CSF treatment.

TUMOURS OF THE SPINAL CORD

Primary tumours of the spinal cord are very uncommon though secondary deposits involving the cord are frequently encountered. Table 11.4 shows the main types of spinal cord tumour. Ependymoma is the commonest glioma to arise from the spinal cord, astrocytoma being much less frequently seen. Schwannomas, vascular tumours and meningiomas are the other relatively common types. Secondary deposits may be intramedullary but are more often extramedullary (usually extradural), frequently resulting from direct spread from the adjacent involved vertebral body. Management of acute cord compression is also dealt with in Chapter 8.

Symptoms

Pain is the usual presenting symptom and is generally felt directly over the cord lesion, though the site of pain can be misleading. More laterally situated tumours (often involving the nerve roots as well) may cause more specific and focally sited pain than centrally placed tumours, for example fusiform intramedullary lesions which can extend in a clinically silent way throughout several segments. Tenderness on palpation of the overlying vertebra is often found though the bone may have to be pressed

Table 11.4 Classification of tumours of spinal cord (with % frequency)

Intradural (55%)	Extradural (45%)
Extramedullary	Metastases (25%)
Meningioma (15%)	Myeloma (6%)
Neurofibroma (10%)	Lymphoma (5%)
Congenital and others (7%)	Sarcomas (5%)
	Others (7%)
Intramedullary	
Ependymoma (5%)	
Astrocytoma (5%)	
Angiomas (6%)	
Others (7%)	

firmly or even struck, to elicit this sign. Sensorimotor loss is also frequently present, with defects of both power and sensation at and below the level of involvement. At the site of the lesion, there may be an obvious sensory loss (especially evident in lesions of the dorsal and lumbar spine involving loss of sensation over the trunk). Muscular weakness in the upper limbs is a feature of lesions of the cervical spine. Below the affected area of an incomplete cord compression there may be partial preservation of function with less obvious neurological abnormalities and only patchy sensory loss. When the cord compression is complete a severe paraparesis results. Complete loss of sphincter function is a late sign with a poor prognosis (see Chapter 8), but lesser degrees occur earlier and their significance is often missed.

Tumours situated below the lower end of the spinal cord (vertebral level L_1 or L_2) may produce a typical cauda equina syndrome with sacral anaesthesia, sciatic pain (often bilateral), gluteal weakness and wasting, impotence and bladder dysfunction with retention and overflow incontinence. However, most cases of cauda equina compression are far less symptomatically clear-cut and in practice the diagnosis is often very difficult to establish although MRI scanning has made such cases easier. Even in proven cauda equina compression the myelogram may be normal and cannot therefore reliably exclude the diagnosis. Ependymomas constitute the largest single group of primary tumours at the lower end of the cord (conus medullaris and filum terminale). Lateral compression of the spinal cord may cause a complete or partial Brown–Séquard syndrome with ipsilateral spastic weakness, reduced vibration sense and proprioception together with contralateral insensitivity to pain and temperature change. Tumour progression causes an increasingly florid clinical picture with weakness, sensory loss, hyperreflexia and autonomic dysfunction (Table 11.5).

In general, the clinical picture depends on the site of the tumour rather than its origin, although destructive secondary deposits, which

Table 11.5 Syndromes of spinal cord compression

Complete compression
Sensory level just below level of lesion
Loss of all modalities of sensation — variable in degree at first
Bilateral upper motor neurone weakness below lesion
Bladder and bowel dysfunction

Anterior compression
Partial loss of pain and temperature below lesion
Bilateral upper motor neurone weakness below lesion
Bladder and bowel dysfunction

Lateral compression (Brown−Séquard)
Contralateral loss of pain and temperature (touch much less affected)
Ipsilateral loss of proprioception and vibration
Ipsilateral upper motor neurone weakness

Posterior compression
Loss of vibration and position below lesion
Pain, temperature and touch relatively spared
Painful segmental paraesthesia at level of lesion

more often involve the vertebral column than the spinal cord, produce more local pain and tenderness than some of the less common primary cord lesions. Common primary sites of vertebral or cord metastases include carcinoma of the bronchus (particularly small cell), carcinoma of the breast and myeloma. Less common primary tumours include carcinomas of the thyroid, large bowel and kidney and also malignant melanoma.

Differential diagnosis

Although the clinical syndrome of spinal cord compression usually implies a malignant aetiology, a few non-malignant lesions can produce a similar clinical picture. These include inflammatory cord lesions (particularly transverse myelitis, infectious polyneuropathy or Guillain−Barré syndrome), anterior spinal artery occlusion, abscess of the cord, syringomyelia and haemorrhage into the cord (haematomyelia). Very occasionally an acutely prolapsed intervertebral disc may produce symptoms of cord compression.

Investigation

Radiological investigation is always required. Plain X-rays of the spine may show an obvious lytic secondary deposit in the vertebra(e) at the level of compression, but X-ray changes may be very subtle, with loss of the pedicle of the spine but no other significant features. Myelography either by the lumbar or cisternal route, gives good anatomical demonstration of the spinal cord lesion and will show whether the block is partial or complete (Fig. 11.7) but has now been largely replaced by MRI scanning. With a complete block, it is difficult to be certain of the upper extent of the abnormality and occasionally a cisternal myelogram will also need to be performed if full anatomical definition is considered important for therapy. Metrizamide gives good definition of root pathology but, being water-soluble, is rapidly cleared so that re-examinations require a further lumbar puncture. In tumours with doubtful or difficult physical signs, CT scanning can be invaluable. This investigation can be even more informative when combined with metrizamide myelography.

Management

For primary tumours of the spinal cord, surgical removal is the treatment of choice where possible. Technical difficulties are often encountered and intramedullary tumours are almost always unresectable. At surgery the tumour should be totally removed where possible, reduced in bulk by subtotal excision, or at least biopsied. Surgical decompression is invaluable even where the tumour cannot be removed, and this is generally achieved by laminectomy often encompassing several segments. Occasionally, spinal neoplasms may extend over a considerable length of the cord. Such tumours are usually low-grade gliomas and even these can sometimes be totally excised. Many benign or extramedullary and intradural tumours of borderline malignancy can be totally removed without need for further treatment. This group includes

Fig. 11.7 Radiological changes in spinal cord compression. (A) Complete cord compression; (B) partial cord compression due to multiple deposits from an ependymoma.

meningiomas, low-grade gliomas, neurofibromas and tumours of the coverings of the cord (angiomas, fibromas and lipomas).

For more malignant tumours and in patients with secondary deposits involving the spinal cord, surgical decompression followed by postoperative radiotherapy is usually the treatment of choice. If rapid transfer to a neurosurgical centre is difficult or if the patient is unfit or unsuitable for surgery (perhaps because of widespread malignant disease), intensive radiotherapy can often provide excellent palliation, particularly if the cord lesion is a secondary deposit of a radiosensitive tumour such as small cell carcinoma of the bronchus or lymphoma. In malignant primary cord tumours such as high-grade gliomas, total surgical removal is usually impossible and postoperative radiotherapy mandatory. A high radiation dose will be required since these tumours are not usually very radiosensitive, and most radiotherapists would treat the spinal cord to its tolerance dose (see below). Very careful judgement of anatomical details, field length, fractionation and total dose is always required.

High doses of dexamethasone are invaluable in reducing cord oedema, making intensive radiotherapy safer. The role of chemotherapy is not established and it has no routine place in the management of spinal cord tumours.

TUMOURS OF THE PERIPHERAL NERVES

These are rare tumours, more often benign than malignant. Multiple neurofibromatosis (von Recklinghausen's disease), the commonest peripheral nerve tumour, is most frequently encountered. In 5–10% of cases, sarcomatous change takes places (neurofibrosarcoma). Tumours of the nerve sheath (Schwannomas) can occur in both cranial and peripheral nerves, particularly the acoustic nerve, spinal nerve roots, peripheral nerves and occasionally the V, IX, or X cranial nerves. These may occasionally undergo malignant change. *Neuroepithelioma* is an exceedingly rare malignant tumour of peripheral nerve, sometimes occurring in conjunction with von Recklinghausen's disease.

The histological appearance suggests a neural crest origin, and metastases are frequent.

Treatment of peripheral nerve tumours is by surgical excision where the tumour is producing troublesome pressure symptoms or where there is any suspicion of malignant change. Routine surgical excision of neurofibromas in patients with von Recklinghausen's disease should be discouraged unless there is a sudden increase in size of one of the peripheral lesions. Management of sarcomatous tumours is dealt with in Chapter 23.

RADIATION DAMAGE IN THE BRAIN AND SPINAL CORD

With radical radiotherapy, particularly of midline tumours, the treatment volume may include the spinal cord. For example, in lung cancer a portion of the cord is usually irradiated. The radiation tolerance of the brain and spinal cord is of great clinical importance since it frequently sets the dose limit [32, 33]. Both acute and late damage may occur, the latter being of much greater importance. In the brain, the early effects include headache, nausea, vomiting and lassitude from raised intracranial pressure, both as a result of the tumour itself and also from acute cerebral oedema produced by the radiotherapy. Drowsiness and irritability have been described as side-effects of whole brain irradiation in children (somnolence syndrome) but are transient and self-limiting. An early syndrome of demyelination may develop but is extremely rare. Late changes include haemorrhage, gliosis, demyelination and necrosis of the brain. These complications are especially likely to occur in the cerebral hemispheres and when retreatment has been undertaken. The usual clinical features are those of progressive focal or generalized neurological damage, occurring months or even years after radiation. Damage to the optic chiasm is well recognized in patients treated for pituitary tumours and is clearly dose-related with minimal risk when daily fraction size is kept between 1.8–2.0 Gy. Radiation tolerance of the brain stem is generally thought to be rather lower than that of the cerebral hemispheres.

Early radiation damage to the spinal cord is frequently encountered and is usually transient. The commonest feature is Lhermitte's syndrome, characterized by 'electric shock' sensations in the extremities (usually the feet), and particularly marked on flexion of the neck. It usually occurs a few weeks after the treatment, but may develop several months afterwards. It is usually self-limiting and without long-term effect.

In late radiation damage to the cord, myelopathy can cause progressive motor and sensory changes at the irradiated site, leading to paraparesis, anaesthesia and, in severe cases, a paraplegia with physiological transection of the cord. If less than the total width of the cord has been irradiated, a Brown–Séquard syndrome may result. These changes are due to direct damage to neurological tissue with loss of anterior horn cells, other neurones and oligodendroglia as well as direct vascular damage leading to infarction of the cord. Progressive and chronic radiation myelopathy is usually irreversible and leads to spastic paraplegia with sphincter disturbance. This is fatal in over 50% of cases, particularly where the lesion is in the cervical or upper dorsal cord.

Radiation tolerance of the cord is inversely related to the length of cord irradiated. It is generally accepted that for a 10 cm length of cord, a dose of 40 Gy (4000 rad) in daily fractions over 4 weeks is safe, though this dose may have to be exceeded in patients with relatively insensitive lesions which cannot be completely excised, for example a chordoma. Fraction size is clearly important since treatment to 50 Gy (5000 rad) in daily fractions over 5 weeks is usually safe, whereas many cases of cord damage have been documented following treatment to a dose of 40 Gy (4000 rad) in daily fractions over 3 weeks [32].

REFERENCES

1 Mckeran R.O., Williams E.S., Thornton-Jones H. The epidemiology of brain tumours. In Thomas D.G.T., ed. *Neuro-oncology*. London: Edward Arnold, 1990: 135–40.

2 Eby N.L., Grufferman S., Flannelly G.M. *et al*. Increasing incidence of primary brain lymphoma in the United States. *Cancer* 1988; **62**: 2461–65.

3 Hoshino T., Nagashima T., Cho K.G. *et al*. Variability in the proliferative potential of human gliomas. *Journal of Neuro-Oncology* 1989; **7**: 137–43.

4 Ali-Osman F., Schofield D. Cellular and molecular studies in brain and nervous system oncology. *Current Opinion in Oncology* 1990; **2**: 655–65.

5 Bigner S.H., Mark J., Burger P.C. *et al*. Specific chromosomal abnormalities in malignant gliomas. *Cancer Research* 1988; **48**: 405–11.

6 Russell D.S., Rubenstein L.J. *Pathology of Tumours of the Nervous System*, 4th edn. Baltimore: Williams & Wilkins, 1982.

7 Thomas D.G.T., Darling J.L., Paul E.A. *et al*. Assay of anti-cancer drugs in tissue culture: a relationship of relapse-free interval and *in vitro* chemosensitivity in patients with malignant cerebral glioma. *British Journal of Cancer* 1985; **51**: 525–32.

8 Peterman S.B., Steiner R.E., Bydder G.M. *et al*. Nuclear magnetic resonance imaging of brain stem tumours. *Neuroradiology* 1985; **27**: 202–7.

9 Black P.M. Medical progress: brain tumours. *New England Journal of Medicine* 1991; **324**: 1471–76; 1555–64.

10 Leibel S.A., Sheline G.E., Wara W.M., Baldrey E.B., Nielsen S.L. The role of radiation therapy in the treatment of astrocytomas. *Cancer* 1975; **35**: 1551–57.

11 Bouchard J., Peirce C.B. Radiation therapy in the management of neoplasms of the central nervous system, with a special note with regard to children: 20 years experience 1939–1958. *American Journal of Roentgenology* 1960; **84**: 610–21.

12 Shaw E.G., Daumas-Duport C., Scheithauer B.W. *et al*. Radiation therapy in the management of low-grade supratentorial astrocytomas. *Journal of Neurosurgery* 1989; **70**: 853–61.

13 Cairncross J.G., Laperriere N. Low grade glioma: to treat or not to treat. *Archives of Neurology* 1988; **46**: 1238–39.

14 Taveras J.M., Thompson H.G., Pool J.L. Should we treat glioblastoma multiforme? *American Journal of Roentgenology* 1962; **87**: 473–79.

15 Bleehen N.M., Stenning S.P. (MRC Brain Tumour Working Party) A Medical Research Council trial of two radiotherapy doses in the treatment of grades 3 and 4 astrocytoma. *British Journal of Cancer* 1991; **64**: 769–74.

16 Larson D., Gutin P., Leibel S. *et al*. Stereotaxic irradiation of brain tumors. *Cancer* 1990; **65**: 792–99.

17 Walker M.D., Green S.B., Byar D.P. *et al*. Randomized comparisons of radiotherapy and nitrosoureas for the treatment of malignant glioma after surgery. *New England Journal of Medicine* 1980; **303**: 1323.

18 Levin V.A., Silver P., Hannigan J. *et al*. Superiority of post-radiotherapy adjuvant chemotherapy with CCNU, procarbazine, and vincristine (PCV) over BCNU for anaplastic gliomas: NCOG 6G61 final report. *International Journal of Radiation Oncology, Biology and Physics* 1990; **18**: 321–24.

19 Phillips T.L., Sheline G.E., Boldrey E. Therapeutic considerations in tumours affecting the central nervous system: ependymomas. *Radiology* 1964; **83**: 98–105.

20 Sheline G.E., Boldrey E.B., Karlsberg P., Phillips T.L. Therapeutic considerations in tumours affecting the central nervous system: oligodendrogliomas. *Radiology* 1964; **82**: 84–9.

21 Cairncross J.G., MacDonald D.R. Successful chemotherapy for recurrent malignant oligodendroglioma. *Annals of Neurology* 1988; **23**: 360–64.

22 Pierce S.M., Barnes P.D., Loeffler J.S. *et al*. Definitive radiation therapy in the management of symptomatic patients with optic glioma. *Cancer* 1990; **65**: 45–52.

23 Panitch H.S., Berg B.O. Brain stem tumours of childhood and adolescence. *American Journal of Diseases of Children* 1970; **119**: 465–72.

24 Hughes E.N., Shillito J., Sallan S.E. *et al*. Medulloblastoma at the Joint Center for Radiation Therapy between 1968 and 1984: the influence of radiation dose on the patterns of failure and survival. *Cancer* 1988; **61**: 1992–98.

25 Broadbent V.A., Barnes N.D., Wheeler T.K. Medulloblastoma in childhood: long term results of treatment. *Cancer* 1981; **48**: 26–30.

26 Livesey E.A., Hindmarsh, P.C., Brook C.G.D. *et al*. Endocrine disorders following treatment of childhood brain tumours. *British Journal of Cancer* 1990; **61**: 622–25.

27 Sposto R., Ertel I.J., Jenkin R.D.T. *et al*. The effectiveness of chemotherapy for treatment of high-grade astrocytoma in children: results of a randomised trial. *Journal of Neuro-oncology* 1989; **7**: 165–77.

28 Tait D., Thornton-Jones H., Bloom H.J. *et al*. Adjuvant chemotherapy for medulloblastoma: the first multicentre controlled trial of the International Society for Paediatric Oncology. *European Journal of Cancer* 1990; **26**: 464–69.

29 Bynke O., Hillman J. Role of trans-sphenoidal operations in the management of pituitary adenomas with suprasellar extension. *Acta Neurochirurgica* 1989; **100**: 50–55.

30 Borgelt B., Gelber R., Kramer S. *et al*. The palliation of brain metastases: final results of the first two studies by the Radiation Therapy Oncology Group. *Inter-*

national Journal of Radiation Oncology, Biology and Physics 1980; **6**: 1−9.

31 Twelves C.J., Souhami R.L., Harper P.G. *et al.* The response of cerebral metastases in small cell lung cancer to systemic chemotherapy. *British Journal of Cancer* 1990; **61**: 147−50.

32 Wara W.M., Phillips T.L., Sheline G.E. *et al.* Radiation

tolerance of the spinal cord. *Cancer* 1975; **35**: 1558−62.

33 Constine L.S., Woolf P.D., Cann D. *et al.* Hypothalamic-pituitary dysfunction after radiation for brain tumors. *New England Journal of Medicine* 1993; **328**: 87−94.

Chapter 12
Tumours of the Lung and Mediastinum

CARCINOMA OF THE BRONCHUS

Introduction and aetiology

Carcinoma of the bronchus is by far the commonest cancer in the Western world, having increased steadily in incidence since the 1930s. It had an overall incidence in Britain of 112 per 100 000 males and 27 per 100 000 females in 1978. The incidence is strongly related to age (Fig. 12.1). As a result of the increasing prevalence of cigarette smoking since the First World War, carcinoma of the bronchus has become the leading cause of cancer death in males over the past 50 years. In recent years, more women have become cigarette smokers with the result that lung cancer has become increasingly common in women, and continues to rise [1]. In 1952, the male : female ratio for lung cancer incidence was 13 : 1; in 1984 the figure stood at 4 : 1.

Although several aetiological factors have been implicated, including exposure to radioactivity and possible environmental hazards, these are insignificant compared with the highly carcinogenic effect of prolonged exposure to cigarette smoke. Recent studies have shown that non-smokers married to life-long smokers are at double the expected risk for developing lung cancer. Case–control studies have also suggested an increased incidence in lung cancer in non-smokers who lived in a household of heavy smokers during childhood and adolescence.

A great deal of political debate has followed the demonstration of an incontravertible link between cigarette smoking and lung cancer, in which health education, cost of treatment, possible loss of tax revenue, reduction in productivity resulting from ill-health and freedom of choice have been the principal points for discussion. At an international level, there has been a wide variety of approaches towards the restriction of smoking, stemming from the differing philosophies of different countries. In many Scandinavian countries, for example, it is now almost socially unacceptable to smoke in public places, and cigarettes have become extremely expensive with the result that smoking-related illnesses are beginning to decline. In Britain cigarettes are now relatively cheaper than they were 25 years ago, and restriction of smoking in public areas has been a protracted and uphill battle. There is now a clear inverse relationship both in Britain and the United States between socio-economic status and incidence of lung cancer. The death rate from this disease is disproportionately high in comparison to incidence because of the low cure rates currently achieved (less than 10% at 5 years overall). At present the British Health Education Council has an annual budget of about half a million pounds per annum to spend on its anti-smoking campaign, compared with an estimated seventy million pounds spent on advertising by the tobacco industry. So far, attempts at screening, even in high-risk groups, have met with very little success. In the Third World, cigarette consumption is rapidly rising and high-tar brands which are no longer popular in this country are widely advertised. Despite overwhelming evidence of the dangers of cigarette smoking, major tobacco companies

Fig. 12.1 Cancer of the lung. Age-specific incidence rates for men and women.

are urging Third World farmers to change from production of staple arable crops to growing tobacco.

Fortunately, the carcinogenic effects of cigarette smoke are to some extent reversible. In their classic study of the smoking habits of British doctors, Doll and Hill [2] were able to demonstrate a gradual reduction in mortality of British doctors who gave up smoking. After 12 years of total abstinence from cigarette smoking, the risk of developing lung cancer is almost as low as in non-smokers, except for heavy smokers (more than 20 per day), in whom the risk never falls to that of the non-smoker. In the lower age groups (30–45 years), there is at least some evidence for a slight fall in death rate over the past 15 years (Fig. 12.2). Since there has been little decrease in the number of cigarettes smoked in Britain, this reduction may possibly be due to the wider use of low-tar brands. None the less, insufficient time has elapsed since the introduction of these brands for us to be confident that the risk is indeed lower.

Other aetiological factors, thought or known to have a role, include asbestos exposure, industrial pollution, ionizing radiation, occupational hazards and others (see Chapter 2 and Table 12.1). Of these, asbestos exposure is probably the most critical, both for lung cancer and also mesothelioma (see p. 247). This is particularly important when combined with cigarette smoking: in smokers with occupational exposure to asbestos, the risk of lung cancer is 45 times above that of the normal population.

Table 12.1 Aetiological factors in lung cancer

Cigarette smoking	Air pollution	Occupational
Particulate phase	Coal and tar fumes	Asbestos
Benzpyrene	Nickel	Radioactivity (uranium mines, radon)
Benzofluoranthenes	Zinc	Metal workers (nickel, chromium, iron oxide)
Dibenzanthracene	Benzpyrene	Arsenicals (sheep-dip workers)
Nicotine		
Catechol		
Nickel and cadmium		
Vapour phase		
Nitrogen oxides		
Formaldehyde		
Hydrazine		
Urethan		

Fig. 12.2 Smoking and lung cancer. (A) Trends in lung cancer mortality for men and women of different ages (England and Wales) (From Doll R. *Harveian Oration*. Royal College of Physicians: 1982. With permission.); (B) age-adjusted lung cancer mortality rates (United States); (C) smoking prevalence and lung cancer mortality in men and women (England and Wales) (From Cairns J. *Smoking prevalence and lung cancer*. Copyright © (1975) by Scientific American, Inc. All rights reserved.); (D) relative risk of lung cancer according to daily cigarette consumption.

Pathology of lung cancer

HISTOLOGICAL TYPES

Lung cancer is only rarely a tumour of the true lung parenchyma, arising far more frequently in large and medium-sized bronchi. There are many histological types of lung cancer. It is, however, convenient to consider the commonest varieties in four major groups although there is substantial histological variation within each of these (Table 12.2). There has been considerable debate as to whether the cell of origin is different in the different histological types. There is, however, a great deal of circumstantial evidence to suggest that the cancers arise from a common precursor cell which has the capacity to differentiate into a variety of histological types.

Squamous cell carcinoma

This is the commonest histological type and is characterized by the presence of keratinization and/or intercellular bridging, and is often subdivided on the basis of differentiation. Most of these tumours arise proximally in large bronchi

Table 12.2 Histological classification of lung cancer*

	Frequency
Squamous carcinoma	35—45%
Small cell carcinoma	20%

Adenocarcinoma
  Bronchogenic, acinar
  Bronchioloalveolar
	15—50%†

Large cell carcinoma
  With or without mucin, giant and
  clear cell variants
	10%

Mixed forms	10—20%

Other tumours
  Carcinoid, cylindroma, sarcoma
  and mixed histological types
	2%

* Adapted from WHO classification
† Geographical variation

(though they may also arise peripherally), and tend to be polypoid or infiltrating, often with distinct borders. Since the bronchi at this level are not normally lined by squamous epithelium, it is likely that neoplastic change at this site is preceded by squamous metaplasia, though studies of carcinoma *in situ* have suggested that this may not always occur. Mutations and loss of heterozygosity of the p53 gene have been found in many tumours.

Small cell lung cancer (SCLC)

This is characterized by a diffuse growth of small cells with fine granular nuclei, inconspicuous nucleoli, and scanty cytoplasm. The cells tend to be tightly packed or moulded, with little evidence of supportive tissue. Occasionally, combinations of small cell and squamous cell carcinomas are seen, though many pathologists think that such tumours should be classified as poorly differentiated squamous cell carcinoma. Neurosecretory granules are often present on electron microscopy (Fig. 12.3). These may be the site of origin of the hormones such as ACTH, ADH and calcitonin which are sometimes produced and give rise to ectopic hormone syndromes which may be clinically significant (see Chapter 9). Small cell carcinomas express other markers of neural differentiation. Chief among these is the presence on the cell surface of the neural-cell adhesion molecule (NCAM). The cells secrete autocrine growth factors such as gastrin-releasing peptide (the mammalian homologue of bombesin) which, after secretion, binds to receptors on the tumour cell surface and causes a mitotic stimulus. Numerous other peptide hormones also bind to receptors on the SCLC cell surface and there has been considerable recent interest in the possible therapeutic effects of blocking such autocrine growth mechanisms. The tumours also show over-expression or amplification of one or more *myc*-family oncogenes. Karyotypically, there is an almost universal deletion of part of the short arm of chromosome 3 (bands 14—23), and loss of heterozygosity at the site of the p53

Fig. 12.3 Electron microscopy appearances in small cell carcinoma. Dense neurosecretory granules are shown in cell processes (×52250).

gene (17p). As in non-small cell lung cancer p53 mutations occur frequently. Small cell carcinomas typically develop in proximal large bronchi and are characterized by extensive local invasion associated with early blood-borne and lymphatic metastases, making them almost invariably unsuitable for surgery as a definitive treatment. Many tumours are diagnosed by biopsy of supraclavicular or cervical lymph nodes.

Adenocarcinomas

These show the typical features of neoplastic cells derived from glandular epithelium, with formation of acini, papillae and mucus. Many adenocarcinomas are peripheral in site of origin, frequently invading the pleura. These cancers sometimes arise in scar tissue, and may occur in fibrotic lung disease. Adenocarcinoma is less clearly related to cigarette smoking than either squamous or small cell carcinoma, and was the predominant cell type before the advent of cigarette smoking. Unlike other forms of

lung cancer it is slightly commoner in females. There is some evidence that it is increasing in frequency. In some large series from the United States adenocarcinoma now accounts for 50% of all non-small cell lung cancer. The uncommon bronchioalveolar carcinoma sometimes presents as a multicentric tumour with alveoli lined by neoplastic columnar cells.

Large cell carcinoma

Large cell carcinoma refers to undifferentiated tumours with a variety of appearances. The cells are large, often with featureless cytoplasm and show little tendency towards keratinization or acinar formation. In a proportion of these tumours, there is evidence of mucus production, and there may also be other ultrastructural characteristics which are reminiscent of adenocarcinoma. The tumour borders are generally well defined, and the tumour itself may arise from a subsegmental or more distal bronchus.

Mixed histologies

Approximately 20% of tumours show a mixed histological appearance (small/large cell, adeno/squamous, squamous/small cell). Of interest is the finding that 10–20% of typical adenocarcinomas have some cellular features of neuroendocrine cells such as expression of chromogranin (found in dense core granules), NCAM and neurone-specific enolase. There have been some studies which purport to show that these tumours may, like SCLC, show sensitivity to chemotherapy, but the issue is not settled.

PATHOLOGICAL DIAGNOSIS

In over 80% of patients with lung cancer, malignant cells are found in the sputum, using standard exfoliative cytology techniques. The likelihood of a positive sputum diagnosis increases from 58% with a single specimen, to 78% when four specimens are obtained. This proportion is also increased when specimens are obtained at bronchoscopy either from trap, brush or lavage specimens. The four major categories can be distinguished with an accuracy of 80% by either cytological or histological methods. Occasionally a mixture of cell types is seen, for example mixed small and large cell carcinoma or adenosquamous tumours. About one-quarter of autopsy cases show mixed histologies, although this high proportion may be related to a treatment-induced change in the histology [3]. Cases with mixed histology are one line of evidence suggesting that these carcinomas do not arise from different cells, but that the cancer-inducing event results in cells which can differentiate along more than one pathway.

The clinical distinction between primary adenocarcinoma of the bronchus and secondary pulmonary deposits from primary adenocarcinomas at other sites may be a difficult one, especially if no endobronchial lesion is seen at bronchoscopy. Similarly the clear-cell carcinoma variant of large cell carcinoma can be mistaken for metastatic hypernephroma. One important clinical feature of squamous cell carcinomas is that they may cavitate and can therefore be confused with a lung abscess.

Patterns of local invasion and metastasis

Carcinoma of the bronchus spreads by local invasion and by lymphatic and haematogenous routes (Fig. 12.4). Locally, the tumour may spread into the mediastinum or through the bronchial wall, lung parenchyma and to the pleural space and chest wall. There may be erosion of overlying ribs. Apical tumours typically spread from the apex of the lung to involve the brachial plexus with erosion of upper thoracic ribs and local nerves such as the thoraco-cervical sympathetic chain (Pancoast syndrome). At the hilum of the lung the tumour may damage the phrenic or left recurrent laryngeal nerve. It may also erode posteriorly into the oesophagus or vertebrae.

Lymphatic spread within the chest is chiefly to hilar and mediastinal, subcarinal, tracheo-

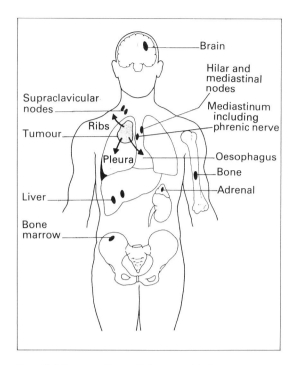

Fig. 12.4 Local and metastatic spread in lung cancer.

bronchial and paratracheal nodes. Beyond the chest, involvement of supraclavicular, cervical and axillary nodes may occur. Lymphatic involvement below the diaphragm is frequent in small cell carcinoma, especially to upper para-aortic nodes.

Blood-borne spread is especially frequent in small cell carcinoma and typically occurs earlier than with other lung cancers. The skeleton is frequently involved, particularly vertebrae, ribs and pelvis and widespread infiltration into bone marrow occurs, especially in small cell carcinoma where estimates of frequency vary from 5–30%, depending on the number of marrow aspirations and the extent of the tumour. Other common sites include the brain (65% of autopsies in small cell carcinoma), liver and adrenals, but secondary deposits can be found in any organ. Early and rapid dissemination is particularly characteristic of small cell carcinoma, which also has the most rapid volume doubling time of any of these tumours.

CLINICAL FEATURES

Most patients with lung cancer present with symptoms directly related to the tumour such as haemoptysis, cough, dyspnoea or chest pain. Since many of these patients are smokers, some of these symptoms (particularly a cough) will already be familiar to them as a result of chronic bronchitis and emphysema. This may well delay them from seeking advice, though a substantial number are sufficiently aware of the increased intensity of their symptoms to give up smoking, often after a lifetime of being unable to do so. The cough is often persistent, nocturnal and may be productive. Sputum may be blood-streaked or persistently discoloured as a result of infection which cannot clear due to atelectasis beyond an obstructing endobronchial tumour. Haemoptyses, though intermittent, usually become increasingly severe. Pain, usually aching, is present in over 50% of patients. It seems to be commoner in patients with mediastinal involvement or atelectasis, and is much commoner than the typical 'sharper' pain of bone metastases.

More peripheral tumours often present rather late, when already of significant size. They may well cause pain in the chest wall by direct extension to the pleura or periosteum of the ribs, often trapping or invading intercostal nerves. Direct tumour invasion of the left recurrent laryngeal nerve may result in hoarseness of the voice, which is a frequent presenting symptom. Pleural effusion, phrenic nerve palsy, and lobar or total lung collapse may all contribute to increasing dyspnoea. Pneumonias that fail to clear should be regarded as suspicious. Dysphagia may result from enlarged mediastinal lymph nodes which compress the oesophagus, usually at its mid or lower third, or by direct invasion. Wheeze and stridor are important signs of obstruction of large airways, generally due to proximal tumours.

Tumours at specific sites may produce typical syndromes. A Pancoast tumour, situated at the apex of the lung, causes severe pain in the shoulder, chest wall and arm as a result of relentless local invasion which destroys ribs and infiltrates the brachial plexus. Weakness of the small muscles of the hand may occur, with paraesthesiae on the inner aspect of the arm, due to C_8/T_1 motor loss. Tumours of the right main or right upper lobe bronchus (often with associated right paratracheal node enlargement) may compress the great veins leading to superior vena cava obstruction (SVCO), producing a typical clinical syndrome consisting of swelling of the face, neck, and upper arms, plethora or cyanosis and rapid development of a visible collateral circulation over the scapula and upper chest wall. In severe cases, conjunctival oedema and chemosis are also seen. The majority of cases of SVCO are caused by small cell carcinomas and prompt treatment may produce a gratifying resolution of these symptoms (see Chapter 8).

Some patients notice a 'mass' in the neck due to lymph node enlargement. In other patients the presenting symptoms are caused by secondary deposits, especially in small cell cancer. Pain in the back may be due to vertebral collapse, and is particularly important since cord compression with paraplegia may develop with great rapidity unless the diagnosis is made and treatment started promptly. Other typical metastatic presentations include neurological symptoms and signs (focal lesions, raised intracranial pressure, cerebellar syndromes) and weight loss and nausea from hepatic involvement.

Constitutional symptoms are also common and most patients with lung cancer complain of anorexia, weight loss, weakness and fatigue. Although many patients do not notice clubbing of the fingers, this is a common manifestation particularly associated with squamous cell carcinoma and rare in small cell carcinoma. Pain in the limbs may result from hypertrophic pulmonary osteoarthropathy which can be severe.

A wide variety of paraneoplastic non-metastatic syndromes have been described in association with lung cancer. These are discussed in Chapter 9. Many of these syndromes are uncommon. Hypercalcaemia (without obvious bone metastases) is most frequently found in squamous cell cancer, and the syndromes of inappropriate antidiuretic hormone secretion (SIADH) and ectopic ACTH production are both commoner in small cell carcinoma. The symptoms and management of hypercalcaemia are discussed in Chapter 8 and of ectopic hormone production in Chapter 9.

TNM staging notation

Although complex, the TNM staging system is becoming increasingly used in non-small cell lung cancer. A staging system based on TNM definitions has been proposed (Table 12.3) and has been shown to be useful prognostically, except in the case of small cell carcinomas, in which the prognosis is so poor that staging systems have little prognostic relevance.

Investigation and staging

Staging of *non-small cell lung cancer* (NSCLC) is important since a crucial distinction between operable and inoperable tumours has to be made. To the surgeon, the most important criteria are the site of tumour, absence of metastases and the general fitness of the patient. Before any consideration of surgery, the maximum amount of information must therefore be obtained. Chest X-ray may indicate that the tumour is inoperable. Findings indicating inoperability include large central primary tumours particularly extending across the midline; widening of the superior mediastinum due to enlargement of paratracheal nodes; intrapulmonary, rib or other bony metastases; pleural effusion; and bilateral tumours. Further assessment is often needed; bronchoscopic evaluation is usually required to make the diagnosis and is essential to assess operability.

Most patients with suspected lung cancer are first seen by a chest physician and the diagnosis made by fibreoptic bronchoscopy. This instrument has the advantage of permitting good access to lobar and segmental bronchi and is especially helpful in evaluating upper lobe tumours out of biopsy range of the rigid

Table 12.3 TNM staging system for NSCLC

T — primary tumour
T_0 Primary tumour not demonstrable
T_X Positive cytology but tumour not demonstrable
T_{is} Carcinoma *in situ*
T_1 Tumour less than 3 cm diameter, no proximal invasion
T_2 More than 3 cm, or invading pleura or with atelectasis, more than 2 cm from carina
T_3 Tumour of any size with extension into chest wall, diaphragm, mediastinal pleura or within 2 cm of carina
T_4 Tumour of any size with invasion of mediastinal organs or vertebral body

N — Regional lymph nodes
N_0 Nodes negative
N_1 Ipsilateral hilar nodes
N_2 Ipsilateral mediastinal and subcarinal nodes
N_3 Contralateral mediastinal or hilar nodes, scalene or supraclavicular nodes

M — Distant metastases
M_0 No metastases
M_1 Metastases present

Stage grouping

Stage I	T_1	N_0	M_0
	T_1	N_1	M_0
	T_2	N_0	M_0
Stage II	T_2	N_1	M_0
Stage III	Any T_3, any N or M		
	Any N_2, any T or M		
	Any M_1, any T or N		

bronchoscope. The rigid instrument is, however, sometimes useful since it may give a better view of proximal bronchi and allows a larger biopsy in doubtful cases.

At bronchoscopy some tumours can be shown to be inoperable. Features indicating inoperability are: endobronchial tumour within 2 cm of the main carina, extrinsic compression and widening of the angle of the main carina indicating mediastinal spread and paralysis of the left vocal cord resulting from recurrent laryngeal nerve palsy.

With very few exceptions mediastinal involvement is a powerful contraindication to surgery.

Assessment of the mediastinum is therefore essential in any patient being considered for operation. Clinical evidence of involvement includes a hoarse voice with a typical 'bovine' cough, resulting from recurrent laryngeal palsy, Horner's syndrome from involvement or the cervical sympathetic chain, pain in the shoulder, SVCO, cardiac dysrhythmia and dysphagia. Further assessment can be made by tomographic views of the mediastinum, and by barium swallow which may show enlarged mediastinal nodes causing extrinsic oesophageal compression. CT scanning is a useful aid in the pre-operative assessment of tumour extent, sometimes demonstrating unexpected lymph node involvement or direct invasion of other structures (Fig. 12.5). Chest wall involvement, for example, usually indicates inoperability. It is, however, important not to rule out surgery on the basis of an equivocal CT scan since not all lymph node enlargement will prove to be neoplastic at thoracotomy.

The mediastinum can be directly visualized by mediastinoscopy (Fig. 12.6). In this procedure the surgeon makes a small incision in the suprasternal notch and the mediastinum is inspected through a mediastinoscope. Biopsies of the nodes are taken where possible. For left-sided tumours an additional mediastinotomy may be necessary, and it is generally performed through the bed of the second intercostal cartilage. In patients whose mediastinoscopy is negative the resectability rate is at least 85% and in over 50% of cases the nodes will not be involved at thoracotomy. In a further 30% the stage will be N_1 only (Table 12.3). Clearly, if the diagnosis has been made from supraclavicular node biopsy or biopsy of metastatic lesions, these patients are unsuitable for surgery. Other evidence of obvious distant spread, such as abnormal liver function tests combined with an abnormal liver scan or hepatic ultrasound, are also obvious contraindications to operation. If

Fig. 12.5 CT scan of thorax, at level of manubrium, in a patient with squamous carcinoma of the lung. The tumour is shown extending through the pleural space into the chest wall, eroding the ribs (arrowed).

Fig. 12.6 The technique of mediastinoscopy.

the liver function tests are normal and there are no neurological symptoms or signs, isotope liver or brain scan will seldom be positive and are therefore not routinely indicated. A bone scan may, however, show unsuspected metastases.

Finally, the surgeon needs to know whether his or her patient is likely to withstand a surgical operation. Routine exercise testing, spirometry and other lung function tests such as ventilation/perfusion scanning can all be valuable. Patients with poor pulmonary reserve may have to be excluded from surgery even though their tumours are operable by other criteria. As a rough guide, patients with FEV_1 (forced expiratory volume/second) less than 1.2 litres do not withstand pneumonectomy though this also depends on age, sex, size and especially height. Patients over 70 years of age also tolerate pneumonectomy poorly (particularly right-sided).

For patients with *SCLC*, the rationale for staging is altogether different. The characteristic early and widespread dissemination of this tumour makes surgical intervention inappropriate in the large majority of cases, although the occasional instance of 'surgically resectable' SCLC is encountered.

In some instances, determination of the degree of spread in SCLC is both logical and necessary. For example, although radiotherapy alone is no longer considered to be the best treatment for this disease (see below), it is sometimes used in patients considered unsuitable for chemotherapy. More commonly, in patients undergoing treatment with chemotherapy, radiotherapy is often given to those with 'limited' disease in whom no metastases can be demonstrated and disease is confined to one hemithorax. If the proposed treatment is only with cytotoxic drugs, irrespective of extent of disease, then routine staging is unnecessary although investigation of specific symptoms is sometimes indicated on clinical grounds.

If staging in SCLC is to be undertaken, the most useful investigations include liver function tests (including measurement of serum albumin), plasma electrolytes and calcium determination, full blood count, bone marrow

aspiration (bearing in mind that aspiration from two sites doubles the yield), isotope bone scanning and liver scanning in patients with abnormal liver function tests. CT scanning of the brain in asymptomatic patients is seldom abnormal and not performed as a routine.

Treatment

The principles of treatment of NSCLC and SCLC are very different. Small cell lung cancer is seldom surgically resectable, usually widespread at presentation and is both more chemosensitive and radiosensitive. For these reasons their management is considered separately.

SURGERY FOR NON-SMALL
LUNG CANCER

For NSCLC, surgical resection offers the best hope of cure. The percentage of operable cases varies with the philosophy of the surgeon, but the criteria for operability are not usually met in more than about 30% of cases. Approximately 50% of tumours are obviously unresectable by chest X-ray or bronchoscopic criteria. Physiological evaluation, biochemical testing and mediastinoscopy raises the unresectability rate still further (see above).

For patients in whom surgery is possible, the choice of operation depends on the location of the tumour and the patient's respiratory capacity. If the tumour is peripheral with no evidence of local extension, a wedge or segmental resection may occasionally be sufficient, particularly in patients whose pulmonary reserve is poor. In patients with more centrally located tumours contained within a single lobe, lobectomy is the usual procedure, provided the hilar nodes are clear. An adequate margin of normal looking lung should be removed where possible. Pneumonectomy is necessary for tumours originating within the main stem bronchus, where the primary tumour involves more than one lobe, or where the hilum is involved. Clearly, these patients should undergo particularly careful measurement of respiratory function before such an operation can be contemplated.

Although patients with evidence of local spread are usually considered to have inoperable lesions, many surgeons are prepared to undertake an operation in Pancoast tumour since cancers at this site (superior sulcus) may be biologically more favourable. Despite local invasion of pleura and ribs, they can sometimes be removed surgically, and regional lymphatic metastases appear to be unusual.

The mortality (5%) and morbidity associated with pneumonectomy are of course greater than with a lesser operation such as a lobectomy (2% mortality); many surgeons do not operate in patients over the age of 70 years, since mortality rises steeply with advancing age.

Results of surgical treatment

The results of surgical treatment depend largely on the degree of patient selection; surgeons using the most stringent criteria for operability will have the best results. A large retrospective survey by Mountain of over 800 patients undergoing thoracotomy [4] showed that histological type and stage of the tumour were important prognostic criteria. Patients with squamous cell carcinoma had the best survival, 37% of all patients surviving 5 years (Fig. 12.7). Patients with adenocarcinoma or large cell carcinoma did less well, and the 5-year survival was 27%. The importance of tumour stage is shown in Fig. 12.8. For patients with Stage I disease, the 5-year survival rate was over 50% for all histologies (but approaching 80% for T_1 squamous carcinomas), suggesting that in NSCLC tumour stage is more important than histology in determining survival. One additional finding was that in patients with squamous cell carcinoma, the presence of local nodal involvement did not necessarily imply early death from blood-borne metastases. In these patients, radical surgery, in the absence of other effective curative measures, seemed the most fruitful approach if the mediastinal node involvement was limited. This is why some surgeons feel that early

Fig. 12.7 Prognosis in relation to histology after curative resection for lung cancer. (From Mountain C.F. *Annals of Thoracic Surgery* 1977; **24**: 365–373. With permission.)

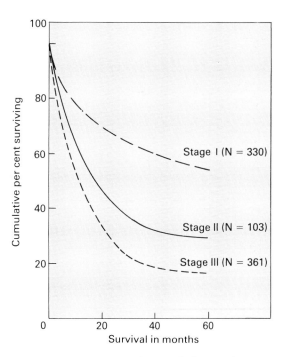

Fig. 12.8 Tumour stage and survival after curative resection for lung cancer. (From Mountain C.F. *Annals of Thoracic Surgery* 1977; **24**: 365–373. With permission.)

mediastinal nodal involvement should not be regarded as an absolute contraindication to surgery, although in general, the presence of mediastinal involvement is an unquestionably adverse feature. In this series, the effectiveness of surgery for local control was further emphasized by the finding that approximately three-quarters of patients who developed recurrent disease first recurred outside the initial site of the tumour (usually brain, bone or contralateral lung). None the less, despite modern operative techniques and more careful case selection, the data shown in Figs 12.7 and 12.8 are only slightly better than those obtained in the 1950s.

RADIOTHERAPY FOR NON-SMALL CELL LUNG CANCER

Although patients with NSCLC have always formed a large part of the radiotherapist's work there is continued debate regarding the indications for its use. In judging which patients are suitable for treatment, the radiotherapist has to decide whether his intention is radical or palliative. In the majority of cases, palliation is the only realistic expectation, though long-term survival is occasionally seen in patients irradiated only with palliative intent.

Palliative radiotherapy

The majority of patients with NSCLC have inoperable disease. Radical radiotherapy with curative intent is usually inappropriate and the decision facing the radiotherapist is whether and when to treat. Over half of these patients are clearly inoperable on bronchoscopic grounds, though a significant minority will have come to thoracotomy, the tumour having initially been thought to be resectable. Although criteria for treatment are difficult to define, palliative radiotherapy is often recommended for patients with loco-regional disease considered unsuitable for surgery but without evidence of distant metastases. Such patients include those with tumours of the main stem bronchus within 1 cm of the carina, those with invasion of important

mediastinal structures such as the recurrent laryngeal or phrenic nerves, and those with troublesome symptoms including haemoptysis, obstruction of a major bronchus, severe cough and pain. In this latter group, radiotherapy produces clinical benefit in the majority of cases. Finally, in patients in whom obstruction to a bronchus is imminent or where SVCO is present, radiotherapy is indicated whether the patient is symptomatic or not.

Relative contraindications to treatment with radiotherapy include metastases beyond the loco-regional nodes, multiple lesions, bronchial fistula, supraclavicular node involvement, or a large tumour mass. Even under these circumstances, palliative treatment may still offer benefit, if the patient's symptoms demand it. If the patient is symptomatic, treatment should be given as soon as possible.

When should treatment be used in asymptomatic patients with inoperable disease? In an early study radiotherapy, chemotherapy or both, was compared to no initial treatment. Survival was the same in all groups (approximately 8.5 months), with no advantage for active treatment unless specific symptoms were present. Delaying radiotherapy until the onset of a specific symptom frequently allowed a patient 4 or 5 months before treatment proved necessary, and this group had the best palliation of all. Many radiotherapists in the United Kingdom therefore delay palliative treatment. However, the trial was much too small to be confident of the result. Increasingly, palliative radiotherapy schedules have become shortened and simplified without apparent loss of benefit [5].

Radical radiotherapy

Occasionally, patients with operable lung cancer are referred to a radiotherapist either because of refusal to undergo an operation, or because of co-existent medical conditions which would make surgery hazardous. In these operable cases and other inoperable localized tumours where the tumour is encompassed by the radiation fields, radiotherapists treat the patient radically with the intention of cure. Even in carefully selected patients the 5-year survival following radiotherapy alone is probably no greater than 10%.

From this rather minimal information, it seems likely that radiotherapy can occasionally cure patients with carcinoma of the bronchus, particularly in patients with small, technically operable tumours. In these patients, a radical approach should be employed if for any reason surgery is refused or considered inappropriate. This requires treatment to a higher dose than is generally employed for palliation of symptoms, in the region of 50−60 Gy (5000−6000 rad) over 5−6 weeks in daily fractions or equivalent (see Chapter 5, Fig. 5.8). However, such treatments are frequently accompanied by side-effects including dysphagia, pericarditis and skin reactions. In addition, irradiation of a portion of spinal cord is unavoidable even with the most sophisticated planning techniques. However, with careful tumour imaging and the use of multifield techniques this problem can almost always be minimalized. Radiation damage to the spinal cord is discussed on pp. 74 & 223.

Outside controlled clinical trials there is no place for routine pre-operative radiotherapy in operable lung cancer. Occasionally a patient with Stage III disease, with mediastinal involvement, may show a rapid and striking clinical regression with a relatively low dose of radiotherapy. However, even in such cases, it is exceptional for surgery to become a practical proposition. Combined treatment with surgery and pre-operative radiotherapy is often recommended for Pancoast tumour (see above), but overall the results are not dramatically better than those of surgery alone.

CHEMOTHERAPY FOR NON-SMALL CELL LUNG CANCER

A variety of single agents has been shown to have some activity in NSCLC (Table 12.4). The response rates are low and no survival advantage has been shown for any of these drugs used as a single agent. Attempts have therefore been made to try and improve response rates by using drugs in combination. Typical combinations are shown in Table 12.4.

Of the various combination regimens that of mitomycin, ifosfamide and cisplatin appears to be among the most active, but is associated with considerable toxicity. Most of the active regimens include cisplatin with its concomitant nausea and vomiting.

In advanced, metastatic disease the value of chemotherapy is questionable. The survival benefit, compared with best supportive care, is small but this oversimplifies the issue. Against the toxicity of chemotherapy must be considered the improvement in symptoms which accompanies response, the fact that responses are more frequent, long-lasting and complete in patients who are fit, and the psychological need of many patients for active treatment [6].

In recent years there has been renewed interest in the combination of chemotherapy before surgery in localized, initially inoperable, tumours and in chemotherapy before radical

Table 12.4 Chemotherapy in NSCLC

Agent	Response rates (%)
Single agents	
Cisplatin	12
Cyclophosphamide	5−10
Doxorubicin	12
Etoposide	10−12
Ifosfamide	15
Methotrexate	5−15
Mitomycin	15
Vincristine	5
Vindesine	17
Combination therapy	
Mitomycin, ifosfamide, cisplatin	45−60
Cisplatin, vindesine	25−35
Cisplatin, doxorubicin, cyclophosphamide	20−35
Methotrexate, doxorubicin, CCNU, cyclophosphamide	15−20

radiotherapy for localized tumours. There is no doubt that pre-operative chemotherapy is associated with a higher response rate (up to 60%) than in metastatic disease, that some tumours are rendered operable and there may even be no viable tumour at resection. The impact on survival is unknown since very large-scale trials (100 patients) will be necessary to determine this. Chemotherapy before or after radical radiation has been assessed in several randomized trials but all were too small to be confident of any survival difference [7,8]. A recent meta-analysis of all data from these trials indicates a potential benefit of 2–7%. It seems that a similar benefit of chemotherapy is present in all stages of localized NSCLC treated with surgery or radiotherapy. Such small differences are nevertheless very important in such a common disease.

Treatment of small cell lung cancer

The majority (two-thirds) of patients present with extensive disease. That is, thoracic disease involving more than one hemithorax or with metastatic spread. In these patients radiotherapy has a palliative role only and even with modern chemotherapy the prognosis is very poor. In patients with limited disease (confined to one hemithorax) chemotherapy is the mainstay of treatment.

RADIOTHERAPY FOR
SMALL CELL LUNG CANCER

Small cell lung cancer is much the most radio-sensitive histological type with complete radiological response of the primary tumour in over 80% of cases. Even large primary lesions associated with massive hilar and mediastinal lymphadenopathy may regress completely, following moderate doses of radiotherapy, 40–50 Gy (4–5000 rad) over 4–5 weeks. In one of the earliest comparative cancer trials, the Medical Research Council demonstrated that in 'operable' cases of SCLC, radiotherapy produced better long-term results than surgery with a

mean survival time of 7 months and a small number of long-term survivors [9].

Although the initial response to radiotherapy is usually gratifying, recurrence in the irradiated area is frequent and long-term local control of the disease is not always achieved. As might be expected, there is evidence that more durable local control may be obtained by higher radiation dosage although at the cost of greater toxicity, particularly if chemotherapy is also used. The combination of radiotherapy and chemotherapy is discussed below.

CHEMOTHERAPY FOR SMALL CELL
LUNG CANCER

It has long been apparent that SCLC is a rapidly dividing tumour, usually metastatic at the time of presentation. For this reason a systemic approach to treatment is essential. Many studies have shown that SCLC is relatively sensitive to cytotoxic agents and chemotherapy has become the mainstay of treatment. A randomized prospective study comparing radiation alone versus radiation and combination chemotherapy [10] showed a clear short-term survival advantage for the patients treated with both chemotherapy and radiation compared with radiation alone, although the toxicity was greater in the chemotherapy treated patients.

Many single agents have been shown to have activity. Cyclophosphamide is the single most useful alkylating agent. Many other drugs such as etoposide, methotrexate, nitrosoureas, vinca alkaloids, cisplatin and anthracyclines are effective in treatment of the disease (Table 12.5).

Single-agent chemotherapy has largely been discarded except under special circumstances which are discussed below.

In the past 15 years numerous trials of combination chemotherapy have been carried out, using a wide variety of regimens and schedules (Table 12.6).

The duration of conventional chemotherapy has been assessed in three large studies. In that of the MRC [11], no survival advantage was found in continuing chemotherapy for 12 cycles

Table 12.5 Single-agent chemotherapy in SCLC (the data should be regarded as approximate especially in previously treated patients)

Agent	Response rates (%)
Carboplatin	60
Etoposide	40–70
Cyclophosphamide	35
Ifosfamide	35
Cisplatin	35
Doxorubicin	30
Methotrexate	20
Vincristine	15
CCNU	10

Table 12.6 Combination chemotherapy in SCLC

Regimens	Response rates (%)
Cyclophosphamide, methotrexate, CCNU	70
Vincristine, doxorubicin, cyclophosphamide	80
Cisplatin and etoposide	80
Cisplatin, doxorubicin, etoposide	85
Doxorubicin, cyclophosphamide, etoposide	85

compared with 6. In that of the Cancer Research Campaign [12], 4 cycles were slightly inferior to 8 unless chemotherapy was given on relapse. The EORTC trial showed no advantage of 12 over 7 cycles. The balance of evidence therefore suggests that 6 cycles of conventional chemotherapy is adequate.

In recent years there have been attempts to increase the intensity of chemotherapy by giving drugs weekly, or by giving very high dose chemotherapy with autologous bone marrow transplantation (ABMT) after the induction of remission. While the overall response rates with these approaches is high, there is as yet no evidence to suggest that long-term survival is improved.

The toxicity of chemotherapy is considerable and the gains in survival are as yet modest. With limited disease it is now possible to achieve survival of 2 years in 15% of patients. A survey of survival in SCLC [13] has shown that 8% of limited disease (LD) patients will be alive at 2 years and 2.2% of patients with extensive disease (ED). Relapse of SCLC occurs for 6 years, at which point only 2.6% of all patients are alive. Even though there is a chance of long survival and possibly cure with chemotherapy, the morbidity of treatment is sufficient to raise serious doubts about the advisability of chemotherapy in every case. Etoposide given orally as a single agent may be an acceptable means of inducing remission without excess toxicity in elderly or infirm patients.

There are certain factors which are known to be associated with a poor prognosis in SCLC, and these are listed in Table 12.7. Of these, the most important are ED, poor performance status, low plasma albumin and sodium, and abnormal liver function tests (Fig. 12.9). In elderly patients, in whom these poor prognostic factors are often present, it is unwise to persist with chemotherapy beyond the first two or three cycles unless there is a clear improvement in the tumour and in the patient's well-being. For younger patients with LD and in whom there are no adverse prognostic features, intensive combination chemotherapy offers the best chance of long-term survival. There will be many patients who fall between these two extremes and here the physician must decide individually what appears to be the best policy.

The combination of chemotherapy and radiotherapy for the primary tumour has been investigated in several randomized trials in which patients treated with chemotherapy were assigned either to receive thoracic irradiation or not. These studies have given conflicting results, but the majority showed some benefit in survival at 2 years. The studies were too small to detect a moderate difference reliably, but a recent overview [14] in which all the studies have been re-analysed has shown a 5% benefit in survival at 3 years (from 7% to 12%) — a 60% relative improve-

Table 12.7 Adverse prognostic factors in SCLC

Poor performance status
Extensive disease
Low plasma albumin and sodium
Abnormal liver function tests
Brain metastases
Marrow infiltration or anaemia

ment relatively speaking. The morbidity of thoracic irradiation may be considerable in combination with chemotherapy. Nevertheless, thoracic irradiation now has an established role in patients with limited disease who are fit enough to receive it and who are responding to chemotherapy. New approaches include synchronous radiotherapy and chemotherapy, and hyperfractionated radiation. The optimum timing of radiation is still uncertain.

In summary, the place of routine thoracic irradiation in SCLC is still not fully determined.

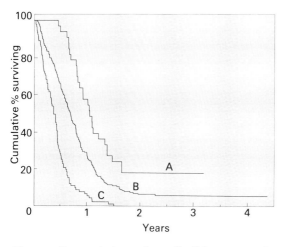

Fig. 12.9 Prognostic factors in small cell lung cancer. In A all patients had good performance status and normal biochemistry (see Table 12.7). In C patients had poor performance status and more than two biochemical abnormalities. Group B is by exclusion. (From Souhami R.L. *et al. Cancer Research* 1985; **45**: 2878. With permission.)

Its use should be considered under the following circumstances:

1 in patients with LD, where there is an incomplete response to chemotherapy but no evidence of distant disease;
2 in patients with LD who are responding to chemotherapy;
3 for local recurrence;
4 for SVCO unresponsive to chemotherapy.

Radiotherapy is of great palliative value in SCLC, and is the treatment of choice for painful bone metastases, and for brain metastases. Clinical evidence of brain metastases occurs in 25% of patients with SCLC and is demonstrable in about two-thirds of patients at autopsy. Treatment with radiotherapy to the whole brain to a total dose of 20 Gy (2000 rad) in 5 fractions in a week is often effective and well tolerated; there seems to be no advantage for more prolonged regimens. Similar fractionation is usually satisfactory for painful bony deposits.

Because symptomatic brain metastases are frequent many groups now routinely offer treatment with prophylactic cranial irradiation (PCI) in SCLC. Routine use of PCI has decreased the clinical frequency of brain metastases from 25% to less than 10%, and the autopsy frequency from 65% to 25%, though it does not appear to increase survival. Prophylactic cranial irradiation may therefore have a role in reducing the undoubted morbidity of brain metastasis. On the other hand PCI is itself associated with short-term toxicity (confusion, unsteadiness, memory loss) and a possible, but as yet unquantified, long-term neurological morbidity. Its value is therefore questionable. A common policy is to offer PCI only to patients who have had a good response to chemotherapy, thereby avoiding unnecessary cerebral irradiation in non-responding patients whose survival time will be short. Attempts at prolonging survival by prophylactic irradiation at other sites (liver, adrenal and para-aortic nodes) have so far proved unsuccessful.

In view of the radiosensitivity of SCLC, several groups have investigated the use of systemic irradiation in SCLC, using either total body or hemi-body radiation. The results have not been encouraging, particularly where low doses have been given. In one study hemibody irradiation seemed to be as effective as combination chemotherapy in patients with limited disease [15]. 'Debulking' surgery has been advocated in patients responding to chemotherapy, but it is not yet clear if there is benefit from this radical approach. Randomized trials are in progress. The major problem in SCLC is still the control of systemic disease.

Immunotherapy of lung cancer

Early reports suggested that BCG instilled intrapleurally after resection prolonged survival. However, this result was not confirmed when the trial was repeated, and the toxicity of intrapleural BCG was considerable. BCG vaccination and intravenous *Corynebacterium parvum* have both been used in SCLC and NSCLC, and conflicting claims for their effectiveness have been made. The same is true for both levamisole and interferon. As with most cancers, there is little to justify these methods as part of current treatment.

TUMOURS OF THE MEDIASTINUM [16]

The mediastinum lies at the centre of the chest and is bordered by the thoracic inlet superiorly, the diaphragm inferiorly, the vertebral column posteriorly, the sternum anteriorly and the pleural reflections laterally (Fig. 12.10). A great variety of tumours can arise in the mediastinum and tend to occur at different sites within it.

The *anterosuperior compartment* of the mediastinum is bounded inferiorly by the diaphragm, anteriorly by the sternum and posteriorly by the vertebral column down to the 4th thoracic vertebra, and then by the anterior pericardium. It contains the upper trachea and oesophagus, the aortic arch and the thymus and may also include a retrosternal portion of a normal thyroid gland, with parathyroid structures and embry-

onic cell rests. The *middle compartment* of the mediastinum is bounded anteriorly by the anterior pericardium and posteriorly by the oesophagus, and extends downwards to the diaphragm. It contains the heart, ascending aorta, main bronchi, hila and carina, and the subcarinal and other closely related tracheobronchial lymph nodes. The *posterior mediastinum* lies between the vertebral column and posterior pericardium and contains the oesophagus, the descending thoracic aorta and the sympathetic nerve chains. The pattern of tumours arising in the mediastinum reflects these anatomical divisions (Table 12.8).

ANTEROSUPERIOR MEDIASTINUM [17]

The commonest malignant tumours are thymomas and germ cell tumours including teratomas of various types and also seminomas. In addition, thyroid and parathyroid adenomas occur at this site and can cause diagnostic difficulties, and carcinomas of the thyroid may occasionally arise from the retrosternal portion of the gland. Symptoms from superior mediastinal tumours are usually caused by pressure on local structures such as the oesophagus, trachea and laryngeal or phrenic nerves. Dysphagia, dyspnoea, stridor, cough and superior vena caval obstruction are relatively common, and vocal cord palsy and/or diaphragmatic paralysis are sometimes seen. These symptoms occur less frequently with slowly growing tumours (such as retrosternal goitre and some thymomas).

Thymoma

Thymic tumours form a mixed histological picture often including more than one population of cells. Lymphocytes, epithelial cells and spindle cells tend to predominate and 'typical' thymomas may contain lymphocytic and epithelial components as apparently distinct populations. Unfortunately, thymic tumour histology is a poor predictor of the behaviour of the tumour, though the macroscopic appearance is more valuable. Some thymic tumours grow

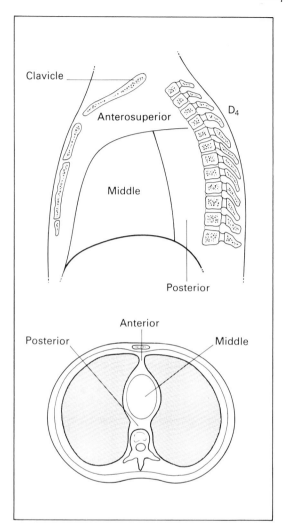

Fig. 12.10 A simplified anatomy of the mediastinum.

Table 12.8 Tumours of the mediastinum

Antero-superior
Thymoma
Teratoma
Thyroid and parathyroid tumours
Sarcoma (haemangiosarcoma, haemangiopericytoma)
Mesothelioma
Lipoma

Middle
Malignant lymphoma
Tumours of the heart
Secondary lymph node involvement
Pericardial tumours

Posterior
Neurofibroma, neurilemmoma, Schwannoma
Neuroblastoma
Neurofibrosarcoma
Phaeochromocytoma
Chordoma
Paraganglioma

very slowly over many years. Others grow more rapidly with local invasion and pleural spread.

The criteria for malignancy are difficult to define in thymomas, and most authorities divide these tumours into invasive and non-invasive. Distant metastases are unusual. Occasionally, Hodgkin's disease can arise from thymic tissue, without the evidence of lymphadenopathy elsewhere. In these cases

surgical excision is less important than with other types of thymic tumour. Thymic *carcinomas* are rare tumours which show clear histological features of malignancy. Many variants have been described (squamous, clear cell, spindle cell, small, mucoepidermoid, adenocystic).

A variety of clinical syndromes are associated with thymomas. The commonest is *myasthenia gravis* which occurs in 44% of patients. Myasthenia may be the presenting feature of the tumour which is benign or malignant. Myasthenia gravis is associated with antibodies to acetylcholine receptors but its relationship to the tumour is not well understood. Removal of the thymoma results in remission of the myasthenia in approximately 30% of cases. *Red cell aplasia* occurs in 4% and may be associated with leucopenia and/or thrombocytopenia. A spindle cell thymic tumour is the commonest pathology. The red cell aplasia may be due to an antibody to red cell precursors in the bone marrow. Occasionally the aplasia recovers after removal of the tumour. Other syndromes include hypogammaglobulinaemia, connective tissue diseases, pernicious anaemia and auto-immune thyroiditis. Together, associated diseases occur in 80–90% of thymomas, with myasthenia gravis and cytopenias being the commonest.

Investigation includes chest X-ray (Fig. 12.11) and CT scan of the chest which may show pleural metastases. Treatment is by surgical removal whenever possible. Complete removal is usually achieved if the tumour is encapsulated and in such cases local recurrence is unusual. Capsular invasion, direct extension to the pleura or pericardium or incomplete resection are all indications for postoperative radiotherapy which reduces the local recurrence rate. A dose of 35–45 Gy (3500–4500 rad) in 3–5 weeks is commonly employed. More distant spread of recurrence after radiotherapy is sometimes treated by chemotherapy although experience is limited and the results are often poor. Prednisolone may induce remissions, but the most active agents appear to be ifosfamide and cyclophosphamide. Cisplatin-containing regimens have been used (usually with cyclo-phosphamide and doxorubicin) and responses occur in 80% of cases, 40% being complete. Responses usually last from 6–24 months.

Encapsulated thymomas have an excellent prognosis and 60% of patients are alive 20 years later. Invasive thymomas have a much worse prognosis, and only 50% of patients are alive after 5 years.

Carcinoid of the thymus

This occurs occasionally and probably develops from APUD cells within the thymus (see Chapter 15). These rare tumours may give rise to Cushing's syndrome by producing ACTH and causing adrenal hyperplasia. They are occasionally malignant and are much more common in men. Although they may be completely resected, they often recur locally and metastasize. They do not cause carcinoid syndrome. The prognosis is not good, with 5-year survival as low as 15% in some series.

Fig. 12.11 Typical PA chest X-ray appearance in a patient with a thymic tumour. There is a well demarcated tumour mass and the lung fields are clear.

Germ cell tumours

Primary germ cell tumours of the mediastinum are uncommon but are potentially curable. Although teratomas and mixed tumours are the commonest, pure seminoma is also described. The tumours may produce βHCG and AFP as do testicular tumours (see Chapter 19). As with thymomas, the usual clinical presentation is with local pressure symptoms, chiefly dysp-noea, cough and dysphagia. Occasionally, gynaecomastia is the presenting feature. Haematogenous metastasis is unusual, lung and brain being the commonest sites. Local lymphatic invasion may occur. Any young male with an unexplained superior mediastinal tumour of uncertain origin should have plasma tumour markers (AFP and βHCG) measured since histological interpretation can be difficult even in experienced hands and these tumours can be misdiagnosed as adenocarcinoma. There is an association between Klinefelter's syndrome (XXY) and mediastinal germ cell tumours.

Plain chest X-ray, tomography and CT scanning are essential to delineate the tumour and for following progress after treatment. CT lung scanning will occasionally reveal unsuspected metastases. The principles of management are essentially as for testicular germ cell tumours (see Chapter 19). Primary treatment is with combination chemotherapy (currently using combinations including cisplatin, bleomycin, vinblastine and etoposide). Seminomas are in some cases curable by local radiotherapy; 40 Gy (4000 rad) in 20 daily fractions over 4 weeks is the usual dose, although chemotherapy is now considered an essential component of treatment.

In mediastinal teratomas, the role of radiation for residual disease is uncertain. Surgical removal of suspicious residual masses should always be considered, ideally when tumour markers have returned to normal. Previous treatment with large doses of bleomycin may lead to pulmonary toxicity with stiff lungs and poor lung compliance, which may make the post-thoracotomy period particularly hazardous. Recent reports of combined chemotherapy and surgical treatment have been encouraging, with several long-term survivors, probable cures, by contrast to earlier reports in which cure was rare.

MIDDLE MEDIASTINUM

In the middle compartment of the mediastinum, lymphomas are the commonest malignant tumours, and both Hodgkin's disease and non-Hodgkin's lymphomas occur. The differential diagnosis includes an important group of non-malignant conditions — pericardial and broncho-genic cysts, mediastinal lipoma, tuberculosis, sarcoidosis and infectious or malignant causes of hilar and/or mediastinal lymphadenopathy. In the absence of palpable lymphadenopathy in an accessible site, the diagnosis is usually made by mediastinoscopy or limited thoracotomy. Tissue diagnosis is essential and examination of fresh (unfixed) tissue is valuable for the histopathologist since the use of immunocyto-chemical stains can help distinguish difficult lymphomas from each other and from anaplastic carcinomas (see Chapter 3).

Staging and management of mediastinal lymphomas follows similar principles to those at other sites (see Chapter 26). Surgical excision has no place in the routine management of these tumours which are sensitive both to chemotherapy and radiotherapy. Occasionally, mediastinal lymphoma causes severe SVCO which requires emergency treatment (see Chapter 8).

Two particular characteristic non-Hodgkin's mediastinal lymphomas occur. The first is T cell convoluted, lymphoblastic, diffuse lymphoma (previously termed Sternberg's sarcoma). It is seen predominantly in adolescent males. The second is a sclerosing B cell lymphoma occurring most frequently in young women (Chapter 26). Hodgkin's disease of the mediastinum, usually in association with obvious lymphadenopathy in the neck and/or axilla, occurs in about 30% of all supradiaphragmatic cases, but the mediastinum may occasionally be the sole site of involvement.

POSTERIOR MEDIASTINUM

Tumours of the posterior mediastinum are chiefly neurogenic in origin, and usually arise from the thoracic sympathetic chain or inter-costal nerves (Table 12.8). They are frequently asymptomatic but may cause back pain, dysphagia or ptosis due to Horner's syndrome. Neurofibromas are the commonest, and can usually be removed surgically. They can arise sporadically or in patients with von Reckling-hausen's disease. Other neurogenic tumours include Schwannomas (both benign and malignant) and neurofibrosarcoma. These neurogenic tumours may extend through the intervertebral foramina (dumb-bell tumours) and cause cord compression. This is suggested by vertebral erosion on lateral chest X-ray. Ganglioneuromas are probably the commonest of the sympathetic nerve tumours and are generally well-differentiated, encapsulated and surgically resectable. In some cases, urinary VMA may be raised and can be useful for monitoring progress. A less well-differentiated form (ganglioneuroblastoma) is also encountered, and has a worse prognosis because of local recurrence and metastases. Phaeochromocytoma, another hormonally active tumour, frequently presents with symptoms of catecholamine excess rather than with pressure symptoms, such as paroxysmal hypertension, headache, palpitation, chest pain and excessive sweating. They should be surgically excised where possible. In children, neuroblastoma is a common cause of posterior mediastinal tumour accounting for about one-fifth of all childhood neuroblastomas. The management of neuroblastoma is discussed in Chapter 24.

Of the rare tumours, chordoma occasionally presents as a posterior mediastinal tumour and its management is discussed in Chapter 11. Paraganglioma (chemodectoma) is rare and may be locally invasive, usually involving the great vessels.

Diagnosis of posterior mediastinal tumours requires careful radiological assessment (sometimes with contrast studies such as aortography or contrast CT scanning) as well as precise tissue diagnosis, which usually requires thoracotomy. Management is by surgical removal of the tumour wherever possible. For incompletely excised malignant tumours, postoperative radiotherapy is usually recommended.

MESOTHELIOMA [18]

This relentlessly progressive malignant tumour arises from the surface of the pleura, occasionally remaining well localized at the primary site but more often spreading diffusely and involving a substantial area of the pleura including the inner surface of the visceral pleura, thereby encroaching onto the pericardium. Pleural effusion is common, and the disease is occasionally bilateral. Primary peritoneal mesothelioma, without pleural involvement, is well described and peritoneal disease occasionally develops in patients in whom the pleura is the main or primary site of disease. Most patients with mesothelioma give a history of asbestos ex-

Table 12.9 Staging for mesothelioma

Stage	Site involved
I	Ipsilateral pleura, lung, pericardium, diaphragm
IIA	Chest wall, mediastinum intra-thoracic lymph nodes
IIB	Opposite pleura
III	Through diaphragm
	Extra-thoracic lymph nodes
IV	Distant metastases

posure though there is characteristically a delay of 20 years or so before the disease becomes apparent. The incidence of mesothelioma is apparently rising, presumably because of the widespread use of asbestos products. However, the past 10 years have seen increasingly stringent constraints on the use of asbestos, and we are probably now at the 'peak' of asbestos-related lung disease. Crocidolite is thought to be the most carcinogenic fibre. A staging system is shown in Table 12.9.

PATHOLOGY

Pathologically the tumours may appear sarcomatous, often with both fibrous and epithelial elements which may be so anaplastic as to be almost indistinguishable from a poorly differentiated carcinoma. The degree of anaplastic change correlates poorly with clinical behaviour. In other cases the distinction from adenocarcinoma may be very difficult. Direct extension is characteristic and mesotheliomas typically invade ribs and chest wall. Early and widespread involvement of intercostal bundles probably accounts for the severe pain so typical of this tumour. In addition, extension through the diaphragm, invasion of local lymph nodes and distant blood-borne metastases are all commonly found.

CLINICAL FEATURES

Patients typically complain of increasing chest

pain, which can be very severe, coupled with shortness of breath on exertion. The dyspnoea tends to be progressive and unremitting, often leading to severe incapacity even at rest. On examination there are signs of diminished chest movement and pleural effusion. Radiologically the most typical feature of asbestos exposure is the pleural plaque, often multiple, and usually associated with pleural effusion (Fig. 12.12).

Fig. 12.12 Mesothelioma. (A) Typical X-ray findings, including pleural shadowing with nodulation behind the heart, in the costophrenic angle and along the lateral chest wall, together with partial destruction of ribs. Courtesy of Dr M.E. Hodson. (B) Typical CT scan appearance with involvement of the whole of the pleura of the left lung with complete sparing on the right.

In mesothelioma there is extensive pleural infiltration extending into the mediastinum and causing 'crowding' of the ribs on the affected side because of contracture caused by the tumour.

DIAGNOSIS

The diagnosis can usually be confirmed by pleural biopsy. In cases with such widespread involvement that surgical resection is impossible, diagnostic thoracotomy should be avoided, particularly since tumour seeding of thoracotomy scars is common and can produce additional severe pain. CT scanning is of great importance for definition of the tumour anatomy, particularly with respect to the juxtapericardial reflection of the pleura, and the adjacent pericardium, which are often poorly visualized by plain X-ray of the chest.

TREATMENT

Treatment of mesothelioma is highly unsatisfactory. Surgery is possible only in a very small minority of cases with localized involvement, though surgical cures are well documented. Local recurrence is common, and most surgeons favour wide excision where possible, including sacrifice of part of the chest wall, diaphragm, pericardium and adjacent lobe of lung where necessary.

Radiotherapy is of very little value, though pain relief and apparent reduction in the rate of tumour growth occasionally occur. Adequate irradiation of the whole pleural surface is technically difficult because of the proximity of the lung, but new methods of tangential arc irradiation may allow this technique to be explored further. A wide variety of chemotherapeutic agents has been used in mesothelioma but with no long-term success although responses to doxorubicin, cisplatin and other agents occasionally occur. Responses to α-interferon are also reported. Combinations of cisplatin and interferon produce responses in about 20% of patients and some responses last for many months. Intrapleural chemotherapy is occasionally attempted for control of the malignant pleural effusion, but the results are discouraging [19].

The very poor results of treatment argue strongly for rigid control of the use of asbestos products, and patients with mesothelioma and a clear history of industrial asbestos exposure are usually considered by independent tribunals to be strong candidates for compensation.

REFERENCES

1 Loeb L.A., Ernster V.L., Warner K.E., Abbotts J., Laszlo J. Smoking and lung cancer: an overview. *Cancer Research* 1984; **44**: 5940−58.

2 Doll R., Hill A.B. Mortality in relation to smoking: ten years' observation on British doctors. *British Medical Journal* 1964; **1**: 1399−410.

3 Abeloff M.D., Eggleston J.C., Mendelsohn G., Ettinger D.S., Baylin S.B. Changes in morphologic and biochemical characteristics in small cell carcinoma of the lung. A clinico-pathologic study. *American Journal of Medicine* 1979; **66**: 757−64.

4 Mountain C.F. The relationship of prognosis to morphology and the anatomic extent of disease. In Israel L., Chahinian A.P., eds. *Lung Cancer*. New York: Academic Press, 1976. pp. 108−41.

5 Inoperable non-small cell lung cancer (NSCLC): A Medical Research Council randomised trial of palliative radiotherapy with two fractions or ten fractions. *British Journal of Cancer* 1991; **63**: 265−70.

6 Splinter T.A.W. Chemotherapy in advanced non-small cell lung cancer. *European Journal of Cancer* 1990; **26**: 1093−99.

7 Dillman R.O., Seagreen S.L., Propert K.J. *et al.* A randomized trial of induction chemotherapy plus high-dose radiation versus radiation alone in stage III non-small-cell lung cancer. *New England Journal of Medicine* 1990; **322**: 940−45.

8 Weiden P.L., Piatadosi S. Pre-operative chemotherapy (cisplatin and fluorouracil) and radiation therapy in stage III non-small-cell lung cancer: A Phase II study of the lung cancer study group. *Journal of the National Cancer Institute* 1991; **83**: 266−72.

9 Fox W., Scadding J.G. Medical Research Council comparative trial of surgery and radiotherapy for primary treatment of small or oat celled carcinoma of bronchus. Ten year follow up. *Lancet* 1975; **ii**: 63−65.

10 Medical Research Council Lung Cancer Working Party. Radiotherapy alone or with chemotherapy in the treatment of small-cell carcinoma of the lung: the results at 36 months. *British Journal of Cancer* 1981; **46**: 228−35.

11 Medical Research Council Lung Cancer Working Party. Controlled trial of twelve versus six courses of chemotherapy in the treatment of small cell lung cancer. *British Journal of Cancer* 1989; **59**: 584−90.

12 Spiro S.G., Souhami R.L., Geddes D.W. *et al.* Duration of chemotherapy in small cell lung cancer: A Cancer Research Campaign trial. *British Journal of Cancer* 1989; **59**: 578−83.

13 Souhami R.L., Law K. Longevity in small cell lung cancer. *British Journal of Cancer* 1990; **61**: 584−89.

14 Pignon J-P., Arriagada R., Ihde D.C. *et al.* The meta-analysis of thoracic radiotherapy for small-cell lung cancer. *New England Journal of Medicine* 1992; **327**: 1618−24.

15 Urtasun R.C., Belch A.R., McKinnon S. *et al.* Small cell lung cancer: initial treatment with sequential hemi-body irradiation vs. 3-drug systemic chemotherapy. *British Journal of Cancer* 1982; **46**: 228−35.

16 Harper P.G., Addis B. Unusual tumours of the mediastinum. In Williams C.J., Krickorian J.C., Green M.R., Raghavan D., eds. *Textbook of Uncommon Cancer*. Chichester, Wiley and Sons, 1988: 411−49.

17 Mullen B., Richardson J.D. Primary anterior mediastinal tumours in children and adults. *Annals of Thoracic Surgery* 1986; **42**: 338−45.

18 Pisani R.J. Malignant mesothelioma of the pleura. *Mayo Clinic Proceedings* 1988; **63**: 1234−44.

19 Kraruf Hansen A., Hansen H.H. Chemotherapy in malignant mesothelioma: a review. *Cancer Chemotherapy and Pharmacology* 1991; **28**: 319−30.

Chapter 13
Breast Cancer

INCIDENCE, AETIOLOGY AND EPIDEMIOLOGY

Breast cancer is the commonest of all malignant diseases in women, with an incidence of 21 000 new cases annually in England and Wales and 143 000 new cases in the United States. The incidence appears to have risen steadily, at least in the United States, over the past 50 years. Indeed, over the 10-year period 1968–1978, an 11% increase was noted both in the United Kingdom and the United States. The age-related incidence is shown in Fig. 13.1. One in ten women will develop breast cancer during their lifetime, making it the leading cause of death from malignant disease in Western women. In 1990, approximately 40 000 women died of metastatic breast cancer in the United States alone. Incidence rates vary markedly in different parts of the world, with an average of 65 per 100 000. There is a very high incidence in North America and Northern Europe, and a low incidence in Asia and parts of Africa.

There are a number of known aetiological factors [1,2]. Women with a first degree relative with breast cancer have a 3-fold increase in risk. In particular, a history of breast cancer diagnosed premenopausally confers on the patient's daughters an additional risk of 3–11 times the normal rate. Women bearing their first child over the age of 30 are three times more likely to develop breast cancer than those who do so under 20 years, and there is an increased risk in patients who have a history of benign breast disease, particularly epitheliosis and benign cellular atypia. Early menarche and

late menopause are also know to predispose to a higher incidence whereas oophorectomy, when carried out early in life, does seem to offer some degree of protection. Although the evidence relating to use of oral or long-acting injectable contraceptives has in the past been contentious, it seems likely that breast cancer is not more common in patients who have used these agents [3]. Follow-up of victims of Hiroshima has shown a late increase in incidence of breast cancer. It seems likely that demographical differences are due more to diet, cultural or geographical variability than to racial characteristics, since Japanese or Hawaiian women who settle in the United States have daughters and grand-daughters whose likelihood of developing breast cancer follows the American pattern after as little as two generations.

PATHOLOGY AND MODE OF SPREAD

Almost all breast cancers arise from the glandular epithelium lining the lactiferous ducts and ductules, and are therefore typical adenocarcinomas. Although true intraduct carcinomas are sometimes encountered, particularly in screen detected cases (see below), most primary breast cancers have invaded into the stroma of the breast by the time of diagnosis. The great majority of these present as breast lumps, although a small number have eroded through the skin of the breast by the time they are first seen, presenting as fungating tumours. Lesser degrees of skin involvement lead to skin dimpling or tethering and *peau d'orange* in

Fig. 13.1 Age-specific incidence of breast cancer.

more rational treatment policy; the treatment arms include tamoxifen, radiotherapy, both or neither.

Modes of spread in breast cancer (Fig. 13.2) have been the subject of great controversy. In the past, the main focus of dispute was whether or not breast cancer always spread 'centrifugally' or by direct lymphatic dissemination, prior to more widespread involvement in the bloodstream; or whether the latter route was possible even in the absence of local nodal involvement. It is now clear that blood-borne metastases do occur independently of the 'direct' lymphatic route although lymph node involvement in the axilla is a useful guide to the probability of haematogenous spread. Local dissemination may occur, either to the underlying chest wall and related structures including the ribs, pleura and brachial plexus, or to overlying skin. Lymphatic spread is to axillary lymph nodes and the supraclavicular, internal

which skin infiltration leads to local lymphatic obstruction. The wide variability in histological appearance has led to a number of attempts at classifying these tumours according to their microscopic characteristics (recently with the help of histochemical stains). Descriptive terms are often used, but they are generally unhelpful since they have little bearing on prognosis.

Intraduct carcinomas of the breast (ductal carcinoma *in situ* and lobular carcinoma *in situ*), without evidence of true invasiveness, are increasingly recognized as 'early' lesions though there may be widespread abnormalities within the breast, even when invasive characteristics are histologically absent [4]. With the advent of mass screening these abnormalities are now encountered far more frequently, indeed pure intraduct carcinoma is rightly regarded as a 'new disease'. There is great uncertainty about its natural history, with different centres recommending local excision or mastectomy, with or without radiotherapy. In the United Kingdom, a multicentre study has recently been initiated to attempt to delineate a

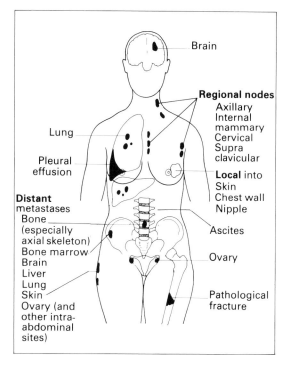

Fig. 13.2 Local, nodal and distant spread in breast cancer.

mammary or contralateral groups. Blood-borne metastasis occurs particularly to bone (especially the axial skeleton), liver, lung, skin and central nervous system (both brain and spinal cord). Intra-abdominal and pelvic metastases, including ovarian and adrenal deposits, are common. Many patients manifest particular patterns of spread and it is not unusual to encounter patients with widespread bone disease but without any evidence of soft tissue disease. Some patients develop relentless local recurrence of disease, cancer *en cuirasse*, without evidence of distant metastasis but with a deep fungating ulcer which may involve a substantial part of the chest wall. The reasons behind these patterns are unclear and they are unrelated to histological characteristics or pathological grade.

Haematogenous spread is of particular importance since patients die from distant metastases rather than from uncontrolled local disease. The likelihood of axillary lymph node metastases correlates closely with the size of the primary tumour. The presence of nodal deposits increases the likelihood of blood-borne metastases, as evidenced by the importance of axillary involvement as a predictor of 5-year survival. There is a quantitative relationship between the number of metastatic lymph nodes and survival [4], see also Figs 4.2 & 13.8. Internal mammary node involvement is an important early site of spread of medially placed tumours. Indeed, such tumours are often considered unsuitable for mastectomy. The finding of supraclavicular lymphadenopathy at diagnosis is a particularly adverse clinical sign.

Recent observations relating to the natural history of breast cancer using evidence from screening programmes has suggested firstly, that breast cancer does indeed behave as a progressive disease; secondly, that time of diagnosis is extremely important in determining outcome; and thirdly, that local treatment can sometimes be totally effective for small tumours whose detection time has been advanced by screening [5].

CLINICAL FEATURES

Most women with breast cancer present to their family practitioner with a lump in the breast, although screen-detected cases are now becoming more important since the widespread adoption throughout Europe and the United States of mass population screening (see below). Most breast lumps are benign and the commonest causes are cysts, fibroadenomas or areas of fibroadenosis. Although a skilled surgeon can often give a correct clinical diagnosis, all breast lumps should be regarded as potentially malignant and firm histological diagnosis is nearly always necessary.

Not all women with breast cancer present with a lump; pain in the breast, discharge or bleeding from the nipple, and pain or swelling in the axilla are also occasionally encountered.

Signs which indicate that a breast lump is likely to be malignant include: an asymptomatic impalpable but radiologically typical lesion, with microcalcification and an opacity with radiating fibrous strands; a change within the breast noticed by the patient herself; or the signs of locally advanced or metastatic disease. These include a large mass, tethering to skin and/or chest wall, axillary or supraclavicular lymph node enlargement, *peau d'orange*, nipple inversion and skin infiltration. Although cancers are typically firm or indurated, this may also be true of a simple cyst. Although women are now presenting more often with relatively early disease, the lump is sometimes deliberately ignored, and can even be present for years before the patient finally presents with a fungating mass of tumour, although this has now fortunately become less common. Alternatively, the patient may present with symptoms from a secondary deposit, for example in the spine or brain. The symptoms may include pain in the back, due to vertebral metastasis leading to vertebral collapse and/or spinal cord compression (see p. 154). Focal neurological signs and raised intracranial pressure are frequent findings in patients with cerebral metastases. General symptoms such as lassitude and anorexia may reflect advanced and widespread disease, particularly liver involvement.

CONFIRMING THE DIAGNOSIS

There are several methods of confirming the diagnosis. Aspiration of cysts is easy and frequently performed. The finding of a cyst with typical greenish fluid and disappearance of the lump after aspiration makes the diagnosis of cancer extremely unlikely. Aspiration cytology from solid lesions is now established as a useful and accurate technique. If there is real doubt, a much larger piece of tissue can be obtained by drill biopsy with a 'Tru-cut' or other percutaneous biopsy needle, which usually yields an adequate core of tissue. If the diagnosis has not been obtained in this way, excision biopsy will be necessary. Most surgeons now feel that it is unjustifiable to proceed to mastectomy without giving their patients an opportunity to consider both the implications of the diagnosis and the alternative approaches for primary control of the tumour.

Mammography, either using conventional X-rays or xeroradiographic techniques, is widely and increasingly used in diagnosis. Although not entirely reliable, carcinomas have a characteristic mammographic appearance, with fine calcification and areas of irregularity; fixation of deep lesions either to chest wall or skin can sometimes be seen. The permissible radiation dose for a mammogram has now been reduced to a mean glandular dose of 3 milliGy (maximum) (the equivalent of 10 standard chest X-rays). There is no longer any need to compromise the exposure time for an individual examination for fear of radiation exposure. Moreover, radiation exposure is generally lower still. In our own hospital, for example, the average exposure dose for a single examination using state-of-the-art equipment is only 0.8 milliGy. Mammography is particularly valuable to exclude synchronous primary cancers within the breast, a finding which would of course have considerable bearing on the choice of operation.

Pre-operative investigation

Before the primary treatment can be properly planned, a number of screening procedures are usually performed in order to ensure that no patient with obvious metastatic disease is needlessly subjected to a major operation. A good deal of controversy has surrounded the question of which investigations are helpful in influencing management. In some centres patients are extensively investigated with isotope bone, liver and brain scans, together with skeletal X-rays, tumour marker analyses and estimations of urinary hydroxyproline. However, the general view at present is that the most valuable tests are a chest X-ray, full blood count, simple assessment of liver function and abdominal (hepatic) ultrasonography. The contribution of isotope bone scanning is not entirely clear, since false-positives are sometimes encountered as a result of previous trauma, arthritis and other conditions. However, this is a valuable investigation occasionally revealing widespread but asymptomatic bony metastases. In the absence of neurological symptoms or signs, isotope and CT brain scanning have a very low diagnostic yield. In short, staging is only important if it defines 'early' breast cancer, distinguishing it clearly from advanced cases which are most unlikely to be surgically curable. Increased scepticism regarding the role of routine staging investigations has led to a reduction in their use.

Staging notation

There have been a number of attempts to devise a simple staging system to describe the degree of advancement of the tumour. Most of these classifications depend on the size of the primary tumour, the presence or absence of axillary node metastases by palpation (and subsequently at operation), and the presence of distant metastases. The Manchester classification (Table 13.1) was successful to the extent that it classified patients into three groups which could be shown to have significantly

Table 13.1 Staging systems in breast cancer

Stage	Description
Manchester staging system	
Stage I	Breast alone involved ± overlying skin
Stage II	Breast as for Stage 1 and axillary nodes involved, but mobile
Stage III	Skin invaded, fixed or ulcerated, or tumour fixed to underlying muscle or pectoral fascia
Stage IV	Fixed axillary lymphadenopathy, supraclavicular involvement and/or distant metastases
TNM staging notation for breast cancer	
T_1*	Tumour less than 2 cm in diameter
T_2*	Tumour 2–5 cm in diameter
T_3*	Tumour >5 cm
T_4	Tumour of any size with direct extension to chest wall or skin
N_0	No palpable node involvement
N_1	Mobile ipsilateral nodes
N_2	Fixed ipsilateral nodes
N_3	Supraclavicular or infraclavicular nodes or oedema of arm
M_0	No distant metastases
M_1	Distant metastases

* T_1, T_2 and T_3 tumours further divide into (a) no fixation and (b) with fixation to underlying pectoral fascia or muscle.

different prognoses. However, this classification is proving increasingly limited because more detailed information has now been obtained concerning the prognostic importance of variables such as the size of the primary tumour and the number of involved axillary lymph nodes (see p. 270). The TNM staging system proposed by the IUCC has become widely accepted for classifying tumours more precisely (Table 13.1). Further modifications are likely, in order to take account of more detailed information regarding the pathological grade of the tumour, and its endocrine receptor status.

Hormone receptors in breast cancer

It is now well recognized that a proportion of breast cancers carry cellular receptors for oestrogen and other steroid hormones (including progestogen) both in their cell nuclei and also the cytoplasm [6,7]. These receptors are present in 65% of cancers in postmenopausal women but only 30% of those premenopausal. Hormone dependence of some breast cancers can be demonstrated clinically by alteration of the hormonal environment (see p. 263). It is now established that the presence of an oestrogen receptor (ER) in a breast cancer cell correlates with the probability of hormone dependence in an individual tumour, making it possible to predict response to hormonal treatments. This has considerable clinical implications. Oophorectomy, for example, can be avoided in patients who are known not to have an ER +ve tumour.

It is not entirely clear whether ER status is the reflection of a genuine and fundamental difference between 'negative' and 'positive' breast cancers or whether there is a continuous distribution from ER-rich tumours to those with no detectable ERs whatever. The evidence at present favours the latter view, and ER 'positivity' is normally used to describe tumours in which the level of ER is greater than a certain defined figure, usually 5 fmol/mg cytoplasmic protein, or 25 fmol/mg nuclear DNA (see Chapter 6).

It seems that ER positivity is associated with well-differentiated tumours (particularly tubular, lobular or papillary types) and with microscopic elastosis in the tumour. Clinically it is apparent that slow-growing tumours tend to be ER +ve. Both primary tumours and metastases show similar ER content, though ER −ve metastases are sometimes encountered from an ER +ve primary tumour. The reverse is rarely true.

How successful have ER measurements been in the prediction of hormone responsiveness? It is now clear that at most 5–7% of ER −ve tumours will respond to hormone manipulation. Conversely, 55% of ER +ve tumours will respond, so ER positivity, although useful, is not entirely reliable. There is, however, a detectable semi-quantitative response; tumours very rich in ERs are clinically hormone dependent in

90% of cases. A probable explanation for the failure of ER +ve tumours to respond to hormone manipulation lies in the observation that the receptor, although present, may not induce a change in cellular growth or metabolism. One result of ER activity is an increase in concentration of progesterone receptors (PR) within the cell. For this reason tumours rich in PRs are usually clinically hormone responsive (more than 80% of cases).

Screening for breast cancer

The general principles of cancer screening are discussed in Chapter 2. At first sight, breast cancer would appear to be an ideal tumour for a screening programme. Firstly, it is relatively common (1–2 cases per 1000 women per year) and secondly, it is relatively accessible to clinical examination by doctors, nurses, paramedical staff and by the patient herself. In addition, mammography often demonstrates a breast cancer before it is clinically evident. Furthermore, there are known groups of patients at relatively high risk: those with a strong family history of breast cancer, those with late first pregnancies or with a history of benign breast disease.

However, unselected mass clinical and mammographic screening has not yet been unequivocally justified by the results. Apart from the substantial cost, it is not clear if the cure rate would be appreciably higher as a result of the earlier detection although several studies have suggested an impressive reduction in mortality in patients over 50 years [8], presumably resulting from detection of the cancer at an earlier stage. However, even low-dose mammography may not be entirely safe if repeated frequently, although the radiation dose of this investigation has fallen sharply in recent years (see above).

Screening of selected high-risk patients may, however, be more worthwhile. In the United Kingdom, the recent Forrest Report recommended regular screening of all women between the ages of 50 and 64 years, since this is the highest risk age group, in line with the results from the Malmö and other studies [9,10] which suggested a possible benefit only for women over the age of 50 years. Taking all age groups together, the overall results so far are not entirely encouraging. The value of screening appears particularly dubious in young women, who, even in the Malmö study, had an overall worse survival than the unscreened group — perhaps due to a more rapid cancer growth rate in the younger patient coupled with a sense of false security between routine scanning appointments. Breast self-examination, though widely practised, cheap and easily repeated, does not appear beneficial.

Several studies have now confirmed an increased rate of mammographic detection of early cancers [5] with a probable survival advantage over unscreened cases, though the false-positive rate is considerable and the anxiety produced is distressing. When a screening programme begins, about 20 (prevalent) cases are detected per 1000 women. When these 'screened' women are followed up, the new (incident) cases are about 2 per 1000 per year; the cost of incident screen-detected cases is therefore between £10 000 and £25 000, and the cost of each life saved as a result of screening is perhaps 2–5 times this figure. Breast screening is clearly not a panacea although it may prove justifiable for certain defined groups. The effectiveness of these programmes depends heavily on the population uptake, and may be more clear-cut in a compliant, well-motivated group than for instance an inner-city population who in any event might be harder to reach because of their much greater mobility. Several important questions relating to screening techniques, interval and management of intraduct non-invasive lesions have yet to be answered.

MANAGEMENT OF THE PRIMARY TUMOUR IN 'EARLY' BREAST CANCER

Surgical operations for breast cancer

In the past — and to some extent, even now — a

good deal of controversy surrounded the choice of operation in patients with 'early' breast cancer. It is worth remembering that the principle of surgery in breast cancer is 'adequate control of locoregional disease'. The classical operation of radical mastectomy, introduced by Halsted over 80 years ago, was designed to ensure local control by removing the breast and, as far as possible, all of the primary lymphatic routes of spread. This might have been a logical approach at a time when lymphatic spread was thought to be of critical importance and dissemination via the bloodstream largely unrecognized, but it is far less justifiable now.

There is no doubt that very good results, in terms of freedom from local recurrence, are achieved by mastectomy even in patients with axillary node involvement. In such patients the additional use of postoperative radiotherapy will reduce the local recurrence rate still further but only by a small degree and at the cost of a much increased risk of arm swelling (lymphoedema). This disabling and often untreatable complication of treatment, which is due to lymphatic and venous obstruction, is much less frequent with simple mastectomy, or when postoperative radiotherapy is withheld.

With increased understanding that patients with breast cancer die not from uncontrolled local disease but from distant blood-borne metastases, there has been an increasing tendency to offer less mutilating procedures than the now out-moded radical operation. In the United States and Western Europe, conservative breast-preserving procedures are increasingly employed and regarded as the treatment of choice (see below) but simple mastectomy with axillary dissection is still required in about 20% of cases — a dramatic difference even from 10 years ago. Patients who are best treated by mastectomy include those with large tumours (especially in a small breast), retroareolar tumours, widespread intraduct carcinoma, and patients with multiple lesions within the same breast. Surgical reconstruction of the breast has advanced considerably over the past 10 years

and there are a variety of techniques now available. The most commonly used are silicone prostheses and myocutaneous flap reconstruction. Many women find that the improved contour is valuable and helps their confidence and self-image. However, the cosmetic result can be mediocre by comparison with the best results from radiotherapy and reconstruction of the nipple is not generally performed, which is a further drawback. There is no doubt that myocutaneous flap reconstruction is the most successful surgical method, but it is a far more lengthy procedure than simple insertion of a silicone prosthesis.

Combinations of surgery and radiotherapy (Table 13.2)

Following treatment by surgery alone, local recurrence of disease in the chest wall, ipsilateral regional lymph nodes or residual breast occurs with a frequency of 7–30%. It is more common with large tumours (above 5 cm) and with axillary node involvement. In patients with disease of an equivalent stage it is considerably less common after radical mastectomy than after simple mastectomy, although the radical operation is performed only rarely nowadays, at least in the United Kingdom. However, postoperative radiotherapy greatly reduces the frequency of local recurrence, particularly in patients with axillary node-positive disease [11].

Unfortunately, most comparative studies have shown no *survival* benefit from the routine

Table 13.2 5-year survival rates in operable breast cancer

Operation	5-year survival rate (%)
Extended mastectomy (Urban)	67
Radical mastectomy (Halsted)	69
Total mastectomy (Patey)	67
Simple mastectomy and radiotherapy (McWhirter)	66
Radical radiotherapy with local excision of tumour (Calle)	74

use of radiotherapy in axillary node-positive cases. These trials have generally been retrospective or uncontrolled. The most important exception is the large Cancer Research Campaign King's/Cambridge study which compared simple mastectomy with simple mastectomy plus local irradiation in patients with early breast cancer who were prospectively randomized to receive one of the two treatment alternatives [12]. This study now has more than 10 years follow-up and the clear result is that local recurrence is indeed reduced by radiotherapy (from 30% to 11% at 10 years) but that survival is unchanged, at least up to 10 years from initial treatment (Fig. 13.3). In some studies, a slight reduction is survival has been encountered in the irradiated group [13] because of an excess of non-cancer deaths, chiefly cardiac in nature, in patients with left-sided tumours. This in turn is thought to be due to the direct radiation effect on the myocardium, with techniques employed in the series at that time (1960–70). Techniques have now substantially altered and greater emphasis is placed on glancing radiation fields which are deliberately positioned to avoid the heart.

This sort of study can of course be interpreted in a variety of ways. One extreme view would be that despite the improvement in local control, radiotherapy should not be routinely applied since survival is not improved and may even be slightly worse in the long term. This approach implies a considerable reliance on radiotherapy as a therapeutic procedure in patients who later develop local recurrence (of whom there would be a substantial number, approaching one-third of all women treated by simple mastectomy alone). The other view would be to advocate routine radiotherapy in all these cases on the grounds that local recurrence is unpleasant, largely preventable and may even be fatal in patients in whom radiotherapy for overt local recurrent disease is unable to deal effectively with the problem. Where simple mastectomy has been performed, it is usual practice to offer postoperative irradiation in the axillary node-positive group,

Fig. 13.3 Local recurrence and survival following simple mastectomy with or without irradiation. (A) The probability of local recurrence. Local recurrence is much more frequent in those not receiving radiotherapy (no RT); (B) the probability of survival. There is no difference between the two groups. (From Cancer Research Campaign Working Party. *Lancet* 1980; **ii**: 55. With permission.)

particularly in high-grade or large tumours where the risk of local recurrence is particularly high. However, the increasing use of adjuvant hormone therapy and chemotherapy may, by reducing the incidence of local recurrence, make postoperative irradiation unnecessary. This point remains unresolved.

Views on the desirability of routine postoperative radiotherapy have altered with changing surgical attitudes. Halsted radical mastectomy, with formal axillary clearance, yielded a very low local recurrence rate, of the order of 4%. However, fewer and fewer surgeons now practise these radical procedures, and in this country the commonest operation is now the simple mastectomy with partial axillary clearance, in which there is no attempt at radical axillary dissection. The proportion of patients referred for radiotherapy is therefore rising, since such an operation cannot be expected to yield the low local recurrence rates achieved in former years by radical mastectomy. Indeed it is the increased confidence that irradiation can produce sterilization of local disease which has led to the greater acceptance of less radical surgical procedures [14].

Techniques of postoperative irradiation vary widely. For example, some authorities omit regional node irradiation entirely (unless there is histological evidence of axillary disease), treating only the chest wall. An example of a field arrangement with dose distribution is shown in Fig. 13.4.

A number of prospectively randomized studies have compared mastectomy with a lesser surgical procedure, usually followed by routine postoperative radiotherapy (Fig. 13.5). In the first, patients at Guy's Hospital, London, were prospectively randomized either to undergo radical mastectomy with postoperative radiotherapy or to wide local excision with radiotherapy to the same dose. This study was widely discussed after its publication in 1972 but was flawed by the over-cautious dose of radiotherapy. The findings from this study, of a clear superiority for mastectomy in patients with axillary node-positive disease, have been negated by later work from Milan [15] and more recently the National Surgical Adjuvant Breast Project (NSABP) in the United States [11]. In the Milan study, patients with small cancers of the upper outer quadrant and no evidence of disease in the axilla were randomized either to radical mastectomy alone or 'quadrantectomy', in which the affected quadrant of the breast is excised, leading to a cosmetically acceptable but far from perfect result. Full axillary dissection and local irradiation were performed in all cases, and after 15 years of follow-up there

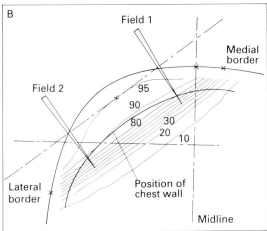

Fig. 13.4 Postoperative irradiation following mastectomy. (A) Use of two wedged fields tangentially applied to irradiate chest wall, axilla and internal mammary nodes. Field 3 irradiates the supraclavicular and lower cervical nodes using a directly applied radiation beam. Many other field arrangements are in common use; (B) transverse view showing isodose distribution from the two tangential fields (1 and 2) in relation to the breast and the chest wall.

have been no major differences in survival or local control. The major treatment-related difference has been a much lower incidence of lymphoedema in the group treated more conservatively.

It has become increasingly apparent that even this form of wide local excision is unnecessary

Fig. 13.5 Survival according to surgical treatment by radical mastectomy or wide local excision. Both groups received postoperative irradiation to a modest dose. These data (from Guy's Hospital, London) suggest that in Stage I disease there is no advantage for radical surgery but that for Stage II disease local treatment may influence survival. However, the results in Stage II disease treated by radical surgery were much better than in most other series.

in the majority of cases. The initial impetus towards minimal surgical excision with breast preservation came from Keynes in London and later, Baclesse in Paris and Crile in the United States. Subsequently, large series from Calle

(Institut Curie, Paris) and others have lent strong support to the safety and effectiveness of these approaches. In Calle's series [16] of over 1000 cases the results of 5 and 10 years are certainly within the range achieved by more traditional surgical approaches, and only the minority of patients in this series later required surgical resection for local recurrence. About half of the patients in the group requiring mastectomy subsequently proved to be long survivors (5 years or more), suggesting that local recurrence following 'adequate' initial treatment may not necessarily be accompanied by widespread metastases. There is, however, considerable difficulty in assessment of the breast, particularly where a high radiation dose has been given to a large volume. A number of patients, subjected to mastectomy for what was judged to be local recurrence, proved not to have disease on histological examination. The presumed recurrence (usually a palpable mass) may be no more than radiation-induced fibrosis of the breast. Other groups rely not only on excision biopsy and external beam irradiation but also on interstitial implantation using ^{192}Ir wires treating the tumour bed to a high radiation dose (Fig. 13.6).

An important American study on the role

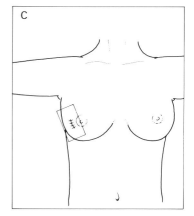

Fig. 13.6 Combined external and interstitial irradiation (Pierquin) for patients undergoing local excision or biopsy alone. (A) Treatment of breast, chest wall and local lymph nodes using ^{60}Co to 45 Gy; (B) boost with electrons to upper internal mammary chain and axilla, to additional 24 Gy; (C) ^{192}Ir — wire implant to tumour bed (25–27 Gy). Comparable results can probably be achieved using external irradiation alone. (From Pierquin *et al*. With permission.)

of breast-conserving primary treatment was initially reported in 1985, and later updated [10,17]. These data, from the NSABP, have given strong support for the concept of breast preservation. Over 1800 patients were randomized to undergo treatment either with simple mastectomy alone, or local excision ('lumpectomy') with or without postoperative radiotherapy. All patients underwent full axillary node dissection and those with node-positive disease were given adjuvant chemotherapy. Five-year disease-free survival after local excision plus radiotherapy was better than with simple mastectomy. Furthermore, overall survival with local excision was if anything also slightly better. Ninety-eight per cent of patients with node-positive disease, treated by local excision, axillary dissection, radiotherapy and adjuvant chemotherapy remained free of local recurrence, compared with 64% of patients not treated with radiotherapy.

The conventional approach for management of early breast cancer has rapidly altered over the past 5 years, in favour of these more conservative treatments. The results from France, the United States and elsewhere suggest that the cosmetic result of radical irradiation of the breast is highly satisfactory in the majority of cases, and is unlikely to be equalled by surgical implant techniques. Now that the psychological and sexual implications of mastectomy are beginning to be understood [18], it is likely that the demand for radiotherapy as an alternative to mastectomy will rapidly increase, although it is also clear that patients treated with local excision and radiotherapy do still face major psychological problems, at least in some cases [19].

The question of whether mastectomy should still be preferred to local excision with postoperative radiotherapy has increasingly been answered both by the changing preferences of surgeons and also by the patients themselves. Long-term follow-up is still essential, especially since features have already emerged which might, in the individual case, argue against local excision with preservation of the breast, rather than mastectomy. These include large primary size, inadequate excision with positive margins, high *in situ* component and high tumour grade.

Adjuvant hormone and cytotoxic therapy are discussed on p. 268.

MANAGEMENT OF THE PRIMARY TUMOUR IN ADVANCED BREAST CANCER

For patients with locally advanced disease (T_3, T_4 and the majority of patients with N_{1B} or N_2 disease) the results of mastectomy have been disappointing. Surgery is contraindicated apart from debulking operations (often referred to as 'toilet' mastectomy) which can be extremely valuable in conjunction with radiotherapy, chemotherapy and hormone treatment in order to give the patient the best possible chance of local control. Such surgical procedures are particularly helpful in patients who present with fungating bulky exophytic cancers.

Radiotherapy is now generally preferred as the major form of treatment. When given cautiously, a high dose can often be safely achieved, with a local control rate as high as 90% at 5 years, although the overall survival in such patients is only 20–25%. The probability of local control is inversely related to the size of the primary tumour [16]; other features such as fixation to the chest wall, fixed axillary lymphadenopathy or involvement of supraclavicular lymph nodes all contribute to inoperability and a higher probability of local recurrence. For radiotherapy to be successful a high local dose is essential. In one recent retrospective series, treatment to a dose of 60 Gy or more resulted in a local control rate of 78% whereas a lower dose achieved local control in under 40%, the addition of chemotherapy reducing the local recurrence rate still further.

In many cases, particularly with elderly patients, radiotherapy can be withheld and the patient treated initially with tamoxifen. This agent can produce remarkable responses even in patients with advanced fungating local disease, and it is usually clear by 6 weeks after starting treatment whether or not it is likely to be successful. In younger women, treatment with chemotherapy may yield even more rapid responses, and even elderly patients should be considered for chemotherapy if other methods are inadequate, since tolerance in this age-group can be surprisingly good, provided great care is given to treatment with anti-emetics and other supportive measures.

Complications of local treatment

SWELLING OF THE ARM

This complication (sometimes called lymph-oedema) is due to lymphatic and venous obstruction. It is a frequent (about 10%) and troublesome sequel to treatment for breast cancer, particularly likely to occur when both radical surgery and radiotherapy have been used, and less common after more conservative procedures. Other factors which contribute to its development include infection and recurrent or persistent disease. If lymphoedema appears years after primary treatment, axillary recurrence of tumour is the likely explanation. Apart from the disfigurement, the swelling can be very uncomfortable, and can also be a focus for spreading subcutaneous infection (cellulitis).

The management of the swollen arm is difficult and often unsuccessful. The patient should be instructed in isometric exercises with the arm elevated, in an attempt to improve the muscle pump. Avoidance of infection is essential, and the patient must take care not to damage the skin of the affected arm, and to wear gloves for tasks such as gardening. Cellulitis must be treated promptly with antibiotics. If a local recurrence of tumour is confirmed it is usually better treated with systemic treatment rather than further radiotherapy, in order to avoid additional radiation damage. Compression sleeves are sometimes helpful in massaging fluid out of the limb but they often need to be used for several hours to be effective. Nocturnal elevation of the arm (for example by

a roller towel arrangement or by resting on pillows) is often recommended if the patient can tolerate it.

STIFF OR FROZEN SHOULDER

Patients undergoing mastectomy should be given a programme of graded exercises post-operatively. These will increase shoulder mobility, prevent stiffness and help to prevent lymphoedema. The movements should begin 3 or 4 days after operation and increase in degree as the wound heals. The aim is to develop normal elevation and rotation in the shoulder joint. Abduction and elevation of the arm are most important. If a frozen shoulder has developed, physiotherapy and short-wave diathermy are helpful.

RESTORING A NORMAL BREAST CONTOUR

Most women adapt well to an external prosthesis. For those who do not, breast reconstruction or an internal implant should be considered. It is often helpful to reassure patients who are about to undergo mastectomy that early breast reconstruction is feasible, and regarded by the surgeon as part of the primary treatment, if the patient so wishes.

PSYCHOLOGICAL DISTURBANCE

Any form of mastectomy is mutilating, especially radical mastectomy. The incidence of depression and psychosexual disorders is about 25% during the first year [14]. These problems are more severe in women who place particular emphasis on their body-image, and this risk constitutes a relative contraindication to mastectomy. Patients can be helped by pre- and postoperative counselling, and the role of patient support and counselling groups is discussed in Chapter 7. Although patients undergoing treatment without losing the breast clearly suffer a range of psychological disturbances, these seem to be different from those encountered in patients who have required mastectomy [19]. Pre-operative counselling is likely to be helpful, and the most difficult period is generally the initial 6 months after primary treatment.

TREATMENT OF METASTATIC DISEASE

In most patients with apparently localized breast cancer it is probable that the disease is in fact systemic or generalized at presentation and that metastatic disease will inevitably develop. This view is supported both by the common occurrence of widespread metastases, often many years after mastectomy has been undertaken, and also by long-term studies of cohorts of patients with breast cancer followed up for periods of 25 years or more (Fig. 13.7). In the classic study by Brinkley and Haybittle, the overall survival was only 20% after 25 years [20]. Even in women deemed suitable for mastectomy (i.e. the 'early' operable group), the survival was only 30%. The clinical appearance of widespread metastases usually results in the

patient's death within 3 years, though many women who respond to treatment live longer. The likelihood of dissemination is strongly linked to the presence or absence of histologically positive axillary lymph nodes at the time of operation, and a quantitative relationship between the number of positive axillary lymph nodes and the probability of metastatic disease has been established (see p. 270).

Hormonal manipulation in breast cancer
(See Chapter 6)

Following the first therapeutic oophorectomy by Beatson in 1896 [21], it has become clear that about one-third of all patients with advanced breast cancer obtain symptomatic benefit from hormonal manipulation. A wide variety of procedures has been used, including oophorectomy, ovarian irradiation (sometimes referred to as 'artificial menopause'), treatment with oestrogens, anti-oestrogens, LHRH antagonists e.g. goserelin, anabolic steroids, glucocorticoids and progesterones, surgical treatment by adrenalectomy or hypophysectomy and 'medical adrenalectomy' with the aromatase inhibitor aminoglutethimide.

The conventional approach is largely based on the menstrual status of the patient. In most premenopausal and perimenopausal patients, surgical or radiation-induced ovarian ablation was traditionally employed for metastatic disease, but the advent of LHRH antagonists has led to these approaches being far less frequently employed nowadays since these agents provide adequate reduction of circulating oestrogen and render most patients hormonally postmenopausal within 2 months of first administration. Goserelin is given monthly by intramuscular injection.

In postmenopausal patients, treatment with additional oestrogen was often recommended, although more recently, tamoxifen, which probably acts as an anti-oestrogen, but perhaps has directly cytotoxic activity as well, has been increasingly preferred because of the relative lack of side-effects and in particular its freedom

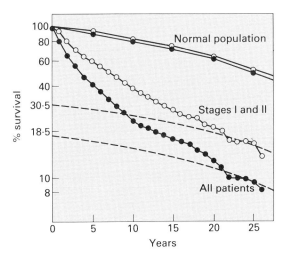

Fig. 13.7 25-year survival of patients with breast cancer. Dashed lines are an extrapolation parallel to the normal population to indicate proportion 'cured' at 25 years. (From Brinkley & Haybittle [20]. With permission.)

from severe cardiovascular and thrombotic complications. The response rate for post-menopausal patients is as good as that obtained with conventional oestrogen therapy, and the dose is 20 mg daily by mouth. The drug is slowly cumulative, and side-effects, although very uncommon, include flushing, nausea, hypercalcaemia, a disease 'flare', thrombocytopenia, fluid retention and menstrual disturbances. Most patients gain a pound or two in weight whilst taking tamoxifen, and some notice changes in the quality of their skin, hair or nails. Interestingly, there is increasing evidence of tamoxifen response in ER −ve patients, raising the possibility that part of the activity of tamoxifen may be independent of its hormonal pathway.

Until recently it was not possible to predict with confidence which patients with metastatic disease were likely to respond to hormonal manipulation. However, it is now clear that patients with ER +ve tumours are very much more likely to demonstrate a significant response to hormonal manipulation [6]; patients with ER −ve tumours rarely respond. This test can be used as a means of identifying patients who are likely to benefit from such treatment. However, the ER status is often unknown at the time when the patient presents with metastases and a trial of hormone treatment is then made without this information. Patients who are ER +ve probably have a different natural history from those who are ER −ve with a longer disease-free interval and overall survival [7]. The fact that 35% of women whose tumours are ER +ve do not respond to hormone therapy may in part be due to a blockage of the pathway of activation induced by oestrogen despite the tumour retaining the ER protein. For this reason attempts are being made to relate response to manifestation of ER *activity*. One such marker is the progesterone receptor (PR) whose synthesis is enhanced by oestrogen activity. Simultaneous measurements of ER and PR appear to give a better determination of the likelihood of response to hormone manipulation than measurement of ER alone

(Table 13.3). PR positivity is also correlated with a longer disease-free interval.

The site of metastatic disease may well influence responsiveness to hormonal treatment. A particular advantage with hormone manipulation is that patients with bony metastases are relatively likely to respond, although the ultimate outcome for such patients is poor, with a mean survival time from confirmation of bone metastases, of only about 12−15 months. None the less, some patients with bone metastases from breast cancer do survive very much longer than this period provided they are sufficiently hormone responsive.

It is unwise to be dogmatic in making recommendations for the correct sequence of hormonal therapies in patients with recurrent disease. In general, most premenopausal patients are treated either by LHRH therapy (goserelin is often preferred) or by radiation-induced menopause in the first instance, whereas postmenopausal patients are more usually treated with tamoxifen if they have not already received it as adjuvant therapy (see below). In each case 30% of patients can be expected to respond, and the exogenous hormone should be continued indefinitely whilst the patient's response persists. Further hormone therapy should generally be reserved for patients who responded to the initial hormonal procedure. Oophorectomy and adrenalectomy are nowadays hardly ever performed, the latter in particular having been supplanted by the aromatase inhibitor aminoglutethimide. This drug, which blocks the formation of oestrogen precursors in the adrenal, and their conversion to oestrogen in peripheral tissues (p. 114), appears to produce responses as frequently as surgical adrenal-

Table 13.3 Response to endocrine therapy

Receptor status	Response (%)
ER −ve PR −ve	10
ER −ve PR +ve	40
ER +ve PR −ve	35
ER +ve PR +ve	70

ectomy. Apart from skin rash, nausea and occasional generalized weakness, it is usually well tolerated, although lethargy, dizziness and other side-effects have also been reported. The chemical adrenalectomy may be enhanced by the additional use of glucocorticoid replacement which depresses ACTH output. Glucocorticoids are also medically necessary because of the adrenal suppression caused by aminoglutethimide, although low doses (without additional glucocorticoids) have also been shown to be effective. A common initial dose regimen is aminoglutethimide 250 mg 2–4 times a day with cortisone acetate 37.5 mg per day. Aminoglutethimide is best employed in postmenopausal patients since suppression of oestrogen production in premenopausal women is only partial. Other more specific aromatase inhibitors are becoming available, although the first (lentaron) is poorly absorbed by mouth and requires fortnightly intramuscular injection.

When relapse occurs following these initial measures, other useful agents include anabolic steroids, progestogens and glucocorticoids. Anabolic steroids are more effective in postmenopausal women and seem to be particularly helpful for bone metastases. Twenty per cent of untreated patients will respond but side-effects of virilization can be troublesome. A convenient preparation is nandrolone decanoate (Deca-Durabolin) 50–100 mg given intramuscularly every 3–4 weeks. Progestational agents can be used if there has been a previous hormone response. The most commonly used drug is medroxyprogesterone acetate (MPA, Provera) which is often given at a dose at 100 mg three times daily by mouth, although higher parenteral doses are also sometimes employed. Recent reports suggest that higher doses may be more effective though excessive weight gain may limit the tolerability of this approach. Another frequently used progesterone, megestrol acetate (Megace), is probably equally effective as MPA.

The use of aminoglutethimide has led to a reduction in the number of patients undergoing surgical adrenalectomy, and there are no longer any indications for this major procedure. Hypophysectomy, however, is a much easier operation for the patient and can easily be carried out by the trans-sphenoidal route. It is sometimes of benefit for relief of bone pain in patients who have become refractory to medical hormonal manipulation. Used selectively, it can be extremely effective.

The question of whether hormone manipulation should still be preferred to cytotoxic chemotherapeutic treatment of first relapse has been widely debated. Although in numerical terms, the choice lies between hormonal manipulation which has a 30% likelihood of response and combination chemotherapy with a response rate of double this figure, this is an over-simplification of what is in fact a very complex decision. Hormone-induced responses tend to be more durable and are usually accompanied by minimal toxicity to the patient. Chemotherapy-induced responses tend to be of shorter duration and are accompanied by a wide spectrum of physical and psychological difficulties. In Britain there is no doubt that most clinicians prefer to employ hormone manipulation first, and this approach is likely to be further refined when oestrogen receptor assay techniques become more widely available.

Chemotherapy

Chemotherapy in breast cancer has become established as one of the major therapeutic modalities. Although introduced much more recently than other treatments, chemotherapy has assumed increasing importance, particularly in the management of patients with metastatic disease.

A wide variety of drugs has been investigated, and responses have been documented to many classes of drug, including alkylating agents, antimetabolites, spindle poisons, antitumour antibiotics and several others (Table 13.4). It may be difficult to measure a tumour response with accuracy. However, the likelihood of objective tumour response coupled

Table 13.4 Responses to cytotoxic drugs in breast cancer

Drug	Approximate response rate (%)
Alkylating agents	
Melphalan	25
Cyclophosphamide	25
Anthracyclines	
Methotrexate	30
5-FU	20
Antitumour antibiotics	
Doxorubicin	40–50
Mitozantrone	30–40
Vinca alkaloids	
Vincristine ⎱	
Vindesine ⎰	20

with frequent improvement in subjective well-being, make these agents well worth considering in the management of metastatic disease. In general, skin, lymph node, and soft tissue metastases respond more readily than deposits in the liver or lung, which in turn are more likely to respond than bony metastases. Previous responsiveness to hormone therapy does not appear to predict the probability of response to chemotherapy.

Following successes with combination chemotherapy in Hodgkin's disease and acute leukaemia, it is now increasingly common to employ cytotoxic drugs in combination in breast cancer, rather than as single agents. Early work using a five-drug regimen of vincristine, methotrexate, cyclophosphamide, prednisolone and 5-FU, suggested that very high response rates could be obtained, but greater experience showed that the response rate was nearer 50%. Since that time a variety of different combination regimens has been used and some of these are shown in Table 13.5.

The most effective combination of drugs is certainly not yet established but it seems likely that combinations of three or four drugs probably offer similar response rates, with more acceptable toxicity, than more complicated

Table 13.5 Responses to some combination chemotherapy regimens in advanced breast cancer

Regimens	Dose and route	Response rate %
CMF		
Cyclophosphamide	$100\,mg/m^2$ p.o. days 1–14	53
Methotrexate	$40\,mg/m^2$ i.v. days 1 + 8	
5-FU	$600\,mg/m^2$ i.v. days 1 + 8 (repeated every 28 days)	
VAP		
Vincristine	2 mg i.v. days 1 + 8	60
Doxorubicin	$40–50\,mg/m^2$ day 1	
Prednisolone	30 mg/day for 7 days (repeated every 21 days)	
AC		
Cyclophosphamide	$1\,g/m^2$ i.v. day 1	60
Doxorubicin	$40\,mg/m^2$ i.v. day 1 (repeated every 21 days)	
M–M–M		
Melphalan	10 mg p.o./day for 3 days	65
Methotrexate	50 mg i.v. bolus day 1 (every 21 days)	
Mitomycin-C	15 mg i.v. bolus (given every alternate course, i.e. every sixth week)	

combinations. Many of the newer combinations include doxorubicin, which is probably the most active single agent for breast cancer. Treatment with intermittent combination chemotherapy has how largely replaced low-dose continuous administration. As with most regimens it is imperative to perform a full blood count before each course of treatment. Toxicity is largely predictable, but is usually no worse than would be expected from the additive use of the single agents chosen. For CMF, for example, the major problems are nausea, stomatitis and cystitis, and for VAP the commonest side-effects are neuropathy and alopecia.

Despite impressive response rates, the expected lifespan for patients with metastatic breast cancer has changed little, if at all, as a result of the more widespread use of these drugs [22]. Although patients who respond live longer than patients who do not, and complete responders have a better prognosis than partial responders, the adverse effects in the non-responders must be weighed against these benefits. This may be one reason for the failure of combination chemotherapy to improve overall survival in patients with metastatic disease. Other reasons are that the responses are often short-lived (sometimes only a few months), and that the responses are perhaps more likely to be patients with an intrinsically better prognosis than non-responders. A central problem, as with so many areas of cancer chemotherapy, is to select those patients who are likely to respond well, and at the same time avoid overtreating patients who are unlikely to be helped. Chemotherapy responses are more likely to be achieved in patients who are fit, who have soft tissue rather than bone metastases, a small number of metastatic sites, and have received no previous chemotherapy. Oestrogen receptor status has little predictive value for chemotherapy response.

Treatment of special problems in metastatic disease

Radiotherapy is the treatment of choice for patients with painful bone metastases offering relief of symptoms in over three-quarters of all cases, although objective radiological evidence of recalcification is much less common. There is no evidence that the particular site of the bone metastasis influences the outcome of treatment though obviously some sites are particularly problematic, such as large cortical deposits in the femur or other weight-bearing bones. In such cases it is often useful to combine radiotherapy with internal orthopaedic fixation before a fracture occurs. Sternal metastases should be treated promptly since, if left untreated, the thoracic cage is unstable leading to a mid-dorsal vertebral fracture which can be life threatening.

Brain metastases are important in breast cancer since some 15% of all patients develop clinical evidence of spread to the brain. Radiotherapy is beneficial in approximately two-thirds of these cases, often with permanent control of symptoms until the patient's death. Spinal cord compression is also common, and its treatment is discussed in Chapter 8.

Pelvic irradiation to a relatively modest dose leads to complete and lasting amenorrhoea in premenopausal patients, and radiation-induced menopause has therefore been used as an alternative to oophorectomy — particularly in patients whose general condition makes surgery inappropriate. The probability of total amenorrhoea is dose dependent and fractionated treatment (12–15 Gy, 5 fractions over 1 week) is usually given. Radiation-induced menopause appears as successful as oophorectomy for relief of symptoms. Clinical problems from metastases at other sites, such as skin, lymph node, pelvic or painful hepatic deposits can often be alleviated by local radiotherapy even when systemic treatments have failed.

Following treatment by surgery alone, local recurrence of disease in the chest wall, ipsilateral regional lymph nodes or residual breast occurs with a frequency of 7–30%. It is more common with large tumours (above 5 cm) and when axillary nodes are involved. In patients with disease of an equivalent stage it is much less common after radical mastectomy than after simple mastectomy. However, postoperative radiotherapy greatly reduces the frequency of local recurrence (see p. 257).

When local recurrence does occur in previously unirradiated patients, radiotherapy is undoubtedly the treatment of choice. However, local recurrence often occurs in the context of systemic metastases, and if after investigation there is evidence of more widespread disease, a systemic treatment may be more appropriate. Even under these circumstances radiotherapy may be the best treatment for a troublesome local recurrence.

If postoperative radiotherapy has previously been given it may be difficult to give further treatment because of the radiation tolerance of local structures such as skin and lung. Treatment by electron beam irradiation can be helpful in this difficult situation.

ADJUVANT HORMONE AND CHEMOTHERAPY

Since patients with breast cancer often die from disseminated disease thought to result from undetectable micrometastases present at the time of initial treatment, increasing attention has been paid to the concept of adjuvant systemic therapy following mastectomy. The aim is to eradicate these deposits before they become clinically apparent. This approach is supported by animal data suggesting that small metastases are more chemosensitive than large tumour masses. A major misconception of the size of the likely difference in mortality with adjuvant hormone or chemotherapy, led to the design of trials which were 10–50 times too small to detect the genuine or probable difference with certainty. This problem, which is of enormous significance for cancer trials, is discussed in Chapter 2 and has been most clearly demonstrated by the overview studies in breast cancer [23,24].

Adjuvant hormone therapy

Following the demonstration that oophorectomy caused regression of advanced breast cancer, several studies of the effect of ovarian ablation as an adjuvant to mastectomy have been performed. Its effect in randomized comparisons has not been convincingly demonstrated but most of these studies were performed before ER status could be determined. In one large study [25] the combination of postoperative ovarian irradiation and oral low-dose prednisone produced in perimenopausal women a prolonged disease-free interval and increased survival time by comparison with mastectomy alone. However, the majority of women (i.e. those who were clearly pre- or postmenopausal) did not benefit. More recently, a large randomized study of adjuvant tamoxifen appears to have shown a prolonged disease-free interval (and possibly survival) in the treated group [26]. The large overview of all prospectively randomized studies [24] of tamoxifen (and adjuvant chemotherapy as well) has now shown unequivocally that there is a real long-term survival benefit in patients given tamoxifen for at least 2 years after initial treatment (Fig. 2.12). The benefit appears to apply to both node-negative and node-positive patients and clearly persists for up to 10 years following therapy. Unexpectedly, the benefit appears to be even greater at 10 than 5 years. There may also be additional benefits from the cholesterol-lowering effect of tamoxifen (with reduction in frequency of death from myocardial infarction) and from the significant protection it appears to produce against postmenopause bone loss [27]. Adjuvant tamoxifen therapy is clearly an important advance, particularly in view of the lack of toxicity of this form of treatment. Recent fears regarding the carcinogenic potential of tamoxifen on the uterine endometrium should not be exaggerated; the complication is extremely rare.

Adjuvant chemotherapy

The earliest study, that of Nissen-Meyer at the Oslo Cancer Institute [28], suggested that cyclophosphamide given immediately after surgery could improve survival at 10 years.

Both the unpredictable nature of breast cancer

and the need for lengthy follow-up have made early interpretation of more recent studies extremely difficult. The trial by Fisher and his colleagues [29] in which melphalan was the agent used has shown a modest improvement in disease-free survival in treated patients (compared with placebo) in premenopausal women only. There was a slight but insignificant improvement in overall survival at 5 years. Further studies from this and many other collaborative groups are in progress (Table 13.6).

Unfortunately several of the studies have been designed without an untreated control group, which will make future interpretation difficult. This situation has arisen because of an excess of enthusiasm aroused by the preliminary results of the studies of Fisher and of Bonadonna *et al.* [30]. The effect on *disease-free survival* in premenopausal women may partly be due to chemotherapy-induced ovarian failure [24].

It is now clear (again from worldwide data generated by the Early Breast Cancer Trialists Collaborative Group) that adjuvant chemotherapy does have a small but real impact on both disease-free survival and overall survival (Fig.

2.12) in node-positive premenopausal patients [24], particularly in women aged 30–40 years. As Peto has pointed out, small improvements in survival may be translated into thousands of lives saved in a condition such as breast cancer where the incidence is so high.

The possible role of adjuvant chemotherapy in node-negative patients has also been tested. In a series of randomized studies reported in 1989, the results demonstrated a clear-cut improvement in disease-free survival, but not so far in overall survival [32] — in contrast to current information for node-positive breast cancer. It seems very likely that within a few years, subgroups of node-negative patients with adverse features such as large or high-grade primary tumour size will increasingly be recognized as likely to benefit from adjuvant chemotherapy. It also seems likely that it will be possible to predict which patients are at higher risk of relapse. Adverse prognostic features include tumour size greater than 3 cm, poorly differentiated tumours, nuclear pleomorphism, hormone receptor negativity, high proliferation rate, and expression of *erb* B2 protein. Some groups already treat young breast

Table 13.6 Results of large-scale randomized prospective trials of adjuvant chemotherapy in operable breast cancer

Source	Drugs	Comments
Nissen-Meyer (1978) (Oslo)	Short course (6 days) cyclophosphamide versus control	Improved disease-free and actual survival (10%) at 10–15 years in pre- and postmenopausal groups
NSABP (1980) (National Surgical Adjuvant Breast Project)	Thiotepa versus control	10-year survival difference (not significant) in premenopausal women with 4 or more nodes
	Melphalan versus control	No survival difference at 5 years. Improved disease-free survival in premenopausal women
Bonadonna (1981) (Milan)	CMF versus control	4% increase in survival at 5 or more years in premenopausal women only
Rubens (1983) (Guy's)	Melphalan versus control	No survival difference
Cancer Research Campaign (1982)	Melphalan and methotrexate versus control	No survival difference at 5 years

cancer patients, diagnosed under the age of 35 years, with adjuvant chemotherapy regardless of node status or other features. More recently, the concept of 'neoadjuvant' therapy for breast cancer has started to be tested in a number of randomized control trials. In this approach, the chemotherapy is given as primary treatment, prior to surgery or radiotherapy. Although an interesting concept in breast cancer, it is clearly far too early to know whether such pre-operative treatment is likely to prove more effective than the conventional sequence of treatment.

The difficulty in assessment of early results of adjuvant therapy is discussed more fully in Chapter 2. The problem is particularly acute in breast cancer, in view of the lengthy follow-up required before firm conclusions can be drawn. It is still not easy to give an unqualified answer to the question, 'Is adjuvant chemotherapy of benefit to patients with early breast cancer?' The advantage is probably confined to sub-groups of patients, and may not be substantially greater than those obtained with adjuvant hormone therapy, generally a far less toxic form of treatment. The toxicity of combination chemotherapy can be considerable (although many patients have little difficulty), and this is clearly an area where a possible benefit must be weighed against the quality of the patient's life (see Chapter 7). Some large study groups, notably the Cancer Research Campaign in the United Kingdom, are currently testing the potential benefit of adjuvant hormone therapy in premenopausal patients, and it is still poss-ible that a benefit could emerge from such treatment which could rival the degree of advantage apparently conferred by adjuvant chemotherapy.

Until about 5 years ago, current practice in the United Kingdom did not generally favour the routine use of adjuvant chemotherapy, even in premenopausal patients with node-positive breast cancer. By contrast, in the United States, current recommendations have for many years included the use of adjuvant chemotherapy for Stage II disease. Adjuvant chemotherapy,

generally with six courses of CMF, has been widely employed in node-positive pre-menopausal patients. Tamoxifen is now rec-ommended for virtually all postmenopausal patients regardless of node status, with the possible exception of those with small (T_1) low-grade tumours. The duration of treatment re-mains uncertain although most specialists recommend at least 2 years of tamoxifen in post-menopausal patients. In the United Kingdom the Cancer Research Campaign is currently ad-dressing the question of how lengthy the tamo-xifen administration should continue, in a large randomized study comparing 2 versus 5 years.

PROGNOSIS OF BREAST CANCER

Very few studies have followed patients with breast cancer for prolonged periods, but there is general agreement that 5- and 10-year sur-vival rates do not give a true picture since relapses may occur well beyond this point (Fig. 13.7). There may even be a few additional deaths from relapse beyond 25 years. Prognosis is dependent on stage of tumour, size of the primary (Fig. 13.8) and tumour grade but prob-ably independent of the extent of initial surgery (see also Fig. 4.2). Axillary lymph node involve-ment is particularly important: of patients with Stage I disease ($T_{1-2}N_0$) 75% are alive at

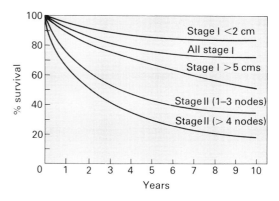

Fig. 13.8 Survival in Stages I and II operable breast cancer. In Stage I disease tumour size is an important prognostic determinant, as is degree of involvement of axillary nodes in Stage II.

10 years whereas with Stage II disease ($N_{1-3}M_0$) the 10-year survival is only 35%. The significance of the age of the patient at diagnosis is uncertain although breast cancer diagnosed during pregnancy has a particularly poor prognosis. Subsequent pregnancy in patients with breast cancer does not appear to have any adverse effect. It has also been suggested that personality factors may have a bearing on outcome [33]. Recent work with molecular markers has suggested that over-expansion of c-*erb*B-2 oncogene may prove to be a further valuable prognostic indicator [34].

Cancer of the male breast

Breast cancer in men is one hundred times less common than in women (Fig. 13.1). Little is known of the aetiology although a few family clusters have been reported, and it is possibly more common in patients who have had bilharzia with consequent liver damage and hyperoestrogenism. It has also been reported in patients with Kinefelter's syndrome, in which gonadotrophin levels are characteristically elevated, and in patients with gynaecomastia.

Most patients present with a tender indurated nipple, often with crusting or discharge, sometimes blood-stained. The disease involves the chest wall early. Routes of spread are similar to the disease in women, as is the pattern of metastasis. Most of the tumours are ER +ve.

Treatment is usually by mastectomy. Many surgeons prefer radical mastectomy because of the paucity of breast tissue in males and the possibility of early direct invasion, coupled with the lesser mutilation of this operation in men. Local irradiation should be given when axillary lymph nodes are involved.

For recurrent disease orchidectomy is generally considered the treatment of choice, with responses in 60% of cases. The value of other endocrine manoeuvres is uncertain but treatment with tamoxifen, progestogens, cyproterone or hypophysectomy have all been employed. There have been few trials of chemotherapy but it is often used when hormone treatments have failed and responses may be seen.

REFERENCES

1 McMahon B., Cole P., Brown J. Aetiology of human breast cancer: a review. *National Cancer Institute Journal* 1973; **50**: 21–42.

2 Gail M.H., Brinton L.A., Byar D.P. *et al*. Projecting individualised probabilities of developing breast cancer for white females who are being examined annually. *National Cancer Institute Journal* 1989; **81**: 1879–86.

3 WHO Collaborative Study of Neoplasia and Steroid Contraceptives. Breast cancer and depo-medroxy-progesterone acetate: a multinational study. *Lancet* 1991; **338**: 833–38.

4 Fisher E.R., Redmond C., Fisher B. Pathologic findings from the National Surgical Adjuvant Breast Project VI. Discriminants for 5-year treatment failure. *Cancer* 1980; **46**: 908–18.

5 Tabar L., Fagerberg G., Day N.E., Duffy S.W., Kitchin R.M. Breast cancer treatment and natural history: new insights from results of screening. *Lancet* 1992; **339**: 412–14.

6 McGuire W.L. Hormone receptors, their role in predicting prognosis and response to endocrine therapy. *Seminars in Oncology* 1978; **5**: 428–33.

7 DeSombre E.R. Breast cancer: hormone receptors, prognosis and therapy. In Furr B.J.A., ed. *Hormone Therapy. Clinics in Oncology*, **1**(1) 191. London: Saunders, 1982.

8 Collette D.J.A., Day N.E., Rombach J.J., de Waard F. Evaluation of screening for breast cancer in a non-randomized study (the Dom project) by means of a case-control study. *Lancet* 1984; **i**: 1224–26.

9 Tabar L., Fagerberg C.J.G., Gad A. *et al*. Reduction in mortality from breast cancer after mass screening with mammography. *Lancet* 1985; **i**: 829–32.

10 Anderson I., Aspegren K., Janzon L. *et al*. Mammographic screening and mortality from breast cancer: the Malmö mammographic screening trial. *British Medical Journal* **297**: 943–48.

11 Fisher B., Bauer M., Margolese R. *et al*. Five years' results of a randomized clinical trial comparing total mastectomy and segmental mastectomy with or without radiation in the treatment of breast cancer. *New England Journal of Medicine* 1985; **312**: 665–73.

12 Cancer Research Campaign (King's/Cambridge) Trial for early breast cancer. A detailed update at the tenth year. *Lancet* 1980; **i**: 1224.

13 Cuzick J. Overview of adjuvant radiotherapy for breast cancer. *Recent Results in Cancer Research* 1989; **115**: 220–25.

14 Tobias J.S. Radiotherapy and breast conservation.

British Journal of Radiology 1986; **59**: 653−66.

15 Veronesi U., Saccozzi R., Del Vecchio M. *et al.* Comparing radical mastectomy with quadrantectomy, axillary dissection and radiotherapy in patients with small cancers of the breast. *New England Journal of Medicine* 1981; **305**: 6−11.

16 Calle R., Pilleron J.P., Schlienger P., Vilcoq J.R. Conservative management of operable breast cancer. Ten years' experience at the Foundation Curie. *Cancer* 1978; **42**: 2045−53.

17 Fisher B., Redmond C., Poisson R. *et al.* Eight-year results of a randomized clinical trial comparing total mastectomy and lumpectomy with or without irradiation in the treatment of breast cancer. *New England Journal of Medicine* 1989; **320**: 491−96.

18 Macguire G.P., Lee E.G., Bevington D.J., Kuchemann C.S., Crabtree R.J., Cornell C.E. Psychiatric problems in the first year after mastectomy. *British Medical Journal* 1978; **i**: 963−65.

19 Fallowfield L.J., Baum M., Maguire G.P. Effects of breast conservation on psychological morbidity associated with diagnosis and treatment of early breast cancer. *British Medical Journal* 1986; **293**: 1331−34.

20 Brinkley D., Haybittle J.L. The curability of breast cancer. *Lancet* 1975; **ii**: 95−97.

21 Beatson G.T. On the treatment of inoperable cases of carcinoma of the mamma. Suggestions for a new method of treatment with illustrative cases. *Lancet* 1896; **ii**: 104−7.

22 Powles T.J., Coombes R.C., Smith I.E., Jones J.M., Ford H.T., Gazet J-C. Failure of chemotherapy to prolong survival in a group of patients with metastatic breast cancer. *Lancet* 1980; **i**: 580−82.

23 Early Breast Cancer Trialists Collaborative Group. Effects of adjuvant tamoxifen and cytotoxic therapy on mortality in early breast cancer. *New England Journal of Medicine* 1988; **319**: 1683−92.

24 Early Breast Cancer Trialists Collaborative Group. Systemic treatment of early breast cancer by hormonal, cytotoxic or immune therapy. *Lancet* 1992; **339**: 1−15 and 71−85.

25 Meakin J.W., Allt W.E.C., Belae F.A., Brown T.C.,

Bush R.S. *et al.* Ovarian irradiation and prednisone following surgery for carcinoma of the breast. In Salmon S.E. & Jones S.E., eds. *Adjuvant Therapy of Cancer*, pp. 95−99. Oxford: North−Holland Publishing Company, 1977.

26 Baum M., Brinkley D.M., Dossett J.A., McPherson K., Patterson J.R., Rubens R.D. *et al.* Improved survival amongst patients treated with adjuvant tamoxifen after mastectomy for early breast cancer. *Lancet* 1983; **ii**: 450.

27 Powles T.J. The case for clinical trials of tamoxifen for prevention of breast cancer. *Lancet* 1992; **340**: 1145−47.

28 Nissen-Meyer R., Kjellgren K., Malmio K. *et al.* Surgical adjuvant chemotherapy. Results with one short course with cyclophosphamide after mastectomy for breast cancer. *Cancer* 1978; **41**: 2088−98.

29 Fisher B., Redmond C., Fisher E.R. and participating NSABP investigators. The contribution of recent NSABP clinical trials of primary breast cancer therapy to an understanding of tumour biology — an overview of findings. *Cancer* 1980; **46**: 1009−45.

30 Bonadonna G., Brusamolino M., Valagussa P. *et al.* Combination chemotherapy as an adjuvant treatment in operable breast cancer. *New England Journal of Medicine* 1976; **294**: 405−10.

31 Howell A., Bush H., George W.D. *et al.* Controlled trial of adjuvant chemotherapy with cyclophosphamide, methotrexate and 5-fluorouracil for breast cancer. *Lancet* 1984; **ii**: 307−11.

32 The Ludwig Breast Cancer Study Group. Prolonged disease-free survival after one course of perioperative adjuvant chemotherapy for node-negative breast cancer. *New England Journal of Medicine* 1989; **320**: 491−96.

33 Dilman V.M. Psychophysiological factors and the progress of breast cancer. In Stoll B.A., ed. *Systemic control of breast cancer*, p. 124. London: Heinemann, 1981.

34 Muss H.B., Thor A.D., Berry D.A. *et al.* C-*erb*B-2 expression and response to adjuvant therapy in women with node-positive early breast cancer. *New England Journal of Medicine* 1994; **330**: 1260−6.

Chapter 14
Cancer of the Oesophagus
and Stomach

CARCINOMA OF THE OESOPHAGUS

Incidence and aetiology

Oesophageal cancer is commoner in males, with a male:female ratio of about 2:1 and a peak incidence in the age group 60−80 years (Fig. 14.1). In the United Kingdom it has become more prevalent in the last 10 years. In some Scandinavian countries, carcinoma of the oesophagus is as common in women as in men. There are marked geographical variations in incidence with very high levels near the Caspian Sea, Central Asia and Far East (Fig. 14.2). The incidence is becoming more common in the Transkei (South Africa) and the disease is more frequently diagnosed in France and Switzerland than in Britain. In the United States it is commoner in lower socio-economic groups and diagnosed three times as frequently in black people as in whites. Aetiological factors include cigarette smoking, excessive alcohol intake and malnutrition. Dietary differences, possibly including specific types of alcohol ingestion, are thought to play a role in the remarkable world variation. Repeated oral infection, development of benign oesophageal stricture or achalasia, and a history of syphilis, are also thought to be contributory. The Plummer−Vinson (Paterson−Kelly) syndrome of a congenital web in the upper oesophagus, with glossitis and iron deficiency anaemia, is a known predisposing factor, and is more common in women. There is a 7% incidence of oesophageal carcinoma in long-standing achalasia. The rare inherited disorder of tylosis

palmaris (see Chapter 3, Table 3.4) is also associated with oesophageal cancer. Barrett's oesophagus should be regarded as a potentially premalignant condition, particularly in patients with dysplasia. Surgical excision is now frequently recommended as a prophylactic measure in this condition.

Pathology

The oesophagus can be conveniently divided into three sections, the cervical oesophagus (distal limit 18 cm from upper incisors), mid third (distal limit 30−31 cm from incisors) and lower third (distal 10 cm of oesophagus). The most frequent sites for oesophageal cancer are the narrowed areas in the cricopharyngeal region, adjacent to the bifurcation of the trachea, and in the lowest part of the oesophagus near the sphincter. The lower third lesions are commonest (40−45%), followed by mid third (35−40%) and cervical oesophageal cancers (10−15%). Both squamous carcinomas and adenocarcinomas occur, the histology varying with the level in the oesophagus. Cervical oesophageal and upper third lesions are always squamous cell in origin. Though adenocarcinomas are very occasionally seen in the mid third and are increasingly common in the lower third, 'true' adenocarcinoma of the oesophagus probably accounts for no more than 2% of tumours, many of the lower oesophageal adenocarcinomas being gastric cancers. Recent evidence strongly supports the view that adenocarcinoma of the oesophagus is indeed rising in incidence [1]. By 1986 it accounted for 23.4% of oesophageal cancer compared with under

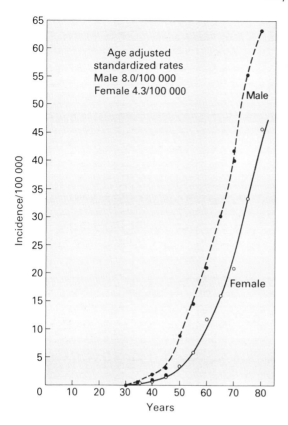

Fig. 14.1 Age-specific incidence of carcinoma of the oesophagus.

Fig. 14.2 Geographical distribution of oesophageal cancer. The shaded area indicates the regions of high incidence. The high-risk belt stretches from the Caspian Sea across Mongolia and Northern China.

7% in 1962. During the same period there was also a rise in the rate of diagnosis of adenocarcinoma of the gastric cardia, against a background of decreasing incidence of gastric cancer at other sites. The 5-fold increase in adenocarcinoma of the oesophagus remains unexplained, the only known predisposing features being Barrett's oesophagus and duodenal ulcer. Other tumour types are very rare and include melanoma and leiomyosarcoma.

Tumour spread (Fig. 14.3) occurs chiefly by direct extension and by lymphatic metastases. Direct extension occurs early in this disease, with rapid invasion within the oesophagus, both in the craniocaudal direction and also circumferentially. Insidious submucosal spread is almost universal and carries important implications for treatment. Direct mediastinal

involvement occurs, usually later in the disease, by penetration of the muscular coat. The pattern of muscular involvement varies with the level of primary tumour. Fistulous connection to the trachea may occur.

Cancers of the upper or cervical oesophagus chiefly drain to the deep cervical nodes either directly or via paratracheal or retropharyngeal lymphatics. Mid and lower third lesions drain to the posterior mediastinal nodes and abdominal nodes, sometimes traversing the diaphragm. Haematogenous spread characteristically occurs later, though unexpected hepatic metastases may be encountered at laparotomy in cases thought to be suitable for radical surgery. The liver is much the commonest site of haematogenous spread, though bone, lung and brain deposits also occur.

Clinical features

Dysphagia is the commonest symptom, and is almost always accompanied by weight loss, often amounting to 10% or more of body weight. The dysphagia is more pronounced for solids than liquids, and patients have often

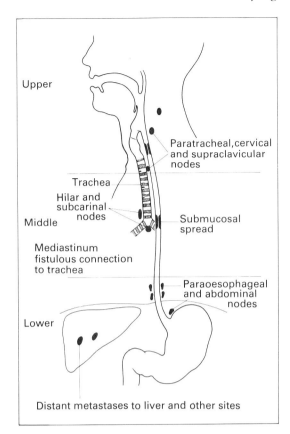

Fig. 14.3 Local and distant spread of oesophageal cancer.

recurrent laryngeal nerve may lead to hoarseness. Haematemesis and melaena are unusual.

On examination there may be no abnormality apart from evidence of recent weight loss and malnourishment. Occasionally, patients present with metastatic symptoms — usually from liver metastases — with only minimal dysphagia. Evidence of metastases may be found on examination with enlarged supraclavicular nodes or an enlarged liver.

Investigation and staging

Patients with dysphagia should be investigated with a barium swallow and meal. Characteristically, carcinoma of the oesophagus is accompanied by an obvious area of irregular narrowing well visualized by contrast radiography (Fig. 14.4). Unlike patients with achalasia of the cardia, there is usually rather minimal dilatation of the proximal oesophagus, presumably because little time has intervened for dilatation to take place. The narrowed segment may be surprisingly long and often there is an irregular 'shoulder' although this may be absent. Patients with severe dysphagia may be difficult to investigate because of the danger of aspiration of contrast material into the lungs. A chest X-ray is essential since paratracheal or other mediastinal node enlargement occurs commonly, and is an absolute contraindication to radical surgery. The chest X-ray may also demonstrate that the cause of the dysphagia is secondary mediastinal lymphadenopathy from a radiologically obvious but clinically silent carcinoma of the bronchus, or that intrapulmonary metastases have occurred.

Direct oesophagoscopy and biopsy are mandatory in all patients who are fit enough to undergo the procedure. At the same time the surgeon may also be able to dilate a malignant stricture or insert a prosthetic tube for palliation of the dysphagia. Oesophagoscopy and biopsy do, however, carry a small risk of oesophageal perforation, with mediastinitis and surgical emphysema which is usually fatal.

discovered for themselves that a soft or liquidized diet is the only means of securing a regular intake of food. Typically the dysphagia becomes more severe and some patients progress to complete dysphagia with inability even to swallow their own saliva, before seeking medical advice. Although many patients are able to point to the site at which the food lodges, a better guide to the level of obstruction is sometimes given by the interval between swallowing and the sensation of food sticking. In other patients, dyspepsia, regurgitation or acid reflux are more prominent clinical features. Pain is a late symptom of oesophageal cancer and is usually felt retrosternally. Spillover of oesophageal contents into the larynx or lung may cause cough, and involvement of the

Fig. 14.4 Barium swallow showing carcinoma of distal oesophagus. A long irregular stricture is shown.

STAGING

No satisfactory staging system has been developed, possibly because of the inaccessibility of this tumour and difficulty in assessing the regional node involvement. At least two-thirds of patients have lymphatic involvement at the time of diagnosis. The extent of the primary tumour may be impossible to determine even under direct vision and it may sometimes be difficult or dangerous to pass the endoscope so that the lower border may be inaccurately determined. CT scanning is extremely useful in demonstrating early mediastinal node involvement in patients with a normal chest X-ray. However, it suffers from the limitation that extramural involvement may be difficult to detect, even with modern equipment – a particularly important drawback in view of the proximity of the thoracic aorta and the surgical implications of inadequate staging. Another valuable technique is intraluminal endoscopic ultrasound, which gives additional internal anatomical detail.

Treatment

It is generally agreed that adenocarcinoma of the oesophagus (almost always lower third lesions) is best treated by surgery. In most other cases, particularly those of the upper third and cervical oesophagus, radiotherapy is probably the treatment of choice, though opinions differ [2]. Before embarking on local treatment, the surgeon or radiotherapist must be clear as to whether the philosophy of treatment is radical or palliative.

RADICAL TREATMENT

When radical treatment is contemplated in patients who are generally fit and with no evidence of distant disease, it is important to determine the extent of the lesion before definitive surgery is attempted. Exploratory laparotomy is often advocated in these cases, and is a routine part of many operations when reconstruction is to be achieved by colonic transposition, creating a viable conduit between pharynx and stomach. Radical removal of the oesophagus, first attempted over 100 years ago by Czerny, is nowadays usually performed as a single-stage procedure with oesophago-gastric anastomosis or colonic interposition. Formerly, operations were performed in which a permanent feeding gastrostomy was left as the means of providing nutrition.

Only a minority of patients with oesophageal cancer are suitable for radical surgery and the commonest indication is a mid or lower third lesion, particularly where the histology is adenocarcinoma, in a fit patient with no demonstrable evidence of metastases. There is no evidence that pre-operative radiotherapy influences resection rate, operative mortality rate or overall survival [3].

In patients with carcinoma of the *upper third of the oesophagus*, radiotherapy is usually considered to be the treatment of choice, though surgical treatment is preferred by some. No randomized comparison has been made. Radiotherapy has several advantages, including wider applicability (most patients are elderly and poorly nourished), avoidance of laryngectomy, significant palliation of dysphagia in most patients, with cure in 5–10% of patients who are able to tolerate high doses: 55–60 Gy (5500–6000 rad) in daily fractions over 5–6 weeks. In addition, surgical treatment by colonic interposition (Fig. 14.5) carries a mortality of about 10% and, unlike radiotherapy, is inappropriate in patients with locoregional spread of disease. Indeed, in a major review of world series, a 29% mortality rate was described, in patients treated during the 1970s [4,5]. Despite poor overall results, surgery has the advantage that palliation is often excellent and that it may sometimes be curative.

The upper third of the oesophagus is technically a difficult area to irradiate, because of the length of the treatment field coupled with the proximity of spinal cord. It is widely accepted that radiation fields should ideally extend for at least 5 cm above and below the known limits of disease, in order to treat adequately the presumed submucosal extension. Sophisticated planning techniques are often required, involving the use of twisted, wedged, oblique, multiple fields, often with compensators, and careful radiation planning at 2 or 3 levels so that a cylinder of tissue is irradiated to a uniform high dose without over-irradiation of the adjacent spinal cord (Fig. 14.6). A similar field arrangement is often employed in postcricoid carcinoma.

For tumours of the *mid third of the oesophagus*, surgery is more frequently performed, using mobilized stomach as the commonest means of reconstruction (Fig. 14.5). The operation is always extensive and carries a substantial mortality. Radiotherapy has been used as definitive treatment, or in combination with surgery; some surgeons feel that the operation is easier and the long-term results better when pre-operative irradiation is given. For pre-operative or radical radiotherapy of tumours of the mid third of the oesophagus, treatment is technically simpler than with tumours of the

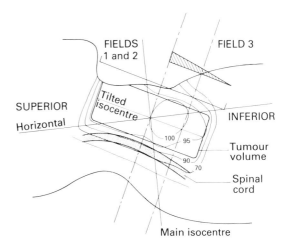

Fig. 14.5 Surgery for oesophageal cancer. (A) Colonic interposition following total oesophagectomy; (B) gastric mobilization and pull-through for carcinoma of the lower third.

Fig. 14.6 Radical radiotherapy for carcinoma of the cervical oesophagus. The irregular anatomy necessitates a complex multifield treatment plan.

upper third. A planned multifield approach will still be necessary in order to deliver a high dose to the tumour and local mediastinal lymph nodes, while at the same time avoiding over-dosage of the spinal cord. Recent studies of chemotherapy as an adjuvant to radiotherapy for these tumours have shown a possible modest benefit for combined treatment [6] but clearly need independent confirmation.

For cancer of the *lower third of the oesophagus*, surgery is preferable and reconstruction, usually employing mobilized stomach (Fig. 14.5), is less difficult. With cancer of the lower third of the oesophagus there is a risk that the stomach will be involved with tumour, making it unsuit-able for reconstruction. Radiotherapy can be useful for inoperable tumours.

At all sites, complications of treatment can be severe, both for radiotherapy and surgery. Radical radiotherapy is always accompanied by radiation oesophagitis, requiring measures such as oral administration of local anaesthetic with alkali or aspirin-containing suspensions to act locally on the oesophageal mucosa. Later com-plications include radiation damage to spinal cord (see Chapter 11) or lung, leading to radi-ation pneumonitis and occasionally dyspnoea, cough and reduction in respiratory capacity. Still commoner is the development of oeso-phageal fibrosis and scarring, which can lead to stricturing of the oesophagus which may re-quire regular dilatation to retain oesophageal patency.

Surgical complications include oesophageal stricture, and anastomotic leak, resulting in mediastinitis, pneumonitis and septicaemia which can be fatal.

PALLIATIVE TREATMENT [7]

Palliative treatment can be very valuable in oesophageal cancer. Palliation can be achieved either by passage of a Celestin or other indwel-ling prosthesis, by radiotherapy or laser treat-ment (or both), or by bypass surgery in which no attempt is made to resect the primary site, but an alternative conduit is created. Patients

unsuitable for radical surgery or radiotherapy should always be considered for palliative treat-ment, particularly if the dysphagia is severe. Modest doses of radiation can result in im-pressive clinical improvements. In experienced hands, passage of a Celestin endo-oesophageal tube is relatively safe and effective, and can be combined with radiation therapy. Common problems associated with tube insertion include migration of the tube, gastro-oesophageal reflux (sometimes associated with lung aspiration of gastric contents) and retrosternal pain or dis-comfort. Complications from palliative irradi-ation should be minimal since dosage is low: treatment to a dose of 30 Gy (3000 rad) in daily fractions over a 2-week period is usually bene-ficial, provided the dysphagia is not total, and high doses are rarely warranted.

In the past 5 years, laser therapy has assumed an increasingly important role [9] and can be used in conjunction with radiotherapy although long-term results are still awaited. It can restore swallowing capacity remarkably quickly, even sometimes after a single session, and is easily repeatable. For patients with unresectable tumours it may offer the best and least traumatic form of palliation.

An interesting addition to the use of laser therapy is the concept of photodynamic therapy (PDT) in which phthalocyamine derivatives are given to the patient prior to laser therapy, and taken up preferentially by the tumour thereby adding to the specificity of the treatment.

CHEMOTHERAPY

There is increasing interest in the use of chemo-therapy as an addition to radiation or surgery. Tumour regression occurs in 60% of cases using combinations which normally include cisplatin and 5-FU. It is still not clear whether this will improve survival, although a small trial has suggested it might [8].

Prognosis

Results of treatment for oesophageal cancer are

Table 14.1 Survival in oesophageal cancer*

Results of surgery
58% of all patients considered operable
39% of total were resectable
29% resection mortality
18% lived 1 year
9% lived 2 years
4% lived 5 years

Results of radiotherapy
51% of all patients offered palliative radiotherapy
18% lived 1 year
8% lived 2 years
6% lived 5 years

* Modified from Earlam [4,5]

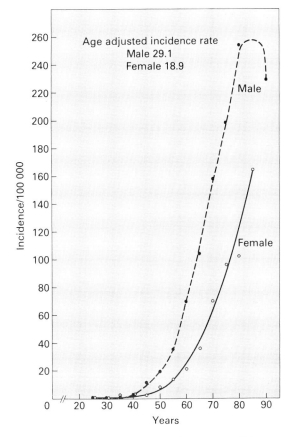

Fig. 14.7 Age-specific incidence of carcinoma of the stomach (England).

very poor (Table 14.1). In at least one series pre-operative irradiation followed by surgical resection appeared to improve the prognosis [10]. Although remarkable figures were claimed by Pearson, who treated 123 patients with radiotherapy alone, with a 19% 5-year survival rate, no other author has produced survival figures as good as this and, with the generally dismal survival statistics, there is an urgent need for careful comparison of current methods of treatment.

Earlam and colleagues have reviewed the results of treatment in 90 000 patients with carcinoma of the oesophagus and arrived at an overall 5-year survival rate of 6% for radiotherapy and 4% for surgery. However, the case selection for surgery and radiotherapy differs and the true advantage of radiotherapy may be greater, since, in general, fitter patients with more localized lesions are likely to have been treated surgically.

CARCINOMA OF THE STOMACH

Incidence and aetiology

Cancer of the stomach is declining in incidence but still remains an important cause of mortality. The age-specific incidence is shown in Fig. 14.7. The overall incidence in Britain is 29 per 100 000 for men and 19 per 100 000 for women. In the United Kingdom, as in the United States, there has been a gradual reduction of death rate in the last 20 years. In other countries the incidence is far higher, for example 80 per 100 000 in Japan and 70 per 100 000 in Chile (Fig. 14.8). Environmental causes are suggested by the fact that Japanese migrants to the United States show a reduction in incidence of the tumour but still retain a higher risk than the indigenous population. The likelihood of developing gastric cancer is also related to social class, the disease being twice as common in social classes 4 and 5 as in classes 1 and 2 (Fig. 14.9).

The causes of carcinoma of the stomach are unknown, but genetic, environmental, infective and premalignant factors have been implicated.

Fig. 14.8 Geographical incidence of stomach cancer. Figures indicate incidence per 100 000 male population. United States figures are for the white population only; rates are approximately double in the black population.

Gastric carcinoma is three to six times commoner in pernicious anaemia which is itself an inherited disorder. The cancer is slightly more common in persons who have blood group A than in the general population, and possibly in patients who have had a Polya partial gastrectomy. Patients with inherited hypogammaglobulinaemia have a greatly increased risk of gastric cancer. Many stomachs resected for gastric cancer show areas of metaplastic change where the stomach epithelium has been replaced by intestinal epithelium. This is associated with well-differentiated tumours and does not generally occur with poorly differentiated carcinomas. The cause of the intestinal metaplasia is not known but dietary factors are possibly important.

There appears to be an increased incidence of carcinoma of the stomach in patients with chronic atrophic gastritis. The increased risk in patients with pernicious anaemia and atrophic gastritis is approximately 3-fold, but gastric cancer is most common in the elderly population, many of whom show areas of atrophic gastritis in the absence of carcinoma. The association is therefore tenuous. Gastric atrophy may be followed by intestinal metaplasia and it has been postulated that dietary carcinogens might provoke this change. A hypothesis for the stepwise causation of gastric carcinoma is shown in Fig. 14.10.

In this process it is postulated that gastric atrophy leads to a rise in pH in the stomach and subsequent bacterial colonization which cannot occur at very low pH. The cause of the gastric atrophy is unknown, but it might be related to malnutrition in some countries where there is a high risk of gastric cancer. Bacterial colonization of the stomach is much more common below 50 years of age in these regions. Pernicious

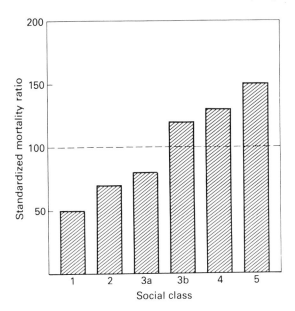

Fig. 14.9 Gastric cancer mortality related to social class. Figures are for men aged 15–64 for the years 1970–72 in England and Wales. (Figures from OPCS data, 1978). Values for each social class are in proportion to 100 which represents all social classes combined.

anaemia is accompanied by gastric atrophy, and hypoacidity may occur following Polya partial gastrectomy — both being situations where the risk of gastric cancer may be increased.

The result of bacterial colonization may be to reduce dietary nitrates (present in water, vegetables and cured meats) to nitrites, which in turn react with amino acids to form N-nitroso compounds. These are carcinogens in animals (causing intestinal metaplasia of the gastric mucosa in rats), and may be so in man.

The recently described association of gastric cancer with the *Helicobacter pylori* infection is exciting much interest [12,13]. The preventive implications of this association, if confirmed, are of great potential importance.

The association with gastric ulcer is uncertain. Much of the apparent association comes from a mistaken diagnosis of benign ulcer in an ulcerating neoplasm. In series where patients with benign gastric ulcer have been followed for several years the incidence of gastric carcinoma appears to be low, though possibly above that in the normal population. The relationship between gastric polyps and malignancy is also contentious. Gastric polyps are relatively common and 10% of them show evidence of carcimona *in situ*. This change has doubtful prognostic significance, and the lesion which seems most likely to be premalignant is the villous adenoma.

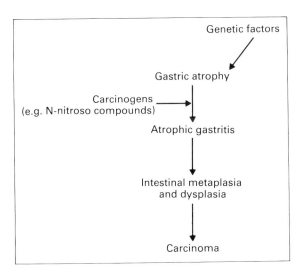

Fig. 14.10 A hypothesis for the causation of gastric cancer.

Pathology

Over 95% of gastric carcinomas are adenocarcinomas. Carcinoid tumours, squamous carcinoma, adenoacanthoma and leiomyosarcoma make up the rest. Early gastric cancer [14] is defined as a tumour confined to the mucosa and submucosa. Histological differentiation from 'precancerous' lesions can be difficult, even with gastric biopsy. The age and sex distribution is similar to advanced gastric cancer. Symptoms are minimal and the diagnosis is often made at endoscopy for screening (see below) or for an unrelated symptom. Macroscopically the lesion may be either elevated or excavated. The lesions are adenocarcinomas with features similar to those for advanced cancers.

The gross pathology takes on different forms. The commonest is a diffuse infiltrating carcinoma which varies in size from 1 cm to a tumour which may occupy most of the stomach. Typically, it has a rolled thickened edge and an ulcerated central portion, and invades the thickness of the stomach wall spreading into the pancreas and omentum. It metastasizes to regional lymph nodes, to the liver and peritoneal cavity. Some tumours exhibit a polypoid growth in which a large fungating tumour projects into the lumen of the stomach, initially growing inside but later invading the stomach wall and adjacent tissues. A less usual type of carcinoma is one which spreads superficially through the mucosa, which does not tend to involve regional lymph nodes until late in the disease and which has a better prognosis. Some cancers of the stomach exhibit a diffuse sclerosis involving the whole of the stomach wall (linitis plastica). The stomach is small and contracted and will not distend. This tumour has a very bad prognosis. Cancers tend to arise in the antrum or lower third of the stomach and are more common on the lesser curvature. Some of the tumours are multicentric. The location of the tumour appears to be changing with time, with an increase in proximal tumours and a decline in those in the antrum, both in the West and in Japan.

Microscopically the most useful division is made between those carcinomas where the cells resemble intestinal cells and there is intestinal metaplasia surrounding the tumour (intestinal type) and those which tend to infiltrate the gastric wall and are surrounded by normal mucosa (diffuse type). Tumours of the intestinal type are associated with a better survival, tend to occur in older patients and are more likely to be preceded by atrophic gastritis. In high-risk populations (such as Japan) most tumours are of this type. The diffuse carcinomas occur more frequently in women, are associated with blood group A, and have a worse overall survival. Infiltrative tumours of the linitis plastica type

are diffuse carcinomas. A recently described variant of gastric carcinoma is the parietal cell tumour which is associated with a better prognosis.

In Japan, screening programmes have resulted in many tumours being diagnosed early, and the term 'early gastric cancer' has been introduced for tumours limited to the mucosa or submucosa. These can be of the intestinal or diffuse types with varying degrees of differentiation. At this stage the prognosis is excellent.

Lymphatic spread of the tumour (Fig. 14.11) is via the superficial lymphatic networks into nodes in the left gastric chain and the splenic and hepatic chains along the lines of major vascular supply to the stomach. Spread is then to nodes in the coeliac plexus, the splenic chain and into the hepatic chain around the porta

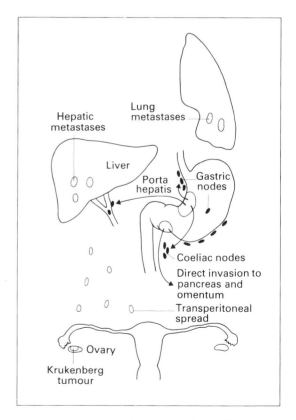

Fig. 14.11 Common paths of spread in gastric cancer.

hepatis. There is sometimes enlargement of nodes in the left supraclavicular region deep to the sternomastoid insertion (Virchow's node). Cancer of the stomach also spreads locally through the stomach wall into the omentum, liver and pancreas. Portions of tumour can break off and seed widely through the peritoneal space causing malignant ascites and Krukenberg tumours on the surface of the ovary. Blood-borne metastases are particularly common in the liver but pulmonary metastases also occur. Bone metastases are uncommon and central nervous system metastases are rare.

Clinical features

One of the great difficulties in diagnosis of carcinoma of the stomach lies in the fact that the initial symptoms are often mild and indefinite. Anorexia, nausea and vague upper abdominal pain are the most notable symptoms, but many patients are only diagnosed at a time when a large epigastric mass is palpable, or when there is malignant ascites making curative resection clearly impossible. Other symptoms include dysphagia, particularly when the tumour involves the cardio-oesophageal junction, and vomiting if there is outflow obstruction from involvement of the antrum. Massive gastro-intestinal bleeding does occur but is unusual. Low-grade bleeding is common and presentation with iron deficiency anaemia not infrequent. Non-metastatic manifestations of malignancy are unusual, but carcinoma of the stomach is one of the commoner causes of acanthosis nigricans (see Chapter 9).

The signs of carcinoma of the stomach are minimal except in the late stages. The patient will usually appear to have lost weight and may be anaemic. Virchow's node may be palpable in the left supraclavicular region and there may be an epigastric mass or hepatomegaly from metastases. Tumour masses may be felt on abdominal or pelvic examination and ascites may be present. All of these signs indicate advanced cancer which is inoperable and incurable.

Diagnosis

The standard diagnostic investigation has been the barium meal examination, and its accuracy has been greatly improved by double contrast techniques. Typically the malignant gastric ulcer shows elevated irregular borders with a poorly circumscribed ulcer crater (Fig. 14.12). In contrast a benign ulcer has sharply defined borders. The mucosal folds are abnormal being fused or tapered next to the carcinoma. Polypoid lesions have a coarse irregular mucosal surface. In antral lesions the resting volume of gastric juice may be large and in linitis plastica the stomach appears small and contracted. Infiltrating lesions give the stomach areas of rigidity which can be seen on screening during the examination. The difficulty with barium meal examination is that it is sometimes difficult to distinguish benign from malignant ulceration and that some small carcinomas are missed.

Endoscopy has led to a great improvement in accuracy of diagnosis. Since the introduction of this technique it has become apparent that 10–30% of carcinomas may be missed in their early stages on barium meal examination. For this reason, if the diagnosis is suspected in a patient with persistent anorexia and weight loss, endoscopy should be performed in addition to the barium meal. At endoscopy, cytological washings are taken and multiple biopsies from the ulcer or tumour. A positive biopsy or cytology is obtained in over 90% of patients, except in the infiltrative forms of gastric carcinoma where the diagnosis can be missed both on endoscopic appearance and on cytological examination. In addition to these investigations liver function tests, full blood count and chest X-ray should be carried out. CT scan may help to define nodal metastases, hepatic metastases and extent of local spread such as involvement of the lesser sac or liver. Hepatic ultrasound may be helpful in the detection of hepatic metastases. Serum tumour markers have not been helpful in gastric carcinomas. Carcinoembryonic antigen (CEA) is sometimes elevated but the relationship to

Fig. 14.12 Barium meal appearances in carcinoma of the stomach. (A) Carcinoma at cardio-oesophageal junction showing tumour infiltration with mucosal irregularity; (B) linitis plastica. The tumour infiltrates extensively (arrowed).

Table 14.2 TNM staging system for gastric carcinoma

T stage
T_1 Limited to mucosa or submucosa
T_2 Extension to serosa
T_3 Extension through serosa
T_4 Invasion of local structures

N stage
N_0 No nodes
N_1 Local node involvement within 3 cm
N_2 Node involvement more than 3 cm, but resectable
N_3 Distant node involvement

M stage
M_0 No metastases
M_1 Distant metastases

Stage grouping

Stage		
I	$T_1 \, N_0 \, M_0$	
II	$T_{2-3} \, N_0 \, M_0$	
III	$T_{1-3} \, N_{1-2} \, M_0$	
	$T_{4a} \, N_0 \, M_0$	
IV	$T_{1-3} \, N_3 \, M_0$	
	$T_{4a} \, N_{1-3} \, M_0$	
	M_1	

tumour mass is too indefinite to be helpful either in diagnosis or in monitoring therapy.

A TNM staging system has been developed and is shown in Table 14.2.

EARLY DIAGNOSIS OF GASTRIC CARCINOMA

Because so many patients present with inoperable disease, programmes have been devised to screen for the disease in countries such as Japan where there is a very high incidence. In Japan, screening with double contrast radiology in asymptomatic patients has led to a detection rate of only 1:1000. A high incidence (31%) of early carcinomas has been found with an excellent survival following surgery. It is not clear if early gastric cancer will always develop into advanced disease but it is reasonable to assume that this will usually occur. Prompt diagnosis is therefore desirable. Screening asymptomatic populations, especially in low-risk countries, has not proved cost-effective. Screening of patients with upper abdominal symptoms has been suggested as a compromise since 50% of cases of early gastric cancer diagnosed by screening had such symptoms. In countries such as the United Kingdom, such an approach is the only practical possibility in view of the declining incidence of the tumour. A recent study [15] has shown that gastric cancer is detected in 5% of such patients and 63% of these had early operable lesions. In addition 75% of all patients had an identifiable cause of dyspepsia (including other cancers), which adds to the value of endoscopy.

Treatment

TREATMENT OF GASTRIC CARCINOMA

Surgical resection is the only curative treatment for gastric carcinoma. A variety of surgical procedures can be performed, depending on the localization of the tumour and the degree of local extension. The most radical surgery involves total gastrectomy, with removal of the entire stomach, part of the duodenum and occasionally even part of the transverse colon if it is involved by local infiltration (Fig. 14.13). For most localized tumours a partial gastrectomy can be performed. At the present time some form of subtotal gastrectomy is the most generally employed surgical procedure. Total gastrectomy involves removal of the entire stomach, the greater omentum, usually removal of the spleen and occasionally of the lower portion of the oesophagus if the tumour is proximal. In a radical subtotal gastrectomy 80% of the stomach is removed with the omentum and part of the duodenum. The spleen is not usually removed unless the lesion is relatively proximal.

The morbidity of total gastrectomy is considerable. There is difficulty in maintaining body weight; it is necessary to eat small, frequent meals, and, if the patient survives, the inevitable production of iron and B_{12}-deficient anaemia requires life-long treatment.

Patients presenting with a large intra-

Fig. 14.13 Operations for gastric carcinoma. (A) Radical subtotal gastrectomy; (B) extended total gastrectomy.

abdominal mass are nearly always inoperable. Other indications of inoperability are malignant ascites, demonstrable nodal deposits or liver metastases. If the tumour is fixed and immobile on barium meal examination it is also likely to be inoperable. Often a decision about the operability can be made only at laparotomy. In inoperable cases bypass procedures are usually unrewarding.

The results of surgery are poor. In European studies only 60% of patients undergoing surgery prove to have resectable tumours. Of these only 20−25% will be alive at 5 years. This gives an overall 5-year survival rate of 10−15% in all operated cases. In Japan the results are much better, with a higher resectability rate

(70–75%). Of those resected 55% are alive at 5 years and the overall 5-year survival rate of all operated cases is about 30%. In Japanese studies 15% of cases have early gastric cancer compared with 2.5% in the West.

RADIATION TREATMENT

Palliation of some of the symptoms of gastric carcinoma can occasionally be achieved with radiation. Treatment is difficult since there are numerous radiosensitive organs in the upper abdomen, namely the small intestine, liver, spinal cord and kidneys. A dose of 40 Gy (4000 rad) can usually be administered safely in 4–5 weeks. Anorexia and nausea are frequent and patients usually lose weight during the procedure. The intention is palliative although occasional long-term survival has been noted.

CHEMOTHERAPY FOR
CANCER OF THE STOMACH [16]

Cancer of the stomach is the gastro-intestinal carcinoma which is most sensitive to cytotoxic drugs. In advanced gastric cancer some drugs are able to produce response rates of greater

Table 14.3 Response to cytotoxic agents in gastric carcinoma

Drug	Response rates (%)
Single agents	
Doxorubicin	15–25
5-FU	15–20
Mitomycin C	25–30
Nitrosoureas	5–15
Alkylating agents	10–15
Cisplatin	20
Combination chemotherapy	
5-FU, doxorubicin, mitomycin (FAM)	30
5-FU, nitrosourea, doxorubicin	25
5-FU, mitomycin, doxorubicin, nitrosourea	25
5-FU, doxorubicin, cisplatin	35–40
5-FU, doxorubicin, methotrexate	35–45

than 30% (Table 14.3). Most of these responses are partial and usually last for only a few months. There is no evidence that survival is prolonged by the use of chemotherapy either as single agents or in combination, even though responders will live longer than non-responders, as in most other tumours.

The single most effective agent appears to be doxorubicin and the usual dose is 60 mg/m^2 every 3 weeks. 5-Fluorouracil has been widely used but the response rate is relatively low. There has been extensive experience with mitomycin C in Japan, and some trials from that country have reported response rates of 40% though the more general experience has been that the response is less than this. Nitrosoureas and alkylating agents are less useful. Cisplatin is active but nausea and vomiting may be a problem.

In advanced gastric cancer several combination chemotherapy regimes have been used and some of these are shown in Table 14.3. One of the most widely used has been the combination of 5-FU, doxorubicin and mitomycin (FAM) with a response rate of about 40% [17]. There is no evidence that patients are ever cured by chemotherapy. Responses may be associated with palliation of symptoms as long as the toxicity of the regimen is not great.

It is possible that the effectiveness of chemotherapy may be improved by the administration as long-term intravenous infusion of 5-FU with the addition of cisplatin and/or epirubicin as brief infusions. Ambulatory infusion has been made practicable by battery and driven infusion pumps. Response rates are high and the toxicity appears acceptable. Excellent palliation is sometimes achieved.

Adjuvant chemotherapy

There has been recent interest in the use of chemotherapy as an adjuvant to surgical removal of the tumour. So far most studies have failed to show an improved survival in the chemotherapy treated group compared with surgery alone. At the present time, therefore, adjuvant chemotherapy is not offered routinely to patients undergoing gastrectomy. Further trials using more effective regimens (such as infusion chemotherapy) are now in progress.

REFERENCES

1 Powell J., McConkey C.C. Increasing incidence of adenocarcinoma of the gastric cardia and adjacent sites. *British Journal of Cancer* 1990; **62**: 440−43.

2 Bancewicz J. Cancer of the oesophagus: find a good surgeon. *British Medical Journal* 1990; **300**: 3−4.

3 Gignoux M., Roussel A., Paillot B. *et al.* The value of pre-operative radiotherapy in oesophageal cancer: results of a study by the EORTC. *Recent Results in Cancer Research* 1988; **110**: 1−13.

4 Earlam R., Cunha-Melo J.R. Oesophageal squamous cell carcinoma. I: A critical review of surgery. *British Journal of Surgery* 1980; **67**: 381−90.

5 Earlam R., Cunha-Melo J.R. Oesophageal squamous cell carcinoma. II: A critical review of radiotherapy. *British Journal of Surgery* 1980; **67**: 457−61.

6 Araújo C.M.M., Souhami L., Gil R.A., Carvalho R. *et al.* A randomized trial comparing radiation therapy versus concomitant radiation therapy and chemotherapy in carcinoma of the thoracic esophagus. *Cancer* 1991; **67**: 2258−61.

7 Bown S.G. Palliation of malignant dysphagia: surgery, radiotherapy, laser, intubation alone or in combination? *Gut* 1991; **32**: 841−44.

8 Herskovic A., Martz K., Al-Sarraf M. *et al.* Combined chemotherapy and radiotherapy compared with radiotherapy alone in patients with cancer of the esophagus. *New England Journal of Medicine* 1992; **326**: 1593−98.

9 Tobias J.S., Bown S.G. Palliation of malignant obstruction − use of lasers and radiotherapy in combination. *European Journal of Cancer* 1991; **27**: 1350−52.

10 Reed P.I. Changing pattern of oesophageal cancer. *Lancet* 1991; **338**: 178.

11 Pearson J.G. Radiotherapy of carcinoma of the oesophagus and post cricoid region in S.E. Scotland. *Clinical Radiology* 1966; **17**: 242−57.

12 Correa P. Is gastric carcinoma an infectious disease? *New England Journal of Medicine* 1991; **325**: 1170−71.

13 Parsonnet J., Friedman G.D., Vandersteen D.P. *et al.* Helicobacter pylori infection and the risk of gastric carcinoma. *New England Journal of Medicine* 1991; **325**: 1127−31.

14 Williams G.T. Early gastric cancer. In: Filipe M.I., Jass J.R., eds. *Gastric Carcinoma*. London: Churchill Livingstone, 1986: 172−96.

15 Hallisey M.T., Allum W.H., Jewkes A.J. *et al.* Early detection of gastric cancer. *British Medical Journal* 1990; **301**: 513−15.

16 Earl H.M., Coombes R.C., Schein P.S. Cytotoxic chemotherapy for cancer of the stomach. *Clinics in Oncology* 1984; **3**(2): 351.

17 MacDonald J.A., Schein P.S., Woolley P.V. *et al.* 5 Fluorouracil, mitomycin C and adriamycin (FAM): A new combination chemotherapy program for advanced gastric carcinoma. *Annals of Internal Medicine* 1980; **93**: 533−36.

Chapter 15
Cancer of the Liver, Biliary Tract and Pancreas

PRIMARY LIVER CANCER

There are four types of primary carcinoma which arise in the liver. The most frequent is hepatocellular carcinoma which, in Britain, is about 10 times more common than cholangiocarcinoma of the intrahepatic bile ducts which in turn is 10 times more frequent than angiosarcoma. Hepatoblastoma is a rare tumour of childhood. The importance of hepatocellular carcinoma is disproportionate to its incidence in the West, because there are now many clues about its aetiology and pathogenesis.

Hepatocellular carcinoma (hepatoma)

INCIDENCE

There are about 1 million cases a year worldwide. In Britain and the United States the incidence is approximately 1.8 per 100 000 for men and 0.7 for women (Fig. 15.1). The tumour can arise in childhood. Worldwide the incidence (per 100 000) varies greatly — 104 in Mozambique, 29 in South Africa, 12 in Nigeria.

AETIOLOGY

In the West, most cases of hepatocellular carcinoma arise in cirrhotic livers. When the disease arises in a non-cirrhotic liver the patient is usually younger than when there is associated cirrhosis. The causes of cirrhosis with the highest risk of developing a hepatoma are chronic hepatitis associated with hepatitis B, and haemochromatosis. Hepatoma is much more common in alcoholic cirrhosis where there

is evidence of previous hepatitis B infection, and is infrequent in patients who have not been infected. Patients with primary biliary cirrhosis and HBsAg −ve chronic active hepatitis are less at risk (although more likely to develop the cancer than the non-cirrhotic population). The carcinoma is much more likely to develop in men (M : F 11 : 1) and in patients with long-standing cirrhosis over the age of 50. The association with cirrhosis is found in both high and low incidence areas. The duration of the cirrhosis is more important than the aetiology. The risk of development of hepatocellular carcinoma in a cirrhotic liver after 20 years is about 5% in women and 20% in men. In studies in patients with well-compensated cirrhosis the yearly incidence rate is about 3−5% [1]. The tumour is more likely to develop in patients with persistently elevated levels of AFP. Few of these patients have operable tumours.

The geographical variations in incidence may reflect different causal factors. Cirrhosis from any cause is associated with hepatoma. In low incidence areas (Europe and North America) alcoholic cirrhosis is a more frequent association than in high incidence areas where macronodular cirrhosis associated with hepatitis B virus (HBV) is the main association. Hepatitis C is an RNA virus with a carrier rate of 0.2% in Northern Europe and 5% in the Far East. It is transmitted by parenteral inoculation, but sexual promiscuity does not seem to be as important as for hepatitis B. It appears to be an important co-factor in the development of hepatoma. Exposure to aflatoxin, derived from the *Aspergillus flavus* mould on stored grain, is

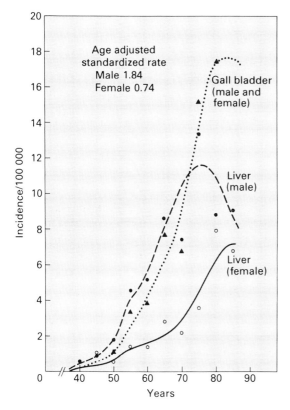

Fig. 15.1 Age-specific incidence of cancer of the liver and gall bladder (United Kingdom figures).

more frequent in areas of high incidence. The toxin may be one of the factors which act as tumour promoters.

Undoubtedly the strongest causal association is with HBV. In high incidence areas 80% of cases are associated with serological evidence of HBV with a risk of 230:1 in HBsAG +ve individuals [2]. In the West 15–20% are HBsAG +ve. Viral DNA sequences have been demonstrated in the genome of liver cells of HBsAG +ve individuals, in hepatoma cells, and hepatoma cell lines [3]. Even in cases where there is no serological evidence of infection, sensitive techniques such as the polymerase chain reaction can often demonstrate viral DNA [4]. Antibodies to hepatitis C are found in 60% of patients and this virus may be another co-factor in production of the tumour.

PATHOLOGY

In 60% of cases the liver contains multiple nodules of cancer. In 30% of cases there is a large single mass of cancer often with surrounding lesions, and, in the remaining cases, the liver is diffusely infiltrated. In 80% of cases the surrounding liver is cirrhotic. In the group of patients where it is not, the sex ratio is equal and the average age is lower. In a small subgroup of the patients without cirrhosis, the tumour forms cords with collagen strands (fibrolamellar carcinoma). In cholangiocarcinoma of the intrahepatic ducts the tumour cells form a tubular pattern usually with extensive fibrosis.

CLINICAL FEATURES

In a cirrhotic patient the development of hepatocellular carcinoma is often accompanied by a rapid deterioration in liver function. Usually the cirrhosis is advanced and long-standing. Presentation is, therefore, with liver failure, jaundice, right upper quadrant pain and ascites. Ascites may be due to cirrhosis, or to the sudden onset of the Budd–Chiari syndrome due to hepatic vein occlusion. In the non-cirrhotic patient the presentation is typically with abdominal pain and a right upper quadrant mass.

On examination the patient is usually gravely ill with evidence of cirrhosis and liver failure. The liver is enlarged with a palpable mass over which there may be a bruit. There may also be a moderate fever.

DIAGNOSIS

Liver function tests have no diagnostic pattern or value but are always abnormal. The tumour may produce erythropoietin and secondary polycythaemia may therefore be present. Hypercalcaemia may occur, in most cases due to bone metastases, but in other cases it is postulated that the tumour produces parathormone-like substances. Other non-metastatic manifestations include hypoglycaemia, gonadotrophin production, ectopic ACTH and elevated plasma calcitonin (see also Chapter 9).

The malignant hepatocytes in most hepatomas produce AFP which can be detected in the serum [4]. With sensitive methods the serum AFP can be of diagnostic help. Levels below 10 ng/ml make the diagnosis very unlikely in a cirrhotic patient, although over half of non-cirrhotic patients do not have an elevated serum AFP. Levels from 10—500 ng/ml make the diagnosis probable but cirrhosis due to chronic hepatitis may be associated with levels of this magnitude (as may metastases from the gastrointestinal tract). In the West, levels above 500 ng/ml in a cirrhotic patient make the diagnosis of hepatocellular carcinoma almost certain.

CT scan and ultrasound liver scans usually show a large lesion or multiple lesions, but in the presence of cirrhosis the appearances may not be diagnostic and care must be taken in interpretation. Angiography may show a tumour circulation but is usually only carried out if there is a possibility of surgical resection of the tumour or if intra-arterial chemotherapy or embolization is considered.

A biopsy of the lesion will help in diagnosis but may not be possible if liver function has deteriorated. If the prothrombin time is prolonged by more than 4 seconds, the procedure is unsafe since the tumours are vascular. Even with a biopsy, the histological distinction from metastatic tumours (such as hypernephroma) may be difficult.

TREATMENT

Resection of the tumour offers a chance of cure. It must be considered particularly in a non-cirrhotic patient because the liver will regenerate even if three-quarters of the organ is removed. In a cirrhotic patient resection will usually precipitate a deterioration of liver function. Resection is therefore applicable to less than 5% of patients.

Embolization or ligation of the hepatic artery has been used, but these procedures also cause deterioration of function in the cirrhotic patient.

Selective hepatic artery embolization may be attempted in a cirrhotic, if the tumour is localized. The value of this technique has not been adequately assessed, but pain may be relieved.

Chemotherapy may produce tumour regression, and the single most useful agent is doxorubicin (Table 15.1). This is usually given at 50—70 mg/m^2 every 3 weeks, but the dose should be halved if the bilirubin is twice normal since the drug is detoxified by the liver. The response to chemotherapy can be assessed by pain, AFP levels, and ultrasound or CT scan. As in gastric cancer, there is increasing interest in infusional intravenous chemotherapy. Intra-arterial treatment may produce considerable shrinkage but is more complex.

RADIOTHERAPY

The liver does not tolerate radiotherapy to high dose since radiation-induced hepatitis occurs with increasing frequency above 25—30 Gy. Fatal hepatic damage occurs when the dose to the whole liver is above 38 Gy. The value of radiotherapy in hepatoma is uncertain since for most patients the prognosis is poor. Regression of the tumour and relief of pain was reported in 50% of cases treated with a total dose of 30 Gy.

PROGNOSIS

When a hepatoma arises in a cirrhotic liver the prognosis is very poor, and 50% of all patients are dead in 3 months with no survivors at 12 months. Without cirrhosis only 10% will be alive at 2 years. The prognosis is better in

Table 15.1 Intravenous chemotherapy of hepatocellular carcinoma

Drug	Approximate response rate (%)
Doxorubicin	20
5-FU (bolus)	15
5-FU (infusional)	30
5-FU, doxorubicin	20

patients who have a complete surgical resection or who show a complete response to chemotherapy. Overall 5-year survival after surgical resection is 15%, although if the tumour is less than 3 cm the figure rises to 50%. These figures have suggested that the results might be improved if patients with cirrhosis are screened regularly with ultrasound and AFP measurement. The impact of such a policy on survival is not known.

Angiosarcoma

These malignant vascular tumours arise in normal livers. They are rare, but of interest since they are known to occur in workers who have had chronic exposure to polyvinylchloride (PVC). The tumours develop 15–20 years after exposure to PVC. They have also been reported in patients who received thorotrast (a radioactive contrast agent used diagnostically in 1930–50). The presentation is of a painful hepatic mass, and diagnosis is made by biopsy. Surgical resection may be possible.

A very rare, indolent, vascular tumour called epithelioid haemangioendothelioma may occur in the liver. Treatment is by local excision if possible.

Hepatoblastoma

This rare tumour occurs in childhood. The tumour is associated with anomalies such as hemihypertrophy, and with storage diseases and the Fanconi syndrome. The pathological features are of immature hepatic epithelial cells or a mixture of these cells with mesenchymal elements.

It usually arises in the right lobe and presents with a visible asymptomatic mass which later causes pain and weight loss. Like hepatocellular carcinoma (which can also occur in children over 5 years of age) the tumour produces AFP. It can be demonstrated by isotopic ultrasound and CT scanning but arteriography gives the best localization and is essential if resection is to be attempted.

The tissue diagnosis is usually made at operation when an attempt at resection is made. The chance of cure is greater if there is complete surgical excision. Up to 75% of the liver can be removed but haemorrhage can be severe and great skill is necessary.

Postoperative chemotherapy is usually given. Doxorubicin is the most effective agent but responses also occur with alkylating agents, 5-FU and cisplatin [5]. It is now clear that unresectable cases can be made to respond to chemotherapy so that surgery can be performed, and there is growing interest in pre-operative chemotherapy in this disease. Combinations of doxorubicin and cisplatin have increased response rates. Although in such a rare disease randomized trials are almost impossible, there is increasing evidence that chemotherapy is increasing the likelihood of surgical care. Serum AFP can be used to assess response.

CANCER OF THE GALL BLADDER AND BILIARY TRACT

Incidence and aetiology

Cancer of the gall bladder and biliary tract has an equal incidence in men and women, most cases occurring after the age of 65 (Fig. 15.1) when it is commoner than hepatocellular carcinoma. Gall-stones are a predisposing cause but the incidence of gall bladder cancer in patients with untreated cholelithiasis is probably not more than 2%, which does not justify surgery for asymptomatic gall-stones. Worldwide, liver flukes are the major predisposing cause (*Clonorchis sinensis*, *Opisthorchis felineus*). These flukes produce a chronic sclerosing cholangitis which appears to be premalignant. Bile duct cancer is also associated with ulcerative colitis, occurring in approximately 0.5% of cases [6].

Pathology

Carcinoma of the gall bladder, which is the commonest cancer of the biliary system, usually arises in the body and only rarely in the cystic duct (4% of cases). The tumours are usually adenocarcinomas (85%) but anaplastic (6%) and squamous (5%) histologies occur.

Half of all bile duct cancers develop in the distal common duct, with carcinoma of the ampulla of Vater being the second commonest biliary cancer. The cancers arise in the proximal duct in 30% of cases and proximal to the porta hepatis in a further 20%. They are almost always adenocarcinomas, usually well-differentiated and sometimes with a fibrous stroma.

All these tumours spread locally and to regional lymph nodes and there may be multiple primary bile duct tumours. From these nodes, lymphatic spread is to the coeliac and aortic nodes. Hepatic metastases are common. Gall bladder cancer may seed into the peritoneum and both types of cancer may directly invade the liver. Carcinoma of the ampulla is usually slow growing and causes obstructive jaundice early before it has spread widely. The tumour often ulcerates and sometimes bleeds and the jaundice may fluctuate if the tumour sloughs. This form of biliary tract cancer has the best prognosis.

Clinical features

Cancer of the gall bladder usually presents with right upper quadrant pain, later with nausea, vomiting, weight loss and obstructive jaundice. Because of pre-existing gall-stones the symptoms may be attributed to this cause at first and the diagnosis delayed.

Cancer of the biliary tree presents similarly but usually causes obstructive jaundice. At this stage the tumour is often advanced. The gall bladder may be enlarged and palpable if the distal duct is obstructed.

Diagnosis

The diagnosis of early gall bladder carcinoma is difficult because the symptoms suggest gall-stone disease. By the time a mass is palpable surgical resection may be impossible. A cholecystogram is often unhelpful, because the gall

bladder is non-functioning. Ultrasound and CT scan may show a mass, but in the majority of cases the diagnosis is only made at a laparotomy for presumed gall-stone disease. In carcinoma of the extrahepatic bile ducts, obstructive jaundice leads to investigation. Percutaneous transhepatic cholangiograms may give an outline of the proximal ducts, and endoscopic retrograde cholangiopancreatography (ERCP) may demonstrate the lower end of the block and provide material for cytological examination (Fig. 15.2), as well as permitting a stent to be inserted. The transhepatic route may also allow a catheter to be placed past the lesion with relief of jaundice either pre-operatively or as a palliative procedure.

Treatment

SURGERY

When a gall bladder carcinoma is found at laparotomy the surgeon must decide if it can be resected. The experience of the surgeon is an important factor in this decision. The results of simple cholecystectomy are not good since the tumour may be locally extensive. Portions of the liver may have to be removed for complete excision. Distant lymph node spread may have occurred and surgical excision deemed unwise, and a palliative procedure is then undertaken, if possible with biliary decompression.

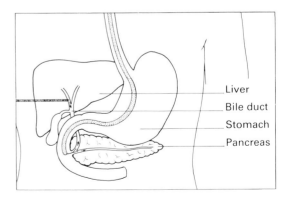

Fig. 15.2 Percutaneous cholangiography and ERCP.

In the surgical management of bile duct cancer it is of great value to have the extent of the tumour defined pre-operatively by radiographic means. Diffuse intraductal spread cannot be resected. Spread into the intrahepatic ducts, invasion of blood vessels and distant lymph nodes and peritoneal and hepatic metastases are also indications of unresectability. Microscopic examination of bile duct carcinomas often reveals intramural spread. In spite of formidable surgical difficulties, tumours at the junction of the right and left hepatic ducts can sometimes be removed as can mid and distal duct tumours, the latter by radical pancreaticoduodenectomy (Fig. 15.3).

In all, only 15% of bile duct cancers will

A Radical pancreaticoduodenectomy

B Total pancreatectomy

Fig. 15.3 Surgical operations for cancer of the bile ducts and pancreas.

be operable and major resections have a high mortality (10−15%). Palliative relief of obstruction may be obtained by bypass operation but internal bile duct drainage by non-surgical procedures is now becoming a preferred method of palliation. Carcinoma of the ampulla has the most favourable prognosis with a 5-year survival of 25−30% after radical pancreaticoduodenectomy.

RADIOTHERAPY

Many patients with biliary tract cancer have a localized but unresectable tumour. In these cases effective control can for a time be achieved with radiotherapy. The dose is usually 40−50 Gy in daily fractions, but the treatment details depend on the volume and site of the irradiation. Relief of pain and obstructive jaundice may be achieved.

CHEMOTHERAPY

There has been little systematic study of the role of chemotherapy in biliary tract cancer. Responses have been reported with 5-FU, mitomycin and doxorubicin, but are usually short-lived. Newer approaches include long-term infusion therapy using 5-FU as for cancer of the stomach (p. 286).

CANCER OF THE EXOCRINE PANCREAS

Incidence and aetiology

The incidence of carcinoma of the pancreas is slowly rising. At present it is 15 per 100 000 in men and 13 per 100 000 in women (Fig. 15.4). The condition has a high mortality, less than 1% of patients surviving 5 years. The disease is twice as common in diabetes mellitus. There is possibly an increased incidence in patients with calcific pancreatitis which is, in turn, associated with excess alcohol consumption.

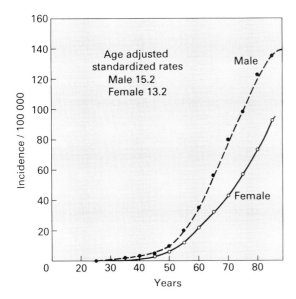

Fig. 15.4 Age-specific incidence of cancer of the exocrine pancreas (United Kingdom figures).

5% of the total. Sarcoma of the pancreas is a rare disease, usually occurring in childhood.

The exocrine pancreas has an extensive lymphatic drainage along blood vessels. Spread to local nodes has usually occurred by the time of presentation in tumours of both the body and tail.

The head of the pancreas is the site of the tumour in 65% of cases, body and tail in 30% and tail alone in 5%. Local spread occurs and accounts for many of the clinical features (Fig. 15.5). Tumours in the head spread into the duodenum, obstruct the bile duct, spread back into the retroperitoneal space and forward into the lesser sac and peritoneal cavity. The portal vein may be infiltrated and tumours of the body and tail may occlude the splenic vein and extend into the transverse colon and spleen. Metastatic spread to the peritoneum, liver and lung are frequent.

Pathology

The great majority of histologically verified tumours are adenocarcinomas (Table 15.2), though in many patients a histological diagnosis is never established. The adenocarcinomas are thought to arise from the ductular epithelium and those arising in large ducts tend to be more often mucin-producing than those originating in ductules. An intense fibrotic reaction often accompanies the tumour. Cystadenocarcinoma (1%) has a particularly good prognosis. Acinar cell tumours constitute

Table 15.2 Pancreatic tumours

Tumours of exocrine pancreas	
Adenocarcinoma	
Acinar cell tumour	
Sarcoma	

Tumours of endocrine pancreas	*Malignant (%)*
Islet cell tumours	20
Gastrinoma	70
Glucagonoma	60
VIPoma	90
Carcinoids	not known
Somatostatinoma	90

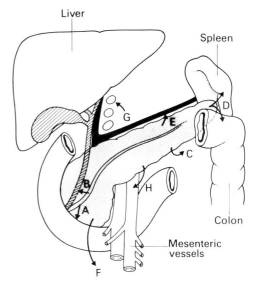

Fig. 15.5 Sites of spread and production of symptoms in adenocarcinoma of the pancreas. (A) To duodenum: pain, vomiting, obstruction; (B) to bile duct and pancreas: jaundice, pancreatitis; (C) to retroperitoneum: back pain; (D) to spleen and colon: left upper quadrant pain; (E) to portal and splenic vein: varices, splenomegaly, hepatic disorders; (F) to peritoneal cavity: ascites; (G) to lymph nodes: obstructive jaundice; (H) to blood stream: distant metastases.

Clinical features

Pain and weight loss are the most frequent symptoms [7]. With tumours of the head the pain is usually epigastric, and with the tail it may be in the left upper quadrant. The pain gradually becomes severe and unremitting, is often nocturnal and extends into the back as retroperitoneal structures are invaded. The patient may get relief by bending forwards. Acute exacerbations may be due to episodes of pancreatitis. Left-sided abdominal pain and altered bowel habit may be caused by infiltration of the colon by tumours of the body or tail. Mental depression is said to be common but it is not clear if this is more marked in pancreatic cancer than in other causes of serious illness. Acinar cell carcinoma may be accompanied by a syndrome of patchy inflammation and necrosis of subcutaneous fat with polyarthralgia and eosinophilia. There are high levels of lipase in serum. The syndrome resembles relapsing panniculitis (Weber–Christian disease). Another non-metastatic manifestation of pancreatic carcinoma is superficial migratory thrombophlebitis (see Chapter 9). Oesophageal varices may develop if the portal vein is occluded and may lead to gastrointestinal bleeding. Diabetes mellitus may be the presenting feature and carcinoma of the pancreas must be kept in mind in elderly patients developing glycosuria.

Obstructive jaundice is frequent and eventually occurs in 90% of patients with tumours of the head. It is usually progressive, although fluctuations may occur if the tumour sloughs. It is much less common in tumours of the body and tail. Fever may occur due to cholangitis. The gall bladder is not usually palpable — unlike a bile duct or ampullary carcinoma. Peritoneal dissemination leads to malignant ascites which is present in 15% of cases at diagnosis.

Investigation and diagnosis

It is difficult to diagnose early pancreatic carcinoma at the stage before obstruction of the bile duct or infiltration of the duodenum. It should be considered in any patient with unexplained continued upper abdominal pain. Barium examinations are usually helpful only when the tumour is large. There may be enlargement of the duodenal loop and displacement of the gastric antrum and posterior wall. The tumour may have infiltrated the duodenal and gastric mucosa and this may be seen as an abnormal pattern on the barium meal.

In recent years diagnosis of smaller tumours and tumours of the body and tail, has become somewhat easier with the use of ultrasound and CT scanning. Ultrasound examination of the pancreas is, however, a procedure requiring considerable experience on the part of the radiologist and false-negative results are not infrequent. CT scanning may show a pancreatic mass or extension of the pancreas into the fat space surrounding it and there may also be evidence of metastatic spread to adjacent nodes and the liver (Fig. 15.5). If a mass is found, fine-needle aspiration may give a cytological diagnosis. Selective coeliac and superior mesenteric artery angiograms may be of diagnostic value but are seldom performed since the advent of CT scanning.

When the disease presents with obstructive jaundice, transhepatic cholangiography [8] and ERCP will usually be performed (Fig. 15.2). The transhepatic approach will show the proximal site of obstruction and help to distinguish the tumour from carcinoma of the gall bladder, ampulla or bile ducts. ERCP may show stenosis of the main pancreatic duct or compression of the common bile duct by tumour. Specimens for cytology can be taken from the pancreatic duct. ERCP has a high diagnostic accuracy (75–85%), but early diagnosis, before biliary obstruction has occurred, remains the clinical problem because symptoms are often late or non-specific. Carcinoembryonic antigen (CEA) is present in the serum of most patients but is also found in other gastro-intestinal diseases and in acute pancreatitis. A pancreatic oncofetal antigen has been described, but, like CEA, is not specific for the disease.

Treatment

SURGERY

Radical surgical resection offers the only hope of cure. Radical pancreaticoduodenectomy and total pancreatectomy are formidable surgical procedures (Fig. 15.3). Preservation of part of the pancreas is desirable but there are considerable problems with fistula formation at the anastomotic site. Total pancreatectomy leads to major problems with diabetes and lack of exocrine function.

Few patients are suitable for surgery, because at the time of diagnosis there is often nodal or distant metastases or a large infiltrating mass which is clearly inoperable. Careful definition of the extent of the tumour pre-operatively is essential. In general only tumours involving the body or tail will prove to be operable. In operable cases the mortality is 15–20% and 5-year survival not greater than 15%.

If the tumour cannot be removed, the obstruction can be relieved by a biliary bypass procedure. This is usually performed surgically, but recently it has become possible to place catheters in the biliary tree by the percutaneous transhepatic route or via the ampulla of Vater.

RADIOTHERAPY [9]

Palliation, especially of pain, can be achieved by radiotherapy. With external beam irradiation the dose required is high (50–60 Gy). Some reports have suggested that a few patients may achieve long-term remission and occasionally cure. Interstitial radiation using ^{125}I implants has also been used, sometimes supplemented with external beam irradiation. Ultrasound and CT imaging are of great help in planning treatment.

CHEMOTHERAPY

Few cytotoxic drugs are effective in pancreatic cancer (Table 15.3). Responses occur with 5-FU, nitrosoureas, mitomycin C and alkylating agents.

Table 15.3 Chemotherapy of pancreatic cancer

	Approximate response rate (%)
Single agents	
5-FU	25
Alkylating agents	?20
Streptozotocin	25
Mitomycin	25
Doxorubicin	10
Nitrosoureas	10
Drug combinations	
5-FU, mitomycin, doxorubicin	40
5-FU, streptozotoxin, mitomycin	35
5-FU, BCNU	30

The criteria for response differ in the various studies and most responses are small in degree and short in duration. Combination chemotherapy has improved the response rate a little [10] but complete responses are rare and the patients are never cured. The toxicity of treatment makes chemotherapy unsuitable for the majority of patients because of ill health and advanced disease at presentation. Intravenous infusional chemotherapy is under investigation.

PALLIATIVE TREATMENT

Pain may be relieved by analgesics, but radiotherapy may be helpful in preventing the need for opiates for several months. Chemical block using alcohol into the coeliac plexus is difficult but sometimes very helpful in relieving pain. Percutaneous drainage of the biliary tree may relieve itching and steatorrhoea due to obstructive jaundice. Steroids may help improve appetite for a while.

CARCINOID TUMOURS

The curious name of these tumours was coined in 1907 to emphasize the benign course which they follow, although they are usually malignant or become so with time.

PATHOLOGY

Localized intestinal carcinoids are present in 0.5% of autopsies, usually near the appendix or along the small bowel or descending colon. There are, however, many other sites at which carcinoids may occur — bronchus, thymus, pancreas as well as any part of the gastro-intestinal tract, ovary and testis [11].

Appendiceal carcinoids are usually near the tip. The tendency to metastasize is related to size; tumours less than 1 cm in size are rarely associated with metastases while 80% of those greater than 3 cm have metastasized. Metastases are much more common with small bowel carcinoids than with appendiceal tumours.

Macroscopically carcinoid tumours are often yellow or orange in colour. Microscopically they consist of densely packed epithelial cells which stain with silver nitrate (argentaffinomas). They are often regarded as being part of the amine precursors uptake and decarboxylation (APUD) series of cells (see p. 231) and contain a variety of substances which, when secreted, give rise to the carcinoid syndrome. The development of this clinical syndrome is related to tumour size, the presence of metastases, and the site of origin (the syndrome being rare with distal colon tumours). Both primary and secondary tumours are usually slow growing. The commonest metastatic site is the liver. Lung and bone are less frequently involved.

CLINICAL FEATURES

Local symptoms

The patient may present with local symptoms due to metastases. Pain in the right upper quadrant, due to distension of the liver by metastases, is a frequent symptom and later, weight loss, anorexia and malaise occur as liver function deteriorates. Primary intestinal carcinoids are seldom diagnosed during life unless they cause obstruction, intussusception or pain in the right iliac fossa leading to appendicectomy.

The malignant carcinoid syndrome

This syndrome occurs in about 50% of all patients with hepatic metastases from carcinoid tumours. A variety of chemicals is produced by the tumour and their release is accompanied by symptoms which may dominate the clinical picture [12]. The syndrome is particularly likely to occur with bronchial carcinoid even without hepatic metastases, since the venous drainage is into the systemic circulation and not via the liver which metabolizes the pharmacological mediators liberated by intestinal carcinoids.

5-hydroxytryptamine (5HT) is produced from tryptophan. A metabolite of 5HT, 5-hydroxy-indoleacetic acid (5HIAA), is excreted in the urine. When present in excess it confirms the diagnosis. 5HT is quickly inactivated in the lungs and liver, so large quantities must be produced to cause symptoms. The release of 5HT is probably responsible for diarrhoea. The diarrhoea is typically episodic, watery and may be explosive leading to incontinence. It is often accompanied by noisy borborygmi and cramping pains. Excess 5HT is probably responsible for endocardial fibrosis which can lead to tricuspid incompetence, which in turn may cause right-sided heart failure with ascites, and deep cyanosis in the flushed face. Bradykinin is produced by some tumours and may be partly responsible for the flushing which is characteristic of the syndrome. The flush is at first intermittent, often being precipitated by emotion and alcohol. The face and neck become red and the patient may perspire. It lasts a few minutes and is reminiscent of the flushing of menopausal women. Later the flushing becomes more frequent and some patients become almost permanently flushed. Telangiectases occur on the face, and skin may become thickened. Prostaglandins are liberated from some tumours and may contribute to both the flushing and the diarrhoea. Bronchospasm occurs and has been variously attributed to histamine, bradykinin and prostaglandins. It is episodic at first but permanent wheezing dyspnoea may develop. Episodes of hypotension are sometimes seen and are thought to be caused by 5HT.

Other clinical features

The tumours are slow growing and the diagnosis is often missed or delayed for months or years. If all the symptoms are present the diagnosis is easy to think of, but if the complaint is of diarrhoea alone, numerous negative investigations for colon cancer or malabsorption may lead to the patient being labelled neurotic or having 'irritable bowel syndrome'. Similarly, late-onset asthma may be diagnosed before the rest of the clinical picture becomes apparent. Bronchial carcinoids usually present with unilateral airways obstructions and haemoptyses. Carcinoids in the bronchus, thymus and pancreas occasionally cause Cushing's syndrome, since in some cases production of ACTH by the tumour leads to bilateral adrenal hyperplasia. The primary tumour may be small and only detectable by CT scanning of the thorax or abdomen.

DIAGNOSIS

In the patients without the carcinoid syndrome the diagnosis is made by the primary tumour in the bowel causing abdominal symptoms leading to laparotomy or, in the lung, symptoms of a bronchial adenoma leading to bronchoscopy or thoracotomy. Secondary deposits in the liver are usually diagnosed by liver biopsy.

In patients with the carcinoid syndrome the 24-hour urinary 5HIAA is usually elevated. False-positive results can be obtained with 5HT containing foods (bananas contain 4 mg 5HT). In some patients the urinary 5HIAA excretion may vary from day to day and this leads to false-negative results and makes 5HIAA excretion an unreliable guide to treatment. Foregut carcinoids may produce 5HT and not 5HIAA. About 60% of tumours take up ^{131}I-MIBG (meta-iodo-benzylguanidine) especially if the tumours are of foregut origin and produce 5HT. The value of scanning is mainly to localize sites of metastasis.

MANAGEMENT

Localized intestinal, bronchial or foregut carcinoids should be removed surgically. In metastatic carcinoid surgery should be considered if liver secondaries are found which are well localized and which are resectable. This may relieve symptoms for months or years because the tumour is slow growing. Another means of reducing the tumour mass is hepatic artery ligation or embolization. All of these surgical approaches may result in a sudden release of large quantities of pharmacologically active agents resulting in hypotension and bronchospasm. Intravenous methysergide may be used to treat bronchospasm during surgery, and methoxamine to treat hypotension. Complications of surgery and embolization include necrosis of the gall bladder and *Clostridium welchii* infections in necrotic tumour.

In patients with metastatic carcinoid syndrome which cannot be treated surgically, the usual approach is to attempt to block the pharmacological effects of the tumours in the first instance. However, this is usually only partially successful since each symptom may be produced by more than one agent and pharmacological antagonists are partially effective against some tumour products and do not exist for others.

Diarrhoea

This may be mitigated by simple measures such as codeine phosphate, diphenoxylate or loperamide. The 5HT antagonist methysergide is sometimes effective. Methysergide may itself cause abdominal cramp and nausea, and prolonged administration carries the risk of mediastinal and retroperitoneal fibrosis. Cyproheptadine antagonizes 5HT and also blocks the histamine (H$_1$) receptor. It may be effective in controlling diarrhoea, and interestingly, may occasionally cause tumour regression. The drug may cause dry mouth and drowsiness. Methyldopa inhibits 5HT synthesis but the results in carcinoid are disappointing.

Parachlorophenylalanine (PCPA) inhibits any

enzyme (tryptophan 5-hydroxylase) which is involved in 5HT synthesis. It will reduce urinary 5HIAA and control diarrhoea. It is toxic causing lethargy, headache, mental changes and allergic eosinophilia, the latter occurring in 50% of patients necessitating cessation of treatment.

Flushing

Bradykinin may be partially antagonized by phenothiazines and, since catecholamines can provoke bradykinin release, α-adrenergic blockade with phentolamine may also have some effect. Prostaglandin effects may occasionally be partly alleviated by indomethacin.

Bronchospasm

Agents that block histamine (cyproheptadine) or bradykinin (phenothiazines) can be tried as can conventional bronchodilators but the results are often disappointing. Isoprenaline may help.

Cytotoxic chemotherapy is usually ineffective. It is the only direct treatment for widespread liver metastases and may be indicated if the carcinoid syndrome is uncontrollable by other means. In this situation sudden destruction of the tumour may lead to release of tumour products with severe asthma, diarrhoea and flushing.

The agents with activity are streptozotocin, 5-FU, doxorubicin and cyclophosphamide. Streptozotocin is the most effective drug. Responses to the other agents are infrequent (10–20%) but combinations of doxorubicin, 5-FU and cyclophosphamide will produce temporary responses in about 30% of patients. Infusions of 5-FU into the hepatic artery may reduce pain and tumour bulk. It is not known if this is more effective than full doses of the drug intravenously. There is no evidence that these regimens prolong survival since the tumour grows slowly if left untreated. They may, however, produce symptomatic benefit. Tumour regression has also been observed with cyproheptadine. The somatostatin analogue octreo-

tide is effective in producing control of the symptoms of carcinoid. The dose range is 200–1500 µg/day. Few tumours show any reduction in tumour size. Response duration is of the order of 6 months.

Responses to α-interferon have been reported in carcinoid tumours. The doses have been $5 \, MU/m^2$ three times a week. Some of the responses have been very durable. The value of interferon is undecided as reports are conflicting [13].

ENDOCRINE TUMOURS OF THE PANCREAS

A variety of endocrine tumours may develop in the pancreas (Table 15.2). Although they are uncommon, they are of importance both because they present with symptoms due to the excess hormone production and can therefore be difficult to diagnose, and because they shed light on the normal function of the endocrine pancreas. It has been postulated that there is a system of cells derived from neural crest of neuroectoderm which have particular biochemical characteristics, namely uptake and decarboxylation of amines such as dopa and 5-hydroxytryptophan. The APUD system was proposed as the cell of origin in medullary carcinoma of the thyroid, carcinoid tumours, small cell lung cancer, endocrine tumours of the pancreas, phaeochromocytoma, neuroblastoma and others. There is debate as to whether the concept can be used to account for the origin of these tumours. The hypothesis does, however, help to explain the syndromes of multiple endocrine neoplasms. About 70% of the tumours are malignant and a similar proportion produce hormone. Metastases are usually to liver and adjacent nodes.

Multiple endocrine neoplasms (MEN)

These inherited syndromes have been the subject of intense genetic studies in recent years. The locus of the MEN I gene is on the long arm of chromosome 11 (11q13) and tumour development is associated with loss of heterozygosity at this site.

Three syndromes are recognized:

1 *MEN 1 (Wermer's syndrome)*. This consists of hyperplasia or adenomas of parathyroids and tumours of islet cells, pituitary, adrenal cortex and thyroid (in order of frequency). Patients usually present with hypercalcaemia. Hypoglycaemia or pituitary tumour are less common. The pancreatic islet cell tumour may be malignant. It is usually an insulinoma but gastrinoma, glucagonoma or VIPoma may occur (see below). The condition is inherited as an autosomal dominant, and usually presents age 20–60 years.

2 *MEN II (Sipple's syndrome)*. This consists of medullary carcinoma of the thyroid, phaeochromocytoma and parathyroid hyperplasia. The phaeochromocytoma is often bilateral. About 10% of all cases of medullary carcinoma of the thyroid are part of the MEN II or MEN III syndrome. The syndrome usually presents with symptoms of a phaeochromocytoma or with a lump in the neck. It can occur at any age. The plasma calcitonin is elevated if medullary carcinoma of the thyroid is present and since C-cell hyperplasia precedes the development of malignancy, siblings of patients should have the plasma calcitonin measured. DNA analysis of potential carriers of MEN IIA (p. 396) provides unequivocal identification prior to symptoms [14]. Treatment of these tumours is discussed in Chapter 20. The condition is also autosomal dominant.

3 *MEN III (mucosal neuroma syndrome)*. In this condition phaeochromocytoma and medullary carcinoma of the thyroid also occur (as in MEN II) but the patients also have neuromas of the lips, tongue, mouth and entire gut. There may be hyperextensible joints, pes cavus and soft tissue prognathism. The management is of the thyroid carcinoma and phaeochromocytoma as in MEN II. Parathyroid hyperplasia is less frequent than in MEN II.

Insulinoma

PATHOLOGY

These are tumours of the β cells of the islets. They produce proinsulin which is converted to insulin. The insulin is secreted with its connecting C peptide (which joins the two chains). The tumours are often small and arise with equal frequency in head, body and tail, and 20% are multiple and an equal number malignant. About 5% are associated with MEN I syndrome. The diagnosis of malignancy is difficult histologically but metastases occur to liver and adjacent nodes in about 10% of cases.

CLINICAL FEATURES

The patient presents with symptoms of excess insulin production: loss of consciousness, dizziness, episodic mental confusion and weakness. As the condition progresses the mental confusion is present most of the time and irreversible dementia may occur. It usually presents in middle life but can occur at any age. Other symptoms of MEN I may be present. The vagueness of the presentation often leads to considerable diagnostic delay.

DIAGNOSIS

A fasting blood sugar of below 2.8 mmol/l is the characteristic finding. The fasting test must be carefully controlled, and blood is taken for both sugar and insulin measurements. In a normal person, fasting lowers the blood sugar (but seldom less than 2.8 mmol/l) but the plasma insulin then falls. By contrast, with insulinoma the plasma insulin is either very high or inappropriately raised or maintained while the blood sugar falls. The main differential diagnosis is from self-induced (factitious) hypoglycaemia which should be suspected particularly in medical staff. Exogenous insulin is, however, associated with a low C-peptide level while insulinoma is not. Surreptitious taking of a sulphonylurea can also cause diagnostic difficulty.

Selective arteriography is helpful in determining whether the lesions are single or multiple. CT and ultrasound scanning are sometimes useful.

TREATMENT

After localization a partial pancreatectomy is performed leaving the head of the pancreas wherever possible. When the tumour has not been localized pre-operatively, it may none the less be palpable at operation. The plasma insulin is monitored during the operation. If no tumour is found, a subtotal pancreatectomy is usually performed. Chemotherapy is discussed on p. 303.

Metastases are uncommon but if they occur they may respond to streptozotocin, 5-FU or doxorubicin. A combination of all three has also been used with response rates of 50–60%. Diazoxide can be used to treat hypoglycaemia. Glucagon is of little value.

Gastrinoma (Zollinger–Ellison syndrome)

INCIDENCE AND PATHOLOGY

These tumours are uncommon. They probably arise from the δ or D cells of the islets and are often malignant [15]. They usually present at the age of 20–45 years and probably account for 0.1% of all peptic ulcer disease. Ninety per cent occur in the pancreas, 5% in the duodenum and others occur in the stomach and, very rarely, in adenomas of the thyroid and ovary. They may be single or multiple and vary greatly in size (less than 5 mm to 15 cm). Gastrinomas are most common in the body or tail and microscopically resemble carcinoids. This resemblance and the fact that occasionally other peptide hormones are produced (ACTH, vasoactive intestinal polypeptide (VIP), glucagon) lend weight to the hypothesis that their origin is from APUD cells. In 60% of patients metastases have occurred at diagnosis usually to adjacent nodes and liver, but more distant spread is not uncommon.

Most of the gastrin produced in the tumour is a 17 amino acid peptide (G-17) but a larger molecule (G-34) is also formed. Circulating gastrin is mainly G-34. The constant stimulation of the gastric parietal cells leads to a great increase in their mass. In some patients other features of the MEN I syndrome are present — usually hyperparathyroidism.

CLINICAL FEATURES [16]

The dominant symptom is peptic ulceration. Usually the ulcer is in the first part of the duodenum or in the stomach. Occasionally there are multiple ulcers which extend down in the proximal duodenum. Recurrence soon after medical treatment, perforation and haemorrhage all occur. The symptoms of ulceration are severe and response to medical treatment is limited although H_2 receptor antagonists are effective for a while.

Diarrhoea occurs in 30–50% of cases, due to the large volume of acid produced by the stomach. Pancreatic lipase is inactivated at low pH leading to steatorrhoea. The low pH also interferes with bile salt function and with the activity of intrinsic factor.

INVESTIGATION AND DIAGNOSIS

The history of recurrent severe peptic ulceration with diarrhoea in a young person should point to the possible diagnosis. There is occasionally a family history of endocrine neoplasia. Acid output is raised, but not necessarily to levels above that found in some patients with duodenal ulcer. The diagnosis is confirmed by finding an elevated plasma gastrin level. Most radioimmunoassay antibodies will detect all types of gastrin molecule produced by gastrinomas.

When the diagnosis has been made, attempts are usually made to locate tumour. CT scanning and ultrasound may be helpful in showing metastases but usually fail to demonstrate the primary, and angiography is little better. Laparotomy is usually required to assess operability.

MANAGEMENT

Pancreatectomy is seldom practicable. The tumours are often multifocal and have frequently metastasized. Histamine antagonists have greatly improved medical management. Before their introduction total gastrectomy was the preferred treatment for intractable ulceration. Death is more a consequence of the complications of ulceration than of malignancy though this may change with the use of cimetidine. About 60% of patients are alive 5 years after diagnosis.

VIPoma (Verner–Morrison syndrome)

This rare syndrome of profuse watery diarrhoea, facial flushing, hypokalaemia, hypochlorhydria and hypertension is caused by the secretion of VIP by tumours of the pancreatic islets [17]. VIP (and the syndrome) can be produced by phaeochromocytomas, ganglioneuroblastomas and bronchogenic (small cell) carcinoma. Hyperglycaemia and hypercalaemia may also occur and can be caused by VIP.

The tumours are usually solitary and can sometimes be shown angiographically. Treatment is by surgical removal. There is a high risk of malignancy.

Glucagonoma

These are tumours of the pancreatic α cell and usually affect postmenopausal women [18]. The clinical syndrome is characterized by a severe skin eruption with migratory erythema, bullous ulceration and scabbing on the legs, trunk, genital area and face (migratory necrolytic erythema). In addition there is normochromic anaemia, stomatitis, diarrhoea and hypokalaemia. Most of the tumours are in the body and tail and are often malignant (60%) but with a slow growth rate. Metastasis is usually to the liver.

The diagnosis is made by the typical rash and the raised plasma glucagon levels. Glucagon causes gluconeogenesis and glycogenolysis, elevating the blood sugar. The mechanism of production of the skin rash is not known. Treatment is by surgical removal wherever possible.

Somatostatinoma [19]

These rare islet cell tumours are usually malignant. The syndrome consists of steatorrhoea and diarrhoea due to suppressed pancreatic exocrine function, gall-stones due to decreased gall bladder contractility, diabetes from suppression of insulin, and hypochlorhydria from suppression of gastrin.

Plasma somatostatin and calcitonin are elevated. Diagnosis is late because the symptoms are not specific. The tumours should be removed if metastases have not yet occurred.

Chemotherapy of advanced endocrine tumours of the pancreatic islet cells

There are few controlled trials of the value of chemotherapy in these diverse tumours. Streptozotocin has been widely used. It produces tumour regression in 30% of advanced cases. Both doxorubicin and 5-FU produce responses in patients who have been treated with streptozotocin and those who are untreated. Chlorozotocin, which like streptozotocin is a nitrosourea-containing agent, has a similar level of activity.

In a recent trial of the Eastern Cooperative Oncology Group [20], streptozotocin appeared to have superior activity when combined with doxorubicin than when combined with 5-FU. Both combinations were superior to chlorozotocin alone when judged by response rate. The doxorubicin-containing combination produced responses in 70% of patients and may have prolonged their survival. Streptozotocin produces severe nausea which chlorozotocin does not, so the latter drug may replace streptozotocin in combination. Hormone responses occur with the somatostatin analogue ocreotide. α-Interferon may also produce regression of islet cell tumours but its value has not yet been defined.

REFERENCES

1 Colombo M., de Franchis R., del Ninno E. *et al.* Hepatocellular carcinoma in Italian patients with cirrhosis. *New England Journal of Medicine* 1991; **325**: 675–80.

2 Beasley R.P., Hwang L.Y. Hepatocellular carcinoma and hepatitis B virus. *Seminars in Liver Disease* 1984; **4**: 113–21.

3 Sharfitz D.A., Shouval D., Sherman H. *et al.* Integration of hepatitis B virus into the genome of liver cells in chronic liver disease and hepatocellular carcinoma. *New England Journal of Medicine* 1981; **305**: 1067–73.

4 Patterlini P., Gerken G., Nakajima E. *et al.* Polymerase chain reaction to detect hepatitis B virus DNA and RNA sequences in primary liver cancers from patients negative for hepatitis surface antigen. *New England Journal of Medicine* 1990; **323**: 80–85.

5 Senzer N.N., Terrell W., Pratt C.B. Evaluation of a chemotherapeutic regimen for primary liver cancer in children. *Cancer Treatment Report* 1978; **62**: 1403–4.

6 Levin B., Riddell R.H., Kirsner J.B. Management of precancerous lesions of the gastrointestinal tract. *Clinics in Gastroenterology* 1976; **5**: 827–53.

7 Coutsofides T., McDonald J., Shibata H.R. Carcinoma of the pancreas and periampullary region: a 41 year experience. *Annals of Surgery* 1977; **186**: 730–33.

8 Pereiras R., Chiprut R.O., Greenwald R.A. Percutaneous transhepatic cholangiography with the 'skinny' needle. *Annals of Internal Medicine* 1977; **86**: 562–68.

9 Dobelbower R.R. The radiotherapy of pancreatic cancer. *Seminars in Oncology* 1979; **6**: 378–89.

10 Smith F.P., Schein P.S. Chemotherapy of pancreatic cancer. *Seminars in Oncology* 1978; **6**: 368–77.

11 Godwin J.D. Carcinoid tumours; an analysis of 2837 cases. *Cancer* 1975; **36**: 560–69.

12 Grahame-Smith D.G. Natural history and diagnosis of the carcinoid syndrome. *Clinics in Gastroenterology* 1974; **3**: 575–94.

13 Oberg K., Alm G., Magnusson A. *et al.* Treatment of malignant carcinoid tumours with recombinant interferon α2b: development of neutralizing interferon antibodies and possible loss of antitumour activity. *Journal of the National Cancer Institute* 1989; **81**: 531–35.

14 Lips C.J.M., Landsvater R.M., Höppener J.W.M. *et al.* Clinical screening as compared with DNA analysis in families with multiple endocrine neoplasia type 2A. *New England Journal of Medicine* 1994; **331**: 828–35.

15 Martin E.D., Potet F. Pathology of endocrine tumours of the GI tract. *Clinics in Gastroenterology* 1974; **3**: 511–32.

16 Regan P.T., Malagelada J.R. A reappraisal of the clinical, roentgenographic and endoscopic features of the Zollinger-Ellison syndrome. *Mayo Clinic Proceedings* 1978; **53**: 19–23.

17 Verner J.V., Morrison A.B. Non-beta islet cell tumours and the syndrome of watery diarrhoea, hypokalaemia and hypochlorhydria. *Clinics in Gastroenterology* 1976; **3**: 595–608.

18 Mallinson C.N., Bloom S.R., Warin A.P., Salmon P.R., Cox B. A glucagonoma syndrome. *Lancet* 1974; **ii**: 1–5.

19 Larsson L.I., Hirsch M.A., Holst J.J. *et al.* Pancreatic somatostatinoma. Clinical features and pathological implications. *Lancet* 1977; **i**: 666–68.

20 Moertel C.G., Lefkopoulo M., Lipsitz S. *et al.* Streptozotocin-doxorubicin, streptozotocin-fluorouracil, or chlorozotocin in the treatment of islet-cell carcinoma. *New England Journal of Medicine* 1992; **326**: 519–23.

Chapter 16
Tumours of the Small and Large Bowel

TUMOURS OF THE SMALL BOWEL

Incidence and aetiology

Small bowel tumours represent less than 5% of all gastro-intestinal tumours and only half of these will prove to be malignant. Their low frequency seems particularly surprising since the small bowel comprises about three-quarters the length of the alimentary tract. Although malignant lesions occur most frequently in the duodenum and jejunum, benign lesions such as adenomas and fibromas occur more frequently in the ileum. The incidence of malignant lesions is approximately 1 in 100 000 (Fig. 16.1) and adenocarcinomas are more common in patients with familial adenomatous polyposis, Peutz–Jeghers syndrome and Crohn's disease. These tumours are more common over the age of 60 years. Long-standing coeliac disease predisposes to the development of small bowel lymphoma (see Chapter 26).

Pathology

There are four major types of malignant small bowel tumours. The commonest are adenocarcinomas (45%), carcinoid tumours (30%), lymphomas (10%) and sarcomas (mostly leiomyosarcomas). Metastatic deposits (most frequently from the ovary and pancreas) are at least as common as primary tumours.

Adenocarcinoma of the small bowel metastasizes to the liver and regional nodes. Histologically these are typical mucin-secreting adenocarcinomas. The characteristic appearance is of an ulcerating neoplasm. Small bowel lymphomas are usually diffuse and poorly differentiated. The small bowel is an important site of non-Hodgkin's lymphoma in childhood. The management of small bowel lymphoma is discussed in Chapter 26.

Carcinoid tumours arise principally in the ileum, caecum, appendix and duodenum. They appear as small yellowish nodules in the bowel wall, arising from the chromaffin cells which probably belong to the APUD system and which secrete small polypeptide hormones and amine. The management of the carcinoid syndrome is discussed in Chapter 15.

Clinical features

Clinical diagnosis is difficult and is not usually achieved before surgery. Patients often present with symptoms of obstruction or intermittent abdominal pain and a history of melaena is sometimes obtained. Intussusception is often the cause of the obstruction and pain.

Chronic anaemia may occur, from gradual blood loss. Weight loss is frequent and diarrhoea and steatorrhoea are occasionally present, particularly with lymphomas. A palpable abdominal mass may also be found, and abdominal distension if there is intestinal obstruction. Commonly, there are no abnormal physical signs. Perforation is rare with adenocarcinoma, but common with lymphoma.

Diagnosis

Contrast X-ray studies are essential in diagnosis, but not always helpful. In proximal tumours, a barium follow-through is required whereas in distal lesions causing ileocolic intussusception, the barium enema is usually

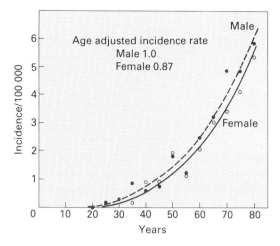

Fig. 16.1 Age-specific incidence of malignant tumours of the small bowel.

more useful. Hypotonic duodenography may give better visualization of duodenal lesions and small bowel enemas are helpful with lower tumours. Occasionally an ultrasound or CT scan is helpful to delineate a mass. Duodenal lesions can usually be seen endoscopically, and biopsy and cytological specimens can be obtained.

Treatment

In the management of small bowel neoplasms, surgical removal is the most important method of treatment. Although benign tumours can usually be removed by simple resection, adeno-carcinomas require a wider excision including, if possible, removal of the lymph node drainage area since lymphatic invasion is common. Only 70% of tumours are resectable. For duodenal cancers, pancreaticoduodenectomy may be required. At the other end of the small bowel, lesions of the terminal ileum are often best treated by hemicolectomy, since better resection of regional lymphatics can be achieved in this way. With leiomyosarcomas, regional node involvement is less frequent and removal of the lymph node drainage area may not be necessary.

For lymphomas of the small bowel, a particu-larly careful search of the abdomen is mandatory since involvement of local lymph nodes, liver or spleen is common. Wide resection of the involved area is necessary, with removal of adjacent nodes. Following resection, treatment with chemotherapy or radiotherapy may be necessary (see Chapter 26).

In resecting small bowel carcinoids, the site and size of the tumour are helpful guides. Carcinoid tumours of the appendix are unlikely to metastasize, and simple appendicectomy is probably sufficient. In any lesion larger than 2 cm a more widespread excision seems justified because of the risk of spread beyond the primary site.

Prognosis

The survival rate for small bowel adenocar-cinomas is poor, only 20% of patients surviving 5 years. For localized carcinoid tumours, 5-year survival rates of up to 90% have been reported. The prognosis for metastatic disease is dis-cussed in Chapter 15. Leiomyosarcomas are discussed in Chapter 23.

Tumours of the appendix

These are uncommon, and 90% of them are carcinoids which are treated by local resection. The remainder are either adenocarcinomas or mucocoeles which contain a gelatinoid mucoid material and can undergo malignant change to become papillary mucinous cystadenocar-cinomas. Rupture of these lesions leads to the condition of *pseudomyxoma peritonei*, a gelati-nous, ascitic implanting tumour which can coat the entire peritoneal surface resulting in pro-gressive abdominal enlargement, and some-times mimicking ovarian carcinoma. Treatment of pseudomyxoma involves surgical evacuation, though repeated operations are usually required. Both whole abdominal irradiation and intraperitoneal or systemic chemotherapy have been advocated, although their effectiveness is uncertain. Cisplatin or carboplatin are the drugs normally used intra-peritoneally.

TUMOURS OF THE LARGE BOWEL

Incidence and aetiology

Cancers of the large bowel (colon and rectum) are amongst the commonest of malignant tumours and represent the second largest cause of death from cancer in the Western world. Cancers of the colon outnumber rectal carcinomas by 3:2 (Fig. 16.2), and the two sites together constitute 10–15% of all cancers. As the age-adjusted incidence has remained constant over the past 30 years, the number of cases has gradually risen due to population growth and increasing age. The disease is uncommon in Africa, Asia and South America, suggesting a possible dietary aetiology. It seems increasingly clear that a high intake of animal fat increases the risk of colon cancer [1]. Substitution of chicken or fish for high-fat red animal meat is possibly now justified by current data. In the United States, the incidence rate amongst black people increased by half between 1947 and 1969, which may reflect an increasingly 'Westernized' diet in this group. A good deal of additional epidemiological data supports this view. Western diets, containing high propor-

tions of meat and animal fats, but little fibre, are quite unlike the typical African diet. Africans have a more rapid stool transit time, which may lead to a reduced exposure to any carcinogen passing down the alimentary canal. Japanese immigrants to the United States show an increasing incidence of colorectal cancer in succeeding generations [2]. Close relatives of patients with carcinoma of the colon have a slightly higher incidence of the disease, possibly suggesting a common genetic factor operating within a background of high dietary risk. Western diet, with a high meat and fat content favours a gut bacterial population which produces enzymes capable of converting sterols to carcinogens in the bowel. The enzyme 7-α-dehydroxylase converts bile acids to deoxycholic and lithocholic acid. It is known that in animal models some bile acids act as promoters of carcinogenesis in tumours initiated by carcinogens such as dimethylhydrazine.

A number of conditions are known to predispose to the development of large bowel cancers. In patients with ulcerative colitis, the risk is greater in patients with a long history and extensive bowel involvement. Patients diagnosed young are at special risk, particularly since modern treatment usually ensures lengthy survival. In the past some physicians recommended total colectomy in patients in whom the disease had been active for more than 10 years, a recommendation which was supported by the fact that these patients tend to develop multicentric and poorly differentiated carcinomas [3]. More recent studies have indicated that a careful 'watch' policy is satisfactory. In some patients with ulcerative colitis, dysplastic mucosal changes appear to precede the development of malignancy.

Familial adenomatous polyposis coli (APC) also predisposes to malignant change. The distal colon tends to be most severely involved and the similarity of symptoms of familial polyposis and true carcinoma makes diagnosis of the development of malignancy extremely difficult. Most surgeons now recommend restorative proctocolectomy, an operation in which a

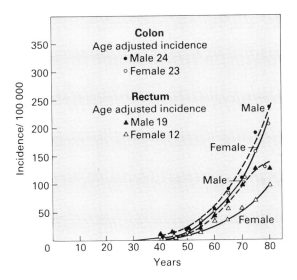

Fig. 16.2 Age-specific incidence of carcinoma of the large bowel.

'pouch' is fashioned from small bowel to replace the rectum, a procedure now considered safe and generally well tolerated.

It is now clear that non-familial (sporadic) adenomatous polyps are premalignant. Most cancers apparently arise from them though not all adenomas become cancerous. Such lesions are found increasingly with age, and in a small percentage of patients with bowel cancer, residual evidence of an adenomatous polyp can sometimes be found. The risk of malignant change increases greatly with increasing size of the polyp [4]. Many surgeons advocate routine removal of polyps found at sigmoidoscopy, particularly since two-thirds of large bowel cancers are found in the rectum and sigmoid colon (see below). Villous adenomas at any site in the bowel are premalignant. The risk relates to size, and villous lesions are more likely to become malignant than are tubulovillous or tubular adenomas. They present with diarrhoea, rectal bleeding or a characteristic picture of fluid and electrolyte loss, often with severe hypokalaemia. The incidence of malignant change is at least 15% and possibly higher, and these lesions should always be removed even if this necessitates an extensive operation.

The last few years have seen a major advance in our understanding of the chromosomal changes which occur in familial adenomatous polyposis. The familial polyposis (APC) gene is located on chromosome 21 (5q). Loss of an allele at this site has been found in 40% of cases of sporadic carcinoma of the colon, implicating the APC gene in the pathogenesis of the disease. Allele loss has also been found for the p53 gene on chromosome 17 and another gene on 18q (called DCC, deleted in colorectal carcinoma). A model of the genetic changes in the development of the adenoma–carcinoma sequence is shown in Fig. 16.3.

SCREENING FOR COLORECTAL CANCERS

Since early or precancerous lesions can be resected if identified, prompt management should lead to reduced incidence and mortality from bowel cancer [4–6]. The prevalence of colorectal cancer in the Western world is sufficiently high for screening to be a realistic proposition, particularly bearing in mind the relatively inexpensive and reliable investigations available — faecal occult blood testing, digital rectal examination and sigmoidoscopy. Moreover, as the disease is strongly age-related, with 94% of all cases in patients over 50 years, a high-risk group should not be difficult to identify. Further, patients with a strong family

Fig. 16.3 The genetic changes in the development of the adenoma–carcinoma sequence.

history or those with familial adenomatous polyposis coli represent additional groups where screening may be worthwhile.

Opinions remain divided as to the cost-benefit of these methods. One study, from Denmark (31 000 subjects), showed no obvious benefit in a trial comparing the death rate in screened and unscreened groups [5] although a large British study showed that over twice this number of subjects would be required if a 20% colorectal mortality difference were to be demonstrated, with a minimum 7-year follow-up period [6]. The present position is that screening may be feasible but has so far shown little success in reducing mortality. It is at least now clear that faecal occult blood testing has a sufficiently high sensitivity to warrant further trial.

Pathology and surgical staging

The distal part of the large bowel is the commonest site of malignancy: approximately 20% of all large bowel tumours occur in the sigmoid colon and 40% in the rectum (Fig. 16.4).

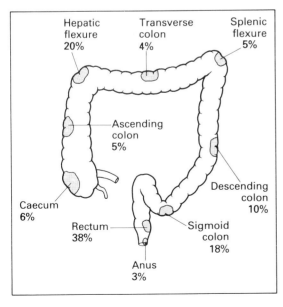

Fig. 16.4 Cancer of the large bowel: proportion of all cases arising at each site.

The typical lesion is either polypoid with a fleshy protuberance on a narrow base, or sessile, with a broader base and a generally flatter appearance. The most characteristic form is a well-demarcated polypoid mass with ulceration in its centre, involving part or all of the bowel circumference. The tumour may have reached the full thickness of the bowel wall although lateral spread beyond 3 cm is unusual. Local lymphatic invasion is common and about one-third of these patients have evidence of nodal metastases at presentation. Blood-borne metastases are usually via the portal vein and the liver is much the commonest site of distant spread. Systemic haematogenous dissemination to the lung, brain and skeleton occurs less frequently. Local recurrence can be a major problem with these tumours often leading to intestinal or ureteric obstruction, or fistula formation.

Surgical staging is of great importance since there is no better guide to prognosis. Although well-localized tumours carry a high probability of surgical cure, over half of all large bowel cancers ultimately prove fatal. The Dukes staging system is widely employed and is easy to apply. It is a valuable predictor of survival in both colonic and rectal lesions (Table 16.1) and extensive regional node involvement has a particularly adverse prognosis. Tumour grade and depth of penetration are also important. Some of these factors are interdependent since the

Table 16.1 Dukes staging system for rectal cancer (with percentage of 5-year survival)

Stage	Description
A	Confined to bowel wall, i.e. mucosa and submucosa, or early muscular invasion (80%)
B	Invasion through the muscle wall but no lymph node involvement (50%)
C1	Lymph node involvement but not up to highest point of vascular ligation (40%)
C2	Nodes involved up to highest nodes at the point of ligation (12%)

higher the tumour grade, the more likely the risk of local nodal metastasis.

Clinical features and diagnosis

The symptoms of colorectal cancer vary with the site of the tumour (Fig. 16.5). In the caecum and right side of the colon, the main complaint is of ill-defined abdominal pain which may be mistaken for gall bladder or peptic ulcer disease. Chronic iron deficiency anaemia from occult blood loss is common and may be the presenting feature. Frank melaena may occur, and episodes of diarrhoea are not uncommon. An abdominal mass may sometimes be felt.

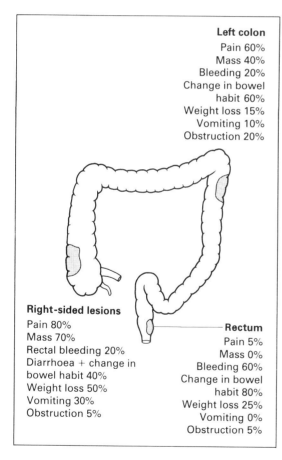

Left colon
Pain 60%
Mass 40%
Bleeding 20%
Change in bowel
    habit 60%
Weight loss 15%
Vomiting 10%
Obstruction 20%

Right-sided lesions
Pain 80%
Mass 70%
Rectal bleeding 20%
Diarrhoea + change in
bowel habit 40%
Weight loss 50%
Vomiting 30%
Obstruction 5%

Rectum
Pain 5%
Mass 0%
Bleeding 60%
Change in bowel
    habit 80%
Weight loss 25%
Vomiting 0%
Obstruction 5%

Fig. 16.5 Symptoms of colorectal cancer according to site.

In left-sided colonic lesions the pain is usually cramping and suggestive of intestinal obstruction. Abdominal distension may be present. Constipation, occasionally alternating with diarrhoea, is a frequent complaint and symptomatic rectal bleeding occurs in 20% of patients. Rectal carcinoma is often accompanied by passage of bright red blood. However, this is a common symptom in the normal population since haemorrhoids are very frequent. Change in bowel habit with tenesmus and constipation are later symptoms.

Rectal examination is the most important single procedure for diagnosing large bowel tumours. Three-quarters of all rectal lesions are within reach and sigmoidoscopy will usually visualize these lesions without difficulty provided care is taken with the details of the examination. Sigmoidoscopy allows examination of up to the distal 25 cm of large bowel and the majority of rectal tumours can be diagnosed in this way. The introduction of flexible sigmoidoscopy and colonoscopy into more general use has led to accurate pre-operative diagnosis of the majority of large bowel cancers, although their use is not yet routine since barium enema examinations are easier, less expensive, more widely available, and relatively efficient as a routine method of diagnosis. The double-contrast enema has improved diagnostic accuracy, giving better resolution of small tumours. Radiologically the tumour may appear as a narrowed or strictured segment or as a mass indenting the contrast medium (Fig. 16.6). On the right side of the colon, the tumour is more easily missed, particularly in the caecum, which may be poorly demonstrated by the examination. In doubtful cases, the investigation should be repeated or colonoscopy performed.

In 1965, Gold and his colleagues demonstrated that colonic and rectal cancers sometimes produced a tumour marker, CEA. Unfortunately, this marker has not proved sufficiently specific to be a reliable indicator of disease in patients with large bowel cancers since it can also be elevated in pancreatitis,

Fig. 16.6 Barium enema appearances in large bowel cancer. (A) Carcinoma of recto-sigmoid; (B) carcinoma of caecum.

inflammatory bowel diseases, and in normal people who are heavy smokers or have a high ingestion of alcohol. It can, however, be useful in monitoring disease in certain patients with bowel tumours who have a raised CEA which is known to have fallen following successful surgery. In these patients, a rise in CEA may be the first sign of recurrence. The question of what to do when recurrence is suggested by a rise in CEA has not yet finally been answered since a postoperative rise may be due to un-resectable metastasis.

The differential diagnosis of large bowel cancer includes other large bowel disorders such a diverticular disease, ulcerative colitis, ischaemic colitis and irritable bowel syndrome. Other causes of rectal bleeding, such as haemorrhoids and polyps, may cause diagnostic difficulty. Abdominal pain may suggest biliary tract disease or peptic ulceration. Radiologically, there may be difficulty in distinguishing left-sided neoplasms from diverticular disease, and benign tumours such as lipomas and neurofibromas may occur at any site though these are extremely rare.

Prognostic factors

Well known adverse prognostic factors include high pathological stage, degree of penetration of the primary tumour, lymph node involvement and age below 40 years. In addition, undifferentiated tumours or those with heavy mucus secretion or 'signet ring' forms, inadequate resection margins, vascular or lymphatic invasion or presentation with large bowel obstruction are also known to be important risk factors. Elevation of pre-operative CEA above 5 mg/ml indicates a high risk of recurrence though CEA levels are usually related to stage and histology. Normal CEA levels in node-positive patients do not obviate the need for consideration of adjuvant therapy (see below). Five-year survival figures are shown in Table 16.1.

Management

SURGERY

Surgery remains the cornerstone of treatment. Radical surgical resection is usually preferred to simple excision, because of the risk of unsuspected node metastases as well as the possibility of multicentric tumours. Wide removal of the involved segment should include resection of the local lymphatic drainage area (Fig. 16.7). Even in patients with evidence of hepatic or peritoneal metastases, surgical tumour removal may offer the best means of palliation. Some surgeons even recommend radical bowel resection in patients with a solitary hepatic metastasis, since hepatic resection can sometimes be accomplished though not at the initial procedure because of the dangers of sepsis. The operative procedure should rest firmly on a knowledge of the anatomy of the vascular supply and lymphatic drainage of the affected bowel segment, and care must be taken to avoid tumour implantation into the operative field at the same time of surgical excision. Anastomotic recurrences have become extremely uncommon, provided that an adequate operation has been undertaken. They are increasingly regarded as a failure of surgical technique.

In rectal cancer the type and extent of the excision depends on the site of the tumour. For lower and middle rectal lesions, the classic abdomino-perineal resection introduced by Miles is widely performed (Fig. 16.7). Sphincter-preserving surgery, first performed in the late 1930s, is now performed on over 50% of surgically resectable rectal cancers. Local resection is sometimes performed for small, mobile polypoid lesions of favourable histological grade. Patients who are unwell through obstruction, cachexia or perforation may benefit from an initial defunctioning colostomy before tumour removal is attempted. Even in totally unresectable lesions, a colostomy should generally be performed since this will at least allow a reasonable quality of life and makes high-dose radiotherapy for the primary tumour a feasible proposition (see below).

Surgical mortality has rapidly diminished in recent years and is now 4% in experienced hands. Complications include anastomotic leaks, postoperative infection and urinary dysfunction, particularly if nerve damage has occured during the operation. Despite radical segmented bowel excision, the incidence of local recurrence is about 10%. High-grade rectal lesions are particularly likely to recur locally, especially where regional node metastases have

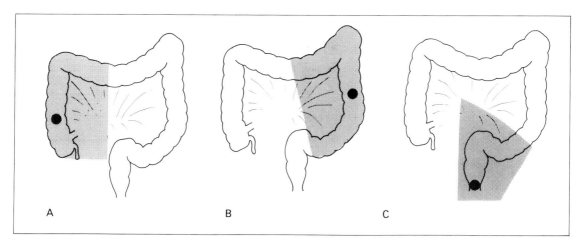

Fig. 16.7 Surgical resection of large bowel cancer. (A) Right hemicolectomy; (B) left hemicolectomy; (C) abdominoperineal resection.

been demonstrated. Detailed pathological description of the surgical specimen is extremely important and should include the gross and microscopic extent of surgical margins, the depth of penetration, the number of nodes removed (and involved) and, in particular, whether the apical node (highest level) is positive. Characteristics such as venous or lymphatic invasion, perineural invasion, histological subtype and grade should also be documented.

RADIOTHERAPY

Although many surgeons feel that radiotherapy has no established place in the primary management of carcinoma of the large bowel, there is increasing evidence to suggest that it is rapidly finding a role in rectal cancer. There is no evidence that it is of value in carcinomas higher than the mid-sigmoid region. As with other abdominopelvic tumours, there seems little doubt that local lymph node involvement is less common in surgical specimens of rectal carcinomas obtained from pre-operatively irradiated patients, suggesting that radiation therapy is sometimes capable of producing histological resolution of lymph node involvement.

Radiotherapy can be useful for inoperable or recurrent cancers. In the majority of patients, troublesome symptoms of pain or rectal bleeding can be palliated and a small number have achieved long survival without further treatment. Perineal, anastomotic or wound recurrences can be extremely painful, particularly if ulceration occurs. In such cases, and indeed when the surgeon is unable to achieve complete operative removal of the primary lesion, radiotherapy is likely to be the most effective treatment. Doses in the range of 40–50 Gy in 4–5 weeks are usually recommended. As a result of this experience, studies of pre-operative irradiation, usually to modest doses, have been carried out, though with conflicting results.

Although it is not yet possible to recommend pre- or postoperative irradiation routinely, several large prospectively randomized trials have now provided evidence which supports its use in high-risk groups (Dukes Stages B and C) [7,8]. For example, a study from the Gastrointestinal Tumor Study Group in the United States showed lower local recurrence rates (though not survival) when radiotherapy was given (40–48 Gy over 4½–5½ weeks); the improvement was greater still when chemotherapy was given as well (see below).

In mobile cancers of the lower rectum, Papillon [9] has developed elegant endocavitary techniques using high-dosage radiation therapy to a limited volume, avoiding the need for surgery. In a carefully selected group of 133 patients, he demonstrated a 78% 5-year survival rate, often in patients whose general condition was poor.

THE ROLE OF CHEMOTHERAPY

5-Fluorouracil has been widely used in patients with *recurrent or metastatic large bowel* cancers for almost 20 years. Despite the occasional impressive symptomatic improvement, objective responses are usually incomplete and transient, and occur in not more than 20% of all patients. There is little evidence as yet to suggest that such treatment prolongs survival in the whole group, though prolongation of life has been claimed in responding patients. A well tolerated drug, 5-FU can be given in a variety of ways, though intermittent intravenous therapy is preferred. The response to 5-FU in metastatic colorectal cancer can be increased by concomitant administration with folinic acid (see Chapter 6) and a synergism with an interferon has been suggested. Other agents, although active, are either less effective or have greater toxicity (Table 16.2). Nitrosoureas (BCNU, CCNU and methyl-CCNU) and mitomycin C have been extensively tested and produce objective responses in about 10–20% of patients.

Various combinations of these and other agents have been employed but with limited success. An increased response rate has been reported using a combination of 5-FU, BCNU, DTIC and vincristine, but at the cost of con-

Table 16.2 Large bowel cancer — response to chemotherapy

	Response rate (%)
Single agents	
5-FU	20
5-FU and folinic acid	35
Nitrosoureas	10
Mitomycin C	20
Combination	
5-FU, methyl-CCNU	15–20
5-FU, methyl-CCNU, vincristine	25

siderable toxicity. The combination is slightly, though not significantly more effective than 5-FU alone. Other studies have shown a similar slight increase in responsiveness to combination chemotherapy. Despite a significant improvement in response rate for patients receiving combination chemotherapy, there is unfortunately no survival benefit. Although 5-FU nitrosourea combinations are marginally more effective in producing responses than single-agent therapy, treatment-related toxicity is undoubtedly greater, myelosuppression can be severe and prolonged, and survival is not improved. In *metastatic disease* pain may be relieved and with combination therapy regressions do occur. With intra-arterial infusion responses may occur even in tumours resistant to intravenous chemotherapy. The complexity of the treatment and the lack of survival advantage reduces the value of this approach. Long-term intravenous infusion of 5-FU is now widely employed for clinically evident metastases. Treatment of hepatic metastases is discussed further in Chapter 8.

Treatment with chemotherapy has been recommended postoperatively as a *surgical adjuvant* and there is increasing evidence that this may be valuable [8,10,11]. It must be appreciated that survival gains of only 5% would save very large numbers of lives in this common disease. Trials to demonstrate these small differences will have to be very large indeed (see Chapter 2,

p. 17). Small trials (thus far the majority) are likely to be misleading.

For patients with rectal carcinoma, in contrast to those with colonic carcinoma, there is a significant risk of loco-regional failure as the only or first site of recurrence following a curative surgical procedure. The best adjuvant therapy for rectal carcinoma (Dukes B or C) is probably postoperative radiotherapy plus chemotherapy. Previously, the use of methyl-CCNU, as recommended by the United States Gastrointestinal Tumor Study Group [7] had not been universally accepted because of the risk of nephrotoxicity and leukaemogenesis. However, the recent large-scale prospectively randomized trial data from Krook *et al.* [8] have again suggested that both radiotherapy and adjuvant chemotherapy may play an important role in the management of high-risk rectal cancer with improvement in 5-year recurrence-free survival from 41.5% (radiation alone) to 62.7% (radiation plus chemotherapy with 5-FU and methyl-CCNU). It may also be possible to achieve equally good results with less toxic chemotherapy. The value of the 'immuno-adjuvant' levamisole still needs to be confirmed.

In studies of patients with *colonic carcinoma* [10], the use of 5-FU/levamisole in combination appeared to reduce cancer mortality in patients with *locally advanced disease* by 33%, though the number of patients studied was limited. In the United States *adjuvant chemotherapy* using 5-FU and levamisole has been recommended as routine treatment for Dukes Stage C colonic lesions. In the United Kingdom and in other European countries the data have been regarded more sceptically since the results are based on subgroup analyses and controls were deficient in that the benefit for levamisole and 5-FU over 5-FU alone was not clearly demonstrated. A large-scale randomized trial of different types of adjuvant chemotherapy in colonic cancer is now in progress which may help to determine if there is a survival benefit compared with no treatment and, if so, which drug combination is most effective.

Hepatic metastases from colorectal cancer can

be treated by infusion of 5-FU into the hepatic vein and the use of this technique is under study at present in a very large-scale trial in the United Kingdom as an adjuvant to surgery in colorectal cancer in patients without visible metastases.

LIVING WITH A COLOSTOMY

Patients faced with the prospect of a permanent colostomy need sympathetic support. Quite apart from worrying about its appearance and the possibility of spillage and smell, most patients are concerned that they will find it impossible to manage the colostomy themselves without skilled help. They may need reassurance that the presence of the colostomy does not imply the residual cancer has been left behind and also that it will be possible to return to a normal active life. Despite enthusiastic help, many patients will develop depressive symptoms and in a proportion, agoraphobia or fear of social contact may become a disability. The value of a skilled stoma therapist cannot be overestimated, and the same is true of the well informed self-help groups such as the *British Colostomy Association*.

It is often valuable for the patient with cancer of the large bowel to meet a colostomy patient before the definitive surgery is performed. In many instances this has been crucial in persuading a hesitant patient to undergo what subsequently proves to be curative surgery.

SCREENING

Secondary prevention (the identification of high-risk groups and early detection of the disease) has been the subject of much investigation. The three methods used have been plasma CEA, sigmoidoscopy and faecal occult blood testing. CEA has proved an insensitive test for early cancer and is no longer used. Studies using sigmoidoscopy have suggested a higher survival rate for those thus diagnosed, and flexible sigmoidoscopes may make the procedure more acceptable to patients. Occult blood

testing of stools (using the guaiac test which turns blue with red cell pseudoperoxidase) has also been used in controlled trials [12]. In one study the rate of positive slide tests was 2.4% and of those who were then investigated 9% had cancer of the colon or rectum, 80% of which were Dukes A or B. The effect of occult blood testing in the general population on the mortality from colorectal cancer is still uncertain, and a longer follow-up period is needed. In high-risk groups such as patients with a family history of polyposis coli, yearly screening with flexible sigmoidoscopy and faecal occult blood testing is recommended.

CARCINOMA OF THE ANUS

Pathology and clinical features

Fortunately these tumours are rare, accounting for about 2% of all large bowel cancers. They are slightly more common in women and may occur in association with carcinoma of the cervix or vulva. Carcinoma of the anus is reportedly more common in male homosexuals and is now recognized as one of the AIDS-related malignancies. The tumour may present as small firm nodules which may be confused with haemorrhoids, the true nature of the lesion becoming apparent only after histological review of the surgical specimen. Rectal bleeding and pain are common symptoms. The diagnosis is often delayed since the symptoms are attributed to haemorrhoids or fissure-in-ano. Other lesions producing occasional diagnostic confusion include leucoplakia, Bowen's disease, or Paget's disease of the anus. Local invasion of the anal sphincter and rectal wall is not uncommon, and more advanced local spread may also occur, to involve the prostate, bladder or cervix. Although mostly squamous carcinomas, other histological types occur including basal cell carcinoma and melanoma. It is important, if possible, to distinguish tumours above the pectinate line from those below since the latter tend to have a better prognosis.

Treatment

Surgical resection is now almost always avoided since non-surgical treatment with radiotherapy (with or without chemotherapy) is generally curative and has become the mainstay of treatment [9,13]. Surgery may, however, be used for very small anal carcinomas or for postradiation recurrence.

In cases initially treated by surgery or radiotherapy but subsequently developing inguinal node metastases, block dissection of the nodes is usually preferable to radiotherapy as a means of ensuring local control, though additional postoperative irradiation can be useful if the dissection is incomplete. Prophylactic block dissection of the inguinal nodes is not usually recommended. In the United Kingdom, a multicentre national study was evaluating the role of adjuvant chemotherapy for anal carcinoma using a combination of 5-FU and mitomycin C. This large study was closed unexpectedly early because of unequivocal superiority (using colostomy requirement as the endpoint) of chemo-radiation over radiotherapy alone. (J. Northover, personal communication).

Care must be taken to avoid, if possible, treating the whole of the anal sphincter in order to avoid extensive fibrosis which might make defaecation impossible.

Prognosis

Prognosis in carcinoma of the anus depends on the location and tumour grade. The 5-year survival rate in patients undergoing abdominoperineal resection is 30–50%. Results from radical radio-chemotherapy are at least as good, with excellent functional preservation in the majority of cases. For tumours of the anal verge, the 5-year survival rate is of the order of 60%. If inguinal nodes are involved at diagnosis, 5-year survival falls to 15%.

REFERENCES

1 Willett W.C., Stampfer M.J., Colditz G.A., Rosner B.A., Speizer F.E. Relation of meat, fat and fiber intake to the risk of colon cancer in a prospective study among women. *New England Journal of Medicine* 1990; **323**: 1664–72.

2 Haenszel W., Correa P. Cancer of the colon and rectum and adenomatous polyps. A review of epidemiologic findings. *Cancer* 1971; **28**: 14–24.

3 Lennard-Jones J.W., Morson B.C., Richie J.K., Shone D.C., Williams C.B. Cancer in colitis. Assessment of the individual risk by clinical and histological criteria. *Gastroenterology* 1977; **73**: 1280–89.

4 Chamberlain J. Is screening for colorectal cancer worthwhile? *British Journal of Cancer* 1990; **62**: 1–3.

5 Kronberg O., Fenger C., Olsen J., Beck K., Sondergaard O. Repeated screening for colorectal cancer with faecal occult blood test. *Scandinavian Journal of Gastroenterology* 1989; **24**: 599–606.

6 Moss S., Draper G.J., Hardcastle J.D., Chamberlain J. Calculation of sample size in trials for early diagnosis of disease. *International Journal of Epidemiology* 1987; **16**: 104–10.

7 Gastrointestinal Tumour Study Group. Prolongation of the disease-free interval in surgically treated rectal carcinoma. *New England Journal of Medicine* 1985; **312**: 1465–72.

8 Krook J.E., Moertel C.G., Gunderson L.L. *et al.* Effective surgical adjuvant therapy for high risk rectal carcinoma. *New England Journal of Medicine* 1991; **324**: 709–15.

9 Papillon J. Intracavitary irradiation of early rectal cancer for cure. *Cancer* 1975; **36**: 696–701.

10 Moertel C.G., Fleming T.R., MacDonald J.S. *et al.* Levamisole and fluorouracil for adjuvant therapy of resected colon carcinoma. *New England Journal of Medicine* 1990; **322**: 352–58.

11 Buyse M., Zeleniuch-Jacquotte A., Chalmers T.C. Adjuvant therapy of colorectal cancer: why we still don't know. *Journal of the American Medical Association* 1988; **259**: 3571–78.

12 Hardcastle J.D., Thomas W.M., Chamberlain J. *et al.* Randomized controlled trial of faecal occult blood screening for colorectal cancer. Results of the first 107,349 subjects. *Lancet* 1989; **i**: 1160–64.

13 Winawer S.J. Radiotherapy in the management of epidermoid-carcinoma of the anal region. *Diseases of the Colon and Rectum* 1982; **17**: 181.

Chapter 17
Gynaecological Cancer

INTRODUCTION

Gynaecological cancers account for approximately one-quarter of all malignant disease in women, although there are striking differences in incidence for each of the major primary sites. (Figs 17.1 & 17.2). After carcinoma of the breast, carcinoma of the cervix is the commonest cancer in women. Tumours of the female genital tract are important not only because of their high incidence, but also because many can be diagnosed whilst still relatively localized. Standard screening techniques are capable of recognizing early and even premalignant stages of disease (see below). Management of these cases often involves the combined skills of surgeons, radiotherapists and medical oncologists, and many women with gynaecological cancer are best treated with a combination of these approaches.

The overall incidence rates of carcinomas of cervix, corpus uteri and ovary are approximately equal, but because curative treatment is much less likely in ovarian carcinoma, the mortality from this disease now exceeds the combined death rate from carcinomas of the cervix and corpus [1,2]. There are a number of known aetiological factors for gynaecological cancer. Important clues have been obtained from epidemiological studies which have shown, for example, that the low incidence of carcinoma of the ovary in Japanese women rapidly rises within a generation or two when they emigrate to the United States — a 6-fold increase which strongly suggests environmental factors predominating over genetic ones. As the aetiology of these malignant diseases becomes better understood, it is clear that the social behaviour of the individual is of considerable importance as a risk factor: good examples would include the relatively high risk of ovarian cancer amongst nulliparous or subfertile women and the close relationship between *in situ* invasive carcinoma of the cervix, and early sexual experience and social class (Fig. 17.3). It is encouraging that screening programmes have undoubtedly helped to reduce the frequency of frankly invasive carcinomas of the cervix [3].

CARCINOMA OF THE CERVIX

Incidence and aetiology

The aetiology of carcinoma of the cervix has been a subject of great interest over the past 20 years. The disease is extremely rare in nuns, and seems clearly related to sexual intercourse and multiple partners. More women with carcinoma of the cervix have been sexually active before the age of 20 than groups of matched controls. Race and social class also seem important, but may not be independent factors since sexual behaviour may differ in these groups. For example, in New York city, the incidence per 100 000 women was 97.6 for Puerto Ricans, 47.8 for black women, 13.5 for white non-Jewish women and 3.6 for Jewish women. It has frequently been suggested that the low incidence of carcinoma of the cervix amongst Jewish women may be the result of male circumcision. However, at least one study has suggested that circumcision of the male partner may be a less important factor than was previously thought.

Many other related aspects of hygiene could be more relevant and it is also likely that such

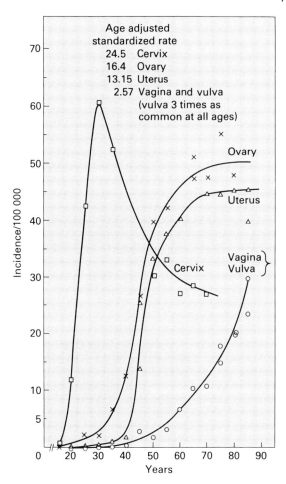

Fig. 17.1 Age-specific incidence of gynaecological cancers. The high incidence of carcinoma of the cervix below the age of 40 is chiefly due to *in situ* cases.

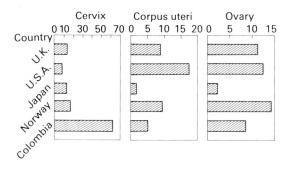

Fig. 17.2 Geographic variation in gynaecological cancer incidence (per 100 000). *Note*: figures for cervix exclude *in situ* cases.

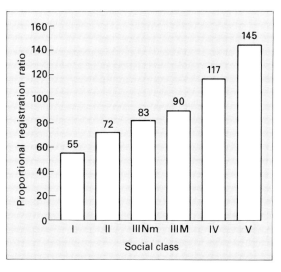

Fig. 17.3 The relationship between carcinoma of the cervix and social class in England and Wales, 1984.

women also start intercourse later in life, and have fewer partners.

There is some evidence that the peak age of onset is falling, possibly because of changes in social habits (see below). In recent years there has been a significant reduction in invasive carcinoma of the cervix, coupled with an increase in micro-invasive or *in situ* disease. Data from the Second (1947) and Third (1969) USA National Cancer Surveys showed a decrease in the annual rate of invasive cervical cancers from 118 to 88 cases per 100 000; invasive carcinomas now account for less than one-third of the total incidence of cervical neoplasia.

The importance of sexual intercourse raises the question of a transmitted agent being responsible. Recent interest has centred around the human papilloma viruses (particularly types 11 and 16) which have been shown to produce morphological changes in human vaginal cells. Apart from the known link with sexual activity and social class, important additional aetiological factors include smoking [4] and a history of cervical dysplasia. Women in developing countries seem also to have a much higher risk of developing cervical carcinoma. Worldwide, this is the second commonest female cancer with some 460 000 new cases annually, 76% occurring in the developing world. Furthermore, it is now clear that insufficient attention has been paid to the substantial incidence of this disorder in women over the age of 65 years who are not routinely eligible for screening in most Western countries [5]. Older women often present with late stages of disease and in the United Kingdom it has been calculated that more active screening of older women would result in hundreds of lives saved annually in the United Kingdom.

Pathology and spread

The widespread application of routine Papanicolaou screening cytology has taught us a great deal about precancerous lesions in the cervix. These changes, collectively known as cervical intraepithelial neoplasia (CIN), can be graded according to the degree of cytological abnormality. Carcinoma *in situ* (now often referred to as CIN 3) represents the most severe of the pre-invasive intraepithelial changes. Though it may remain superficial for up to 20 years, a large proportion, possibly 30–40% of these lesions, will develop into true invasive carcinomas if left untreated [6]. Invasive carcinoma of the cervix probably represents the extreme of a spectrum of cell changes from normality through to carcinoma *in situ*, which is clearly a pre-invasive malignancy.

The usual invasive lesion is a squamous carcinoma which accounts for 85% of all cases. These are typical squamous cell carcinomas, arranged in nests and sheets of abnormal tissue and invading the cervical stroma. Adenocarcinoma accounts for a further 5–10%, and the remainder are much rarer lesions including mixed adenosquamous tumours, adenoacanthomas and sarcomas. There is no firm evidence that adenocarcinomas should be treated differently from squamous cell carcinomas, but surgery has in the past been preferred to radiation therapy. It is thought that the majority of adenocarcinomas of the cervix arise from the endocervical canal.

The major routes of spread are predictable, forming the basis of standard surgical and pathological staging (Table 17.1; Fig. 17.4). Direct and lymphatic spread occur much earlier than haematogenous dissemination. The most important direct routes of spread are downwards into the vaginal vault (often extending microscopically and submucosally beyond the limits of visible or palpable disease) and laterally beyond the paracervical tissues to the parametria, resulting in extension to the lateral wall of the true pelvis.

Lymphatic spread takes place via the paracervical lymphatics and from there to pelvic and para-aortic groups which largely follow the course of the major vessels. Surgical, CT, MRI and lymphographic studies have confirmed a high incidence of nodal spread even in patients with localized disease with tumours apparently confined to the cervix but with no obvious clinical extension into the vagina, uterus or parametria. Nodal metastases can be identified in almost 20% of these 'early' cases. Sites of blood-borne metastases include the lungs, liver and bone (rarely, and chiefly by local extension).

Anterior view   Lateral view

Fig. 17.4 Lymphatic drainage of the cervix. Lymphatic involvement in carcinoma of the cervix generally occurs in an orderly progression. The sequence is (A) obturator; (B) internal, external and common iliac; (C) lateral sacral; (D) para-aortic.

Table 17.1 Clinical staging in carcinoma of the cervix

Stage	Description
Pre-invasive carcinoma	
Stage 0	Carcinoma *in situ*
Invasive carcinoma	
Stage I	Disease confined to the cervix
Ia	Micro-invasive carcinoma
Ib	All other cases of Stage I
Stage II	Disease beyond cervix but not to the pelvic wall. Upper 2/3 of vagina may be involved
IIa	No parametrial involvement evident
IIb	Parametrial involvement
Stage III	Extension to pelvic side wall and/or lower third of vagina. Includes cases with hydronephrosis or non-functioning kidney (unless other known cause exists)
IIIa	No extension to pelvic side wall
IIIb	Extension to pelvic side wall and/or hydronephrosis or non-functioning kidney
Stage IV	Carcinoma beyond true pelvis or involving mucosa of bladder or rectum
IVa	Spread to local organs
IVb	Spread to distant organs

Clinical features

Women with dysplasia or CIN of all grades are invariably free of symptoms though the co-existence of other conditions such as cervical erosion may produce incidental symptoms.

Invasive cancers usually present with vaginal bleeding (80%) and/or discharge, often offensive and discoloured. Many women consider these symptoms a normal feature of their lives and fail to seek advice for many months. Vaginal bleeding often follows intercourse. Abdominal pain, dyspareunia or low back pain may also be present and suggest a bulky or advanced lesion. Urinary and rectal symptoms suggest locally extensive disease.

These tumours are usually visible with simple speculum techniques. *Exophytic* lesions are bulky in character, often forming large friable polypoid growths, making them easy to diagnose. *Infiltrative* tumours can show little in the way of visible ulceration due to a tendency

for abnormal growth to be directed inwards towards the body of the uterus, often replacing the cervix and upper part of the vagina by a large confluent malignant ulcer. If the disease recurs following treatment a characteristic clinical syndrome may develop, with pelvic, back and buttock pain (often with an easily palpable pelvic mass), bowel disturbance, and leg oedema (usually unilateral) due to lymphatic and venous obstruction.

Staging procedures for invasive carcinoma

Careful staging is essential, yielding important prognostic information and facilitating attempts to compare results in centres using different approaches to treatment. The International Federation of Gynaecology and Obstetrics (FIGO) introduced a staging system in 1974 which is still in common use (Table 17.1), and the current TNM system is less widely used. Staging is based on colposcopy, inspection, palpation, curettage and biopsy, together with simple investigations such as chest X-ray and intravenous urography. Colposcopy has become an indispensable staging procedure, capable of diagnosing Stages 0 and Ia cancers which might otherwise escape detection. Wherever possible, examination is performed under anaesthesia. Using these criteria, the reproducibility of assessment is excellent. Unsuspected involvement of the bladder is occasionally found in early cases. Oedema of the bladder mucosa is important since it may be caused by frank invasion of the bladder wall. Intravenous urography is often valuable since hydronephrosis and renal dysfunction are frequently asymptomatic and can occur in patients with clinical Stage Ib disease, placing the tumour into the Stage III category. Lymphography has now largely been replaced by CT scanning but neither is generally regarded as an essential investigation since pelvic nodes are routinely treated either surgically or by external beam irradiation, even in the absence of firm evidence of involvement. Lymphographic studies have shown an increasing incidence of nodal metastases with advancing stage, with involvement in almost 20% of patients with Stage Ib disease, and over 60% of patients with Stage III disease [7].

Other useful investigations include MRI scanning and pelvic ultrasonography, but their value in staging is not yet entirely clear and they have not replaced the other staging procedures.

Management

For patients with CIN 3, therapeutic cone biopsy has been widely employed and usually results in complete excision and cure with preservation of reproductive function. However, newer approaches, particularly laser surgery or cryotherapy, can be expected to cure 70% of cases without cone biopsy. Occasionally, hysterectomy is performed in women beyond the childbearing age or in patients who have no wish for further children. Although hyster-

ectomy is almost always successful, recurrences at the vaginal vault have been reported.

For patients with frankly invasive disease, the most important modalities of treatment are surgery and radiotherapy. Management details vary from one institution to another and it would be unrealistic to deny that local expertise and facilities play an important part in these decisions. Most centres rely on the FIGO staging system to provide guidelines for management.

Stages Ib and IIa cancers are particularly important, now accounting for over half of all carcinomas of the cervix. In some patients, the invasive nature of the disease is more limited than was previously recognized. For this group, with micro-invasive or non-confluent early invasive disease, therapeutic intervention may perhaps be more conservative. It seems important to distinguish true micro-invasive lesions from those with microscopic evidence of lymphovascular involvement. Surgery and radiotherapy are equally effective with high 5-year survival rates (over 85–90% in patients with Stage Ib disease) following either method of treatment [9,10]. Although radiotherapy has become standard treatment in many institutions, few direct comparisons are available from the same source, and no randomized studies have been performed. In general, surgical series tend to be more highly selective — in some series, the operability rate of patients with Stage Ib disease is not much more than half of all patients referred for consideration of surgery. In patients who are suitable, a radical (Wertheim's) hysterectomy is usually recommended. This involves total abdominal hysterectomy with removal of a 2–3 cm cuff of vagina and all supporting tissues within the true pelvis. A complete pelvic lymphadenectomy is performed because 20% of patients have lymph node involvement. Bilateral oophorectomy is often performed but is not mandatory since the tumour rarely metastasizes to the ovary. Indeed, in young women, conservation of the ovaries is one of the advantages which surgery has over radical radiotherapy.

Care must be taken not to damage the ureters, and operations as extensive as this require great skill. It is better for a limited number of gynaecologists to maintain the technique and to practise it frequently than for all gynaecologists to perform this sort of operation infrequently. An important advantage of surgery is the definition of the true state of spread which should allow more accurate overall planning of treatment; the radiotherapist will never have such complete information. A further important advantage is that although early surgical morbidity is greater than that from radiotherapy, there are undoubtedly fewer late complications.

Surgery in skilled hands is a certainly the treatment of choice for young women in whom avoidance of late radiation reactions is particularly desirable. It is often possible to conserve at least one ovary in an otherwise radical operation.

Despite these advantages many centres still recommend that radiotherapy be employed as initial treatment for carcinoma of the cervix, even in early cases with clinical Stage I disease. In older patients, there is little dispute that radical irradiation is the most appropriate form of treatment.

For patients presenting with more *advanced stages of disease (IIb–IV)*, radiotherapy is clearly the treatment of choice. In some centres (mostly in North America), radical lymphadenectomy is performed in selected cases, but its therapeutic contribution is uncertain and it has no place in routine management. The claim that radiotherapy cannot deal with node-positive cases seems unfounded. Rutledge and colleagues studied 500 patients who underwent full pelvic irradiation followed by lymph node dissection [8]. The number of histologically positive nodes was only one-third of that found in a series of patients treated by surgery alone, suggesting that the radiation therapy had been successful in the majority of cases. Several more recent (but mostly smaller) studies have confirmed this important observation.

Radiation technique and dosage

Radiotherapy is the most important single treatment for carcinoma of the cervix, and can cure substantial numbers of patients even including some with advanced disease and a small proportion of those who relapse following surgery. Both internal (intracavitary) and external treatments are used. Intracavitary radium treatment is of considerable historic importance in the evolution of modern radiotherapy techniques, but with improvement in equipment, external irradiation has assumed an increasing role. In general, intracavitary treatment is of greater importance in early disease and external beam treatment makes the greater contribution in advanced cases. Some patients with early disease are initially unsuitable for intracavitary treatment, particularly where there is distortion of local anatomy, where the vaginal vault is narrow or the cervical os is obliterated by tumour, making such treatment impossible in the first instance.

In most centres, intracavitary treatment consists of placement of an intra-uterine source (usually radioactive caesium rather than radium, because of its more suitable characteristics — see Chapter 5) together with radioactive sources placed adjacent to the cervix in the lateral vaginal fornices (Fig. 17.5). Most centres perform these insertions under a general anaesthetic, except for those employing high dose-rate remote after-loading techniques (see below) where local or epidural anaesthetic is generally sufficient. Radiotherapy departments now mostly employ after-loading techniques, whereby the plastic housing for both the intra-uterine and vaginal fornix containers are introduced first and the active source inserted only when the geometrical placement is perfect. These techniques produce a typical pear-shaped isodose distribution (Fig. 17.6). In this way the uterus, cervix and upper vagina all receive a high dose of radiation, with a decreasing but significant dosage to the paracervical and parametrial tissues including at least some of the regional lymphatics. Traditionally, two points,

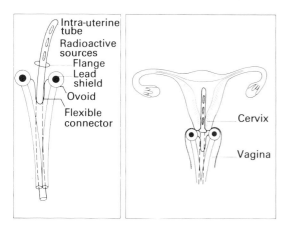

Fig. 17.5 Typical disposable after-loading system of intracavitary irradiation in carcinoma of the cervix. (A) Components; (B) in position. After placement, these sources act as a single irradiation source, and the components are packed into position to retain their location.

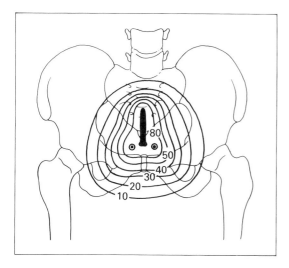

Fig. 17.6 Typical isodose curves following intracavitary placement of caesium sources for carcinoma of the cervix. The numbers refer to the dose in Gy.

designated A and B, are used as a guide to dosimetry. Though variability in gynaecological anatomy necessarily makes dosimetry based on these arbitrary points difficult, they are widely used as a basis for dose calculation. Point A is located 2 cm from the midline of the cervical canal and 2 cm superior to the lateral vaginal fornix. Point B is 3 cm lateral to Point A (i.e. 5 cm from the midline along the same lateral axis).

There is a great variety of applicators, some of which are now disposable. Most low dose-rate techniques employ a relatively short treatment time of the order of 2–3 days, though much longer applications, up to a week or more, are preferred by some. An alternative approach is the use of high dose-rate equipment such as the Cathetron or microSelectron, which allow remote control after-loading of ^{60}Co or ^{192}Ir sources into manually placed applicators. This equipment certainly carries the advantage of a more rapid treatment with minimal hospital in-patient care, without risk of radiation exposure for staff. However, the patient has to accept the discomfort of repeated treatments, and the long-term complications of high dose-rate therapy have yet to be described in detail.

When external beam irradiation is employed in conjunction with intracavitary irradiation, the pelvis is usually treated to a dose of 40–50 Gy (4000–5000 rad) over 4–5 weeks (or equivalent) and supplementary treatment to the parametrial region may also be indicated. Some centres employ higher dosage. Many departments employ a simple anterior and posterior parallel pair of fields with supervoltage equipment, though a multifield arrangement is usually better tolerated. A typical field size of 15 × 15 cm is usually adequate to cover the primary tumour and local nodes. Although some shielding may be possible, irradiation of significant volumes of small and large bowel (including rectum) is unavoidable. In general, it is irradiation damage to these organs which limits whole pelvic dosage. Typical pelvic and parametrial fields are shown in Fig. 17.7. In advanced cases (Stages III and IV), external irradiation is particularly valuable, often controlling pain, haemorrhage and discharge within days. Additionally, intracavitary treatment may be rendered possible as a result of tumour shrinkage. Although some authorities recommend transvaginal or interstitial radiother-

Fig. 17.7 Typical 'whole pelvis' and 'parametrial boost' fields (external beam) used in carcinoma of the cervix. Megavoltage equipment is employed but techniques vary widely. (A) and (B) Whole pelvis. Dotted lines show position of para-aortic field, if used; (C) and (D) parametrial boost, often used if there is palpable residual disease (can be employed bilaterally).

apy for haemorrhage, conventional external beam techniques are probably equally effective.

Combinations of intracavitary and external beam treatment are often employed, though the emphasis may vary in different departments. Fletcher's guidelines (Table 17.2) are based on considerable experience [11] and are widely followed, although they represent a more radical approach in terms of radiation dose, than most British departments would recommend. It is generally accepted that for patients with early stages of disease the intra-

cavitary irradiation is of the greatest importance (additional external irradiation may be unnecessary) and that for more advanced cases, particularly with lateral spread to the pelvic side wall, external radiation therapy to the whole pelvis contributes more to the final probability of cure. When both methods are employed — as in the majority of patients — some radiotherapists prefer the traditional approach of using the intracavitary irradiation first, whereas an increasing number always use external beam treatment initially. Certainly there will be a few

Table 17.2 Radiotherapeutic guidelines for management of carcinoma of the cervix. Values given are for maximum dose. From Fletcher [11]

Stage	Intracavitary irradiation (mg-hour)*	Point A dose (Gy)	External irradiation (Gy) Whole pelvis	Parametrial boost
I (<1 cm)	10 000	62.7	–	–
I (>1 cm) ⎱	6 500–	58.4	0–40	0–40
IIa ⎰	10 000	62.7		
IIb	6 500	58.4	40–50	–
IIIa	6 500	58.4	50	0–15
IIIb	5 000	48.6	60	0–10
IV	4 000	42.6	70	–

* Intracavitary irradiation using radium or (more commonly) caesium is traditionally given on two occasions 1–2 weeks apart though there are many variations both in sources and techniques since the advent of remote after-loading equipment.

Milligram-hour (mg-hr) is simply a convenient measure of radium dosage. It is derived from the product of the number of milligrams of radium multiplied by the number of hours of exposure. For example, a total of 4000 mg-hr could be achieved by an exposure of 40 mg radium for a total of 100 hours. This would generally be attained in two procedures, each lasting 50 hours.

Point A: this radiation dose reference point is measured from the upper surface of the vaginal ovoid (Manchester system) and is situated 2 cm above this level and 2 cm lateral from the midline.

cases in whom the attempt to insert radioactive tubes at the outset is unsuccessful, because of tumour bulk which can to some extent be reduced by treating with external irradiation first. However, the use of intracavitary treatment as primary therapy does allow for central shielding of this treated area when the external beam irradiation is added later — a real advantage in terms of treatment-related side-effects without significantly reducing the overall radiation dosage to the cervix or upper vagina.

Although both early and late complications of irradiation have been reduced substantially by improved technique and understanding of radiation pathology, they cannot be avoided entirely, particularly if effective dosage schedules are rigidly adhered to. Early problems include diarrhoea, anorexia, nausea and vomiting, together with erythema, dry and (less frequently) moist desquamation of the skin. Most of these symptoms are easily controllable with symptomatic measures, and skin problems have been markedly reduced with the routine use of supervoltage equipment. Intracavitary

treatment may produce proctitis and vaginal discharge, although cystitis is less common. Late complications are much more important and include chronic proctosigmoiditis, small bowel damage and rectovaginal or vesicovaginal fistulae, which can require urinary or colonic diversion. Avascular necrosis of the femoral heads was a serious complication before the advent of supervoltage treatment, but is now rarely seen. Chronic skin changes, consisting of excessive fibrosis, depigmentation and telangiectasia, are common though rarely cause serious problems. After radiotherapy, the upper vagina usually becomes stenosed and dry. Sexual intercourse is possible but additional lubrication is often required. Radical surgery leads to a short but normally lubricated vagina. The frequency of radiation sequelae is dependent on dose and technique. When intracavitary irradiation is given before the external beam treatment, central shielding of the external beam can be introduced (Fig. 17.8), to avoid over-irradiation of the primary tumour and midline structures, particularly the rectum.

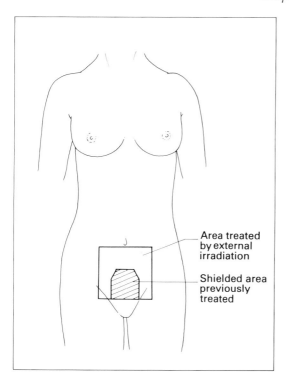

Area treated by external irradiation

Shielded area previously treated

Fig. 17.8 Central shielding of midline structures in external beam therapy of carcinoma of the cervix for use after intracavitary treatment.

This seems reasonable since the dose to central structures is already considerable, because of the effectiveness of intracavitary treatment.

Radiation damage occurs even in the most experienced hands since malignant tumours are only marginally more sensitive to radiation than normal tissues and radiation dosage is therefore limited by the tolerance of surrounding normal tissues such as bladder, bowel, kidneys and skin (see Chapter 5). Fortunately, with increasingly sophisticated planning and treatment techniques, severe complications such as fistulae and bowel necrosis are now seen less frequently.

Treatment of recurrent disease

In patients with recurrent post-irradiation local disease, but no evidence of distant metastases, pelvic exenteration represents the only chance

of cure. This is a major operation with complete removal of the pelvic contents usually including the rectum and bladder, and with a permanent colostomy and ileostomy. Very few surgeons are prepared to undertake this formidable procedure, and careful selection of patients is essential.

Chemotherapy

Although chemotherapy has not proven helpful for prolonging life in patients with advanced or recurrent disease, several agents have now been identified with significant response rates in cervical carcinoma. Cytotoxic drugs with activity in squamous carcinoma of other sites do appear to have similar response rates in cervical carcinoma as well [12]. Increasingly, multi-agent regimens are preferred since the response rates are clearly higher, for example the BIP combination (bleomycin, ifosfamide and cisplatin) has a response rate in previously untreated patients with advanced disease of over 70% [13]. The most promising role for this and other regimens may well lie in their use as 'neoadjuvant' therapy, i.e. before definitive radiotherapy, though, as yet, no clear-cut survival benefit has emerged. None the less, almost all patients enjoy a subjective improvement often including worthwhile relief of pain. The increased number of responses seen in recent years gives some hope that chemotherapy might find a role in initial management.

Prognosis

There was a fall in the overall death rate from carcinoma of the cervix between 1940 and 1960 [14], from 9.8 per 100 000 to 6 per 100 000 white American women, and 21.6 to 16 per 100 000 black American women. This was partly due to the 100% curability of CIN 3, which in recent years has been diagnosed more frequently as a result of routine cervical smear testing. For *invasive* carcinoma there has also been some improvement in overall survival, particularly in older women, in the period 1950–1988 (Fig.

17.9). However, in the increasing proportion of young patients diagnosed during the 1970s and 1980s, the disease appears to be more aggressive and the prognosis worse.

Five-year survival rates reflect the final outcome in the majority of patients, since most, though not all, will recur before five years or not at all. Tumour stage is clearly the most important prognostic factor, and patients with Stage I disease have a 5-year survival rate of 80–90%; the 10–20% who fail are probably those who have occult abdominal nodal disease. For patients with Stage III or IV disease, the 5-year survival rates are of the order of 15–35%, and Stage IV disease has a particularly bad prognosis.

Cancer of the cervix and pregnancy

Diagnosis of cancer of the cervix complicates one in 2500 pregnancies. Moreover, in about 1% of cases of cervical cancer, the diagnosis is made during pregnancy, and this proportion may rise as the mean age of diagnosis of cervical cancer falls. Management depends largely on the stage of disease at diagnosis, but also on the stage of the pregnancy and the mother's wishes regarding termination.

If carcinoma *in situ* is diagnosed in a young woman, it is usually safe to allow the pregnancy to continue, though regular cervical smears and colposcopy should be undertaken throughout the pregnancy. In older women, early surgical treatment (cone biopsy) has in the past been considered advisable though there is a 20% complication rate, particularly from haemorrhage. It is no longer considered necessary, providing regular colposcopy is undertaken.

For invasive carcinoma, treatment during the first and second trimester should generally be undertaken without regard to the fetus, providing the patient is prepared to accept termination. Pelvic irradiation causes fetal death and inevitable abortion within 6 weeks. Following evacuation of the uterus, intracavitary treatments can be undertaken in the usual way. If the diagnosis is made in the final trimester, most authorities agree that treatment can safely be delayed, with elective caesarian section before the 38th week. Treatment is by surgery (sometimes performed at the time of the caesarian section) or by irradiation following healing of the surgical wound. Unfortunately, delayed treatment cannot always be recommended in the third trimester, for example where severe haemorrhage may present a real threat to the mother's health. Provided that diagnosis and treatment are prompt, the results are as good as those obtained in non-pregnant patients.

CARCINOMA OF THE UTERUS

Aetiology

Endometrial carcinoma is commonest amongst women 50–70 years of age. Its incidence has risen slightly in the past 20 years, though the reasons are not entirely clear (see below). There are wide variations in incidence, from a low of 0.6 per 100 000 Nigerian women, to 14 per 100 000 women living in the south of Great

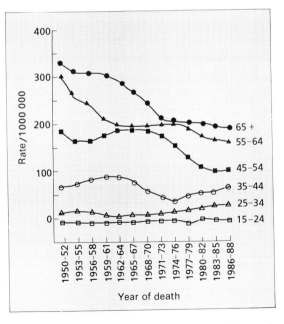

Fig. 17.9 Age-specific mortality of invasive carcinoma of the cervix in England and Wales, 1950–1988.

Britain. It is common in Jewish women. The death rate is low since this is a relatively slow-growing and well-localized malignancy. Obesity, hypertension and diabetes have long been considered to be risk factors and are directly or indirectly associated with excess oestrogen exposure. It seems likely that there is peripheral conversion of oestrogen precursors in fat, which may account at least for the role of obesity. Diabetes and hypertension appear to be risk factors only by virtue of their association with obesity. A widely discussed possible aetiological factor is the presence of endometrial hyperplasia, particularly since the use of exogenous oestrogens for hormone replacement therapy at the menopause frequently produces such change. Of the two major types of endometrial hyperplasia, cystic glandular hyperplasia is generally thought to have a low rate of progression to malignancy, whilst in the other type, atypical adenomatous hyperplasia, at least 1 in 10 patients progress to develop endometrial carcinoma. Late menopause is a risk factor not only because of excess and prolonged oestrogen exposure but also because of the frequency of late anovulatory (oestrogenic) cycles and the presence of metropathia.

A number of studies have suggested an increased incidence of carcinoma of the endometrium in patients taking exogenous oestrogens. In several of these, the risk index for all women receiving oestrogens was over five times that of control subjects. However, there are a number of criticisms of these studies including the frequency with which control cases and patients taking exogenous oestrogen were examined, as well as the possibility that hyperplasia itself can be difficult to distinguish from frank malignancy, even by experienced pathologists. Although there is good evidence therefore that cyclical oestrogen therapy produces endometrial hyperplasia, its role in the development of invasive carcinoma has yet to be fully established. Unopposed continuous oestrogen replacement may be more dangerous in this respect than cyclical oestrogen used in conjunction with a progestogen. Low-dose oestrogen probably carries little risk. Tamoxifen is clearly associated with a small additional risk of endometrial carcinoma (see Chapter 13).

Pathology and staging

By far the commonest of tumours of the body of the uterus is the endometrial adenocarcinoma which constitutes at least 90% of all endometrial neoplasms. The next largest group of endometrial tumours is the adenoacanthoma, which is an adenocarcinoma with areas of benign squamous metaplasia. Mixed mesodermal tumours also occur. Other tumours include adenosquamous carcinoma and a variety of soft tissue sarcomas, chiefly leiomyosarcoma which arises from the muscle wall.

The degree of differentiation of adenocarcinoma of the endometrium can be very variable. Conventionally, three grades or histological differentiations are recognized. The largest single group is the well-differentiated (Grade I) adenocarcinoma.

Lymphatic spread is chiefly to pelvic nodes, particularly the external and common iliac group (and thence to the para-aortic nodes), as well as the paracervical and obturator nodes. Lymph node 'skipping', i.e. with metastatic involvement of para-aortic nodes bypassing the pelvic node groups, is well described. Inguinal node metastases are also encountered. Morrow [15] reviewed a large series of patients with localized carcinoma of the endometrium, noting an incidence of positive nodes of 11% with a particularly high likelihood in patients with Grade III (the most anaplastic) lesions. It was also clear from this and other studies that deep myometrial invasion of tumour is associated with a high incidence of positive local nodes (Table 17.3). As these authors pointed out, this clearly implies that local nodal metastases are almost as common in endometrial carcinoma as in cancer of the cervix.

As with other cancers, the histological grade, depth of invasion, frequency of nodal involvement and likelihood of local recurrence are interrelated variables. For this reason it is diffi-

Table 17.3 Incidence of pelvic lymph node metastases in carcinoma of the endometrium: the relationship to tumour grade and depth of myometrial invasion. Figures refer to the number of patients in whom positive nodes were confirmed (n = 140)

Depth of myometrial invasion	Histological grade			Total number with + ve pelvic lymph nodes (%)
	I	II	III	
<1/3	1/60	4/42	4/14	9/116 (8)
>1/3	1/5	2/8	4/11	7/24 (29)
Total	2/65	6/50	8/25	16/140 (11)

From Morrow [15].

cult to assess the separate contributions of histological grade and tumour stage to prognosis.

Myometrial invasion is important since its depth correlates closely with the incidence of recurrence. Patients whose tumour shows superficial invasion only, have a local recurrence rate of well below 10%, whereas with deep invasion the recurrence rate is approximately 25%. Although more common in patients with high-grade tumours, myometrial involvement is sometimes seen in patients with well-differentiated lesions. Direct spread to the cervix and vagina also occurs though vaginal 'satellite' metastases (i.e. not as part of direct extension) are unusual at presentation. Vaginal deposits are commoner in patients with recurrent disease, and occur predominantly in patients who have not been treated with radiotherapy. Local spread to other pelvic structures such as the broad ligament, fallopian tubes and ovaries also occurs.

Blood-borne metastases are unusual, though more common than with carcinoma of the cervix. Peritoneal involvement, pulmonary deposits and even ascites are features of advanced disease. Late metastases to para-aortic nodes, lung, bone and supraclavicular nodes are increasingly encountered with greater survival time.

The routes of spread and current staging systems are summarized in Fig. 17.10 and Table 17.4. At present both the TNM and FIGO

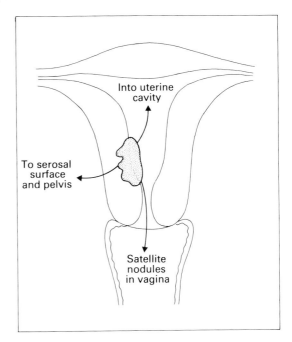

Fig. 17.10 Local spread in carcinoma of the corpus uteri.

Table 17.4 Clinical staging in carcinoma of the endometrium. T-stage (from TNM staging system) shown in brackets, but the staging definitions are essentially those of the FIGO

Stage	Description
Stage 0	Carcinoma *in situ* (T_{is})
Stage I	Carcinoma confined to the corpus uteri (T_1)
Ia	Uterine cavity 8 cm or less in length (T_{1a})
Ib	Uterine cavity >8 cm (T_{1b})
Stage II	Extension to cervix only (T_2)
Stage III	Extension beyond the uterus but disease confined to true pelvis (T_3)
Stage IV	Extension beyond true pelvis, or invasion of bladder or rectum (T_4)

systems are used, though both suffer from the fact that the limits of cancer spread cannot be determined by clinical means as easily as in carcinoma of the cervix. The large majority of patients with endometrial carcinoma have localized disease, and are potentially curable by surgery. For most carcinomas of the uterus, the clinical stage at presentation is Ia or Ib. Surgical staging at laparotomy is particularly important, often dictating which patients require additional treatment, using information which cannot be determined pre-opertively.

Clinical features and treatment

Postmenopausal bleeding is the cardinal symptom of endometrial carcinoma and is an indication for dilatation and curettage even if the bleeding is mild. Twenty per cent of cases occur in perimenopausal patients so intermenstrual bleeding is also an important clinical feature. About 5% of all cases occur in patients below the age of 40 years. Other symptoms such as pain and vaginal discharge are uncommon and suggestive of more advanced disease. The uterus may be enlarged clinically and these patients should be investigated with particular urgency. The diagnosis is established by curettage, and the differential diagnosis includes postmenopausal bleeding from other causes, of which the most common is probably atrophic vaginitis.

Surgery is the most important treatment for endometrial carcinoma. Most gynaecologists agree that a total abdominal hysterectomy with bilateral salpingo-oophorectomy is the operation of choice. Because of the success of surgical treatment in localized cancers, the role of radiotherapy as routine additional treatment has been questioned. There seems little need for irradiation for localized well-differentiated tumours without evidence of myometrial invasion. On the other hand, where the histology is poorly differentiated or anaplastic, many gynaecologists refer such patients for postoperative irradiation because of the risk of local recurrence, particularly in patients with evidence of myometrial invasion beyond one-third of the thickness of the uterine wall. With myometrial penetration, or involvement of the cervix, the risk of node metastases is also high — at least 30% in a high-grade tumour.

Additional radiotherapy treatment can be either pre-operative, usually by means of intra-uterine radioactive caesium insertion, or by external beam irradiation to the true pelvis. Pre-operative intracavitary irradiation reduces the volume of tumour and also reduces the probability of subsequent vaginal metastases. However, pre-operative treatment may be technically difficult because of enlargement of the uterus and/or widespread intra-uterine involvement by the tumour. It may be necessary to pack the uterus with several irradiating sources rather than relying on the arrangement usually employed for carcinoma of the cervix. External beam irradiation may be an acceptable alternative and is also effective for reducing the incidence of vaginal metastases. Such treatment may result in up to 50% of patients being free of disease at the time of subsequent planned hysterectomy.

In Britain, many gynaecologists and radiotherapists advocate pre-operative intracavitary irradiation and a dose of 60 Gy (6000 rad) to Point A (see Table 17.2) is often recommended. However, our own practice is to recommend postoperative external irradiation in selected cases. After total abdominal hysterectomy with bilateral salpingoooophorectomy, supplementary external radiation therapy is best reserved for patients with adverse risk factors such as deep myometrial invasion or poor histology, both of which can be better determined at operation. In most patients, a dose of 45−55 Gy (4500−5500 rad) in daily fractions over 4½−5½ weeks is well tolerated and effective.

In patients with recurrent disease, the use of further irradiation, endocrine therapy with progestogens, or chemotherapy can all be worthwhile. Vaginal recurrences, usually seen in previously unirradiated patients, respond to local therapy with intravaginal caesium loaded in a plastic (Dobbie) applicator, though some radiotherapists prefer to use interstitial radiotherapy (usually with ^{192}Ir).

The most valuable form of systemic therapy is progestogen treatment, which may be beneficial for local recurrence but is particularly valuable for patients with distant metastatic disease. Several large series of patients have confirmed that about one-third show an objective response, and that responding patients have a much longer lifespan than patients who show no response. On the other hand, the use of progestogens as an adjuvant to surgery has not been shown to prolong survival. The most popular drug is medroxyprogesterone acetate, given by mouth at doses of the order of 100 mg t.d.s. Pulmonary metastases seem particularly likely to respond.

In patients who fail to respond to progestogen therapy, chemotherapy has sometimes been of value. The most useful agents appear to be cyclophosphamide, 5-FU, vincristine and doxorubicin. Combination chemotherapy may produce more responses than treatment with single agents, but at the cost of increased toxicity. There is no place for chemotherapy in the routine treatment of early endometrial carcinoma.

For further discussion of uterine sarcomas and their management, see Chapter 23.

Prognosis

In white American women, the age-adjusted death rate is 1.4 per 100 000, with a total death rate of 3300 in 1975. About two-thirds of patients with endometrial carcinoma are cured by current treatments. As previously mentioned, the survival falls with extra-uterine spread, poorly differentiated tumours and those with deep myometrial invasion.

Unfortunately, no prospectively randomized study has been done to assess the value of pre- or postoperative radiotherapy as an adjunct to surgery. Taking together the large series of patients treated with pre-operative radiotherapy and surgery, the 5-year survival rate is over 75%. Indeed the results of radiotherapy alone have often surprised those who feel surgery to be essential. In Kottmeier's classic series of almost 1500 patients treated in Stockholm, the 5-year survival was 63% [16]. The survival of 'operable lesions' (809 patients) was 79%, comparable to or better than many of the surgical series.

The relatively good prognosis of endometrial carcinoma is largely due to the preponderance of localized disease, which itself is probably a reflection of the slow-growing nature of the tumour and the early concern aroused by its major symptom: postmenopausal bleeding.

The increasing incidence of adenosquamous carcinomas is of considerable concern since this particular group of tumours is often thought to have a poor prognosis. The 5-year survival rate is less than 20%, compared to over 70% for well-differentiated adenocarcinomas and adenoacanthomas. Patients with sarcomas of the uterus also do less well, with reported 5-year survival rates between 15% and 32%, but possibly with a slightly more favourable outlook in younger women. Once again, in this group the degree of myometrial invasion is important. If leiomyosarcoma is an incidental finding following removal of a uterine fibroid, the survival rate is over 80% whereas in patients with invasive leiomyosarcomas, survival is very poor indeed.

CARCINOMA OF THE OVARY

Little is known of the aetiology of this disease. It is commoner in women carrying the BRCA1 gene [17], and in nulliparous and subfertile women. There are wide demographic differences in mortality rates; for example, the mortality rate in Denmark is six times as great as in Japanese women. There is both a familial incidence and an increased frequency in women with breast cancer — both also related to nulliparity and possession of BRCA1. In addition there is a 10% risk of ovarian tumours in patients with the Peutz–Jeghers syndrome.

Ovarian cancer has become the most common pelvic malignancy in many Western countries, and is the sixth commonest female tumour in the United Kingdom. In the years 1979–82 3500 cases were diagnosed annually, a crude yearly rate of 17.3 per 100 000.

Clinical features

These tumours usually present late and only one-third are localized at the time of diagnosis. Early ovarian cancer is often asymptomatic.

When symptoms occur they are often vague and are overlooked by the patients even when the tumour is locally advanced and lower abdominal distension has become medically obvious. Lower abdominal pain, bloating and anorexia are common, but often insufficiently specific to raise suspicions which might then lead to further investigation. Signs such as ascites or palpable pelvic masses often indicate advanced disease. Even with more widespread use of cervical smear tests and annual examinations, the proportion of early diagnoses has not risen. At present there is no evidence that routine screening tests are able to uncover a significant number of women with early disease. Possibilities for the future include pelvic ultrasound, which is rapidly improving in its resolving power, as well as transvaginal aspiration with cytology of peritoneal washings and also the increasing use of CA-125, a moderately specific tumour antigen which is elevated in a large proportion of patients with ovarian carcinoma [18] and can be detected by a simple blood test. It has a semi-quantitative relationship with tumour response or progression. So far, rate of diagnosis in asymptomatic women is low but these and other methods may prove valuable in the future, particularly perhaps if used in combination.

Pathology, staging and prognosis

There is great variety in the histological subtypes of ovarian cancer. The World Health Organization lists 27 subtypes for benign and malignant primary ovarian tumours [19]. About 90% of ovarian carcinomas originate from the epithelial surface of the ovary, the remainder comprising the much less common group of germ cell tumours (both teratomas and dysgerminomas), ovarian sarcomas, granulosa cell tumours, thecomas, Leydig and Sertoli cell tumours. Of the epithelial carcinomas, the major types include serous cystadenocarcinoma, mucinous, endometrioid, clear cell (mesonephroid) and undifferentiated adenocarcinomas. For epithelial tumours there is little doubt that the tumour grade, or degree of differentiation, is of prognostic importance, at least in serious tumours. Within this group, the histological grade can vary from those which are barely malignant to highly undifferentiated invasive tumours. In general, tumours which are relatively well-differentiated are more likely to be operable. Mucinous tumours appear to be associated with improved survival by comparison with serous carcinomas.

Clinical staging is of considerable importance in ovarian cancer and is often considered the most important indicator of prognosis [20]. The FIGO staging system is now widely accepted (Table 17.5), and Table 17.6 shows the relation between FIGO stage and prognosis. Patients with disease localized to the ovaries have an overall survival rate of 60%. However, even within this group, further risk factors have been identified. For example, in a large series from the Mayo clinic, patients with intracystic tumours had a 5-year survival rate of 98%, whereas in those with adherence of the tumour to surrounding structures, the 5-year survival was reduced by half. When the disease has spread outside the ovary but is still confined to the pelvis, there is an important distinction

Table 17.5 FIGO staging system in carcinoma of the ovary. From Tobias and Griffiths [19]

Stage	Description
Stage I	Growth limited to ovary (26%)*
Ia	One ovary involved
Ib	Both ovaries involved
Ic	Ascites present, or positive peritoneal washings
Stage II	Growth limited to pelvis (21%)
IIa	Extension to gynaecological adnexae
IIb	Extension to other pelvic tissues
Stage III	Growth extending to abdominal cavity — including peritoneal surface seedlings, omentum etc. (37%).
Stage IV	Metastases to distant sites (including hepatic parenchymal disease) (16%)

* Figures in brackets refer to proportion of total cases presenting with each particular stage.

Table 17.6 Relationship between FIGO stage and prognosis in carcinoma of the ovary. From Tobias and Griffiths [20]

Stage	Number of patients	5-year survival rates (%)
Stage I	751	61
Ia	528	65
Ib	130	52
Ic	80	52
Stage II	401	40
IIa*	40	60
IIb	205	38
Stage III	539	5
Stage IV	101	3

* The distinction between Stages IIa and IIb is a particularly important one prognostically, the 5-year survival of patients with Stage IIa disease being similar to that of patients with Stage I disease.

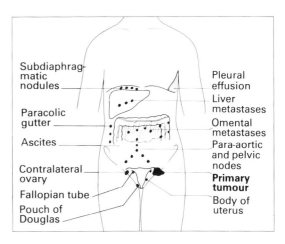

Fig. 17.11 Common sites of metastasis in carcinoma of the ovary.

between tumours with minimal local spread to adjacent gynaecological organs (Stage IIa) which carry a 5-year survival rate almost as good as Stage I tumours, and those which have spread more widely (Stage IIb) and which carry a very much poorer prognosis.

Once the tumour has disseminated beyond the pelvis into the peritoneal cavity, the outlook is very much worse, particularly in patients with bulky abdominal disease. Common sites of intra-abdominal tumour include the omentum, the peritoneal surface (often the site of multiple seedlings) and the undersurface of the diaphragm, a particularly important area for inspection at the initial operation (Fig. 17.11). Beyond the peritoneal cavity, important sites for metastasis include liver, lungs and occasionally the central nervous system. Lymph node spread is chiefly to pelvic and para-aortic nodes, and less commonly to supraclavicular, neck and inguinal nodes. Bone marrow dissemination is extremely unusual.

For women below the age of 65 years, ovarian cancer is a significant cause of death, particularly since the majority of patients with this disease present with advanced stages of disease

(Table 17.5). Survival has improved little if at all in recent years, with over 4000 deaths in the United Kingdom in 1989 (OPCS data) making it the fifth most lethal female cancer and accounting for 1000 more deaths than cervix and corpus uteri combined. The average 5-year survival for cases diagnosed during 1970–80 was only 25% and overall, death from ovarian cancer accounts for 4.4% of all cancer deaths in women aged 35–60 years (exceeded by lung and breast cancer). The age-specific mortality increases from 0.8 (per 100 000) for ages 25–34 to 17.7 for ages 45–54 and to 35.0 at ages 55–64 years. Survival is closely related to stage (Table 17.6) and there is also evidence that younger women may survive better, possibly related to improved diagnosis or, possibly, use of oral contraceptives.

Surgical management

Operative treatment has always been the cornerstone of successful management in ovarian cancer. The initial operation has a greater bearing on outcome than any subsequent therapy, and the success of postoperative treatment largely depends on careful operative assessment and adequate removal of tumour.

Careful inspection of the whole of the abdominal cavity is an essential part of the initial procedure before removal of tumour. In particular, the infradiaphragmatic surfaces and paracolic gutters should be carefully inspected, since these are common but often overlooked sites of spread. Even when subdiaphragmatic seedlings are not visible, peritoneal lavage may reveal malignant cells from this and other sites. The importance of such inspection cannot be overestimated since a substantial proportion of patients initially thought to have localized disease have evidence of more widespread dissemination, making local treatment entirely inappropriate.

For Stage I disease, surgery is often the only treatment recommended and usually consists of total abdominal hysterectomy and bilateral salpingo-oophorectomy. Even with unilateral tumours, the opposite ovary is normally removed as there is a 20% frequency of bilateral tumours or occult metastases. In young women, particularly those anxious to retain fertility, conservative operations are occasionally performed, though the safety of this approach is uncertain. In tumours of borderline malignancy, conservative operations can be recommended with greater confidence though most gynaecologists understandably prefer to perform a full operation unless the patient is particularly anxious to become pregnant.

In patients with more advanced disease (Stages II−IV) the consensus of opinion favours excision of as much tumour as possible at the time of initial operation. Good palliation may be achieved by the reduction of a heavy tumour burden but there is little evidence that surgical debulking procedures substantially improve survival unless all or nearly all of the tumour can be excised. Many of the technically operable tumours are of relatively low grade which will itself imply a more favourable prognosis. None the less, Griffiths and others have shown that the size of the largest postoperative residual tumour nodule is a good predictor not only of responsiveness to the subsequent postoperative treatment, but also of the ultimate outcome [21]. Using a multiple linear regression equation with survival as the dependent variable, only histological tumour grade and size of the largest postoperative residual mass were factors of real importance; the operation itself contributed nothing to survival, unless it reduced the size of the largest tumour mass below an upper limit of 1.6 cm in diameter.

Postoperative chemotherapy or radiotherapy in patients with residual palpable masses is extremely unlikely to be curative. For this reason many radiotherapists and oncologists recommend a second operative procedure by an expert gynaecologic-oncologist in selected patients in whom the initial laparotomy did not include any attempt at removal of tumour. It therefore seems likely that expert surgeons will be needed to perform the definitive operation, wherever possible. Gynaecological oncologists have become increasingly radical in their surgical approach, and lengthy operations including removal of pelvic contents, omentectomy, bowel resection and excision of the entire parietal pelvic peritoneum, are now performed more frequently [21].

Quite apart from the critically important first operation, the gynaecologist may have a role in 'second-look' procedures. Despite the advent of abdomino-pelvic ultrasonography, lymphography, CT scanning and other imaging procedures, there is no reliable guide to the effectiveness of treatment in advanced ovarian cancer short of a further exploratory procedure. Such information may be useful for several reasons. First, it indicates whether postoperative treatment has been successful in eradicating residual tumour. Secondly, it may be possible to perform further surgery at the second procedure. Finally, in patients who have achieved a complete remission confirmed by a second-look procedure, it may be reasonable to discontinue chemotherapy. Laparotomy may not be required in all such cases, since laparoscopic re-evaluation sometimes shows residual disease even in patients who have achieved a complete clinical remission. Laparotomy is justifiable in cases where laparoscopic examination has failed to show residual disease and peritoneal washings have been negative. None the less, it is difficult to demonstrate beyond doubt that second-look laparotomy has contributed to improved survival in ovarian cancer, although treatment decisions have become more logical as a result. It is now widely accepted that second-look laparotomy only has a role where it could reasonably be expected to influence further treatment. If no further therapeutic options are felt suitable — for example in patients who have relapsed after multiple courses of combination chemotherapy — then second-look laparotomy cannot be justified on grounds of academic interest alone. It is fair to say the second-look (and subsequent) laparotomy is more widely practised in the United States and parts of Europe than in the United Kingdom.

In summary, the role of the gynaecological surgeon in the management of ovarian cancer has changed and continues to evolve. The initial assessment and operative procedure is a critically important part of management, both for localized and generalized disease. The surgeon also has an important role in the assessment of response. Although second-look laparotomy is the most reliable means of judging response, there remains considerable doubt about its therapeutic value in patients with residual disease.

Radiotherapy

Radiotherapy has been used in several distinct ways: as definitive therapy, as an adjuvant to surgery, for recurrent disease and occasionally as pre-operative treatment. It has often been recommended as postoperative treatment for patients with disease confined to the pelvis, though evidence for its routine use is unconvincing [16]. The two main techniques which have been used are first, pelvic irradiation (for patients with Stage I or II disease) usually to a dose of 40–50 Gy (4000–5000 rad) over 4–5½ weeks, using either anteroposterior or multifield techniques (Fig. 17.12); and secondly, whole abdominal

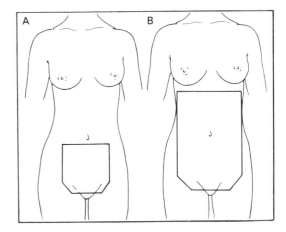

Fig. 17.12 Commonly used radiotherapy treatments in carcinoma of the ovary. (A) Pelvic field; (B) whole abdominal irradiation.

irradiation. The latter is technically one of the most difficult techniques in clinical radiotherapy, and is always difficult to achieve, in view of the very large treatment volume (Fig. 17.12). Adequate irradiation including the subdiaphragmatic areas results in a treatment volume extending from the pelvic floor to the domes of the diaphragm. The dose rate has to be low (usually 1 Gy/day) for patients to be able to tolerate this treatment without developing severe nausea and myelosuppression. It is especially difficult to deliver after chemotherapy because of the risk of radiation nephritis and hepatitis. The kidneys and liver are shielded after doses of 15–20 Gy and the total elsewhere has to be limited to doses of the order of 25 Gy (usually taking about 5 weeks daily treatment) together with boosting of the pelvis alone to a dose of 40–50 Gy (4000–5000 rad).

In FIGO Stage I disease, retrospective studies of surgery alone versus surgery with postoperative irradiation have suffered from the usual difficulty that the two study groups may not have been similar enough for comparison to be valid.

In many of these retrospective studies, the group receiving postoperative radiotherapy did less well than the group receiving surgery alone, implying that patients selected for postoperative irradiation were, in general, a higher risk group, because of cyst rupture at operation or other unspecified features. Five-year survival rates in patients with Stage I disease vary from 50 to 65%, regardless of whether or not radiotherapy is given. Survival figures from prospective studies of surgery alone versus surgery plus local irradiation are beginning to emerge, though no clear differences have so far been demonstrated. There may possibly be a role for adjuvant chemotherapy in Stage I disease particularly with high-grade or adherent tumours (see below).

In Stage II disease, there seems to be a genuine benefit from the use of postoperative pelvic irradiation [19]. In almost all series, admittedly retrospective, the 5-year survival rate was improved (Table 17.7), particularly where adequate surgery had already been undertaken (see p. 334). Since these studies were performed before careful operative staging was a routine part of the initial assessment, many of these patients would in fact have had Stage III disease. For this reason the results of postoperative radiotherapy in true Stage II disease may be even better than these figures

suggest. In patients with more advanced disease (Stages III–IV) the value of postoperative irradiation is equivocal; although postoperative whole abdominal irradiation has been claimed to produce modest improvement in 5-year survival from about 5% to 10%, the evidence is unconvincing. In the 1970s, work from Toronto reawakened interest in radiation therapy for ovarian carcinoma [22]. Patients undergoing surgery (total hysterectomy, bilateral salpingo-oophorectomy and omentectomy) were randomized to receive either chemotherapy with chlorambucil, pelvic irradiation alone, or radiotherapy to the whole abdomen with a boost to the pelvic region. There was a clear survival advantage for patients receiving abdomino-pelvic irradiation (Stages IIa–III) despite the difficulties in achieving more than a low dose of irradiation to such a large area (Fig. 17.13). There seems little doubt that the superior results from this study largely reflected the adequacy of initial surgical treatment. There was a highly significant survival difference in favour of patients without palpable postoperative tumour, regardless of whether chemotherapy or radiotherapy was used as the postoperative treatment. It is also possible that the 'moving

Table 17.7 Adjuvant radiotherapy in FIGO Stage II disease. From Tobias and Griffiths [19]

Number of patients		5-year survival rates (%)	
Operation alone	Operation + irradiation	Operation alone	Operation + irradiation
8	22	25.0	36.4
27	91	33.0	48.0
32	36	28.2	52.8
16	61	0	40.0
4	12	55.0	63.0
6	51	16.7	31.4
—	18*	—	72 †
—	6‡	—	33 †
—	13	—	69
13	16	23.1	25

* Palpable disease after operation
† 4-year follow-up results only
‡ No palpable disease after operation

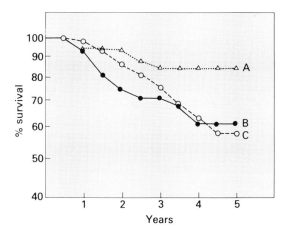

Fig. 17.13 Survival in Stages Ib and II carcinoma of the ovary treated with pelvic irradiation after surgery. (A) Additional whole abdominal irradiation; (B) pelvic irradiation alone; (C) Additional chlorambucil. (From Dembo *et al.* [21]. With permission.)

strip' technique of radiotherapy employed by this group allowed a reasonable radiation dose to be delivered without undue toxicity though later data discount this view. As expected the radiation dosage was limited by renal, hepatic and bowel tolerance. Most radiotherapists feel that the gastro-intestinal dysfunction and partial bowel obstruction so commonly associated with advanced ovarian cancer makes many patients poor candidates for whole-abdominal irradiation, with its high likelihood of additional gastro-intestinal side-effects. Unfortunately the incidence of recurrent sub-acute bowel obstruction appears to be increased by the use of abdominal radiation therapy [20].

An alternative form of radiotherapy is the use of intraperitoneal radioactive colloids such as gold (^{198}Au) or phosphorus (^{32}P). Originally used for treatment of malignant effusions, they have gradually been replaced by systemic treatment with chemotherapy. This approach is now more commonly used as adjuvant therapy in patients with small superficial intraperitoneal tumour implants, particularly when recurrent ascites, not controlled by cytotoxic drugs, is a clinical problem. It has also been claimed that radioactive colloids are of value in patients with Stage I disease either incompletely removed, or resected with intra-operative spillage from rupture of a malignant cyst [23].

Chemotherapy

For patients who present with disease outside the true pelvis (FIGO Stages III and IV) the initial treatment after surgery is usually with chemotherapy. In addition, chemotherapy is increasingly offered to selected patients with Stage I disease notably those with high-grade tumours, adherence or incomplete resection. Although no convincing randomized studies have yet confirmed a survival benefit, increasingly effective anti-emetic and other support techniques have made single-agent chemotherapy widely acceptable to this group of patients at high risk of postoperative relapse. Ovarian cancer is moderately sensitive to cyto-

toxic agents but for most drugs, information regarding response rates to single agents was gained at a time when no attempt had been made to reduce tumour bulk before starting treatment. Since massive disease so clearly reduces responsiveness (see Chapter 6), the reported response rates to many agents may be lower than those which could be achieved under more favourable conditions. Stringent criteria of assessment were seldom used; complete response therefore usually meant no more than the clinical disappearance of disease, artificially raising the response rate. Nowadays response rate data should be based on careful pre- and post-treatment assessment of tumour size, including, where necessary, the use of imaging techniques and, if appropriate, second-look laparotomy.

SINGLE AGENTS

The response rates to the most useful single agents are shown in Table 17.8. Alkylating agents have been widely employed [20]. Chlorambucil, cyclophosphamide and melphalan

Table 17.8 Response to single-agent chemotherapy in advanced ovarian carcinoma

Agent	Response rate (%)
Alkylating agents	
Cyclophosphamide	50–60
Chlorambucil	50
Melphalan	45
Antimetabolites	
Methotrexate	25
5-FU	25
Others	
Cisplatin*	40–60
Doxorubicin*	30–40
Hexamethylmelamine	30–40
Paclitaxel*	25

* Since much of the data regarding response rates of newer drugs has been obtained in patients already resistant to alkylating agents, the true single-agent response to cisplatin, doxorubicin, paclitaxel and others may be higher.

have been used most frequently, with response rates for each in the range of 40%. Recent studies have not altered this figure. There is, however, some evidence that response rates are higher when the dose is given in high dose in a pulsed intermittent form. Of the antimetabolites, 5-FU and methotrexate have some activity but complete responses are rarely seen. The vinca alkaloids have not been tested extensively in ovarian cancer but reported response rates are low. Hexamethylmelamine is a drug with activity, though its side-effects are considerable (see Chapter 6) and it is not widely used at present. Although introduced more recently, cisplatin and its derivatives — notably carboplatin — have rapidly become established as the most important agents in ovarian cancer. Response rates of 25—60% have been recorded, but the schedules of administration have varied widely. There is evidence that higher doses may be associated with increased response rates, though of course this incurs the penalty of increased toxicity. It is now clear that cisplatin is more effective than alkylating agents such as cyclophosphamide. Cisplatin is a toxic drug though recent advances in anti-emetic therapy, particularly with $5HT_3$ antagonists such as ondansetron, have made it far more acceptable. The newer analogues appear to have similar activity to the parent compound, but reduced toxicity [24]. Unfortunately, despite the lesser degree of gastro-intestinal toxicity, carboplatin is a more myelosuppressive agent than cisplatin and is less easy to use in combination regimens. Doxorubicin has some activity (30% response rate) but is not useful in patients who have relapsed after failure with alkylating agents. The recent interest in paclitaxel (Taxol), the first in a group of taxane cytotoxic agents, arises from its unequivocal activity in cisplatin-resistant disease [29]. The overall response rate, however, is under 25% with fewer than 5% complete responders.

In ovarian cancer attempts have been made to predict tumour responsiveness *in vitro* using colony formation (see Chapter 6). It is too soon to assess the potential of these techniques. At present it seems that they will only provide negative evidence — if a drug is inactive *in vitro*, it will be ineffective *in vivo* [25].

COMBINATION CHEMOTHERAPY

As in other malignancies, there has been an increasing tendency in recent years to use combinations of drugs for advanced ovarian cancer. In previously untreated patients, higher response rates have been achieved than with single agents (Table 17.9). However, where studies have been carried out in patients who have relapsed after treatment with a single agent, responses to the combinations have usually been poor.

Most of these studies have not made any formal comparison with a single agent so that an advantage in *survival* over simple alkylating agent therapy has not been shown. In the widely quoted study of Young *et al.*, an early advantage was observed for combination chemotherapy over single-agent treatment [26], but the toxicity was much greater. In a study from the Mayo Clinic a similar advantage for a two-drug regimen (cyclophosphamide and doxorubicin) was seen only in patients with minimal residual disease after surgery [27]. A large Italian study [28] suggested an improvement with combined use of cyclophosphamide and cisplatin (compared with cisplatin alone) although the addition of a third drug, doxorubicin, was unhelpful.

In future studies of combination chemotherapy, it will be essential to compare effective combinations with single-agent therapy after 'debulking' surgery has been carried out. It is important to establish whether aggressive chemotherapy increases the chance of cure in patients who have had effective surgery. Studies which include a majority of patients with a poor prognosis (including those in whom the operation did not attempt any worthwhile removal of bulk disease) may obscure the potential benefits of intensive chemotherapy in the other patients. For patients with a poor prognosis, the substantial toxicity of combination

Table 17.9 Novel and combination chemotherapy in advanced ovarian cancer*

Drug	Dose	Response rate (%)
Paclitaxel	$135\,mg/m^2$ by i.v. infusion over 24 hours every 3 weeks	25†
Doxorubicin Cyclophosphamide [A−C]	$40\,mg/m^2$ day 1 } every 4 weeks $500\,mg/m^2$ day 1	55
Hexamethylmelamine Cyclophosphamide Methotrexate 5-FU [Hexa-CAF]	$150\,mg/m^2$ daily × 14 } $150\,mg/m^2$ daily × 14 $40\,mg/m^2$ day 1, 8 } every 4 weeks $600\,mg/m^2$ day 1, 8	75
Cyclophosphamide Doxorubicin Cisplatin [CAP]	$300\,mg/m^2$ daily 1 } $30{-}40\,mg/m^2$ day 1 } every 3 weeks $50\,mg/m^2$ day 1	60−75
Cyclophosphamide Hexamethylmelamine Doxorubicin Cisplatin [CHAP]	$300\,mg/m^2$ day 1 } $150\,mg/m^2$ daily × 14 $40\,mg/m^2$ day 1 } every 4 weeks $50\,mg/m^2$ day 1	65−80

* Schedules and administration vary widely. Reported response rates also differ and figures are approximate.
† In cisplatin-resistant patients.

chemotherapy may not be justified by the few extra months of life. The current position is that surgical removal of as much of the tumour mass as possible, followed by an effective single agent, usually cisplatin or carboplatin, or combination chemotherapy regimen, will result in a minority of patients being free of tumour 1−2 years after the initial treatment, as judged by subsequent laparotomy or laparoscopy. The ultimate prognosis of these patients remains to be determined but there now seems little doubt that cure is possible though in a disappointingly small proportion.

Unresolved controversies in epithelial ovarian cancer

Several important issues in management remain contentious.

1 The contribution of debulking surgery both to improving response rates to chemotherapy, and to overall survival.

2 The role of radiotherapy in Stage II disease, in Stage III disease after cytoreductive surgery, and in patients with minimal residual disease after second-look laparotomy.

3 The contribution of second-look laparotomy to treatment. It seems clear that there is no useful therapeutic contribution of second-look laparotomy though its value as a staging procedure remains uncertain. In selected cases, where further treatment decisions might depend initially on the presence of microscopic disease, it may still be valuable.

4 Definition of the place of combination chemotherapy compared with the best single-agent therapy. Assessment of the role of new platinum analogues in combination.

5 Is second-line chemotherapy of any value in patients who fail to achieve complete remission or who relapse after treatment?

6 Might paclitaxel or semi-systemic analogues be more effective than standard regimens for primary treatment?

Table 17.10 Germ cell tumours of the ovary

Tumour	Percentage of all malignant germ cell tumours
Benign (20% of all ovarian tumours)	
Dermoid cyst — mature cystic teratoma	
Malignant (3% of all ovarian tumours)	
Dysgerminoma	50
Endodermal sinus tumour or yolk sac tumour	20
Embryonal carcinoma	3
Malignant (immature) teratoma (includes malignant monodermal teratomas and carcinoids)	20
Mixed germ cell tumours	7
Choriocarcinoma	Rare
Gonadoblastoma	Rare

GERM CELL TUMOURS OF THE OVARY

A pathological classification of germ cell tumours of the ovary is shown in Table 17.10. Benign dermoid cysts are relatively common and are cured by surgical excision. Occasionally they consist largely of thyroid tissue, *struma ovarii*, which may even be functioning. Less than 5% of strumas are malignant — so-called *monomorphic* or *monodermal teratomas*. Rarely they may show secondary malignant change, most commonly squamous carcinoma.

Of the malignant tumours, *dysgerminoma* is much the commonest and histologically is a uniform clear cell tumour resembling seminoma in males. Lymphocytic infiltration is common. The endodermal sinus tumour (*yolk sac tumour*) is a highly malignant tumour which produces AFP which can be demonstrated in the tumour and is detectable in the blood. Rupture of the tumour occurs early. *Embryonal carcinoma* consists of glandular and papillary masses, often with trophoblastic elements which secrete HCG. It may occur in childhood and produce

sexual precocity. AFP may also be produced by yolk sac elements in the tumour. *Immature teratoma* is a mainly solid tumour containing a multiplicity of different tissues. Primitive neuro-ectoderm often predominates but monomorphic forms consisting of thyroid tissue or malignant carcinoid also occur. Even when the tumour has not metastasized, carcinoid syndrome may occur because of the large size. The *mixed germ cell tumour* contains mixtures of the previous histological types. *Gonadoblastoma* is a small tumour arising in childhood, usually composed of several of the elements of the developing gonad. It may calcify, rarely metastasizes, but might cause virilization as it may contain functioning Leydig cells.

Clinical features

In dysgerminoma, as with other malignant ovarian tumours, the presentation is with an abdominal mass and pain, but the mean age is far lower; 75% of patients are between 10 and 30 years old (median 20 years). They do not usually produce marker hormones unless teratomatous elements are present, and they not infrequently present during or shortly after pregnancy. Other germ cell tumours (yolk sac, endodermal sinus tumours, teratoma, mixed germ cell tumour) are also tumours of adolescents and young women. Many of these patients have precocious puberty, menstrual disturbance and a positive pregnancy test (with pregnancy as a differential diagnosis of the pelvic mass!). These tumours grow rapidly causing abdominal pain.

Management

In dysgerminoma, management depends on stage. Ninety per cent of patients with FIGO Stage I are cured by unilateral oophorectomy but the recurrence rate is higher with large tumours, positive peritoneal washings at operation, or if the tumour contains mixed germ cell elements. If recurrence occurs, or if there are metastases, patients are usually treated with whole abdominal irradiation, often extending into the mediastinum and left supraclavicular region. The routine use of postoperative radiotherapy is questionable and more advanced stages of disease might well be better treated with chemotherapy as for teratoma (see below) but experience is very limited. Yolk sac, endodermal sinus and mixed germ cell tumours have a much worse prognosis with surgical treatment than dysgerminoma, even in Stage I disease. The use of serum AFP and βHCG as markers has greatly improved the monitoring of chemotherapy, which is now an essential part of treatment for most patients (exceptions are discussed below).

The use of platinum-based regimens has followed the outstanding success achieved in testicular teratoma. Since the tumours are unilateral they can be managed by unilateral salpingo-oophorectomy followed by chemotherapy, with the possibility of preservation of fertility. Exceptions to the use of chemotherapy include teratomas which contain low mitotic activity, those with no embryonal or trophoblastic elements and where there are no detectable tumour markers after surgery. Such patients can be treated by surgery alone, but need careful follow-up. Ovarian choriocarcinoma is usually treated with chemotherapy as for other non-dysgerminomatous ovarian germ cell tumours.

At present, chemotherapy for these tumours consists of combination treatment with cisplatin, vinblastine and bleomycin, in a regimen identical to that used for testicular non-seminomatous germ cell tumours (see Chapter 19). Epipodophyllotoxin (VP-16213) is an active agent and is sometimes given as a substitute for vinblastine with the advantage of lesser toxicity.

Ovarian carcinoids and struma ovarii are treated by unilateral oophorectomy.

Granulosa cell tumours of the ovary

These tumours account for 3–5% of malignant ovarian tumours. The cell of origin is unclear. They are frequently hormone-producing. The granulosa-theca tumour is composed of cells which resemble the normal granulosa cell of the follicle. It may be difficult to decide whether the tumour is malignant or not because it often lacks the typical cellular features of malignancy. Capsular invasion and cellular atypia are the most reliable signs of malignancy, and probably influence prognosis. Granulosa-theca cell tumours produce oestrogen (mainly from theca cells), androgens and progesterone. Oestrogen-related symptoms include postmenopausal bleeding, menorrhagia and breast tenderness. Virilizing symptoms, which are rarer, include hirsutism and oligomenorrhoea.

The prognosis of these tumours is excellent as they are mostly cured by conservative surgery (unilateral salpingo-oophorectomy). Responses to chemotherapy have been recorded in patients with recurrence of tumour.

Sertoli–Leydig cell tumours of the ovary

These rare tumours, representing 0.5% of ovarian cancers, are seen at the ages of 20–40 years and are sometimes termed *arrhenoblastomas*. Eighty per cent of them are associated with virilization. The histological appearance varies and some are poorly differentiated though all contain Leydig cells identical to the male testicular cell. Occasionally, teratomatous elements are present.

Following surgical removal, the prognosis is excellent and over 90% of patients are alive at 10 years. The tumours are rarely bilateral so unilateral oophorectomy is usually adequate.

CARCINOMA OF THE FALLOPIAN TUBE

This uncommon gynaecological malignancy is sometimes considered as a 'variant' of ovarian carcinoma since the two diseases share the common aetiological feature of low fertility or nulliparity, with adenocarcinoma (solid, cystic or mixed) as the commonest histological type. Clinical symptoms include pelvic pain and vaginal discharge which is sometimes profuse and often blood-stained. Other symptoms, similar to those found in ovarian carcinoma, include abdominal distension, altered bowel habit or, in occasional cases, dyspareunia.

Both staging and treatment are similar to the recommendations for ovarian cancer (see above). Where a carcinoma of the fallopian tube is encountered at the initial laparotomy, it is much more likely to be due to secondary involvement from a carcinoma of the ovary than a true primary fallopian tube cancer. As for ovarian cancer generally, stage is an important prognostic determinant.

CARCINOMA OF THE VULVA

This uncommon tumour accounts for about 5–6% of all gynaecological cancer (1% of all cancer) with about 1000 new cases annually in Britain, chiefly affecting the older age group. Invasive carcinoma is distinctly uncommon in patients under 50 years of age (Fig. 17.1) while carcinoma *in situ* (now generally referred to as vulval intraepithelial neoplasia, VIN (3) — analogous to CIN 3) occurs in younger women (average age 50 years).

Aetiology and pathogenesis

Leucoplakia and other dystrophic changes in vulval skin can predispose to carcinoma. These skin changes can be hypoplastic including lichen sclerosus and atrophic vulvitis, or hyperplastic, including leucoplakia as well as hypertrophic vulvitis. The hypoplastic form of dystrophic change is not usually regarded as premalignant although there are certainly instances on record where this appears to have been the case. These changes are distinct from true intraepithelial neoplasia, which is a group including carcinoma *in situ* (often multifocal), and Paget's disease. Most vulval cancers are squamous cell carcinomas, though other histological types are occasionally seen, including adenocarcinoma (usually arising in a Bartholin's gland), melanoma, basal cell carcinoma, fibrosarcoma and adenoid cystic carcinoma. Diabetes is not infrequently associated with carcinoma of the vulva.

Diagnosis

Most patients present with pruritus, vulvae, pain, ulceration, bleeding or discharge although some patients are unaware of any vulval problem and seek advice about a lymph node in the groin. The most common sites of origin are the labia majora, although the labia minora and clitoris can be primary sites. All thickened, fissured, ulcerated or sloughing lesions should be viewed with great suspicion, particularly in elderly patients, and biopsied. The histological distinction between premalignant lesions (particularly leucoplakia and lichen sclerosus et atrophicus) and frank invasive carcinoma can be difficult, particularly since intraepithelial cancer can occur in areas of hypertrophic leucoplakia. Vulval carcinomas are almost always visible so careful follow-up of suspicious lesions should not be difficult. Clinical photographs are useful to document slowly evolving changes.

Benign lesions can cause diagnostic confusion. These include chronic vulvitis, vulval condylomas of tuberculous, syphilitic, viral or unknown aetiology, lymphogranuloma inguinale, lymphogranuloma venereum (chiefly in younger patients) and vulval abscesses. The vulva is occasionally a site of secondary spread

Table 17.11 FIGO staging in carcinoma of the vulva

Stage	Description
Stage 0	Carcinoma *in situ*
Stage I	Tumour confined to vulva (<2 cm) No palpable nodes
Stage II	Tumour confined to vulva (>2 cm) No palpable nodes
Stage III	Tumour spread to urethra, vagina, or perineum. Palpable mobile nodes
Stage IV	Tumour infiltrates bladder or rectum. Fixed nodes

from carcinoma of the endometrium, cervix and large bowel.

Patterns of spread and clinical staging

The FIGO system is widely used (Table 17.11) and is based on the predictable behaviour of vulval carcinoma. Dissemination is chiefly via direct and lymphatic routes, and haematogenous spread is very unusual. Local spread occurs to contiguous areas of the vulva, vagina and urethra, or to the perineum and/or anus (Fig. 17.14). Local pubic tenderness results from infection and periostitis, though malignant bone erosion has been described. Nodal involvement may be unilateral or bilateral, first to the inguino-femoral group, then more deeply (including to contralateral node sites). Clitoral lesions may spread to either groin but do not directly involve deeper node groups without superficial node involvement in the first instance. Overall, nearly half of all vulval cancers have evidence of local lymphatic involvement.

Investigation and management

Routine investigation should include full blood count, chest X-ray, blood urea and electrolyte estimation. Lymphography can be useful in delineating pelvic and para-aortic nodes, particularly in patients where there is doubtful clinical evidence of involvement and the gynaecologist is uncertain whether to proceed with surgery. Unfortunately the advanced age of many patients and the presence of gross infection with reactive lymphadenopathy limits the applicability and reliability of this technique, and a negative lymphogram cannot exclude microscopic nodal involvement. Needle aspiration of enlarged superficial nodes may occasionally help to decide whether surgery is appropriate though a positive result is more reliable than a negative one. CT scanning of the pelvis may also be useful in delineating suspicious areas of nodal or direct spread.

Treatment

Treatment is by surgical excision, preferably of the primary carcinoma and lymphatic drainage *en bloc* [30]. Even in patients who are elderly or have advanced local disease, surgery is generally the treatment of choice. Wide excision of vulval skin has been considered necessary since contiguous subdermal lymphatic spread is common; however, many gynaecologists are now less radical in their approach. Both superficial and deep node dissection are advocated by some surgeons although this need not be so extensive in Stage I disease, and deep node dissection is now less frequently performed. Removal of the lower part of the urethra may also be necessary in more advanced stages. Because of the laxity of skin and subcutaneous tissue in this area, primary closure is usually possible despite the wide excision. Although

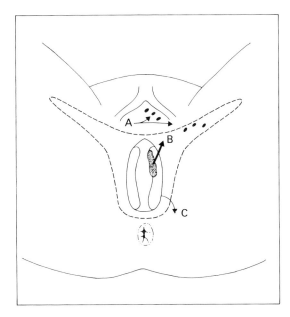

Fig. 17.14 Local and nodal spread in carcinoma of the vulva. (A) Nodal involvement: inguinal, femoral, deep pelvic and common iliac nodes. Bilateral spread is common; (B) anteriorly to contiguous parts of the vulva, clitoris, vagina, urethra and bladder; (C) Posteriorly to posterior vulva and rectum. Dotted line shows incision and resection in radical vulvectomy.

postoperative infection is not uncommon and is the major surgical complication, most patients rehabilitate well. Surgical excision is clearly the treatment of choice although a few patients are unfit for these procedures, and palliative local irradiation can be valuable, particularly in those with pain and ulceration. Radiation tolerance in these elderly patients is limited by bladder, bowel and other local structures. It is usually possible to achieve a total dose of at least 45–55 Gy (4500–5500 rad) in 4–5½ weeks, to the perineum and/or nodal sites. Treatment to a radical dose of 60 Gy should be attempted in younger, fit patients. Where there is obvious local extension to the anus or rectum (Stage IV) local irradiation is probably best preceded by a defunctioning colostomy which can sometimes be closed after completion of treatment. In some patients with extensive nodal disease, a combination of primary resection with groin exploration and postoperative radiotherapy (to the nodal areas) represents the best means of achieving local control. Very occasionally in patients with extensive local spread, primary exenteration will be required.

Prognosis

The survival rate largely depends largely on whether or not there is nodal involvement. About 75% of operable patients without lymphatic metastases are alive and free of disease at 5 years, whereas the 5-year survival of patients with inguinal or femoral node deposits is 30–40%, and less than 20% in patients with pelvic node involvement, even where pelvic lymph node dissection has been performed. Very occasionally further surgery (including pelvic exenteration) may be considered for patients with recurrent disease, though the end results are generally poor.

CARCINOMA OF THE VAGINA

This is a rare tumour [31] accounting for less than 1% of all gynaecological malignancy (i.e. about one-fiftieth as common as carcinoma of

the cervix) and chiefly occurring in the 50–70-year-old age group (Fig. 17.1). Little is known of the aetiology, but prolonged irritation from a vaginal ring pessary sometimes appears to predispose to malignant change. Vaginal carcinoma is almost invariably a squamous cell carcinoma, most frequently arising in the upper vagina, sometimes extensively involving the vaginal wall. Clear cell adenocarcinoma of the vagina has been reported in girls and young women whose mothers were taking exogenous stilboestrol in pregnancy — an example of a transplacental carcinogen [32] with a latent period of 15–30 years. Secondary deposits are occasionally encountered in the vagina, usually as a result of lymphatic spread from endometrial carcinoma (often thought to occur at operation); vaginal deposits from malignant melanomas are also well recognized and rarely the vagina is the primary site of a melanoma. Direct extension may occur from carcinoma of the cervix or bladder.

Symptoms and mode of spread

Blood-stained vaginal discharge is the commonest symptom, and is often unaccompanied by pain. In view of the typical age group, vaginal bleeding, when it occurs, is usually postmenopausal. Urinary complaints (chiefly frequency, nocturia and haematuria) or rectal discomfort occur with advanced disease.

As with carcinoma of the cervix, spread of the disease tends to take place chiefly by direct and lymphatic invasion (Fig. 17.15). Direct extension occurs to the parametria, pelvic side wall, and bladder. The lymphatic route varies with the site of the lesion. Lymphatic drainage of the upper part of the vagina is similar to that of the cervix, i.e. via the external, internal and common iliac nodes. Lesions placed lower in the vagina drain to pelvic, inguinal and femoral nodes. Posteriorly placed lesions may spread towards the rectum because the lymphatic drainage of the posterior vaginal wall is to deep pelvic nodes (sacral, rectal and lower gluteal). As with carcinoma of the cervix, haemato-

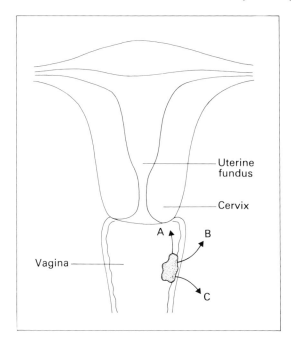

Fig. 17.15 Local and lymph node spread in carcinoma of the vagina. (A) Submucosal spread to adjacent parts of vagina and cervix; (B) parametrial tissues, bladder, rectum and eventually to pelvic side wall; (C) lymphatic spread: upper vagina as for cervix (Fig. 17.4). Posterior vagina as for rectal lymphatics. Anterior wall: towards lateral pelvic wall nodes. Lower vagina: to pelvic and inguino-femoral nodes.

genous spread is uncommon, and local control of disease tends to be the major clinical problem.

Diagnosis and staging

Careful vaginal examination should always be performed in patients presenting with vaginal bleeding and discharge, with direct inspection using a vaginal speculum. Colposcopy and biopsy can be extremely valuable, particularly where the speculum examination is inconclusive. Cytology of vaginal smears can be diagnostic. Where there is no obvious visible lesion, but definite cytological abnormalities are present, carcinoma *in situ* (now often termed vaginal intraepithelial neoplasia, VAIN) of the

vagina must be suspected. This condition should also be considered where cervical cytology has yielded malignant cells but colposcopy-directed biopsy of the cervix has proved negative — particularly where subsequent high vaginal smears are still abnormal.

Important investigations include examination under anaesthetic with cystoscopy, cervical dilatation and uterine curettage and biopsy of the cervix to exclude a primary carcinoma of the cervix. CT or MRI scanning, lymphography, sigmoidoscopy and peritoneal cytology may help to confirm the extent of spread in doubtful cases.

A FIGO staging system is generally used. This clinical staging system (Table 17.12) has been in use for over 10 years.

Treatment

Both radiotherapy and surgical removal can be effective though the surgical operation has to be very radical to stand a real chance of success and it is not often employed as a primary procedure. Total vaginectomy, pelvic lymphadenectomy and abdominal hysterectomy would be necessary, with reconstruction of the perineum and vagina where possible. This operation is only suitable for early lesions (Stage I) or in a few highly selected cases following radiation failure. For most patients, radiotherapy is considered to be the treatment of choice.

CARCINOMA IN SITU

The whole of the vaginal mucosa is usually

Table 17.12 FIGO staging of carcinoma of the vagina

Stage 0	Carcinoma *in situ**
Stage I	Vaginal wall only
Stage II	Subvaginal tissue involved
Stage III	Extension to pelvic side wall
Stage IV	Spread beyond true pelvis —
IVa	to adjacent organs
IVb	to distant organs

* Vaginal intraepithelial neoplasia, VAIN.

irradiated using a vaginal applicator containing radioactive sources (often termed Dobbie applicators after their originator). The intravaginal mould can be differentially loaded to treat the area at greatest risk to a higher dose, but irradiation of the whole mucosa is usually advised as there may be more than one neoplastic site. Complications of treatment include vaginal stenosis, lack of lubrication and proctitis. A radical dosage of at least 60 Gy (6000 rad) mucosal dose is usually recommended.

Alternatively, laser therapy with colposcopy may be adequate for well-localized lesions. Occasionally, treatment by topical chemotherapy (generally with 5-FU) may be valuable, sometimes in conjunction with local irradiation.

INVASIVE CARCINOMA OF THE VAGINA

For Stage I tumours, surgery, as described above, is occasionally recommended, particularly in younger patients with more distal lesions (lower third of vagina). For the large majority of patients, treatment by intracavitary caesium insertion is combined with external beam irradiation as for carcinoma of the cervix (see above). This applies particularly to tumours of the upper part of the vagina. In tumours of the lower third, it may be more difficult to deliver adequate local irradiation by intracavitary applications. Irradiation of the whole pelvis, using external beam multifield techniques, may be the best means of achieving adequate and homogeneous treatment to the primary site and local node groups. In patients with more advanced disease (FIGO Stages II−IV), a pelvic nodal dose of 45−50 Gy (4500−5000 rad) given in daily fractions over 4½−5 weeks is usually well tolerated and generally considered adequate for sterilizing *microscopic* direct or local lymphatic extension, though it is essential to give additional irradiation to the primary site and to any area which is obviously clinically involved. This is achieved either by intracavitary treatment or by additional external beam radiotherapy to encompass the whole of the vagina, treating the primary site if possible

to a total of 60 Gy (6000 rad) in daily fractions over 6 weeks.

Despite the use of lead shielding techniques to minimize the rectal dose, acute proctitis must be expected in a substantial proportion of patients, and late radiation-induced rectal stricture may result. Other complications include increased urinary frequency with cystitis (often sterile and poorly responsive to antibiotics) and as later complications, local fistula formation, proctitis or sigmoid colitis, any of which may require bowel diversion, although local intra-rectal steroid preparations may relieve symptoms. In view of the poor results and high complication rate when treating patients with very advanced (Stage IV) disease, the treatment of these patients is usually palliative and lower doses, consistent with symptom relief, are generally felt to be more appropriate. Overall, the results of treatment are disappointing. Even with a radical approach, the 5-year survival rate falls from 75% for patients with Stage I disease, to 25% with Stage II disease and less than 5% for patients with Stage IV tumours.

CHORIOCARCINOMA

This rare tumour has received considerable attention because of its extreme chemosensitivity, placing it in the small group of solid tumours which can be cured even when metastatic. In addition, the secretion of a tumour marker, HCG (see Chapter 4) in 100% of cases of choriocarcinoma, permits a logical treatment approach based on a reliable index of tumour bulk.

The tumour most frequently follows pregnancies which have resulted in a hydatidiform mole (occurring in approximately 1 in 1400 normal pregnancies in Britain), though it may rarely accompany a normal or ectopic pregnancy, or even a termination. It is more common in Asia than Europe or the United States, and following pregnancy in 'elderly' subjects (i.e. over 40 years).

Pathology

Histopathologically, the tumour consists of malignant syncitio- or cytotrophoblast cells, which can be shown immunocytochemically to contain HCG. Following successful evacuation of a hydatidiform mole, sequential determination of plasma HCG provides reliable information as to the completeness of the evacuation. In some cases, the HCG level falls more slowly to normal than would be predicted by the half-life of HCG (24–36 hours), suggesting that spontaneous regression of a tumour may have occurred. In other cases, local or distant invasion of tumour supervenes and the HCG level remains elevated.

The traditional classification of trophoblastic tumours was based on morphology: *hydatidiform mole*, *invasive mole* or *true choriocarcinoma*. However, the availability of the quantitative HCG assay has largely supplanted these terms, since the diagnosis is made as a result of persistently raised HCG and tissue is now rarely available. It is probably better to use the term 'gestational trophoblastic tumour' instead. Abnormalities such as mitotic activity, degree of cellular atypia and local invasiveness appear to correlate fairly closely with prognosis.

Although the tumour may remain localized within the uterus, local extension into myometrium or even the serosal surface or vagina may take place, sometimes causing severe intrauterine or intraperitoneal bleeding. More distant blood-borne secondary deposits occur, chiefly to lung, liver and brain, with a frequency which depends on the antecedent history; possibly as many as 1 in 20 molar pregnancies, but excessively rarely following normal or ectopic pregnancy.

Diagnosis and staging

Vaginal bleeding during or after pregnancy should be regarded with suspicion. Some patients appear to suffer from particularly marked symptoms of pregnancy, or pre-eclampsia. Ultrasound examination may lead to an almost certain diagnosis of a molar pregnancy before delivery. Evacuation of a hydatidiform mole and/or persistent elevation of postpartum HCG levels should result (in Britain) in registration of the patient with the Royal College of Obstetrics and Gynaecology. In the United Kingdom, the reference centres are Charing Cross Hospital in the South and Sheffield in the North. The patient will then be followed closely, sending regular samples of blood and/or urine to one of these designated centres. Staging investigations include repeat estimations of βHCG, with chest and abdominopelvic CT scanning. Isotope bone scanning is not routinely performed as less than 1 in 1000 cases involve bone. Pelvic ultrasound may be valuable since it is easier and safer for repeated estimations than CT scanning.

Risk classification is important since optimal treatment is different for patients at varying risk of drug resistance [33]. Clinical staging systems are no longer used. Important prognostic factors include age (older patients do worse), interval between antecedent pregnancy and start of chemotherapy, height of initial HCG level, number and sites of metastases (the brain is a particularly adverse site) and previous administration of chemotherapy.

Treatment

Patients with *low-risk* disease are treated either by chemotherapy (generally single agent chemotherapy with methotrexate) or hysterectomy in older patients who have no wish for further children. Where surgery is performed, it is often recommended that the hysterectomy be 'covered' by administration of methotrexate. If methotrexate is the definitive method of treatment it is usually given daily or every other day for one week, the response assessed by serial HCG measurement, and treatment repeated until the marker has been undetectable in the serum for 6–8 weeks. Patients should be advised to avoid further pregnancy for at least 1 year.

Patients with more advanced *moderate-risk*

disease are treated with combination chemo-therapy, once again using serial HCG assays as a means of monitoring response. Surgery (hysterectomy) may be necessary if vaginal bleeding is troublesome.

Most drug regimens include methotrexate, actinomycin D and an alkylating agent (cyclo-phosphamide or chlorambucil). Higher doses of methotrexate (with folinic acid rescue) are generally given for patients with early disease. Newer regimens include vinca alkaloids, cis-platin and etoposide. One hundred per cent of patients in this category respond to combi-nation chemotherapy, usually resulting in cure, and a small number of patients who develop drug resistance to 'conventional' combination regimens respond to newer drugs [34].

In patients with pulmonary metastases but no other adverse features, single-agent chemo-therapy with methotrexate and folinic acid remains the treatment of choice. For patients with involvement at other distant sites (or other features placing them in the *high-risk* cat-egory), intensive multi-drug combination chemotherapy should be given, together with local irradiation, for example to the brain, if indicated.

Prognosis

Prior to treatment with chemotherapy, patients with localized disease were treated by surgery and/or pelvic irradiation and the cure rate was 40%. Patients with more advanced disease were virtually never cured. With current treatment, 100% of patients with localized disease should be cured, as are over 70% of all patients with more advanced stages. Even with Stage IV disease, the majority of patients survive, and the number of tumour deaths in England and Wales is now under 10 per annum. For the most part, fertility of choriocarcinoma survivors is well maintained, and these patients do not appear to be at increased risk of second tumours [35].

REFERENCES

1 Cancer statistics: registrations, England and Wales (1984) MBI N° 16 HMSO, 1988.
2 Silverberg E., Lubera J. *Cancer Statistics (USA), 1988.* **38**: 5–22.
3 DiSaia P.J. The cervix. In Romney S.L., Gray M.J., Little A.B. *et al.*, eds. *Gynaecology and Obstetrics — The Health Care of Women.* p. 1017. New York: McGraw Hill, 1981.
4 Barton S.E., Maddox P.H., Jenkins D. *et al.* Effect of cigarette smoking on cervical epithelial immunity: a mechanism for neoplastic change? *Lancet* 1988; **ii**: 652–54.
5 Fletcher A. Screening for cancer of the cervix in elderly women. *Lancet* 1990; **335**: 97–99.
6 Peterson O. Spontaneous course of cervical precan-cerous conditions. *American Journal of Obstetrics and Gynecology* 1956; **72**: 1063–71.
7 Piver M.S., Wallace S., Castro J.R. The accuracy of lymphangiography in carcinoma of the uterine cervix. *American Journal of Roentgenology* 1971; **111**: 278–83.
8 Rutledge F.N., Fletcher G.H., MacDonald E.J. Pelvic lymphadenectomy as an adjunct to radiation therapy in treatment for cancer of the cervix. *American Journal of Roentgenology* 1965; **93**: 607–14.
9 Perez C.A., Camel H.M., Kao M.S. *et al.* Random-ized study of preoperative radiation and surgery or irradiation alone in the treatment of stage IB and IIA carcinoma of the uterine cervix: final report. *Gynae-cological Oncology* 1987; **27**: 129–40.
10 Brunschwig A. The surgical treatment of cancer of the cervix stage I and II. *American Journal of Roentgen-ology* 1968; **102**: 147–51.
11 Fletcher G.H. Cancer of the uterine cervix. *American Journal of Roentgenology* 1971; **111**: 225–42.
12 Buxton J., Tobias J.S. Does neoadjuvant chemother-apy have a role in cervical cancer? *Clinical Oncology* 1994; **6**: 352–53.
13 Blackledge F., Buxton E.J., Mould J.J. *et al.* Phase II studies of ifosfamide alone and in combination in cancer of the cervix. *Cancer Chemotherapy and Phar-macology* 1990; **26** (suppl): S12–16.
14 Cutler S.J., Myers M.H., Green S.B. Trends in survival rates of patients with cancer. *New England Journal of Medicine* 1975; **293**: 122–24.
15 Morrow C.P. Endometrial carcinoma stages I and II: is surgery adequate? *International Journal of Radiation Oncology, Biology and Physics* 1980; **6**: 365–66.
16 Kottmeier H.L. Carcinoma of the corpus uteri — diagnosis and therapy. *American Journal of Obstetrics and Gynecology* 1959; **78**: 1127–40.
17 Ford D., Easton D.F., Bishop D.T., Norad S.A., Coldgar D.E. Risks of cancer in BRCA1-mutation carriers. *Lancet* 1994; **343**: 692–95.
18 Bast R.C., Klug T.L., St.John E. *et al.* A radioimmuno-

assay using a monoclonal antibody to monitor the course of epithelial ovarian cancer. *New England Journal of Medicine* 1983; **309**: 883–87.

19 Serov S.F., Scully R.E., Solvin L.H. *Histological Typing of Ovarian Tumors*. International histological classification of tumours, No. 9. Geneva: World Health Organization, 1973.

20 Tobias J.S., Griffiths C.T. Management of ovarian carcinoma: current concepts and future prospects. *New England Journal of Medicine* 1976; **294**: 818–23; 877–82.

21 Griffiths C.T. Surgical resection of bulk tumor in the primary treatment of ovarian carcinoma. *National Cancer Institute Monograph* 1975; **42**: 101.

22 Dembo A.J., Bush R.A., Beale F.A. *et al.* Ovarian carcinoma: improved survival followed abdomino-pelvic irradiation in patients with a completed pelvic operation. *American Journal of Obstetrics and Gynecology* 1979; **134**: 793–800.

23 Keettel W.L., Fox M.R., Longnecker D.S., Latourette H.B. Prophylactic use of radioactive gold in the treatment of primary ovarian cancer. *American Journal of Obstetrics and Gynecology* 1966; **94**: 766–79.

24 Adams M., Kerby I.J., Rocker I. *et al.* A comparison of the toxicity and efficacy of cisplatin and carboplatin in advanced ovarian cancer. *Acta Oncologica* 1989; **28**: 57–63.

25 Alberts D.S., Chen H.S.G., Salmon S.E. *et al.* Chemotherapy of ovarian cancer directed by the human tumor stem cell assay. *Cancer Chemotherapy and Pharmacology* 1981; **6**: 279–85.

26 Young R.C., Chabner B.A., Hubbard S.P. Prospective trial of melphalan (L-PAM) versus combination chemotherapy (Hexa-CAF) in ovarian adenocarcinoma. *New England Journal of Medicine* 1978; **299**: 1261–66.

27 Edmondson H.J., Fleming T.R., Decker D.G. *et al.* Different chemotherapeutic sensitivities and host

factors affecting prognosis in advanced ovarian carcinoma versus minimal residual disease. *Cancer Treatment Reports* 1979; **63**: 241–47.

28 Gruppo Interegionale Cooperativo di Oncologia Ginecologica. A randomized comparison of cisplatin with cyclophosphamide/cisplatin and with cyclophosphamide/doxorubicin/cisplatin in advanced ovarian cancer. *Lancet* 1987; **ii**: 353–59.

29 Trimble E.L., Adams J.D., Vena D. *et al.* Paclitaxel for platinum-refractory ovarian cancer: results from the first 1000 patients registered to NCI treatment referral center 9103. *Journal of Clinical Oncology* 1993; **11**: 2405–10.

30 Podratz K.C., Symmonds R.E., Taylor W.F. *et al.* Carcinoma of the vulva: analysis of treatment and survival. *Obstetrics and Gynecology* 1983; **61**: 63–74.

31 Manetta A., Pinto J.L., Larson J.E. *et al.* Primary invasive carcinoma of the vagina. *Obstetrics and Gynecology* 1988; **72**: 77–81.

32 Robboy S.J., Woller K.L., O'Brien P. *et al.* Increased incidence of cervical and vaginal dysplasia in 3980 diethylstilbestrol-exposed young women: Experience of the National Collaborative Diethylstilbestrol Adenosis Project. *Journal of the American Medical Association* 1984; **252**: 2979–83.

33 Rustin G.J.S., Bagshawe K.D. Gestational trophoblastic tumours. *Critical Reviews in Oncology and Haematology* 1985; **3**: 103–42.

34 Newlands E.S., Bagshawe K.D. Activity of high-dose cis-platinum (NCI 119875) in combination with vincristine and methotrexate in drug resistant gestational choriocarcinoma. *British Journal of Cancer* 1979; **40**: 943–45.

35 Rustin G.J.S., Rustin F., Dent J., Booth M., Salt S., Bagshawe K.D. No increase in second tumours after cytotoxic chemotherapy for gestational trophoblastic tumours. *New England Journal of Medicine* 1983; **308**: 473–76.

Chapter 18
Genito-urinary Cancer

Cancers of the kidney, bladder, prostate and testis represent an important group of tumours which together constitute over a quarter of all male cancer. Due to important advances in the management of testicular tumours this topic is dealt with separately in Chapter 19. Other rare sites of cancer include the urethra, penis and epididymis.

Non-testicular genito-urinary cancers present many challenges in their management and although surgery has traditionally been the cornerstone of treatment, both radiotherapy and cytotoxic chemotherapy are assuming an increasing importance. These tumours are currently the object of a good deal of study since surgical and radiotherapeutic techniques have changed markedly during the past 20 years.

TUMOURS OF THE KIDNEY

Incidence and aetiology of renal tumours

Tumours of the kidney account for about 2% of all cancers (Fig. 18.1) and represent particular problems of management both to surgeons and others since their developments. Clinical evolution and pattern of dissemination is sometimes measured over many years, with apparent success followed by late recurrence, often several years later. In adults, the commonest type of renal tumour is the *renal cell carcinoma (hypernephroma)* which accounts for 75% of adult renal cancer. Tumours of the renal pelvis are uncommon (10%) and are discussed later. In children, *nephroblastoma (Wilms' tumour)* is amongst the commonest of malignant paediatric

tumours, and is discussed in Chapter 24.

Renal cell carcinoma is about three times as common in men as in women, and there is increasing evidence that it is aetiologically related to cigarette smoking [1]. Little else is known about its pathogenesis, though it is common in patients with von Hippel–Lindau syndrome (characterized by haemangioblastomas in the cerebellum and retina, associated with phaeochromocytoma). Stone formation in the renal pelvis, carcinogenic derivatives of aromatic amines or tryptophan, and phenacetin abuse, are all thought to be important in the aetiology of renal pelvic tumours.

Renal cell adenocarcinoma (hypernephroma, Grawitz tumour)

PATHOLOGY AND STAGING

Although Grawitz considered that the tumour arose from cell rests of adrenal tissue, this view is no longer held, particularly since electron microscope studies have revealed the presence of brush border characteristics, making it almost certain that these tumours arise from the epithelium of the renal tubules themselves. For this reason, the term *renal cell adenocarcinoma* is now increasingly preferred to hypernephroma.

Local, lymphatic and haematogenous spread are all relatively common, making surgery unwise or technically impossible in about one-third of all cases [2]. Direct invasion into perirenal tissues occurs in over 20% and local lymph node metastases in 8%. Renal vein invasion is also common with cords of tumour cells sometimes growing directly into the inferior vena

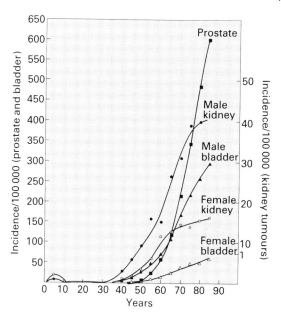

Fig. 18.1 Age-specific incidence of renal, bladder and prostatic cancer.

Table 18.1 Renal carcinoma — TNM staging system

T_0	No evidence of primary tumour
T_1	Small tumour surrounded by normal kidney
T_2	Large tumour with deformity and kidney enlargement
T_3	Perinephric or renal vein involvement
T_4	Invasion of neighbouring structures (diaphragm and abdominal wall)
N_0	No involvement
N_1	Ipsilateral node involvement
N_2	Contralateral or bilateral nodes
N_3	Fixed node involvement
M_0	No distant metastases
M_1	Distant metastases

TNM Stage Grouping

	T	N	M
Stage I	1	0	0
II	2	0	0
III	3	0 or 1	0
IV	4	0–3	0 or 1

cava, although this is not usually detectable pre-operatively. The likelihood of local or lymphatic spread correlates with histological differentiation. In patients with low-grade carcinoma the incidence of metastatic disease at presentation is very low.

A number of staging systems have been proposed, chiefly relying on the information obtained at operation. A straightforward TNM staging system has been suggested which is both reproducible and also yields important prognostic information (Table 18.1). Prognosis is closely related to stage (see p. 356).

CLINICAL FEATURES OF RENAL CELL ADENOCARCINOMA (HYPERNEPHROMA)

These tumours present with a wide variety of symptoms. Approximately 50% of all patients have haematuria, which may be very slight but occasionally is sufficiently severe to produce anaemia. Loin pain and a palpable mass are classical features, and a large mass may be palpable even when the tumour is confined to the kidney, without extracapsular spread. Apart from these local symptoms, many patients initially present with complaints resulting from metastases, such as pathological fracture through a bone deposit, dyspnoea and cough from mediastinal, hilar or lung metastases, or epilepsy from an intracerebral deposit. Renal cell tumours are a well known cause of pyrexia, and fever without other symptoms is not uncommon. Hypertension, polycythaemia and hypercalcaemia also occur in about 5% of patients. Liver function tests may be abnormal even in patients without metastatic disease, although they are unreliable as tumour markers.

Even when a renal cell carcinoma is suspected, the diagnosis can be difficult. Intravenous urography (IVU) usually demonstrates a space-occupying mass in the renal cortex, often with distortion of the calyceal system (Fig. 18.2A), although a negative IVU is unreliable since these tumours can be small. IVU with tomography may help in these cases, and can usually distinguish a solid tumour from a renal cyst. This distinction is particularly well made by ultrasound examination of the kidney (Fig.

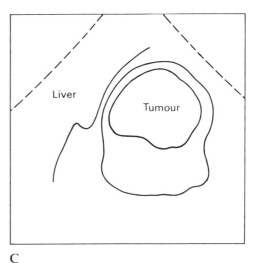

Fig. 18.2 (A) Intravenous urogram in renal carcinoma. The left kidney contains a tumour (arrowed) which displaces the calyces. (B) Transverse ultrasound scan showing a large renal carcinoma below the liver. (C) Line drawing of (B).

C

18.2B), which is a useful examination in iodine-sensitive patients in whom IVU would be hazardous. Renal calcification particularly if 'rim-like' is a common finding. In difficult cases, further radiological investigations using CT or MRI scanning (or very occasionally, ascending ureterography) may give additional information (Fig. 18.3). These techniques, coupled with cyst puncture and aspiration cytology, have reduced the need for renal angiography as a routine investigation, although some urological surgeons still request a pre-operative angiogram in order to obtain the maximum anatomical detail. Before surgery, a chest X-ray must always be obtained in case pulmonary metastases are already present. There may be a place for routine whole-lung tomography or CT scanning, since pulmonary metastases have to be at least 2 cm in diameter to be visible on a standard chest X-ray. Isotope bone scanning may reveal unsuspected bony metastases particularly in patients whose primary lesion is palpable. Biochemical tests of renal and liver function are important, and it is also wise to perform isotope renography pre-operatively, to assess the function of the contralateral kidney.

Fig. 18.3 Renal arteriogram (late arterial phase). (A) A tumour circulation is seen due to a large carcinoma occupying the upper two-thirds of the kidney. (B) CT scan of the abdomen (with contrast) in a patient with a carcinoma of the right kidney.

MANAGEMENT OF RENAL CELL CARCINOMA

Surgical resection is unquestionably the most effective method of treatment, although over 25% of renal carcinomas are technically unresectable. Many surgeons recommend *en bloc* resection of the kidney with as little disturbance as possible, coupled with wide lymphatic dissection of local nodes from the aortic bifurcation to the diaphragm, and with prevention of tumour dissemination by early ligation of the renal artery and vein. Although still controversial, lymph node dissection seems advisable since it has been noted that the incidence of regional lymph node involvement can be as high as 15%. In general, an aggressive surgical approach is usually justifiable since other methods of treatment are at best palliative. In cases where the tumour is large, or difficult to remove, it may be necessary to perform nephro-ureterectomy, with removal of part of the bladder if indicated. Where evidence of involvement of the renal vein or inferior vena cava is apparent (about 10% of patients),

attempts at radical surgical removal are often justified, since renal vein involvement without other evidence of extra-renal extension appears to have little effect on the prognosis at 5 and even 10 years [3]. Difficulties arise where a renal carcinoma occurs in a solitary or horseshoe kidney, and the commonest approach is to perform a partial nephrectomy. Occasionally, if the tumour is too large for a conservative resection, total nephrectomy is unavoidable, with transplantation of an allogeneic kidney (if available) at a later procedure.

In patients with obvious clinical or radiological evidence of metastases elsewhere, the choice of initial treatment is more difficult. The primary lesion may be technically operable, and providing the patient's condition is reasonably good, nephrectomy is by far the most effective and simplest means of securing control of the primary, particularly when there are troublesome symptoms such as renal pain or haematuria. Although there are sporadic case reports of regression of secondary lung deposits following resection of the primary tumour, this phenomenon is in fact very rare and the possibility of its occurrence should never be used as the sole rationale for surgery. Since this capricious tumour can remain quiescent for many years (even decades) before metastases become apparent, it is sometimes recommended that solitary metastases should be surgically removed. In symptomatic patients with obvious widespread metastatic disease in whom nephrectomy seems unwise, renal artery embolism or occlusion is worth considering since it leads to partial or complete infarction of the kidney and offers a reasonable chance of temporary control of the tumour. It should probably be used only in symptomatic patients since it can be painful and indeed hazardous, though some urologists use this technique routinely as a pre-operative adjunct to nephrectomy. Several other methods of occlusion are currently in use, including intra-arterial balloon catheter occlusion, induction of an autologous local thrombus, or insertion of foreign material such as gelatine sponge or polyacrylamide gel.

Radiotherapy (Fig. 18.4) has a limited role in renal cell cancer, even in cases where complete surgical removal is technically impossible. Renal cell adenocarcinomas are only marginally sensitive to radiotherapy, and radical irradiation of the kidney in totally inoperable cases does no more than delay the onset of local progression of disease. There is clearly no survival advantage from the routine use of adjuvant radiotherapy for renal carcinoma. In operable tumours, the routine use of postoperative irradiation remains controversial but is probably unwise. Several years ago, in a prospective study of postoperative irradiation following apparently successful nephrectomy, Finney was unable to demonstrate any useful benefit, even in the incidence of local recurrence [4]. In another trial using pre-operative irradiation (which may be expected to lead to a lower rate of dissemination of viable tumour cells at operation), no survival advantage was seen, although the proportion of technically complete operations was higher in patients undergoing radiation therapy [5]. On the other hand, Rafla [6] demonstrated an improvement in survival following radio-

therapy for patients where capsular invasion was noted at surgery with no other evidence of distant disease — the one group in whom postoperative radiotherapy might be expected to be beneficial. A more recent randomized Danish study gave far less encouraging results, in a trial comparing radiotherapy with no additional treatment following nephrectomy [7]. No difference in relapse rate could be demonstrated although overall, 19% of the treated (radiotherapy) group experienced severe side-effects, including a few treament-related deaths (Fig. 18.4).

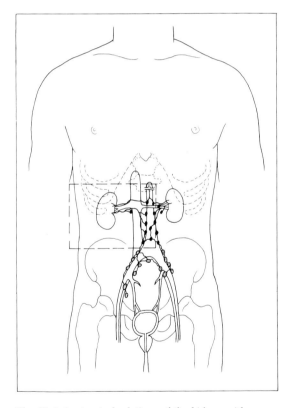

Fig. 18.4 Anatomical relations of the kidney with lymphatic drainage pathways and typical volume treated when irradiating the renal bed. In most cases the kidney will have been surgically removed. Particular care must be taken with right-sided tumours because of the risk of radiation hepatitis. Commonly affected lymph nodes are shown in black.

In spite of early reports of response to hormone preparations, the overall response rate to progestogens and androgens is very low, of the order of 5%. Despite this disappointing figure, these agents are non-toxic and therefore worth considering in patients with widespread metastases. Medroxyprogesterone acetate is widely used (100 mg t.d.s. by mouth). Other hormonal agents such as flutamide and tamoxifen probably have similar response rates [8].

CHEMOTHERAPY

Chemotherapy has had little success. The most widely used agents are vinblastine, CCNU, doxorubicin, cyclophosphamide and hydroxyurea. None of these agents has high activity on its own and in combination the response rate is still very low (20%). Dissatisfaction with these poor results has led to the increasing investigation of newer therapies in metastatic renal cancer, notably immunotherapy using cytokines and other agents [9]. In 1983 human interferon was first reported to show activity and more recently an overview of some 1500 patients treated with α-interferon showed an overall response rate of 16% although sadly a complete response rate of only 2% [10]. Median response duration was, however, short and the experimental use of interferons together with chemotherapy does not appear promising. Use of interleukin-2 (IL-2), lymphokine activated killer (LAK) cells, and other types of interferon seems less encouraging than the initial euphoria aroused by Rosenberg's contention [11] that metastatic renal cell carcinoma was frequently responsive. Although there are now more potentially valuable treatments available to such patients, the outlook in general remains bleak, with an overall median survival of approximately 9 months. Moreover the toxicity of IL-2 (with or without LAK cells) remains considerable [12].

Although cytotoxic and cytokine drugs have no established role in palliation, treatment with radiotherapy may be very successful, particularly in the relief of bone pain. Bone metastases are very common and internal orthopaedic fixation of long bones is invaluable in prevention or treatment of pathological fractures, thereby allowing early mobility.

Prognosis

The prognosis in renal cell cancer depends on the stage and grade of the tumour, and the completeness of surgery (Fig. 18.5). For Stage I tumours, the 5-year survival is over 60%, whereas if the regional nodes are involved this falls to 30%. For Stage IV tumours, there are very few 5-year survivors. With high-grade tumours, only 30% of patients are alive at 5 years whilst with low-grade tumours, 80% of patients survive.

Carcinoma of the renal pelvis

These tumours are uncommon (about 7% of all renal carcinomas) and are usually transitional

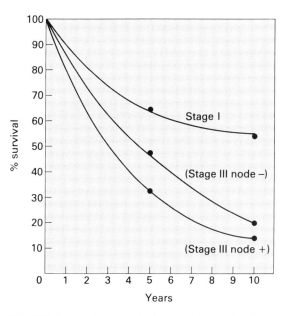

Fig. 18.5 Prognosis of renal adenocarcinoma related to stage and lymph node involvement.

cell carcinomas (80%) or squamous cell carcinomas, which may be more common in women. Clinical symptoms include haematuria (90%) and loin pain due to obstruction of the renal pelvis. On examination, in advanced cases, there may be a palpable loin mass.

Investigation includes an IVU, which usually shows a filling defect in the collecting system and occasionally demonstrates non-function where there has been long-standing post-renal obstruction by tumour. Fifty per cent of all patients have malignant cells in the urine and cytological examination of the urine is therefore a mandatory investigation.

For tumours of the renal pelvis, surgery is again the most important method of treatment. Nephro-ureterectomy is usually required; for transitional tumours a part of the bladder wall is also usually removed since as with all such cell tumours, a wide area of epithelium is at risk. As the histology of the renal pelvic tumour is not usually known pre-operatively, the operation is the same for both transitional cell and squamous carcinomas. However, local ureteric stump recurrence is reportedly less frequent with squamous carcinomas.

Radiotherapy may be worth considering for inoperable or recurrent cases but there is little evidence that it is ever curative in these situations. It may, however, temporarily retard the local progression of disease. In the follow-up care of patients with renal pelvic tumours, the possibility of a contralateral lesion must always be borne in mind. Repeated cystoscopy and cytological examination of the urine are both important, since 50% of patients will later develop a carcinoma of the bladder at some stage. About 10% of patients with transitional cell carcinoma of the renal pelvis have a synchronous bladder carcinoma as well.

CARCINOMA OF THE URETER

This rare tumour is usually a transitional cell carcinoma although sarcomas are occasionally encountered. Typically, the disease presents with frequency and dysuria. Ureteric colic is unusual.

The diagnosis is usually made by IVU which shows ureteric dilatation or distortion, or a non-functioning kidney. Retrograde pyelography demonstrates the site of the block. Urinary cytology may also be helpful in diagnosis.

Treatment is by nephro-ureterectomy, but occasionally the kidney may be preserved. In removing the ureter a cuff of bladder should be taken. Radiotherapy has occasionally been employed in patients with inoperable tumour, but with little success.

The prognosis depends largely on the cellular differentiation of the tumours. The 5-year survival is 80% with well-differentiated tumours but only 10% with the most anaplastic forms.

CANCER OF THE URINARY BLADDER

Aetiology and incidence

Bladder cancer is now the fifth most common cancer in men in Western countries, with 45 000 new cases in the United States annually [13]. Its incidence is clearly rising. At the end of the 19th century it was recognized that workers in the aniline dye industry had a higher incidence of bladder cancer than expected, and the active carcinogen to which they were exposed was later identified as β-naphthylamine. Workers in the rubber industry form another group (see also p. 11 and p. 27) and there are clearly others as well. Chronic bladder infection or infestation also predisposes to malignant change; worldwide, the most important of these causes is schistosomiasis. There is no doubt that bladder cancer is more frequent amongst cigarette smokers, and this may partially explain its much higher incidence in males. It has been estimated that at least 50% of cases in males, and 25% in females may be causally related to cigarette smoking. In both sexes the rate appears to be related to duration of smoking, and decreases comparatively rapidly in ex-smokers. In the

United States, the disease is reportedly four times as common in white men as in black and is commoner in urban than in rural areas. Other probable aetiological factors in bladder cancer include multiple urinary infections and previous exposure to cyclophosphamide [15]. In one retrospective study of non-Hodgkin's lymphoma, several patients developed carcinoma of the bladder after long-term chronic oral cyclophosphamide [15].

Screening for bladder cancer has been increasingly attempted, indeed bladder cancer was probably the first solid tumour in which a systematic screening programme was seriously considered [16]. In low-risk groups (the general population), screening has generally been performed by dipstick testing for occult haematuria — a technique with high predictive accuracy but in this group, low yields of the order of 2.5% in unselected males aged 21–72 years. In higher risk groups the approach is clearly more logical although even in men working in the rubber industry, it is nowadays difficult to confirm excess death rates, in contrast to studies performed in former years. At present the cost and low yield appear to argue against the wide introduction of screening programmes although careful investigation of even a single episode of haematuria (or occult haematuria) is mandatory.

Pathology and staging

Over 90% of bladder tumours are derived from transitional cell epithelium. In Western countries, transitional cell carcinoma (TCC) of the bladder is at least five times as common as squamous cell carcinoma, although in Egypt where schistosomal infestation is common, the squamous carcinoma is more frequent. Other histological types such as adenocarcinoma, leiomyosarcoma and rhabdomyosarcoma are rare. TCCs may be single or multiple, and are sometimes pedunculated, whereas squamous carcinomas are usually sessile and often necrotic in appearance. Multiple papillomatous tumours are often of low grade, although there is general

agreement that they should be regarded as pre-malignant lesions. Fortunately, the majority of patients (70%) with bladder cancer present with superficial disease only.

In TCC, pathological grading is of considerable importance, though pathologists may differ in their methods of classification. Well-differentiated tumours clearly carry a better prognosis than anaplastic ones, quite independent of the stage of the tumour. Further important prognostic information can be obtained from a knowledge of the depth of infiltration of the bladder wall, with a direct correlation between pathologically-verified depth of penetration (P-stage) and survival.

The TNM staging notation (Table 18.2) allows a convenient shorthand description of bladder tumours, based largely on the degree of local

Table 18.2 TNM and P-staging for bladder cancer

T_{is}	Pre-invasive carcinoma (carcinoma *in situ*)
T_a	Papillary non-invasive carcinoma
T_0	No evidence of primary tumour
T_1	Tumour limited to the lamina propria (P_1) Bimanual examination may reveal a mobile mass which cannot be felt after TUR
T_2	Tumour limited to superficial muscle (P_2) Mobile induration of the bladder wall may be present, but should be impalpable following TUR
T_3	Invasion of deep muscle layer of the bladder wall (P_3). On bimanual palpation a mobile mass is felt which persists after TUR
T_{3a}	Deep muscle invasion
T_{3b}	Invasion through the muscle wall
T_4	Invasion of prostate or other local structures (P_4); tumour fixed or locally extensive
T_{4a}	Tumour infiltrates prostate, uterus or vagina
T_{4b}	Tumour fixed to pelvic and/or abdominal wall
N_0	No regional lymph node involvement
N_1	Involvement of a single ipsilateral regional node group
N_2	Contralateral, bilateral or multiple regional node involvement
N_3	Fixed regional lymphadenopathy (i.e. a fixed space between this and the tumour)
N_4	Involvement of juxta-regional nodes
M_0	No distant metastases
M_1	Distant metastases

spread at presentation (Fig. 18.6). The most important distinction lies between T_2 and T_3 tumours, since over 50% of all patients with T_2 tumours will be alive at 3 years from diagnosis, whereas less than 25% of patients with T_3 tumours (i.e. with invasion of the deep muscle of the bladder) will survive. In 1988, the UICC staging criteria for bladder (and prostate) cancer altered to parallel the United States based systems more closely. However, the resulting staging system has not been welcomed as superior since it takes far less account of clinical information. For this reason the previous TNM and P-stage criteria continue to be widely used.

Important prognostic factors are shown in Table 18.3. In addition to TNM stage, pathological grade and histological type, the size, location and number of bladder tumours will influence the management. Multiple bladder tumours are so frequently encountered that the whole of the transitional cell epithelial surface may be considered to be at risk, and in some

instances where tumours are widespread throughout the bladder, total cystectomy may be required even though the local invasiveness of each one may be unimpressive. The major sites of distant metastasis are lymph nodes, lung, liver and bone.

Much has been learnt in recent years of the molecular biology of bladder cancer. It is now clear that patients with an abnormal chromosome complement have a poor prognosis. There appears to be a strong correlation between DNA content (ploidy) and level of invasion (pathological grade), depth of tumour invasiveness and response to certain types of therapy [13]. We also now know that tumours expressing A, B or H blood-group antigens are associated with a better prognosis.

The development of a bladder cancer from normal or premalignant urothelial tissue may relate to the presence of transforming oncogenes, particularly those of the *ras* family which are known to be present on chromosomes 1, 11 and 12. There may be an association between *ras* expression and high histologic grade.

Clinical features

The majority of patients with bladder cancer complain of haematuria, usually painless, although other symptoms such as urgency of micturition, nocturia, and frequency or reduction of the urinary stream may also be present. Loin or back pain may be a feature, particularly if tumour obstruction has led to hydronephrosis or if large intra-abdominal lymph node metastases are present. Even single episodes of haematuria should be fully investigated by cystoscopy. Fortunately, the majority of patients with superficial bladder tumours do not develop invasive disease, indeed it is probably true that superficial and deeply-invasive bladder carcinomas are distinctly separate disorders [13].

Definitive diagnosis usually requires cystoscopy with biopsy, which gives a clear indication of the site, size, general appearance and multiplicity of bladder tumours. This procedure

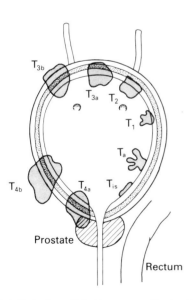

Fig. 18.6 T staging of bladder cancer. T_{is}: *in situ* carcinoma; T_a: non-invasive papillary carcinoma; T_1: limited to lamina propria; T_2: superficial muscle involvement; T_{3a}: deep muscle involvement; T_{3b}: full thickness of bladder wall; T_{4a}: invading neighbouring structures (prostate, vagina); T_{4b}: involvement of rectum, fixed to pelvic wall.

Table 18.3 Survival of patients with deeply invasive carcinoma of the bladder treated (a) by surgery (total cystectomy with or without pre-operative irradiation); or (b) by radical irradiation alone, using external beam treatment

(A) Present status of all patients (%)

	Group I (137 cases)	Group 2 (109 cases)	Group 3 (119 cases)	Group 4 (86 cases)
Alive and no evidence of disease after 5 or more years	10	28	27	38
Dead with no evidence of disease in <5 years	18	25	18	18
Dead with no evidence of disease in >5 years	22	7	11	2
Dead of disease in <5 years	48	32	39	2
Dead of disease in >5 years	1	3	5	41
Lost to follow-up in <5 years	1	5	0	1

Treatment details
Group 1   Radical cystectomy alone
Group 2   Radical radiotherapy (60 Gy) with 'salvage' surgery for local failure
Group 3   Planned pre-operative irradiation (40 Gy) followed by radical cystectomy
Group 4   Planned intensive 1-week pre-operative irradiation (20 Gy) followed by radical cystectomy

(B) Urinary bladder cancer (radiotherapy 1957−1970) corrected survival rates (Karolinksa Hospital)

Category (T stage)	Interval (years)	Number of patients	Survival rate (%)
$T_{1/2}$	5	188	31
	10	151	22
T_3	5	283	20
	10	220	14
T_4	5	129	10
	10	103	4

Data for (A), from Whitmore *et al.* [19] and for (B), from Edsmyr [21].

is normally performed under general anaesthesia, permitting a full examination including thorough rectal and bimanual palpation which are essential for accurate staging. Urinary exfoliative cytology is a valuable addition to diagnosis and is currently being evaluated as a means not only of diagnosis but also of monitoring response to treatment.

An intravenous urogram should routinely be performed, giving essential information regarding the anatomy and functioning of the kidneys and ureters, and often some degree of information as to the site and extent of the primary tumour. Renal function should also be assessed by measurement of blood urea and creatinine clearance (or other form of assessment such as DTPA clearance). Very few centres now perform pelvic arteriography, but MRI and CT scanning

are extremely valuable particularly for accurate assessment of extravesical spread (Fig. 18.7). The technique is less satisfactory in visualizing enlarged lymph nodes, since the nodes of the external and internal iliac/paravesical-obturator groups are less well surrounded by adipose tissue than the regional lymph nodes higher within the abdomen. None the less, CT scanning has rapidly become established as an important investigation in patients with deeply invasive bladder cancer, and is particularly valuable if radical irradiation is being contemplated.

Management of carcinoma of the bladder

Management of superficial bladder tumours is almost entirely the province of the surgeon.

Fig. 18.7 CT scan in advanced bladder cancer. The tumour (arrowed) is shown extending posteriorly to the rectum and laterally to the side walls of the pelvis. We are grateful to Dr Janet Husband for this figure.

Small papillary tumours can be repeatedly treated by cystodiathermy, often for many years, although other methods such as cryo-surgery or laser treatment are becoming more widely used. Intravesical chemotherapy using thiotepa, mitomycin C, doxorubicin and other cytotocins is receiving increasing attention, since these agents are sometimes able to prevent or treat small recurrences of superficial bladder tumours. Thiotepa is far less used nowadays since it may cause considerable local discomfort. Although such tumours are rarely fatal, up to 10% of patients will develop widespread intravesical recurrence after repeated cystodiathermy, necessitating further treatment either with radiotherapy or even by total cystectomy. In these, intravesical chemotherapy may prove helpful in avoiding or delaying such treatment, thereby improving the quality of survival.

Because superficial bladder cancers can progress to more deeply penetrating lesions, both external radiotherapy and intravesical chemotherapy have now been tested as means of preventing this development. BCG has been assessed in this way and also for recurrent carcinoma *in situ* [17]. No long-term benefit

from these approaches has yet been shown. More recently, intravesical chemotherapy with and interferon has shown promise in at least one preliminary study. Photodynamic therapy has also been attempted, using haematoporphyrin derivatives taken up by the malignant urothelium followed by cystoscopy to reveal areas of fluorescence which correlate with areas of histologically proven tumour. The haematoporphyrin derivative can be used as a sensitizing agent for argon-dye or other types of laser treatment.

In patients with invasive carcinoma of the bladder (T_2-T_3), the choice usually lies between a surgical procedure, radiation therapy, or a combination of both. In some patients with small lesions located in a mobile portion of the bladder, partial cystectomy is possible. An adequate cuff of normal bladder must be removed, and the procedure is usually only recommended where the initial capacity of the remaining bladder is likely to be greater than 300–400 ml. Surgical technique is important in order to avoid implantation tumour nodules developing at the anastomosis, and the operation is less widely used than formerly. Interstitial irradiation is an alternative to partial cystectomy in patients with T_2 and early T_3 lesions. A large study from van der Werf-Messing [18] gave a 5-year survival rate of 40% (T_2) and 25% (T_3), using interstitial (intravesical) irradiation with radium implants (sometimes with low-dose external irradiation).

The introduction in the 1950s of a satisfactory method of total cystectomy led to rapid acceptance of this operation as the treatment of choice for many patients with deeply invasive (T_3) tumours without extravesical or distant spread. This major procedure involves complete removal of the bladder, prostate and seminal vesicles (or bladder and urethra in the female), although some surgeons prefer a still more radical approach which combines total cystectomy with a pelvic lymph node dissection. Urinary diversion is usually achieved by fashioning a conduit from a section of resected ileum into which the ureters are implanted and which opens onto the abdominal wall (ileostomy), or by implanting the ureters directly into the sigmoid colon or rectum (Fig. 18.8).

One of the largest series of patients treated by surgery alone was reported by Whitmore *et al.* [19]. Of 137 patients treated by surgery alone, the operative mortality was 14% with an overall 5-year survival of 10% (Table 18.3). In three further groups of patients, pre-operative irradiation was used in an attempt to improve these results; three different techniques and dose schedules were employed, and in each group the 5-year survival rate was at least

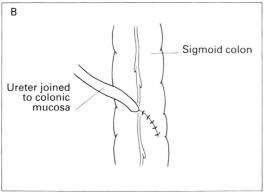

Fig. 18.8 Common procedures for ureteric diversion following total cystectomy. (A) Formation of an ileal conduit; (B) implantation into sigmoid colon.

doubled. Although this study was not randomized, these data have persuaded most urologists that combinations of surgery and radiotherapy offer superior results to the use of total or radical cystectomy alone. In recent years, important surgical advances have included more acceptable methods of urinary diversion including 'continent' forms in which the patient controls the emptying of the urinary conduit by self-catheterization or other techniques, allowing more normal urinary function. A further important advance has been the possibility for the first time of continued sexual potency through careful sparing of critical neurovascular structures [20].

More recently, several large radiotherapy groups have reported the results of treatment with radical radiotherapy alone, which increasingly seem comparable to those achieved by surgery [13]. A large series of over 500 patients was reported by Edsmyr [21] with similar results to those obtained by Whitmore (Table 18.3). In patients who later suffered local recurrence it was often possible to perform a total cystectomy, with successful 'salvage' (i.e. a significant additional recurrence-free period, or even a cure) in a substantial proportion.

In view of the effectiveness of radical radiotherapy for carcinoma of the bladder, it seems reasonable to ask whether cystectomy as primary management can be avoided altogether. A large co-operative study based at the Royal Marsden Hospital attempted to answer this question. Nearly 200 patients were allocated either to receive radical radiotherapy alone (60 Gy (6000 rad) over 6 weeks) or pre-operative irradiation (40 Gy (4000 rad) over 4 weeks), followed by radical cystectomy a month later [22]. At 5 years, there was a trend in favour of the group of patients undergoing both radiotherapy and surgery, with a survival rate of 38% compared with 29% for the group undergoing radical radiotherapy. Although the overall result did not reach statistical significance, the combination of pre-operative irradiation and surgery seemed more effective in younger patients and in males. The difference between the two groups may also have been exaggerated because 20% of patients randomized to radiotherapy and surgery could not complete the treatment as planned. After local recurrence with radiotherapy alone, it was possible to perform salvage cystectomy with the impressive result of a 52% 5-year survival post-cystectomy.

The biological effectiveness of radiotherapy for bladder cancer is also shown by the phenomenon of post-irradiation tumour 'down-staging'. Several groups have shown that after radiotherapy, the pathological (P) stage of the excised surgical specimen is frequently lower than the initial tumour (T) staging would suggest. For example, in the study mentioned above, almost half (47%) of the bladder specimens excised after radiotherapy demonstrated this effect [22]. Sterilization of locally involved lymph nodes can also be achieved by radiotherapy, the same study showing an incidence of node metastasis of 23% (the expected proportion would be 40–50% with unirradiated T_3 tumours). Only 8% of patients who had been judged to be good responders to radiotherapy had histologically positive local nodes and required cystectomy, suggesting that pre-operative irradiation may be particularly useful for patients with limited or microscopic regional or local lymph node deposits. Perhaps the most important result of all was that where down-staging could be demonstrated, the 5-year survival rate was 51% whereas in patients who showed no such change, the survival at 5 years was only 22%.

Although cystectomy remains a widely practised treatment for T_3 tumours, these and other data suggest that radiotherapy may be its equal, with considerable advantages in terms of morbidity. The quality of life with an ileal conduit is of course less satisfactory than for patients who micturate by the usual route. Common additional difficulties include odour, leakage, psychological adjustment to the stoma, and feelings of loss of sexual attractiveness. Many of these problems can be reduced by careful surgical technique and support but these patients naturally require a great deal of explanation and support pre- and postoperatively.

Radical external beam irradiation of bladder cancer should always be carried out using supervoltage equipment and requires a multi-field technique employing 3 or 4 fields (Fig. 18.9). There is considerable debate as to whether it is essential to treat the local pelvic nodes as well as the bladder itself. Although it is difficult to show any evidence of improved survival when the pelvic nodes are treated, the demonstration of down-staging as described above certainly strengthens the case. Treatment-related morbidity is of course greater when the pelvis is treated, even to the relatively modest dose of 40 Gy (4000 rad). Data from surgical series suggest that with nodal involvement, overall 5-year survival is less than 10%, suggesting that the disease is usually disseminated at diagnosis in node-positive cases. Current studies mostly favour the use of neoadjuvant chemotherapy programmes (including randomized trials by the MRC, EORTC and other international groups) with small-volume irradiation — probably a more logical approach. Chemo-responders may well be the same type of patients who 'down-staged' with pelvic irradiation.

Apart from the importance of radiation treatment with curative intent, symptoms such as pain, haematuria and frequency usually respond well, and radiotherapy is the most valuable palliative treatment even in advanced (Stage IV) tumours where there is virtually no prospect of cure.

CHEMOTHERAPY IN CARCINOMA OF THE BLADDER

The value of systemic chemotherapy for advanced bladder cancer remains controversial. Cyclophosphamide, doxorubicin, mitomycin C, 5-FU, methotrexate and cisplatin all produce responses of the order of 20–30%. Many groups have attempted to improve the results still further with combination regimes [13], but no clear-cut survival advantage has yet been demonstrated although there are recent encour-

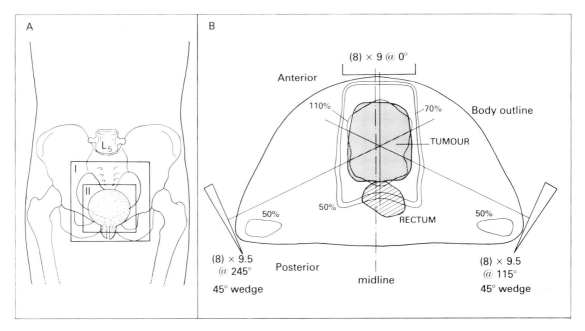

Fig. 18.9 Typical external irradiation treatment technique for invasive (T_3) carcinoma of the bladder. (A) Vertical representation of treatment volume. I: for first phase of treatment bladder and pelvic nodes are treated; II: for second phase of treatment the bladder is boosted to radical dose. Phase I is treated with the bladder full to minimize radiation damage to the small bowel. (B) Typical treatment plan in phase II of radical treatment (field sizes in cm).

aging early reports. Cisplatin is often regarded as the most active agent, yet the results of combination regimes including cisplatin seem to be almost identical with those of cisplatin therapy alone [23]. Further studies will be required to determine whether any groups of patients really benefit from such intensive treatment. At present, chemotherapy for advanced bladder tumours cannot be considered as conventional or established therapy, particularly since these patients tend to be in poor health and often have impaired renal function. There is considerable interest in the concept of neoadjuvant chemotherapy in carcinoma of the bladder. In the largest study so far reported, 376 patients were treated by radiotherapy or cystectomy, with or without neoadjuvant and adjuvant methotrexate [24]. No benefit was seen, indeed the chemotherapy, though relatively simple, proved too toxic for many patients to tolerate. A further British study in patients

prospectively randomized to receive neoadjuvant cisplatin (versus no chemotherapy) was also disappointing [25].

PROGNOSIS

About 50% of all patients with invasive bladder cancer survive for 5 years. Important prognostic determinants include histological grade, tumour stage and presence of nodal spread. T_1 tumours have a 5-year survival of about 75% with surgery alone. In T_2 and early T_3 lesions the 5-year survival is 35% while with more advanced disease, particularly where there is nodal involvement at diagnosis, only 10–15% will survive. There are virtually no long-term survivors when distant metastases are present at diagnosis. The use of adjuvant chemotherapy has not so far contributed to an improvement in these long-term results.

CARCINOMA OF THE PROSTATE

Incidence and aetiology

Carcinoma of the prostate is among the commonest of all cancers in men (Fig. 18.1), and in the United Kingdom is the third largest cause of death from cancer in males, exceeded only by deaths from cancer of the lung and large bowel. In the United States, the mortality rate is almost twice as high in black men as in white men and in 1977, 57000 new cases were registered, with over 20000 deaths (American Cancer Society figures). In the United States, England and Australia there is strong evidence to suggest an increasing incidence and mortality during the past 50 years [26,27] and the current death rate is $15-20$ per 100000 men. The positive autopsy rate for unexpected prostatic cancer is of the order of 30% in men over 50 years.

Little is known of the aetiology of prostatic carcinoma. It does not occur in castrated men and is also thought to be less common in hepatic cirrhosis which is accompanied by impaired oestrogen degradation.

Because of the frequency of prostatic carcinoma and its clear age relation, screening amongst unselected elderly males has increasingly been attempted, generally employing clinical examination by digital rectal prostatic palpation [28]. The detection rate is of the order of 1%, but the majority of cases are confined to the prostate, strengthening the rationale for this approach. Apart from digital rectal examination, common techniques include rectal ultrasonography and assay for prostate-specific antigen (PSA). These methods clearly increase the sensitivity although they are of course more costly. At present, despite the high incidence and detection rate, no series has convincingly shown a survival in screen-detected cases. Since the risk of developing prostate cancer is high, for example $0.37\%/\text{year} \times 25 = 8\%$ in a 50-year-old male, further studies are clearly warranted [27].

Pathology and staging

Adenocarcinoma is overwhelmingly the most common cell type, although transitional cell carcinoma may arise in the large prostatic ducts. Seventy-five per cent of all prostatic cancers arise in the posterior or peripheral part of the prostate, and about 10% of these tumours are discovered during prostatectomy for an apparently benign prostatic hypertrophy. Such cases tend to be more localized than when the diagnosis of carcinoma is suspected clinically.

Histological grading is of considerable importance, though the majority of prostatic cancers are moderately well-differentiated. The incidence of lymph node metastases increases with the degree of anaplasia and there is no doubt that patients with low-grade lesions survive substantially longer (60% 5-year survival, compared with 5% 5-year survival for patients with high-grade lesions).

No clinical or surgical staging system has yet found universal acceptance. The pattern of local invasion is shown schematically in Fig. 18.10. The TNM system is increasingly employed (Table 18.4), but can be difficult in practice, particularly in determination of the T-stage of the tumour. As with bladder tumours, the more recent TNM system has not found wide accept-

Table 18.4 TNM staging system for cancer of the prostate

T_0	No palpable tumour
T_1	Intracapsular tumour surrounded by normal prostatic tissue
T_2	Tumour confined to the gland but with deformity and with minimal capsular invasion.
T_3	Tumour extends locally beyond the capsule (including invasion of seminal vesicles)
T_4	Tumour fixed or involving local structure
N_0	No lymph node involvement
N_1	Regional lymph node involvement (single)
N_2	Regional lymph node involvement (multiple)
N_3	More widespread nodal involvement
M_0	No known metastases
M_1	Distant metastases (usually bone)

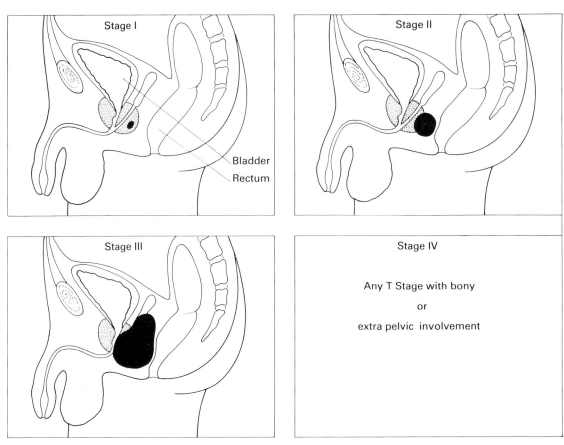

Fig. 18.10 Local extension and clinical staging in carcinoma of the prostate.

ance. The American system [29] is simpler and correlates fairly closely with the TNM staging. In this classification, the stages are defined thus:

Stage I carcinoma: microscopic cancer arising in a prostate gland which is not indurated on rectal examination. There are no metastases present.

Stage II carcinoma: a well-defined nodule or area of induration is present, confined to the prostate on rectal examination and without evidence of metastatic disease.

Stage III carcinoma: there is local extension beyond the confines of the prostate gland, usually with involvement of the bladder neck or seminal vesicle, but without clinical evidence of distant metastases.

Stage IV carcinoma: metastatic disease is

present, usually in the bones or in other extrapelvic sites.

There is some evidence that clinical staging is an accurate reflection of the true degree of spread. Where radical prostatectomy has been performed and the specimen carefully analysed, close agreement between surgical and clinical findings is discovered in about three-quarters of all cases, although sometimes with unsuspected local invasion — usually of the seminal vesicles. Invasion of pelvic lymph nodes may be clinically silent but is increasingly likely with advanced stages of disease as the prostate has an unusually rich lymph node network. Drainage is most commonly to the obturator-hypogastric group and then to the external and common iliac nodes. Distant metastases are predominantly osseous, particularly to the pelvic and lower lumbar vertebrae though ribs, dorsal spine and skull are not uncommonly involved. The bone metastases are typically osteosclerotic, as a result of the relatively slow clinical evolution of disease, although the pattern may be chiefly lytic or mixed.

Clinical features and investigation

Prostatic carcinoma is often asymptomatic, and is increasingly diagnosed at routine rectal examination. The typical finding is a firm, indurated or craggy gland which is usually enlarged. There may be obliteration of the median sulcus or spread to the lateral pelvic walls. Many patients present with bone pain from secondary deposits particularly in the back and pelvis. In patients with local prostatic symptoms, the commonest complaints are urinary infection or obstruction, with changes in the urinary stream including hesitancy or urgency of micturition.

Histological diagnosis is always required and transrectal biopsy is widely favoured. If fragments from a transurethral resection of a hypertrophic gland show evidence of malignancy, further confirmation is not usually necessary. Other methods of biopsy include the perineal or retropubic routes.

It is important to assess the local extent of disease as well as the presence of distant metastases in order to decide on the correct treatment, and to identify cases in which a local approach to treatment could be curative. Serum acid phosphatase is valuable, although now largely superseded by the use of PSA (see below). An isotope bone scan should always be done since bone metastases are often asymptomatic, particularly in the skull, ribs and upper part of the vertebral column. Skeletal X-rays give further details of these deposits but are not usually essential to management decisions unless local therapy for the metastasis is being considered. Routine tests of renal function are often revealing, and an IVU may show prostatic irregularity and back-pressure on the kidneys.

For patients who are candidates for surgery or radiotherapy of the primary tumour (with curative intent), it is essential to determine the full extent of local disease. Despite initial enthusiasm, routine lymphography has not become an established part of pretreatment investigation, since false-positive and false-negative results are not uncommon. CT scanning is more useful for detecting unsuspected nodal metastases, and also gives more detailed information regarding local extent of disease, particularly with respect to the degree of periprostatic invasion. It is not, however, generally considered to be as valuable an investigation as it is with bladder cancer.

Prostate specific antigen has increasingly been employed as a valuable tumour marker. Several groups have now shown a correlation between PSA level and extent of disease. If patients with localized disease are treated by radical prostatectomy, the PSA level should fall to zero, the PSA level then proving extremely valuable if serially measured.

Of the various features of prostate cancer analysed for their relative prognostic importance, a number of important characteristics have emerged including initial performance status using standard scales such as Karnofsky or ECOG, initial acid phosphatase/PSA level and T category. Some of these factors apply even in patients with unequivocal evidence of advanced disease at diagnosis [30]. The rapidity of reduction in PSA levels after therapy may also be relevant, and there is some suggestion that in patients with extensive disease, soft-tissue secondary sites may possibly be more responsive than bony sites to some types of hormone manipulation.

Management of prostatic cancer

There are few areas in clinical cancer management today where such diversity of opinion exists, even amongst experts [27,31]. Most would agree that in patients with clinically localized prostatic cancer, and without evidence of bone or extrapelvic metastases, some attempt at curative therapy should be made. However, some urologists believe (rightly or wrongly) that the true incidence of early (T_1) disease is so low that a localized approach is never really justifiable, preferring palliative methods of treatment in every case. In support of the 'no treatment' option, the study by Adolfsson and colleagues (61 patients with T_0-T_2 lesions, aged below 70 years), median follow-up at 8 years confirmed a death rate from prostate cancer of only 2% at 5 years and 8% at 10 years, although 23% had developed metastatic disease by the 10th year [31]. The cancer deaths were related to the tumour grade, allowing further speculation as to which patients might be deemed suitable for no initial active therapy [32]. More aggressive surgeons are prepared to consider radical surgical techniques even in patients with local periprostatic extension (i.e. up to Stage III disease), sometimes using hormonal treatment in an attempt to produce tumour shrinkage pre-operatively.

There are only two possible approaches for patients in whom radical treatment with curative intent is considered justifiable: radical prostatectomy or radical radiotherapy. The radical surgical approach has evolved since the turn of the century, and consists of *en bloc* resection of the prostate, prostatic urethra and seminal vesicles with part of the surrounding connective tissue (Denonvillier's fascia). Only patients with disease confined within the prostatic capsule and without lymph node metastasis can be considered suitable, and the operation has always been more popular in the United States than in Britain. The surgical approach can be either retropubic or perineal. The suprapubic approach also allows for pelvic lymphadenectomy, if this is considered appropriate. Complications are discussed below.

Radical radiation therapy, though more recently introduced, is certainly more widely applicable than surgery since minimal extracapsular extension or periprostatic invasion do not represent contraindications to treatment. Although any form of radical treatment should be considered with care since the majority of these patients are over 65 years of age, there

seems no doubt that radical surgery demands a greater general level of medical fitness than the radiotherapeutic approach. It is known that the normal prostate tolerates high dosage of radiation without prostatic symptoms developing, although excessive irradiation of surrounding tissues (bladder, prostatic urethra or large bowel) can cause serious problems (see Chapter 5).

In patients suitable for radical radiotherapy, a high dosage has to be given to the whole of the gland and periprostatic area. Although interstitial approaches using radium implants into the gland were initially employed by early workers, external beam irradiation is now usually preferred (but see below).

There is general agreement that a total dose of at least 60 Gy (6000 rad) over 6 weeks (or equivalent over a shorter period) is required for eradication of prostatic cancer and even higher doses have been recommended. In addition, the pelvic contents are often irradiated (Fig. 18.11), to a dose of 40 Gy (4000 rad) over 4 weeks, because of the possibility of unsuspected peri-

Fig. 18.11 Typical treatment volume for radical irradiation of carcinoma of the prostate using external beam therapy. (A) First phase of treatment (to 40 Gy/4 weeks) treats prostatic lymph node drainage as well as prostate and prostatic urethra; (B) prostate and periprostatic area boosted to total of 60 Gy/6 weeks. Field arrangement similar to Fig. 18.9.

prostatic or lymphatic spread; some radio-therapists recommend a minimum of 50 Gy (5000 rad) to the whole pelvic contents, with a final boost to the periprostatic and prostatic region when the pelvic irradiation has been completed. As with bladder cancer, the appropriate choice of volume for treatment of prostatic cancer remains contentious. Many radiotherapists avoid treatment of the pelvic contents because of increased morbidity in an an elderly population, and point to the lack of survival advantage in patients in whom prophylactic pelvic node irradiation has been undertaken. A variety of techniques has been used to achieve these high dosages. Multifield arrangements are invariably required, often employing three or four fields of treatment as for treatment of bladder cancer, always using supervoltage equipment.

An alternative approach, receiving increasing attention, is the use of permanent interstitial implants, usually employing ^{125}I seeds, to the prostate (and periprostatic area if necessary), (Fig. 18.12). This treatment delivers a very high local dose (>100 Gy, 10 000 rad) with remarkably low morbidity, and clearly warrants further trial, possibly in conjunction with external irradiation of the pelvic lymph nodes.

RESULTS OF RADICAL TREATMENT

It is difficult to assess the results of treatment in carcinoma of the prostate, because of its uncertain and often indolent natural history and the high death rate in any group of elderly men. Among the best results of radical surgery is a large recent series from Leandri and colleagues [33]. Despite careful selection, the operation failed to control the local disease in a significant minority of cases. Complications of treatment included stress incontinence, urinary frequency and loss of erectile function. Several centres have reported large series of patients treated by radiotherapy, in whom a proportion appear to have been cured [34,35] although 'cure' is difficult to define in this elderly population. In following up these patients, it is

Fig. 18.12 Transperineal interstitial implantation of the prostate. ^{125}I seeds are used to obtain a high local dose (in excess of 100 Gy (10 000 rad)). Intra-rectal ultrasound is used for localization of the gland avoiding the need for open operation.

important to realize that in the irradiated prostate, subsequent biopsy may show evidence of persistent malignant cells for up to a year, without any supportive clinical suggestion that the treatment has failed. In one series, 60% of patients with locally advanced disease had positive biopsies up to 9 months after treatment, falling to only 24% at 12–30 months, without further treatment [36].

One of the largest radiation series, by Bagshawe and colleagues [37], provided results in over 400 patients (Fig. 18.13) showing a difference in survival between patients whose disease was limited to the prostate and those who had extracapsular extension. Survival at 5 years approached 60%, with 40% of patients alive at 10 years. Although these results were published nearly 20 years ago, few departments could claim better results today.

Complications of radical surgical treatment include an operative mortality rate of up to 5%, permanent impotence in at least 90% of

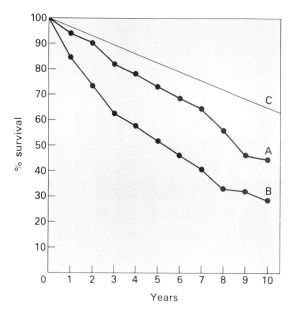

Fig. 18.13 Results of radical radiation therapy for carcinoma of the prostate. (A) Disease limited to prostate; (B) extracapsular extension; (C) expected survival, adjusted for age. (From Bagshawe *et al.* [36] With permission.)

patients (unless treated by nerve-sparing procedures, see below), and urinary incontinence in at least 5%. Rectovesical fistula and ureteric damage may also occur. Important complications of radical radiotherapy include side-effects of diarrhoea, dysuria and perineal skin reaction (sometimes severe), commonly occurring during the latter part of treatment. Long-term sequelae also occur, and a degree of subcutaneous fibrosis, urethral stricture and fibrotic reduction of bladder capacity may have to be accepted. Treatment with a full bladder will help to keep the small bowel out of the irradiated volume. The avoidance of impotence as a side-effect is a valuable advantage since with either radical surgery or hormonal treatment for prostatic cancer, impotence is almost certain unless specific nerve-sparing surgical techniques are used [34]. However, even with radical prostatic irradiation, impotence rates of up to 50% have been reported. The introduction

of the nerve-sparing radical prostatectomy has led during the past decade to an enormous increase in the popularity of surgical treatment for localized carcinoma of the prostate, at least in the United States.

HORMONAL THERAPY
IN PROSTATIC CANCER

In 1941, Huggins discovered that prostatic cancers were almost always hormonally dependent [38]. Both oestrogen therapy and orchidectomy were found to be useful for palliation, particularly in patients with bone metastases. Since the majority of patients are unsuitable for radical surgery, the use of oestrogen derivatives or orchidectomy (sometimes both) became increasingly widespread as part of standard therapy both for early and advanced cases.

Hormonal manipulation has been increasingly widely used as definitive treatment for advanced disease (Stages III and IV), although many radiotherapists prefer to offer local irradiation to patients with Stage III disease who have no evidence of metastases elsewhere, and whose clinical condition warrants an attempt at radical treatment.

The increasing availability of newer forms of androgen-ablating hormone therapy has fuelled still further the controversy regarding optimal timing for introduction of such treatment, particularly since their side-effects and acceptability differ from those of oestrogen therapy. Furthermore, it remains unclear whether the type of hormone therapy critically influences overall outcome, and also whether combined anti-androgen therapy may prove superior to single-agent or sequential treatment [27]. Considerable interest has followed the demonstration that analogues of gonadotrophin-releasing hormone (so-called LHRH agonists) may interfere with gonadotrophin release, leading to a fall in circulating testosterone. Recently introduced agents include goserelin (Zoladex), a depot form of gonadotrophin-releasing hormone analogue, and flutamide, a pure anti-androgen compound which interferes with testosterone binding to the androgen receptor. Both of these agents, together with the more traditional forms of hormone therapy (oestrogen derivatives, orchidectomy), appear to have similar response rates though the analogue agents have very few cardiovascular complications and appear superior to diethylstilboestrol [38]. Flutamide is probably similar in its mechanism of action to cyproterone acetate, which was introduced earlier (1973) and is also widely used. One valuable advantage of treatment with flutamide and other nonsteroidal pure anti-androgens over stilboestrol is the potential for preservation of potency. Unlike the progesterone-like cyproterone acetate, these agents do not lead to central inhibition of LH release. Since they block negative testosterone feedback, increased serum levels of testosterone occur.

Total androgen blockage, using combinations of hormonal agents in an attempt to block both testicular and adrenal output, has also been tested in randomized controlled studies [38]. In patients with advanced disease there may be some benefit, and combinations of a gonadotrophin-releasing hormone analogue together with an anti-androgen such as flutamide are generally employed. Such treatment is clearly more costly and toxic but may be justifiable [27].

In palliative treatment of metastatic prostatic cancer, radiotherapy has an important role since the majority of the metastases are bony, and likely to be painful. These deposits generally respond well to moderate doses of radiotherapy. In recent years, single fraction hemi-body irradiation has been shown to be valuable, particularly since widespread metastases in the lower spine are so common. Treatment of the lower half of the body to a single fraction dose of 7.5−10 Gy (750−1000 rad) is well tolerated and often dramatically effective for pain relief.

In patients with widespread metastatic problems unresponsive to oestrogens or palliative irradiation, there is every reason to consider bilateral orchidectomy since worthwhile responses certainly occur. However, patients with hormone-resistant prostatic carcinoma have particular problems [40]. Long-term survival is unlikely once the disease is refractory to hormone therapy though it seems important to continue to keep the patient androgen-depleted. If anti-androgen treatment is withdrawn, testosterone levels may rise and survival may be shortened, especially in patients receiving gonadotrophin-releasing analogues.

Chemotherapy for prostatic carcinoma has been disappointing although a number of agents show modest levels of activity, including cyclophosphamide, methotrexate, 5-FU, nitrogen mustard and cisplatin.

In patients with unresponsive widespread bone pain, treatment with radioactive phosphorus may be of value, and up to 75% of all patients have been reported to benefit, though remissions tend to be short. ^{89}Sr has recently been marketed as a superior radionuclide for use in this way. It may be preferentially taken up in metastases rather than treating the whole bone marrow. Hypophysectomy is sometimes effective and can be done without craniotomy using a trans-sphenoidal approach.

Overall, it has been estimated that patients with carcinoma of the prostate lose, on average, almost a decade of life; the disease is now claiming 9000 lives annually in the United Kingdom [41].

CANCER OF THE URETHRA

Male urethra

This very rare tumour may arise in the prostatic, bulbar or penile urethra, and is thought to be commoner in patients with a history of chronic inflammation or stricture. In the prostatic urethra, the tumour is a transitional cell carcinoma but in the penile urethra, squamous carcinomas are more common. The tumour spreads by direct invasion into the perineum and penile tissues.

The penile urethra drains to inguinal lymph nodes, and the prostatic urethra to pelvic nodes.

Urethral carcinomas present with a urethral

mass, obstruction, fistula, pain and haematuria. The age range is 50–80 years. Prostatic urethral tumours are treated either by radical prostatectomy or cystoprostatectomy, or by radical radiotherapy. This latter method is increasingly employed, using doses of the order of 60–70 Gy (6000–7000 rad) to the prostate. Radiation technique is similar to that employed for carcinoma of the prostate (Fig. 18.11).

Distal penile urethral carcinomas are usually treated by amputation of the distal part of the penis. Lesions of the bulbomembranous urethra are generally treated by radical excision.

Female urethra

The tumour is twice as common in females, and the histological pattern is more varied. Squamous carcinoma is the predominant form in the distal two-thirds, and transitional cell carcinoma in the proximal third. Adenocarcinoma may arise from the periurethral glands, and melanoma and sarcoma occasionally occur. Leucoplakia of the urethra is regarded as a premalignant change, as are urethral papillomas and polyps.

The tumour typically presents with a mass or with bleeding and offensive discharge. Lymphatic involvement occurs late, tumours of the distal urethra draining to the inguinal nodes and those of the proximal urethra to the iliac nodes.

Tumours of the anterior urethra are sometimes treated by partial urethrectomy but there is a high risk of local recurrence and nodal spread frequently occurs. There is increasing interest in the use of radical radiation therapy since surgical control of the more extensive tumours is hard to achieve and the results are very poor. Interstitial radioactive implants are sometimes used for small tumours, and external beam radiation therapy for larger lesions. The usual tumour dose is of the order of 60 Gy (6000 rad), carefully fractionated to avoid stricture formation.

CANCER OF THE PENIS

Incidence and aetiology

Carcinoma of the penis is uncommon in Britain and the United States. Worldwide, its incidence is only 0.6–1.0 per 100 000 population accounting for less than 0.2% of all male cancer deaths in Britain. It is, however, much more frequent in South East Asia, and in parts of India and Africa. It is thought that general hygiene has a bearing on its incidence, and early circumcision is known to be associated with a very low risk. Men with phimosis also appear to be at higher risk. At present, a viral origin seems likely to explain at least a proportion of cases [42]. At least one married couple have been described with co-existent penile and vulval carcinoma, and the viral hypothesis is strengthened by the observation that many patients with penile cancer also harbour condylomata acuminata. There is slight concordance between the incidence of penile and cervical carcinomas in sexual partners. In addition, there are several premalignant conditions which predispose to the development of the tumour. These include Bowen's disease (intraepithelial carcinoma), erythroplasia of Queyrat, leucoplakia and Paget's disease. Leukoplakia may co-exist with an invasive carcinoma. These premalignant lesions should be treated by local excision. The carcinoma is almost always a squamous cell lesion although melanoma, basal cell carcinoma and Kaposi's sarcoma have all been described.

Clinical features

Presentation is usually with an exophytic, or occasionally an excavating, ulcerated lesion, most commonly arising in the glans or the inner surface of the prepuce. There is often wide surface extension before deeper invasion to the urethra and corpora cavernosa. Some carcinomas of the penis are clinically obvious with a circumferential exophytic necrotic tumour, whereas in other cases only careful inspection with retraction of the prepuce will allow the tumour to be visualized. Local invasion to the inguinal nodes is common, but lymph node enlargement may be due to local infection rather than to metastasis. The superficial inguinal nodes drain the prepuce and most of the penile skin, whereas the glans and corpora cavernosa drain chiefly to the deep inguinal nodes. A biopsy should always be performed since non-malignant conditions, such as lymphogranuloma venereum, trauma, penile warts (condylomata) or leucoplakia can cause diagnostic confusion.

A TNM staging classification has been proposed (Table 18.5), but can be difficult to apply in practice, particularly since palpable inguinal lymph nodes are often due to local infection. Though relatively unlikely to disseminate widely, the commonest sites of blood-borne metastases (M_1) are the lungs and bone, and a chest X-ray should always be performed as part of the investigation. The value of lymphography is limited by the frequent concurrent infection.

Treatment

For very localized lesions, cryosurgery or laser excision may be adequate; for more extensive tumours wider excision has traditionally been considered the treatment of choice, although amputation of the penis has never been a popular method of treatment and radical local

Table 18.5 TNM staging for cancer of the penis

T_0	No evidence of primary tumour
T_{is}	Carcinoma *in situ* (include Bowen's disease and erythroplasia of Queyrat)
T_1	Superficial tumour <1 cm diameter
T_2	Larger tumour but remains superficial
T_3	Tumour invades underlying tissues
T_4	Tumour invades local tissues including corpora cavernosa, urethra or perineum
N_0	No regional lymphadenopathy
N_1	Unilateral regional node involvement
N_2	Multiple unilateral node groups involved, or bilateral nodes
M_0	No distant metastases
M_1	Distant metastases present

irradiation has increasingly been used as an alternative. As the tumour is uncommon, few surgeons or radiotherapists have a large experience. Treatment is often individualized: a small non-infiltrating tumour, which can be surgically excised without amputation, is probably best treated by surgery, with local irradiation given wherever there is doubt about the adequacy of the resection edge of the specimen. Many radiotherapists are disinclined to offer radical irradiation in bulky lesions because of the probability of hypoxia within the necrotic part of the tumour which limits the prospect of radiocurability; such tumours are probably best dealt with surgically, particularly if partial amputation will suffice. More proximal lesions would require total amputation, but many surgeons are prepared to agree to radical irradiation in the first instance, with surgery if there is local recurrence.

A variety of radiotherapy techniques has been described, including superficial X-rays (with single or opposed direct fields), treatment by radium mould, or by orthovoltage or supervoltage irradiation using photons or electrons. A wax block can be used to improve dose homogeneity. Interstitial implants with radioactive iridium or other sources can also be used. The total dose of external irradiation is usually 60 Gy (6000 rad) in daily fractions over 6 weeks, or the equivalent over a shorter treatment period. With mould treatments using iridium wire or radium, the treatment can usually be completed within 10 days (the patient wearing the mould for 8–10 hours per day), to a total dose of the order of 60 Gy. The major complications of radiation therapy for carcinoma of the penis include urethral stricture (10–12% of patients), fibrosis, ulceration and local recurrence (10–40% depending on the size of the tumour). For larger and more infiltrating tumours, surgery is probably the treatment of choice, particularly where the inguinal nodes are obviously involved by tumour. Where the inguinal nodes are mobile, block dissection is generally preferable to local irradiation although it is probably wise to perform aspiration cytology to confirm that the nodes are indeed metastatic. Before the advent of aspiration cytology, delay in inguinal block dissection was often advocated to allow infected palpable nodes to settle. Where the inguinal nodes are clearly fixed and surgery is not possible, local irradiation of the inguinal node groups can be useful as a palliative procedure. Although remissions have been documented in such cases, survival is poor. The majority of patients with Stage I (T_1 or T_2, N_0) tumours are free of inguinal metastases but the incidence in Stage II (T_3, N_0 or N_{1a}) is well over 50%, and it is these patients who probably benefit most from block dissection.

Prognosis

Early carcinoma of the penis has an excellent cure rate with surgery and/or radiotherapy. Although few large series of patients have been reported, it seems probable that T_1 and T_2 N_0 cases are equally well treated by surgery or radiotherapy. In one series, 18 out of 20 patients treated by radical irradiation were free of disease at 3 years [43], which compares closely with surgical figures. Patients with deep involvement of penile structures or inguinal node involvement do far less well, and the survival rate is approximately 50%. Where there are inoperable inguinal metastases or distant involvement, the 5-year survival rate is well under 10%.

REFERENCES

1 Doll R., Peto R. *The Causes of Cancer: Quantitative Estimates of Avoidable Risks of Cancer in the United States Today.* Oxford University Press, 1981.

2 Selli C., Hinshaw W.M., Woodard B.H., Paulson D.F. Stratification of risk factors in renal cell carcinoma. *Cancer* 1983; **52**: 899–903.

3 Skinner D.G., Colvin R.B., Vermillion C.D., Pfister R.C., Leadbetter W.F. Diagnosis and management of renal cell carcinoma. *Cancer* 1971; **28**: 1165–77.

4 Finney R. An evaluation of postoperative radiotherapy in hypernephroma treatment — a clinical trial. *Cancer* 1973; **32**: 1332–40.

5 Van der Werf-Messing B. Carcinoma of the kidney. *Cancer* 1973; **32**: 1056–61.

6 Rafla S. Renal cell carcinoma: natural history and results of treatment. *Cancer* 1970; **25**: 26–40.

7 Kjaer M., Frederiksen M.D., Engelholm S.A. Postoperative radiotherapy in Stage I and II renal adenocarcinoma. A randomized trial by the Copenhagen Renal Cancer Study Group. *International Journal of Radiation Oncology, Biology and Physics* 1987; **13**: 665–72.

8 Ahmed T., Benedetto P., Yagoda A. *et al.* Estrogen, progesterone and androgen-binding sites in renal cell carcinoma. *Cancer* 1984; **54**: 477–81.

9 Waxman J., Thomas H. Is the outlook changing for patients with renal cell cancer? *European Journal of Cancer* 1990; **26**: 860–61.

10 Horoszewicz J.S., Murphy G.P. An assessment of the current use of human interferons in therapy of urological cancers. *Journal of Urology* 1989; **142**: 1173–80.

11 Rosenberg S.A., Lotz M.T., Muul L.M. *et al.* Observations on the systemic administration of autologous lymphokine-activated killer cells and recombinant interleukin-2 to patients with metastatic cancer. *New England Journal of Medicine* 1985; **313**: 1485–92.

12 Anon. Biological therapy for metastatic renal cell cancer. *Lancet* 1991; **337**: 522–23.

13 Raghavan D., Shipley W.U., Garnick M.B. *et al.* Biology and management of bladder cancer. *New England Journal of Medicine* 1990; **322**: 1129–38.

14 Wallace D.M.A. Occupational urothelial cancer. *British Journal of Urology* 1988; **61**: 175–82.

15 Bjergaard J.P., Ersboll J., Hansen V.L. *et al.* Carcinoma of the urinary bladder after treatment with cyclophosphamide for non-Hodgkin's lymphoma. *New England Journal of Medicine* 1988; **318**: 1028–32.

16 Plail R. Detecting bladder cancer. *British Medical Journal* 1990; **301**: 567–68.

17 Lamm D.L., De Haven J.I., Shriver J. *et al.* Prospective randomized comparison of intravesical with percutaneous BCG versus intravesical BCG in superficial bladder cancer. *Journal of Urology* 1991; **144**: 738–40.

18 Van der Werf-Messing B. Cancer of the urinary bladder treated by interstitial radium implant. *International Journal of Radiation Oncology, Biology and Physics* 1978; **4**: 373–78.

19 Whitmore W.F., Batata M.A., Ghoneim M.A., Grabstald H., Unal A. Radical cystectomy with or without prior irradiation in the treatment of bladder cancer. *Journal of Urology* 1977; **118**: 184–87.

20 Brendler C.B., Steinberg G.D., Marshall F.F. *et al.* Local recurrence and survival following nerve-sparing radical cystoprostatectomy. *Journal of Urology* 1990; **144**: 1137–41.

21 Edsmyr F. Radiotherapy in the management of bladder carcinoma. In Oliver R.T.D., Hendry W.F., Bloom H.J.G., eds. *Bladder Cancer*, pp. 139–49. London: Butterworths, 1981.

22 Bloom H.J.G., Hendry W.F., Wallace D.M., Skeet R.G. Treatment of T3 bladder cancer: controlled trial of pre-operative radiotherapy and radical cystectomy versus radical radiotherapy. Second report and review (for the Clinical Trials Group, Institute of Urology). *British Journal of Urology* 1982; **54**: 136–51.

23 Yagoda A. Chemotherapy of metastatic bladder cancer. *Cancer* 1980; **45**: 1879–88.

24 Shearer R.J., Chilvers C.E.D., Bloom H.J.G. *et al.* Adjuvant chemotherapy in T3 carcinoma of the bladder: a prospective trial. *British Journal of Urology* 1988; **62**: 558–64.

25 Wallace D.M.A., Raghaven D., Kelly K.A. *et al.* Neo-adjuvant (pre-emptive) cisplatin therapy in invasive transitional cell carcinoma of the bladder. *British Journal of Urology* 1991; **67**: 608–15.

26 Lu-Yao G.I., Greenberg E.R. Changes in prostate cancer incidence and treatment in the USA. *Lancet* 1994; **343**: 251–54.

27 Scher H.I. Prostatic cancer: are we closer to rational treatment selection? *Current Opinion in Oncology* 1992; **4**: 442–54.

28 Gerber F.S., Chodak G.W. Routine screening for cancer of the prostate. *Journal of the National Cancer Institute* 1991; **83**: 329–35.

29 Rubin P. Cancer of the urogenital tract: prostatic cancer. *Journal of the American Medical Association* 1969; **209**: 1695–96.

30 Ernst D.S., Hanson J., Venner P.M. Analysis of prognostic factors in men with metastatic prostate cancer: Uro-oncology group of Northern Alberta. *Journal of Urology* 1991; **146**: 372–76.

31 Adolfsson J., Cartensen J. Natural course of clinically localised prostate adenocarcinoma in men less than 70 yrs old. *Journal of Urology* 1991; **146**: 96–98.

32 Chodak G.W., Thisted R.A., Gerber G.S. *et al.* Results of conservative management of clinically localised prostate cancer. *New England Journal of Medicine* 1994; **330**: 242–48.

33 Leandri P., Rossignol G., Gautier J. *et al.* Radical retropubic prostatectomy: morbidity and quality of life: experience with 620 consecutive cases. *Journal of Urology* 1992; **147**: 883–87.

34 Fuks Z., Leibel S.A., Wallner K.A. *et al.* The effect of local control on metastatic dissemination in carcinoma of the prostate: long-term results in patients treated with ^{125}I implantation. *International Journal of Radiation Oncology, Biology and Physics* 1991; **21**: 537–47.

35 Kaplan I.D., Prestidge B.R., Bagshawe M.A. *et al.* Importance of local control in treatment of prostatic cancer. *Journal of Urology* 1992; **147**: 917–22.

36 Cox J.D., Stoffel T.J. The significance of needle biopsy after irradiation for stage C adenocarcinoma of the prostate. *Cancer* 1977; **40**: 156–60.

37 Bagshaw M.A., Ray G.R., Salzman J.R., Meares E.M. Extended-field radiation therapy for carcinoma of the prostate: a progress report. *Cancer Chemotherapy Reports* 1975; **59**: (Part I), 165–73.

38 Huggins C., Hodges C.F. Studies on prostatic cancer. I: The effect of castration, of estrogen and of androgen injection on serum acid phosphatase in metastatic carcinoma of the prostate. *Cancer Research* 1941; **1**: 293–97.

39 Crawford E.D., Eisenberger M.A., McLeod D.G. *et al.* A controlled trial of leuprolide with and without flutamide in prostatic carcinoma. *New England Journal of Medicine* 1989; **321**: 419–24.

40 Scher H.I., Curley T., Yeh S. *et al.* Therapeutic alternatives for hormone refractory prostatic cancer. *Seminars in Urology* 1992; **10**: 55–64.

41 Dearnaley D.P. Cancer of the prostate. *British Medical Journal* 1994; **308**: 780–84.

42 Boon M.E., Schneider A., Hoegewonig C.J.A. *et al.* Penile studies and heterosexual partners: peniscopy, cytology, histology and immunochemistry. *Cancer* 1988; **61**: 1652–59.

43 Duncan W., Jackson S.M. The treatment of early cancer of the penis with megavoltage X-rays. *Clinical Radiology* 1972; **23**: 246–48.

Although testicular tumours are uncommon, with a frequency of just over 2 per 100 000 males per year, they have an importance well beyond their low incidence. Firstly, they represent the most common malignant disease of young men between the ages of 25 and 35 years; secondly, they are exceptionally chemosensitive tumours with a high cure rate even with disseminated disease; and thirdly, they often manufacture tumour markers which can be used to monitor treatment and to predict recurrence before it is clinically evident. Furthermore, their incidence has risen considerably over the past decade. Some 800 cases are now diagnosed annually in the United Kingdom, and 5000 in the United States. During the same period there has been considerable progress in the management of these conditions and death from testicular tumours is now extremely uncommon.

GERM CELL TUMOURS

Aetiology and incidence

Over 90% of testicular tumours are *germ cell tumours* which are believed to arise in the pluripotent germ cell. This cell, when malignant, can give rise to tumours which have either somatic or trophoblastic features, or both. Somatic differentiation results in the mixture of tissues typically found in teratomas while choriocarcinoma comes from trophoblastic differentiation. *Non-germ cell tumours* are discussed on p. 391 and include lymphomas, metastatic deposits and Leydig and Sertoli tumours. Although most male germ cell tumours arise in

the testis they may occasionally be *extragonadal* in origin, and these are described on p. 390.

The presence of an undescended testis (cryptorchidism) is associated with a 10-fold increase in the incidence of testicular tumours. About 10% of all patients with a testicular germ cell tumour have a history of maldescent. Orchidopexy reduces, but does not abolish, this risk. Data from North America suggest that testicular tumours are rarer in black than in white Americans. Teratomas of the testis (about 50% of all germ cell tumours) present at an earlier age (peak age 20−30 years) than seminomas (peak age 30−50 years). The age-adjusted incidence in Britain is 3.8 per 100 000; incidence at different ages is shown in Fig. 19.1. Teratoma and seminoma are the usual tumours at 10−40 years, but in older age groups lymphoma is the commonest tumour. Familial instances of testicular germ cell tumour have occasionally been described.

The mechanism of carcinogenesis has attracted considerable attention. It seems likely that atrophy of the germinal epithelium with loss of feedback inhibition of the pituitary may be the common aetiological factor. This increase in pituitary-driven hormonal stimulation of the remaining testicular germ cells might then result in neoplastic change. There may even be a higher risk of relapse with total aspermia (i.e. the greatest degree of atrophy) than in patients with similar stages and pathology of their disease but with some residual degree of active spermatogenesis [1]. This mechanism might also account for the worrying possible association with vasectomy − in which the risk of testicular neoplasia may possibly be higher,

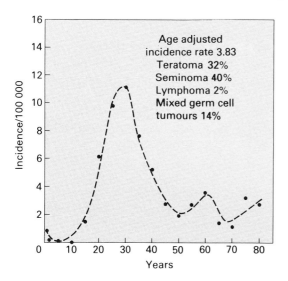

Fig. 19.1 Age-specific incidence of testicular tumours.

Table 19.1 Pathological classification of testicular tumours

British Testicular Tumour Panel
Seminoma
Malignant teratoma undifferentiated (MTU)
Malignant teratoma intermediate (MTI)
Malignant teratoma trophoblastic (MTT)
Teratoma differentiated (TD)

Dixon and Moore [3]
Pure seminoma
Embryonal carcinoma (pure or with seminoma)
Teratoma (pure or with seminoma)
Teratoma with embryonal carcinoma, choriocarcinoma
  or seminoma
Choriocarcinoma pure or with seminoma embryonal
  carcinoma (or both)

World Health Organization
1 Tumours of single cell type
  Seminoma
  Embryonal carcinoma
  Teratoma
  Choriocarcinoma
2 Mixed histological appearances
  Embryonal carcinoma with teratoma
  Embryonal carcinoma with teratoma and seminoma
  Embryonal carcinoma with choriocarcinoma
  Teratoma with seminoma
  Choriocarcinoma with any other cell type

particularly in patients whose operation was complicated by haematoma or infection. Testicular atrophy following mumps orchitis may also result in neoplastic change via the same general mechanism. The long-standing uncertainty of the role of testicular trauma has recently been more fully investigated and cannot confidently be excluded as an unimportant factor [2].

Pathology

A variety of different systems of classification are in current use (Table 19.1). In Britain, the commonest classification is that of the British Testicular Tumour Panel, whilst in the United States, the Dixon and Moore classification is widely used [3]. Each is the result of a review of a large number of patients, and both are traditionally based on light microscopic criteria, and attempt to identify the predominant cell type. A major problem with all classifications is that the tumours are often heterogeneous, the teratomas displaying pleomorphism and a tendency to multiple cell types. Future classifications may depend increasingly on histochemical criteria, particularly in those tumours which produce tumour markers.

Most testicular tumours are of germ cell origin (Fig. 19.2). These can usually be classified into seminomas (40%), teratomas (32%), or combined tumours with elements of both (14%). Non-germ cell tumours are discussed more fully on p. 391. In the past 10 years there has been increased recognition that carcinoma *in situ* (CIS) may occur in the testis, and may, after several years of apparent dormancy, develop into an invasive carcinoma. These tumours appear particularly common in patients with a history of testicular maldescent, with a probable frequency of 2% [4]. The changes of CIS are frequently widespread within the testis [5].

Although the precise histological type of germ cell tumour previously carried great prognostic significance, particularly in the distinction between seminoma and the teratomas (non-seminomas), the recent dramatic improvements

Fig. 19.2 Histological appearances of testicular germ cell tumours. (Original magnification ×200). (A) Pure seminoma; (B) malignant teratoma differentiated, showing cartilage and smooth muscle (arrowed); (C) malignant teratoma intermediate, showing differentiated epithelium and embryonal carcinoma (arrowed); (D) malignant teratoma undifferentiated, showing embryonal carcinoma; (E) yolk sac tumour, showing a Schiller–Duval body (arrowed); (F) choriocarcinoma, showing syncytiotrophoblast (arrowed) and cytotrophoblast.

in treatment (particularly of teratomas) have reduced these disparities. Apart from the cell type, the most important prognostic feature, available from the operative specimen at orchidectomy, is the presence of tumour cells either at the cut end of the cord or within its vessels (intravascular invasion). Such tumours have an adverse prognosis. The level of initial tumour marker values (see below) also carries prognostic significance.

The relationship between *in situ* carcinoma and invasive testicular cancer is now increasingly well recognized, although testicular biopsy is still of course unacceptable to many.

None the less, a high-risk group can be recognized by presence of *in situ* change and this is of practical importance because low-dose irradiation of an affected testis can prevent the later development of invasive testicular tumours without lowering testosterone levels or affecting sexuality.

Chromosomal analysis has indicated a remarkable consistency in the finding of a single abnormality (iso chrome 12p) which is almost as common in testicular tumours as the Philadelphia chromosome in chronic myeloid leukaemia. Other cytogenetic studies have suggested that seminomas may be an 'intermediate' step in the progression towards the most malignant forms of testicular teratoma since the chromosome number in seminoma cases is intermediate between precursor *in situ* cell change and histologically more advanced disease [6].

SEMINOMA

Seminomas tend to be encapsulated and firm, with the cut surface pale grey and often featureless, and with little or no necrosis or haemorrhage. The microscopic appearance shows large round cells with distinct cell borders, clear cytoplasm, and large nuclei often with conspicuous nucleoli (Fig. 19.2). Lymphocytic infiltration is frequently seen. When spread beyond the testis occurs, it is almost invariably to pelvic and para-aortic lymph nodes followed by involvement of mediastinal and supraclavicular nodes. Although chiefly testicular in origin, primary extragonadal seminomas are occasionally encountered in the retroperitoneal region, mediastinum, and suprasellar region or pineal area of the brain.

TERATOMA (NON-SEMINOMATOUS GERM CELL TUMOURS)

Malignant teratoma undifferentiated (MTU, embryonal carcinoma)

This is the commonest non-seminomatous germ cell tumour. These are often firm and nodular, showing areas of haemorrhage and necrosis. Microscopically, large anaplastic cells are usually seen, with less distinct cell borders and an eosinophilic cytoplasm containing nuclei of widely varying shapes. Some form of differentiation may occur, often with a glandular pattern (Fig. 19.2).

Teratoma differentiated (TD)

Occasionally, a fully mature or differentiated testicular teratoma is encountered, in which mature bone, bone marrow and cartilage, and other tissues may all be present. Even these tumours should be regarded as 'potentially malignant'.

Malignant teratoma intermediate (MTI or teratocarcinoma)

This usually shows characteristic differences from MTU, with a nodular appearance which, on sectioning, frequently feels gritty because of the presence of cartilage and/or bone. There is often a wide variety of germ cell types, including cells derived from all three of the primitive germ cell layers, including bone, cartilage, connective tissue and smooth muscle as well as cells suggestive of respiratory or gastrointestinal epithelium.

Malignant teratoma trophoblastic (MTT, choriocarcinoma)

This is very much less common, and is histologically distinct because of the typical elements of cytotrophoblast and/or syncytiotrophoblast cells. These tumours are highly malignant, metastasizing early and widely. It is extremely unusual to encounter a true trophoblastic testicular tumour which is confined to the testis. They tend to be bulky tumours at presentation and are more often associated with brain metastases than other types of teratoma. They may develop drug resistance early, and should probably be treated with regimens containing methotrexate. A prognostic distinction can be drawn between MTT and the commoner teratoma types (MTI and MTU). MTU probably has a more rapid doubling time than MTI, more commonly presents with lung deposits, seems more responsive to chemotherapy, and carries a somewhat better prognosis.

Spread

A. Along lymphatics of cord
B. Iliac and retroperitoneal (para-aortic) nodes including renal hilar nodes
C. Mediastinal and supraclavicular nodes
D. Lung
E. Liver, brain and other sites
Sequence is usually A to E

Fig. 19.3 Pathways of spread of testicular germ cell tumours.

Patterns of metastases

Clinical staging is based on a relatively predictable pattern of progression (Fig. 19.3). Typically, the mode of spread is lymphatic, along the lymphatics of the spermatic cord to the para-aortic lymph nodes, and thence to the retroperitoneal and retrocrural nodes, thoracic duct, posterior mediastinum and supraclavicular nodes (usually left-sided, although bifid or right-sided thoracic ducts occur in a small percentage of the population). Blood-borne spread frequently occurs, especially in MTT and MTU. In over 90% of cases this is associated with demonstrable nodal spread; in the remainder, metastases develop in the lungs, in the absence of abdominal lymphatic disease. Although liver involvement is not frequent, it is exceptional in patients without lung deposits. Intracerebral and bone metastases are occasionally encountered. MTU is more commonly associated with locally invasive primary tumours and with haematogenous spread than MTI.

Clinical features

Patients typically present with a painless swelling of the testis, although pain may be a feature in about 25% of cases, particularly with rapidly growing tumours. There seems to be a great difference in level of concern, some young men presenting with a tumour of only 2–3 cm whilst others are unaware of the change until the testis is well over twice its normal size. Some patients insist that a traumatic injury to the testis preceded its enlargement. Although small hydroceles are frequently present, invasion of the scrotal skin is extremely unusual and the tunica albuginea is rarely breached. Occasionally a spermatocele or varicocele may cause diagnostic difficulties.

The lymphatic drainage of the testis can be traced to the original embryonic site of origin in the abdomen (pelvic, common iliac and para-aortic nodes), rather than to adjacent nodes. Dissemination of tumour into these lymph node groups is common and may cause low back pain (about 10% of all patients). Patients may also notice lymphadenopathy in other sites, particularly the left supraclavicular nodes. In patients with a previous history of inguinal or testicular surgery (usually herniorrhaphy or orchidopexy), inguinal lymph node involvement may occur due to interference with the normal lymphatic pathways. Occasionally, abdominal swelling may occur as a result of massive nodal deposits from an unsuspected primary testicular tumour. The presenting symptoms will then be different and may include ureteric obstruction, acute abdominal pain or retrograde ejaculation as a result of pressure on the presacral plexus.

When patients present with obvious abdominal lymph node disease, it is sometimes the case that the only sign of the primary tumour is testicular atrophy rather than a mass. Gynaecomastia may also occur (in up to 25% of patients with advanced disease), presumably due to ectopic hormone production by the tumour. Rarely, patients present with symptoms due to secondary spread in lung or brain or other sites. Infertility, due to azoospermia, may be the presenting complaint and clinical examination of the testes should be a routine procedure in the infertility clinic.

When considering a diagnosis of testicular cancer, other causes of testicular swelling may cause diagnostic difficulty. These include cystic swellings (hydrocele if involving the testis, varicocele if clearly separate) and solid masses such as a testicular torsion or haematoma. Scrotal inguinal hernias may also occasionally lead to diagnostic problems. The commonest mistake, however, is to confuse epididymo-orchitis in the young male, so often the cause of an important delay.

Tumour markers

An important advance in the management of these tumours was the recognition that they manufacture tumour markers of which AFP and βHCG are the best known [7]. AFP is synthesized by the fetal yolk sac, and plasma levels are elevated in about 70% of patients with MTU or MTI. It is never raised in patients with pure seminoma, and detection of AFP in such cases must be assumed to be due to foci of occult teratoma. βHCG, which is produced by trophoblastic elements in the tumour, is detectable in the plasma of about 50% of patients with testicular teratoma and can also be modestly raised in patients with pure seminoma. With current radioimmunoassay techniques it is possible to measure these hormones at nanogram levels. The levels of these markers vary independently, reflecting their differing cell of origin. This may be confusing since treatment may lead to a fall in one marker without affecting the other.

In patients whose tumours manufacture a marker, repeated measurements give a quantitative indication of tumour responsiveness and activity, and have become an established part of management. At presentation it is essential to obtain a pre-operative plasma sample for measurements of tumour markers.

In patients with marker-producing tumours, these levels will fall after orchidectomy to within the normal range provided the patient has no metastases (Fig. 19.4). If the pre-operative levels of AFP and/or HCG are very high, the return of these values to normal may not be complete for several weeks since the half-life of AFP is 6–7 days, and that of HCG is 16 hours. For this reason single, elevated postoperative marker level does not always imply that there is residual disease. It is now clear that the level of both AFP and HCG at diagnosis gives an indication of prognosis. Patients with levels of AFP above 500 ng/ml and/or HCG above 10 000 ng/ml have a worse prognosis.

Tumour markers are also of great importance in the early diagnosis of relapse (Fig. 19.4). Almost all patients with marker-producing tumours will develop elevated plasma levels as the first and most sensitive indication of relapse. Occasionally patients with recurrent disease will develop raised levels of only one marker even though both may previously have been elevated. This can be due either to the

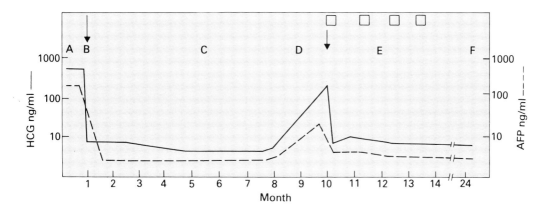

Fig. 19.4 Serum markers in testicular teratoma. (A) Presentation with left testicular swelling: HCG = 623 ng/ml, AFP = 246 ng/ml; (B) orchidectomy: HCG falls in 6 days to 10 ng/ml, AFP falls more slowly ($t_{1/2}$ = 6 days) to 4 ng/ml; (C) no rise in markers, clinical remission; (D) HCG and AFP rise, CT scan confirms enlargement of para-aortic nodes; (E) cyclical intermittent combination chemotherapy produces rapid fall in HCG and slower fall in AFP, both to normal values; (F) two years after presentation: normal markers, clinical remission, probable cure.

differing sensitivity of components of the teratoma to chemotherapy or to a differential metastatic potential of the various elements of the primary tumour. Tumour markers are particularly valuable in the diagnosis of extragonadal primaries since the differential diagnosis from other causes of a retroperitoneal, mediastinal or intracranial suprasellar mass is so wide.

Other tumour markers elaborated by testicular germ cell tumours include placental alkaline phosphatase (PLAP) and lactate dehydrogenase (LDH). Although they are of far less value for disease monitoring than AFP and βHCG, LDH in particular can provide useful prognostic information and is particularly useful in patients who are otherwise marker-negative. Although about 90% of cases of pure seminoma have elevated PLAP levels, it is an unreliable marker since it is also raised, for example, in smokers.

Staging

Clinical staging systems vary widely, but all depend on the anatomical extent of spread at diagnosis (Table 19.2). In Britain a simple system analogous to that used for Hodgkin's disease and other lymphomas (see Chapter 25)

is often used. Greater detail can be incorporated into this system, to take account of the importance of tumour volume both in the abdomen and lungs, since these characteristics are recognized as crucial to the outcome.

Increasingly sophisticated non-surgical staging methods such as lymphography, CT and MRI scanning have helped our understanding of the natural history of these tumours. For example, the frequency of spread to the mediastinum was not appreciated until the advent of CT scanning and it is now recognized that nearly 30% of patients with testicular teratomas have evidence of involvement. This technique has also led to much more accurate diagnosis of pulmonary deposits. Other important investigations include lymphography (less frequently used since the wider availability of CT), intravenous urography, and testicular ultrasonography. These are particularly important in seminoma where irradiation of the para-aortic nodes may still be an important part of treatment at some centres, so that care must be taken to avoid irradiation of the kidneys as far as possible. Ultrasonic scanning of the liver can occasionally be helpful. The staging notation in Table 19.2 is based on investigations including lymphography, CT and MRI scanning.

In the United States retroperitoneal lymph

Table 19.2 Staging of testicular tumours

UK Notation

Stage I   Tumour confined to testis
                 (Tumour markers not elevated after
                    orchidectomy, all investigations
                    negative)

Stage II   Tumour in pelvic and abdominal
                    (retroperitoneal) nodes. (Tumour
                    markers may be persistently elevated.
                    Positive lymphogram or CT scan of
                    abdomen)

          IIa   Nodes <2 cm diameter
          IIb   Nodes 2−5 cm diameter
          IIc   Nodes >5 cm diameter

Stage III   Mediastinal and/or supraclavicular nodes

Stage IV   Distant metastases*
                 L_1 <3 metastases, maximum diameter
                    <2 cm
                 L_2 >3 metastases, maximum diameter
                    <2 cm
                 L_3 maximum diameter >2 cm

TNM Staging Notation

T_1 Confined to testis and adjacent spermatic
              cord
T_2 Tumour detected in spermatic cord at level
              of inguinal ring
T_3 Testicular capsule breached (or scrotal
              orchidectomy)

N_0 No pathological involvement
N_1 Normal size nodes, microscopic
              involvement
N_2 Enlarged nodes but no extranodal
              extension
              (A: less than 2 cm and less than 5 nodes)
              (B: more than 2 cm and more than 5
              nodes)
N_3 Extranodal extension
N_4 Retroperitoneal nodes with residual
              disease after surgery

M_0 No distant metastases
M_1 Distant metastases

* The number and size of lung metastases should be
noted, in view of the prognostic importance of this
observation.

node dissection is still frequently performed,
partly for its value in staging and partly for its
possible therapeutic effect. The TNM system is
therefore partly surgically based (Table 19.2). In

Britain a greater emphasis is placed on non-
surgical approaches and the operation is rarely
performed. The accuracy of lymphography and
CT scanning are demonstrated by comparison
with American data which indicate that about
25% of lymph node dissection specimens in
patients clinically thought to be free of extratesticular spread are indeed positive — a figure
remarkably similar to British data from non-
surgical series.

Management of testicular tumours

The last 20 years have seen major changes in
the management of testicular tumours. Increased
understanding of the importance of scrupulous
staging, coupled with the advent of highly
effective chemotherapy and the routine use of
tumour marker studies have led to widespread
acceptance that this is a tumour best treated
by a multimodal approach. Expert surgeons,
tumour pathologists, radiotherapists and medical oncologists all play an important and
complementary role. Since these tumours are
uncommon and expert attention is so crucial,
they are best treated in special units, or at least
by study groups which will ensure some uniformity of approach.

SURGERY

For patients with a suspected testicular tumour,
the correct operation is a radical inguinal
orchidectomy. Scrotal procedures, although still
sometimes performed, should never be considered since trans-scrotal orchidectomy carries
a real risk of scrotal recurrence or later development of inguinal node involvement. The
spermatic cord should be excised as high as
possible to provide information regarding the
possibility of direct or intravascular spread of
tumour, which will have important implications
for both management and prognosis. Before
orchidectomy it is essential that the surgeon
request AFP and HCG levels, for the reasons
described above.

Surgery in seminoma

If the tumour proves to be a pure seminoma, it is generally accepted that the surgeon has no further part to play, except perhaps for biopsy procedures if, for example, a supraclavicular node is discovered. Although American authorities sometimes recommend surgery in seminomas with bulky abdominal lymph node metastases or seminomas in which the HCG level is modestly raised, this is not usual practice in Britain. Radiotherapy alone will usually cure even bulky disease, and the addition of chemotherapy will increase this cure rate still further (see below).

Surgery in teratoma

For malignant teratomas there has been an important difference of opinion between British and American authorities. For patients with no evidence of abdominal node involvement, or evidence of only minimal node deposits (usually detected at lymphography or CT scanning), standard British practice has in the past been to recommend treatment by irradiation (or more recently, by careful surveillance, see below).

In the United States most of these patients would be treated by extended retroperitoneal lymphadenectomy, removing all lymphatic and connective tissues along the great vessels from the diaphragm to the level of the iliac vessels, a formidable surgical procedure. Many American urologists claim that a lymph node metastatic rate of 25% fully justifies radical lymphadenectomy in all cases. In Britain it is generally felt that combinations of radiotherapy and chemotherapy (or chemotherapy on relapse, if it occurs) can effectively sterilize small volume metastases in abdominal lymph nodes, and that the potential postoperative problems of aspermia (dry ejaculation) render such surgery unjustifiable.

Although it has been claimed that results of treatment by lymphadenectomy are superior to those in patients treated more conservatively, careful study of the literature does not bear this out. Comparisons are difficult since British patients are staged by clinical investigation while most American urologists rely on lymphadenectomy as a staging operation as well as a potentially therapeutic procedure. In malignant teratomas the lymphogram (if performed) is positive only in about one-third of cases and it seems inescapable that many patients undergoing radical lymphadenectomy will have done so unnecessarily, in addition to having to face the undesirable sexual difficulties that the operation may bring. Reasonable comparison is possible between patients where lymphadenectomy confirms histologically positive para-aortic nodes and those from British series who have obviously positive lymphographic appearances (Stage II). Comparison of such cases confirms similar overall survival rates, regardless of treatment.

Over the past 10 years, this debate has largely become historic since the recognition that many patients with early disease, well staged and without adverse features, can be safely followed up by post-orchidectomy surveillance [7,8]. This requires serial marker studies and CT scanning, but does not include immediate postoperative treatment. Although approximately 20% of these patients relapse, close monitoring ensures that the relapse is almost always of small volume, and 99% of patients are curable by modern chemotherapy. Almost 80% of Stage I surveillance cases require no post-orchidectomy treatment whatever — i.e. are cured by this simple operation. Surgery is, however, being used increasingly after initial chemotherapy has been completed in order to reassess the state of residual intra-abdominal disease. This approach is discussed further on p. 389.

RADIOTHERAPY

Radiotherapy in seminoma

For patients with testicular seminoma radiotherapy can be curative, even in patients with

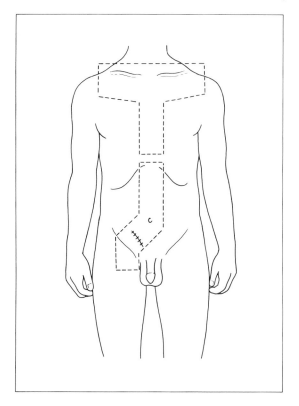

Fig. 19.5 Widely used radiation fields in seminoma. The fields are designed to cover the lymph node groups illustrated in Fig. 19.3. Seminoma is highly radiosensitive and a dose of 30 Gy over 3–4 weeks is generally sufficient.

advanced disease. For patients with Stage I seminoma, modest dosage of irradiation to bilateral para-aortic nodes and the ipsilateral common iliac chain is routinely performed (Fig. 19.5) since there can be no guarantee that orchidectomy alone will have cured these patients. Seminoma is among the most radio-sensitive of all tumours; a dose of 30 Gy (3000 rad) delivered by anterior and posterior fields over a 3-week period (daily fractions of treatment) is normally considered adequate and leads to few, if any, symptomatic acute or chronic side-effects. Infertility is not normally a problem provided that the contralateral testis is protected from scattered irradiation by means of lead shielding. For this and other reasons,

supervoltage radiotherapy is often regarded as essential, although a number of specialized centres now adopt a 'watch-and-wait' policy (i.e. without any radiotherapy at all) for patients with Stage I seminoma since as with teratoma, a substantial proportion of patients are cured by orchidectomy alone.

In the Royal Marsden series, for example [8], the relapse rate at a mean follow-up interval of 2 years was only 13% — probably all curable by chemotherapy or radiotherapy since careful radiological surveillance was mandatory. In other words, despite the relative absence of circulating tumour markers, the policy proved feasible and 87% of the Stage I seminoma group avoided unnecessary radiotherapy.

Where a scrotal operation such as orchid-opexy, trans-scrotal biopsy or scrotal orchid-ectomy has been performed, the scrotal sac and ipsilateral inguinal nodes must also be treated. Some authorities also irradiate the inguinal nodes if there has been a herniorrhaphy. Although preservation of fertility cannot be guaranteed, an attempt at shielding the contra-lateral testis should once again be made.

Prior to the availability of effective chemo-therapy, many radiotherapists previously adopted a policy of 'keeping one step ahead' of known nodal involvement from a seminoma. In patients with Stage II disease, this included para-aortic and pelvic node irradiation, fol-lowed by radiotherapy to the mediastinum and supraclavicular nodes. Although this approach can be curative, such wide field irradiation can be a real drawback if chemotherapy is sub-sequently required for recurrent disease, since a large volume of bone marrow will have been treated, thus compromising haematological tolerance. In patients with abdominal node involvement at presentation, the relapse rate is closely dependent on tumour bulk (less than 10% for small volume disease, over 50% for bulky node involvement). For this reason in some centres (including the authors') patients with bulky abdominal disease are now routinely treated with chemotherapy prior to irradiation. Indeed some centres omit irradiation entirely, relying on chemotherapy for patients with bulky abdominal disease. It is not yet clear whether this approach will prove superior.

The same alternative approaches also apply in patients with Stage III disease, although one would now recommend chemotherapy as unequivocally the better treatment. In Stage IV disease, chemotherapy has been increasingly accepted as representing the best opportunity of cure, although some centres have reported encouraging results with total body irradiation.

Occasionally patients with 'pure' seminoma have an elevated serum βHCG, and HCG can be demonstrated immunocytochemically [10]. This does not appear to be associated with a worse prognosis. An elevated serum AFP is usually regarded as an indication for treatment as for non-seminomatous germ cell tumours (see below).

Although seminoma is a highly curable tumour, many questions of management remain unanswered. These have recently been fully reviewed [11] and many important trials are currently continuing, under the auspices of the MRC and others. Treatment of early stage disease by orchidectomy alone (without adjuvant radiotherapy) is becoming increasingly popular since the early results from major treatment centres are holding up well [12].

Radiotherapy in teratoma

For non-seminomatous germ cell tumours, radiotherapy is now much less widely employed than in the 1950s and 1960s. In the first place, surveillance of patients with Stage I disease is associated with a high cure rate — at least 75%. Secondly, chemotherapy is almost always curative in the minority who do require treatment. Thirdly, previous treatment with abdomino-pelvic radiotherapy is a positive hazard in such cases, because of increased myelosuppression. In patients with Stage II disease of small volume (less than 2 cm maximum diameter, radiologically demonstrable but non-palpable lymph-adenopathy) radiotherapy will be curative in about 80% of patients. However, chemotherapy is curative in over 90%, although there has been no formal comparison of these two treatments. Radiotherapy in Stage II disease is compatible with normal fertility [13] which is an important advantage over radical lymph node dissection. With bulky Stage II disease, control by radiation is much less certain and the case for chemotherapy is well established. Patients with Stages III and IV disease are treated, and often cured, with chemotherapy, although radiotherapy may still have a role in the control of bulky abdominal disease (see below).

CHEMOTHERAPY

The emergence of chemotherapy for testicular teratoma has been one of the most exciting advances in cancer medicine over the past 25 years. In the early 1960s one or two agents were available with known but limited activity. Li and colleagues [14] described a combination regimen comprising actinomycin D, chlorambucil and methotrexate, which was the first major advance in the treatment of widespread testicular teratoma. Mithramycin was introduced at about this time and, although no longer widely used, is capable of producing regression of metastases particularly in patients with MTU (embryonal carcinoma) with long-term survival in a small number of patients.

The next important step was the recognition of further agents of quite different classes, each of which had major activity (Table 19.3). Vinblastine, bleomycin, and later cisplatin and its derivatives have all been identified as independently effective. Samuels and colleagues investigated combinations of vinblastine and bleomycin, demonstrating very high response rates even in patients with advanced disease, particularly when the bleomycin was given as an infusion [15].

This effective but highly toxic regimen was a major advance but it was replaced by a regimen which added cisplatin to the two-drug combination. Cisplatin is not only a highly effective agent, the most powerful of all the cytotoxics for this condition, but is also relatively free

Table 19.3 Cytotoxic drugs in germ cell testicular tumours

	Response rates (complete and partial)
*Single agents**	
Actinomycin D	40%
Vinblastine	20%
Cisplatin	>60%
Methotrexate	20%
Bleomycin	40%
Etoposide	40%
Alkylating agents	30%
Combination therapy	
Cisplatin, bleomycin, vinblastine (PVB)	98% (70% CR)
PVB and etoposide (see text)	100% (70% CR)
Vinblastine, bleomycin	75% (50% CR)

PVB regimen
Cisplatin 20 mg/m^2 i.v. daily for 5 days every 3 weeks
Vinblastine 0.3 mg/kg i.v. every 3 weeks
Bleomycin 30 mg i.v. three times weekly (four complete courses are usually given)

BEP regimen
As for PVB, but substituting etoposide at a dose of 120 mg/m^2 i.v. for 3 days for vinblastine, which is omitted

* Of historical interest. No longer employed singly for non-seminomatous tumours.

from toxicity to the bone marrow, making it particularly suitable as part of a combination regimen. Twenty years ago Einhorn and colleagues at Indiana developed a combination of cisplatin, vinblastine and bleomycin in patients with advanced disease [16]. This regimen is still sometimes used although newer less toxic combinations, for example BEP (in which the vinblastine is replaced by the podophyllotoxin etoposide) have now largely replaced it. At many major centres both in the United States and Europe, BEP is regarded as the 'gold standard' chemotherapy for testicular cancer (L.H. Einhorn, personal communication).

Despite the remarkable results of modern therapy for metastatic testicular germ cell tumours, the toxicity of all these regimens is a serious problem, with gastro-intestinal disturbance, granulocytopenia and infection, nephrotoxicity and pulmonary fibrosis as the major hazards, particularly with PVB. In Einhorn's earlier series four patients died in complete remission and two of these deaths were clearly drug-related. Reduction of vinblastine dosage led to a significant improvement in tolerance without jeopardizing responsiveness. Bleomycin is used in large doses in these regimens and as haematological toxicity has diminished, pulmonary toxicity from bleomycin has become the main toxicity (see Chapter 6). Although carboplatin is less toxic to the gastro-intestinal tract than cisplatin, it is more myelotoxic and thus more difficult to use in combination with vinblastine and bleomycin.

Some patients are now recognized as having a particularly poor prognosis. Adverse features include: presence of liver, bone or brain metastases, AFP at presentation of more than 1000 ng/ml, βHCG more than 10000 ng/ml, mediastinal node mass more than 5 cm or greater than 20 pulmonary metastases. Such cases are probably better treated by a still more intensive chemotherapy regimen, and about two-thirds of this group appear curable.

There is rarely, if ever, any justification for giving more than four courses of similar chemotherapy. Although most patients are cured, it is important not to assume failure if after this time there is radiological evidence of residual disease — for example, visible lung metastases. Such patients should not be retreated immediately with further chemotherapy since lung metastases can fade radiologically over several months. For retreatment of later recurrences, or treatment of truly refractory disease, the introduction of ifosfamide-based regimens has, for the first time, given durable responses and a small proportion of cures. The VIP regimen (containing vincristine, ifosfamide and cis- (or carbo-) platin) is probably the most useful choice at present, particularly since with BEP as the primary choice, patients treated with VIP will not previously have been exposed to vinblastine.

The use of chemotherapy for patients with less advanced disease needs further exploration, particularly where there is modest para-aortic involvement (Stages IIa and IIb). It is also clear that seminoma is a highly chemosensitive disease. Most cases of seminoma present early, at a radiocurable stage, but for the few patients that have advanced disease or later develop recurrence, there was little effective chemotherapy until the advent of cisplatin-based regimens. Current practice includes combinations of drugs similar to those used for teratoma, with radiotherapy sometimes still given to sites of bulk disease. However, the use of single-agent cisplatin may be as effective for metastatic seminoma as the more complex combination regimens, and is still undergoing evaluation in this setting.

SURGERY AFTER CHEMOTHERAPY AND RADIOTHERAPY

As survival times lengthen, surgery has become increasingly aggressive in selected young patients, particularly where there is evidence of residual disease after orchidectomy. Abdominal 'debulking' surgery, and even excision of pulmonary metastases by repeated thoracotomy, are frequently performed. Combinations of chemotherapy and surgery are increasingly used [17], and it is now clear that chemotherapy should precede surgery [9]. Postponing surgery to the end of treatment, after administration of repeated courses of combination chemotherapy, gives both an accurate histological picture of the effect of preceding treatment, as well as removing tumour in patients with residual disease. Ideally, such surgery should be performed only after tumour markers have fallen to undetectable levels and at least one additional course of chemotherapy given beyond this point.

In a large proportion of these cases there is evidence of treatment-induced differentiation into mature teratoma, and although this observation is encouraging, its significance and implications for long-term survival are not yet entirely clear. Most of such patients appear to be cured, showing no evidence of relapse after several years' follow-up.

Prognosis of testicular tumours

Stages I and II seminoma are nearly always curable by radiotherapy (Stage I, more than 95%; Stage II, 85–90%). The prognosis of bulky Stage II (Stage IIc) and Stages III and IV is improving with chemotherapy (Fig. 19.6A) and the majority of patients are now cured even in these more advanced stages [18].

In non-seminomatous germ cell tumours the prognosis is excellent for Stage I and early Stage II disease. Approximately 70% of all patients

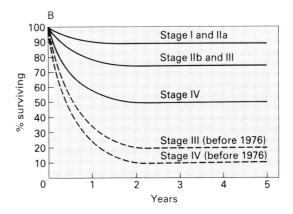

Fig. 19.6 Prognosis of testicular germ cell tumours related to stage. (A) Seminoma; (B) teratoma (all types). These survival curves illustrate the dramatic improvement with advanced stages since the introduction of combination chemotherapy.

with Stage III disease will be cured, but bulky disease and Stage IV patients are still at risk of incomplete drug response and relapse. Nevertheless the last decade has seen a great improvement even in this poor prognosis group (Fig. 19.6B). Results from large centres in Britain are amongst the best reported, with overall survival of 80 to 90% following treatment with combination regimens containing cisplatin, bleomycin, vinblastine, etoposide and/or other drugs. Poor prognosis patients clearly require special attention [19]. At present, the major effort in poor prognosis patients lies in generating new chemotherapy programmes to improve on the established three-drug regimens, notably BEP. In the United States, the current multicentre study developed at the University of Indiana is a randomization between BEP and a combination of cisplatin, etoposide and ifosfamide. Since only 65% of poor prognosis patients are curable by BEP, it should be feasible to demonstrate a possible improvement from the new regimen with a study of only a few hundred patients.

EXTRA-GONADAL GERM CELL TUMOURS

Primary extra-gonadal germ cell tumours are extremely uncommon, but have been described in a variety of sites including the retroperitoneum, anterior mediastinum, suprasellar or pineal area and in the presacral region. Although the pathogenesis is not entirely clear, it is possible that these tumours result from malignant change in primordial germ cells which have migrated incompletely (cell 'rests') or in cells displaced during embryogenesis. There appears to be a genetic predisposition at least in some cases, since Klinefelter's syndrome is a well-described predisposing feature.

The commonest site is probably the anterior mediastinum, followed by the retroperitoneum. In occasional cases, an associated congenital or developmental abnormality is present. The tumours comprise only 1% of all mediastinal tumours. The largest single group are mixed tumours, but pure seminomas are more common than pure teratomas or choriocarcinomas. Since primary testicular tumours can be small and impalpable, one should always be wary when diagnosing a germ cell tumour apparently arising from an extratesticular site, since metastasis from an occult primary is an alternative diagnosis.

Both teratomas and seminomas are encountered and in general show the same radiosensitivity and chemosensitivity as primary testicular tumours. For mediastinal seminomas, surgery followed by radiotherapy appears effective, with long-term survival rates of about 50%. However, in bulky disease chemotherapy can be extremely effective at reducing tumour volume thus eliminating the need for wide field irradiation of the lungs. Although long-term effectiveness and morbidity of chemotherapy has yet to be fully determined, this approach is clearly extremely valuable. At present, treatment with cisplatin, bleomycin and either vinblastine or etoposide seems most effective, although more complicated regimens have been used.

For primary mediastinal non-seminomatous germ cell tumours, radiotherapy is relatively ineffective. Several reports have appeared showing a dismal prognosis with no cures and an average survival of only 5 months from diagnosis. However, recent reports show good response to modern chemotherapy, usually including cisplatin, vinblastine, etoposide, bleomycin, and actinomycin D. Primary germ cell tumours of the brain are treated quite differently. Most of these are pineal or suprasellar tumours, and both teratomas and seminomas occur. These can sometimes be cured by wide field irradiation (especially the pure seminoma group), including full irradiation of the whole central nervous system. The 5-year survival rate in children with radiosensitive pineal tumours (usually not biopsied but assumed to be seminoma or the less common pinealoblastoma) is 50%. With proven pineal teratomas (i.e. biopsy-proven or where the AFP or βHCG are clearly raised) the outlook is less good, although response to chemotherapy can be dramatic. For these rare tumours which are only partly or doubtfully radiosensitive, combination chemotherapy has now become the standard form of primary management.

The apparent rarity of extra-gonadal germ cell tumours may have to be revised in the light of recent reports describing patients originally thought to have undifferentiated carcinomas but with a clinical course and response to chemotherapy much more suggestive of extra-gonadal germ cell tumours. This has been described as the 'atypical teratoma syndrome' and none of these patients have clinically apparent testicular tumours. In the majority of cases serum markers (AFP and βHCG) are raised, and subsequent staining of tissue sections by immunoperoxidase techniques shows intracellular AFP and βHCG. Treatment with cisplatin, vinblastine and bleomycin is effective, with a high proportion of complete responders. In young men with mediastinal tumours which on biopsy prove to be 'poorly differentiated carcinoma' it is therefore essential to consider this diagnosis and to measure plasma βHCG and AFP. Even if these are negative, it is so important not to overlook this potentially curable tumour that response to platinum-based regimens should be fully assessed.

MANAGEMENT OF NON-GERM CELL TUMOURS OF THE TESTIS

Orchidectomy alone is usually sufficient for Leydig and Sertoli cell tumours since these rarely metastasize. Lymphomas of the testis are usually large cell centroblastic B cell neoplasms. As they are frequently bilateral, irradiation of the contralateral testis is usually recommended even if the disease appears localized. These patients need careful staging as for other lymphomas (see Chapter 26). With paratesticular rhabdomyosarcomas occult metastasis is so frequent that adjuvant combination chemotherapy is an essential part of management (see Chapter 24).

REFERENCES

1 Ondrus D., Hornak M., Vrabec J. Low sperm counts as a prognostic factor of progression in stage I non-seminomatous germ cell testicular tumours. *British Journal of Urology* 1988; **62**: 82–84.

2 Swerdlow A.J., Huttly S.R.A., Smith P.G. Testicular cancer and antecedent diseases. *British Journal of Cancer* 1987; **55**: 97–103.

3 Dixon F.J., Moore R.A. Testicular tumours: a clinico-pathological study. *Cancer* 1953; **6**: 427.

4 Giwercman A., Grinsted J., Hansen B. *et al.* Testicular cancer risk in boys with maldescended testis: a cohort study. *Journal of Urology* 1987; **138**: 1214–16.

5 Berthelsen J.G., Skakkebaek N.E. Distribution of carcinoma *in situ* in testes from infertile men. *International Journal of Andrology* 1981; **4**: 172–84.

6 Oliver R.T.D. Testicular cancer. *Current Opinion in Oncology* 1990; **2**: 529–32.

7 Lange P.H., McIntire K.R., Waldmann T.A. *et al.* Serum alphafetoprotein and human chorionic gonadotrophin in the diagnosis and management of non-seminomatous germ-cell testicular cancer. *New England Journal of Medicine* 1976; **295**: 1237–40.

8 Peckham M.J., Brada M. Surveillance following orchidectomy for stage I testicular cancer. *International Journal of Andrology* 1987; **10**: 247–54.

9 Williams S.D., Stablein D.M., Einhorn L.H. *et al.* Immediate adjuvant chemotherapy versus observation with treatment at relapse in pathological stage II testicular cancer. *New England Journal of Medicine* 1987; **317**: 1433–38.

10 Javadpour N., McIntire K.R., Waldmann T.A. Human chorionic gonadotrophin (HCG) and alphafetoprotein (AFP) in sera and tumour cells of patients with testicular seminoma: a prospective study. *Cancer* 1978; **42**: 2768–72.

11 Horwich A. Germ cell tumour chemotherapy. *British Journal of Cancer* 1989; **59**: 156–59.

12 Duchesne G.M., Horwich A., Dearnaley D. *et al.* Orchidectomy alone for Stage 1 seminoma of the testis. *Cancer* 1990; **65**: 1115–18.

13 Smithers D.W., Wallace E.N.K., Wallace D.M. Radiotherapy for patients with tumours of the testicle. *British Journal of Urology* 1971; **43**: 83–92.

14 Li M.C., Whitmore W.F., Golbey R., Grabstald H. Effects of combined drug therapy on metastatic cancer of the testis. *Journal of the American Medical Association* 1960; **174**: 1291–99.

15 Samuels M.L., Johnson D.E., Holoye P.Y. Continuous intravenous bleomycin therapy with vinblastine in stage III testicular neoplasia. *Cancer Chemotherapy Reports* 1975; **59**: 563–70.

16 Einhorn L., Donohue J.P. Cisdiamminechloroplatinum, vinblastine and bleomycin combination

chemotherapy in disseminated testicular cancer. *Annals of Internal Medicine* 1977; **87**: 293—98.

17 Motzer R.J., Bosi G.J., Geller N.L. *et al*. Advanced seminoma: the role of chemotherapy and adjunctive surgery. *Annals of Internal Medicine* 1988; **108**: 513—17.

18 Steinfeld A.D. Testicular germ cell tumors: review of contemporary evaluation and management. *Radiology* 1990; **175**: 603—06.

19 Einhorn L.H. Complicated problems in testicular cancer. *Seminars in Oncology* 1988; **15**: (suppl.) 9—15.

Chapter 20
Thyroid and Adrenal Cancer

Thyroid cancer is exceptional in many ways. First of all, some thyroid cancers are very indolent with a long natural history, often over many decades, even where complete control of the tumour has not been achieved. Secondly, because most thyroid cancers take up iodine, the administration of oral radioactive iodine — a highly specific therapy — results in sterilization of both normal and neoplastic thyroid cells and may be used for total ablation of the tumour, usually resulting in excellent 20-year survival rates. Thirdly, in the majority of patients with metastases from well-differentiated thyroid carcinomas, the metastatic lesions retain the important characteristic of radio-iodine uptake, so that even patients with metastatic disease at presentation can still be treated successfully. If necessary, these treatments can be repeated several times, using whole-body isotope scanning as an accurate method of assessment of progress and to determine whether further therapy is required.

There are important histological and behavioural differences between the major types of thyroid cancer and these differences help to determine treatment strategy (Table 20.1). Although these tumour subgroups are well defined, several types of thyroid carcinoma have been recognized only recently, and further histopathological refinements seem likely. The clinician needs a complete histopathological description of the tumour which should include not only the tumour type but also the degree of differentiation. If a thyroidectomy specimen is available, the degree of local invasion into blood vessels, local structures and adjacent lymph nodes should also be described.

AETIOLOGY AND INCIDENCE

A number of aetiological factors have now been described. Like other thyroid diseases it is commoner in women than in men (Fig. 20.1), with a bimodal age distribution. The lower age peak of incidence is due to papillary and follicular tumours, and the rise in incidence in older patients is chiefly due to anaplastic cancers. Both thyrotoxicosis and Hashimoto's thyroiditis share a similar age distribution with well-differentiated thyroid carcinomas. It has been described as being more frequent in survivors of the atomic bomb, and has also been reported following irradiation of the neck, usually with a latent period of 10–30 years. Therapeutic neck irradiation, usually to the thymus or tonsils, was generally taken to only a low dose. The risk of carcinogenesis is higher in females, or where the radiation exposure occurred in very young children, and also increases with increasing length of follow-up. Medullary thyroid carcinoma has both a familial and a sporadic incidence and may form part of the syndromes of multiple endocrine neoplasia (see Chapter 15).

PATHOLOGY

Papillary carcinoma

The commonest type of cancer is papillary carcinoma (Fig. 20.2), which comprises about 60% of all thyroid cancers, and a slightly greater proportion of those occurring in childhood. In at least 20% of cases the tumour appears to be multifocal in origin, and in older patients tends

Table 20.1 Clinical characteristics and survival in thyroid tumours

Histological type	Response to radio-iodine	Clinical behaviour	10-year survival (%)
Papillary	+++	Young patients. Often slow to evolve. Metastases usually lymphatic	95
Follicular	+++	Young, middle-aged patients. Metastases often haematogenous (bone, lung)	90
Medullary	−	Young patients. Familial. Produces calcitonin as marker. C cell tumour. Often a rapid clinical evolution. Surgery very important as radioresponsiveness variable	40
Anaplastic	−	Elderly patients. Predominantly local invasion with pressure symptoms	5
Small cell	−	Rapid but very radiosensitive. Usually localized	5
Lymphoma	−	Middle-aged group (highly radiosensitive)	40

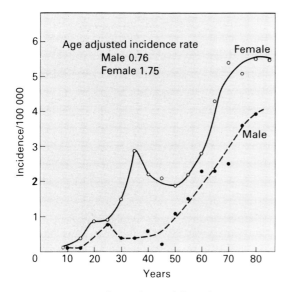

Fig. 20.1 Age-specific incidence of thyroid cancer.

to have a more aggressive clinical course, with correspondingly poorer survival than in children and young adults. Papillary carcinomas are almost three times as common in women as in men [1], with a peak incidence in the 3rd and 4th decades. Any differential thyroid tumour that contains neoplastic papillae is by definition a papillary carcinoma, regardless of the presence of neoplastic follicles. The tumour is made up of cuboid cells and often contains psammoma bodies. A characteristic feature of papillary tumours is large empty nuclei — so-called 'orphan Annie' nuclei. Over 90% of these tumours appear to be encapsulated, but lymph node invasion is common, although this finding is thought to be prognostically unimportant. Occasionally, papillary microcarcinomas (even up to 1 cm in size) are discovered in thyroidectomy specimens where a neoplasm was not suspected pre-operatively. It is generally accepted that these small clinically undetected tumours can be ignored (from the point of view

Fig. 20.2 Histological appearances in thyroid cancer. (A) Follicular carcinoma showing follicle formation (×200); (B) papillary carcinoma showing characteristic 'empty' nuclei (×200); (C) medullary carcinoma showing small cells with masses of amyloid (×200); (D) anaplastic carcinoma (×200).

of further treatment) unless a tumour is found adjacent to one of the resection margins of the specimen. Larger tumours, with evidence of extrathyroid invasion and/or invasion of the thyroid capsule, are associated with a worse prognosis, particularly in older patients. However, in general this is a slowly growing tumour, usually completely resectable and with a low overall mortality.

Follicular tumours

Follicular tumours (Fig. 20.2) are much less common, accounting for about 15% of all cases and often found in patients with a long history of goitre. The increased frequency with which follicular cancers are diagnosed in the United States and Canada (see, for example, [1]) is probably due to a difference in histopathological criteria from European cities. These tumours are unusual in children and are seen in a rather older age group than the papillary carcinomas, again with a slight female predominance. The mean age of diagnosis is approximately 10 years older than for papillary cancers (52 versus 41 years for patients with resectable disease [1]). Overall prognosis is good (Table 20.1). Lymph node involvement is uncommon, as the main route of dissemination is via the bloodstream with lung and bone as the commonest sites of metastasis. This is often reflected in the histological appearance of the tumour, since microangioinvasion can frequently be demonstrated even though, as with papillary carcinomas, over 90% of these tumours appear macroscopically to be encapsulated. The presence of plugs of tumour within the lumen of the capsular venous sinusoids is associated with a higher risk of dissemination, as is permeation of extrathyroidal veins. These are important adverse prognostic features. The tumour can be difficult to distinguish histologically from atypical adenomas, since the presence of nuclear pleomorphism and even bizarre nuclear forms is not necessarily tantamount to true malignancy, in the absence of evidence of microangioinvasion.

Medullary thyroid tumours

Medullary thyroid tumours (Fig. 20.2) have a quite different derivation and are thought to arise from the parafollicular or C cells. The disease is often familial (see below). Typically, the stroma of the tumour has an amyloid appearance and the tumour itself may be bilateral. Medullary thyroid tumours tend to have a high metastatic potential both to lymph nodes and also the bloodstream. The large majority secrete calcitonin, a particularly important tumour marker in view of the familial incidence of the disease and the obvious importance of identifying affected family members as early as possible [2]. Equally important is the use of the calcitonin assay for monitoring results of therapy.

In the past most patients reached the age of

30 years by the time of diagnosis. The mean age at diagnosis is expected to drop in the future, since the familial nature of the tumour is well understood and the use of the calcitonin assay has now become widespread.

In some familial forms of the disease other abnormalities have also been noted, particularly phaeochromocytoma and hyperparathyroidism — the so-called *multiple endocrine neoplasia (MEN)* syndromes. These can be associated either with the sporadic or the familial form of medullary thyroid cancer. The disorders are inherited as an autosomal dominant with a high degree of penetrance but variable expression. The commonest variant of MEN, *Wermer's syndrome*, can involve the thyroid and parathyroid glands as well as the pancreatic islets, pituitary and adrenal cortex (see Chapter 15). Two-thirds of these patients have tumours of at least two of the endocrine glands. The second type of MEN, *Sipple's syndrome*, includes more patients with medullary thyroid carcinoma; approximately 50% of these patients have parathyroid hyperplasia and/or phaeochromocytoma. Medullary thyroid cancer may be associated with ectopic hormone production from the thyroid tumour itself, and may produce ACTH, VIP and also prostaglandins and serotonin.

Multiple endocrine neoplasia

The gene for MEN IIA (medullary thyroid cancer, phaeochromocytoma and parathyroid hyperplasia) is inherited as an autosomal dominant trait with incomplete penetrance so that 40% of carriers do not present with symptoms until 70 years of age [3,4]. Detection of presymptomatic carriers by provocation of calcitonin release identifies 90% by the age of 25 years, but DNA analysis is more reliable still, permitting unambiguous identification of MEN IIA gene carriers [5]. The gene is located in the pericentromeric region of chromosome 10. Several markers of this region have now been identified and studies using DNA restriction fragment polymorphism now allow a more accurate identification of the carrier state. A recent consensus statement from the European Community medullary thyroid carcinoma group has laid down guidelines for a combined biochemical and genetic screening programme for MEN type II [3]. This should lead to a rapid improvement in early detection and cure rates.

Anaplastic carcinoma

Anaplastic carcinoma of the thyroid (Fig. 20.2) is the predominant form of thyroid cancer in elderly people, and approximately 75% of patients with this disorder are over 60 years old at the time of diagnosis. These tumours form about 15% of all thyroid cancers, and are seen more frequently in women, in the ratio of 3:2. Unlike well-differentiated thyroid cancer, they are generally rapidly growing tumours, often painful and with pressure symptoms as an early feature. In some cases the tumour appears to arise in a long-standing goitre. The course of these tumours is quite different from that of the more slowly growing varieties commoner in younger patients, and several histological subtypes of anaplastic carcinoma have been recognized, including spindle and giant cell carcinomas in which there may be areas of well-differentiated carcinoma, supporting the suggestion that these tumours may sometimes arise from transformation of pre-existing well-differentiated thyroid cancer.

A very small number of 'anaplastic' carcinomas are characterized by infiltration with small lymphocyte-like cells, and are generally known as *small cell* carcinomas of the thyroid. These are typically found in elderly patients and are rapidly growing and locally invasive. *Thyroid lymphomas* are discussed in Chapter 26.

DIAGNOSIS AND INVESTIGATION

Patients may present with a firm mass in the neck, due either to the primary thyroid mass or to an involved cervical lymph node. It is sometimes possible to classify the thyroid mass on clinical grounds as obviously benign, sus-

picious of cancer, or 'probable' [6,7], although rather few thyroid cancers present with symptoms or signs which are of real prognostic value. The most one can say clinically is that most cases prove not to be malignant. In making these distinctions, useful clinical criteria include the size and position of the mass, its mobility, and the presence of signs of compression of vital structures in the neck.

Non-malignant conditions can simulate thyroid cancer; these include benign adenomas and multinodular goitres, as well as less common causes such as thyroglossal or colloid retention cysts. These may cause particular difficulty since they also produce the 'cold' nodule on thyroid isotope scanning so characteristic of malignant neoplasms (Fig. 20.3). Ultrasound scanning will distinguish between cystic and solid lesions but rarely contributes significantly to the diagnosis beyond this point. It is useful, however, if it is decided to undertake follow-up alone — e.g. for a colloid nodule. The circulating thyroglobulin level may be elevated, but the

Fig. 20.3 ^{123}I scan of thyroid, showing a cold nodule in the enlarged right node.

test is still regarded by many as an unreliable marker of malignancy. Evidence of micro-calcification in a soft tissue X-ray, although rarely seen, is strongly suggestive of papillary carcinoma, and is due to the psammoma bodies. Apart from the mass itself, and the pressure-effects such as stridor or recurrent laryngeal nerve involvement, patients with medullary carcinoma may occasionally present with systemic endocrine symptoms from an associ-ated MEN syndrome. The great majority of patients with thyroid cancer are clinically euthyroid. Autoimmune thyroiditis can usually be identified by the presence of a high level of anti-thyroglobulin antibodies as well as a low ^{131}I uptake and diffuse glandular enlargement. This clinical syndrome is quite different from de Quervain's subacute thyroiditis, in which the thyroid is often painful or tender.

In general, patients with thyroid scans sug-gestive of a 'cold' nodule, i.e. one which fails to take up radio-iodine, should be regarded as potentially malignant. The diagnostic scheme for thyroid nodules has now moved towards fine needle aspiration cytology (rather than open surgical biopsy) as the initial investi-gation. In the first place, this will immediately identify a thyroid cyst, to the great relief of the patient. Secondly, cytological examination by an expert will generally reveal the nature of the malignant lesion, with accurate prediction of the neoplastic cell type. One limitation, how-ever, is that with follicular carcinoma the dis-tinction between benign and malignant may be impossible, in which case surgical biopsy is essential. At most, only 20% of these patients will prove to have a malignant neoplasm. In order to make the diagnosis, hemithyroidec-tomy may sometimes be necessary, or, in the case of larger lesions, partial or subtotal removal of the gland. For papillary (the largest single subtype), medullary and anaplastic cancers, needle aspiration may be sufficient, whereas in follicular carcinoma, important histological features may not be recognizable in such small specimens.

Surgical management of thyroid cancer

In making the diagnosis of thyroid cancer a substantial thyroid resection may have been undertaken consisting of unilateral thyroid lobectomy (hemithyroidectomy) with resection of the isthmus. However, there is no clear agree-ment, once the diagnosis has been established, as to whether the surgeon should then consider a further operation to complete a total or near total thyroidectomy. The risk of surgically-induced hypoparathyroidism is low — prob-ably about 3% in experienced hands. Repeated operations by inexperienced surgeons un-doubtedly increase this hazard.

In small cancers, completely enclosed by normal tissues, it may seem unjustifiable to advocate further surgery in view of the risk of a second operation in a difficult site. Nonetheless, routine total thyroidectomy has sometimes been recommended, even for *well-differentiated papillary tumours*, because of the high incidence of microscopic foci in the contralateral lobe [1,6]. A common recommendation in British centres is that a near-total or subtotal thyroidec-tomy be performed. However, the use of serum thyroglobulin for follow-up has in recent years tended to modify this view. Younger patients under the age of 40 years, with histopathology confirming a well-differentiated tumour, ap-parently completely removed, can be given suppressive T4 so as to reduce TSH to an un-detectable level (0.2 mU/l on current highly sensitive IRMA assays) and follow-up is then undertaken with serum thyroglobulin (see below). The increasing use of this marker, coupled with a move towards more conservative surgery, has in the past decade led to a con-troversy in selection of treatment options which has yet to be resolved.

For *follicular carcinomas* total thyroidectomy is usually best even in cases where metastases are present at the time of diagnosis, though this carries a risk of permanent hypoparathyroid-ism. In cases of papillary and follicular car-cinomas, any obviously enlarged lymph nodes should be removed at the initial operation. *En bloc* resection of the thyroid gland and pathological nodes should be attempted even if bilateral lymph nodes are present. Despite the high incidence of histologically confirmed malignancies in clinically impalpable lymph nodes (probably of the order of 50%), prophylactic lymph node dissection is not usually recommended since recurrence after subsequent postoperative treatment with radio-iodine will occur in less than 30% of patients.

In *papillary carcinoma* it is important to remember that the presence of palpable lymph nodes at diagnosis does not affect the prognosis. There is no difference in outcome between patients treated by prophylactic neck dissection in whom lymph node involvement is confirmed histologically, and those with a later nodal recurrence who may then be treated by therapeutic lymph node dissection (and possibly other methods as well). This is particularly true of the largest group of low risk patients, i.e. women under 40 years of age with well-differentiated tumours.

With *medullary carcinomas* routine neck node dissection is sometimes recommended, in addition to total thyroidectomy [6], a view substantiated by the high local recurrence rate in the order of 25%. For *anaplastic carcinomas* surgical removal of the tumour should be attempted wherever possible, although this is often technically difficult since early direct extension is the rule and tissue planes may be hopelessly destroyed. These tumours are only partly responsive to external beam irradiation so surgical removal of as much tumour as possible is increasingly performed even where this involves cutting directly across tumour. Because of the frequency of compression of the oesophagus, pharynx and trachea, maintenance of the airway by tracheostomy is often required.

For true *small cell carcinomas* and *lymphomas* of the thyroid, thyroidectomy is unnecessary although it is occasionally performed for biopsy purposes. Where these tumours are suspected, 'Tru-cut' or other needle biopsy procedures are now more often employed in order to avoid

thyroidectomy wherever possible. They are highly radiosensitive and surgery plays a correspondingly small part in the management.

The role of radiotherapy in thyroid cancer

RADIO-IODINE THERAPY (^{131}I)

Postoperative management depends on the histological findings, the extent of disease and the completeness of surgery. In most cases of well-differentiated thyroid cancer (both papillary and follicular), ablation of residual thyroid tissue, together with neck and whole body scanning should be carried out postoperatively, using oral radioactive iodine. This is particularly important if there is any doubt as to the completeness of surgery. About half of all follicular carcinomas fall into this category, and rather fewer of the papillary group. Treatment with ^{131}I is not necessary for all of the well-differentiated tumours [8], since occult and intrathyroid carcinomas have an excellent prognosis following surgery alone, and high doses of radioactive iodine can generally be avoided with safety in these predominantly young patients for whom radiation dose is a particularly important consideration.

For patients in whom ^{131}I treatment is required, a moderately large dose should be given, of the order of 80 mCi (approximately 3 GBq) so as to ablate the residual thyroid tissue which always takes up iodine more avidly than the tumour, making therapeutic use of ^{131}I impossible in the presence of a significant volume of active residual thyroid tissue (Fig. 20.4). If thyroxine (T4) has been administered postoperatively, this must be discontinued well before (usually 4 weeks) any attempt at thyroid ablation with radio-iodine, in order to ensure that the TSH rises. It is the rise in TSH rather than the hormone withdrawal that is important. After the ^{131}I radio-ablation has been performed, a short 6-week course of tri-iodothyronine (T3) is then given (in preference to T4 which has a much longer duration of action and

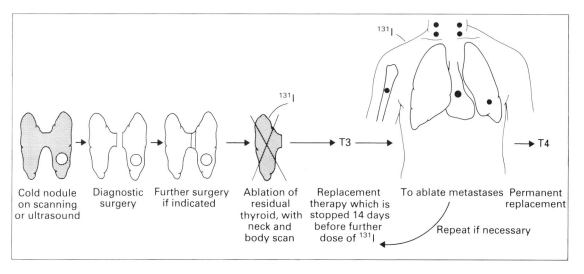

Fig. 20.4 The use of ^{131}I in management of thyroid cancer.

is therefore less flexible). After withdrawal of T3 for 10 days, neck and whole body scanning is once again performed, and residual uptake in the neck or elsewhere provides evidence of metastatic or unresected primary cancer. If this is demonstrated a therapeutic dose of ^{131}I (150–200 mCi or 5.5–7.0 GBq) is indicated. This can be repeated at approximately 3-monthly intervals (discontinuing exogenous T3 10 days beforehand) for as long as the repeat scans confirm residual active disease, i.e. until the metastases are totally eradicated or treatment fails.

Despite the dangers of significant radiation doses to the neck, marrow, gonads and other sites, it is important to realize that this specific and cytotoxic form of irradiation has produced many cures even in patients with widely metastatic disease. These patients (indeed most patients with thyroid cancer) need life-long T4 replacement since all thyroid tissue will have been ablated long before the final therapeutic dose. In a proportion of patients no longer responsive to radio-iodine but with residual or metastatic disease, hormone replacement with T4 may produce further regression of disease (particularly in those under 40 years old) since many of these tumours retain at least a partial

dependency on TSH, which is suppressed by exogenous T4. Occasionally it is necessary to give treatment with therapeutic doses of ^{131}I when the patient has only just discontinued taking T3 or T4. In these cases TSH should be given for 2–3 days (by injection) before the ^{131}I is administered.

Although routine use of postoperative ^{131}I ablation is now regarded as overtreatment of many surgically treated cases of papillary carcinoma, the indications for use of radio-iodine in selected patients were well demonstrated by Mazzaferri and colleagues in Italy and Tubiana [9,10]. Adverse features include age 40 years or over, a large primary tumour, and extracapsular extension. Local recurrence is more than twice as common after subtotal as after total thyroidectomy and, more importantly, may result in increased mortality. In addition, the use of radio-iodine ablation is often recommended where adequate uptake can be demonstrated in patients with multiple, locally invasive, or large primary tumours, as well as those with distant metastases. Finally, the routine use of T4 seems to be of value even in patients who have not undergone total thyroidectomy and who do not require it for physiological replacement.

Follow-up investigation and examinations

are particularly important in these patients. They may develop recurrences many years after apparent cure. Apart from careful clinical palpation of the thyroid, follow-up should include regular chest radiography (about once every 3 years since pulmonary metastases and mediastinal nodes are particularly common areas of recurrence), together with serum thyroglobulin measurements. Radio-iodine tests are now much less used, and serum thyroglobulin can and should be measured when the patient is taking thyroxine [11]. This should be undertaken yearly for the first 5 years after the patient is regarded as disease-free, and every second year of follow-up thereafter. [131]I tests (185 MBq dosage is accepted as a safe out-patient procedure), with scanning 3–5 days afterwards, are increasingly used only in patients with an abnormal thyroglobulin level or in those who are known to have residual tumour postoperatively.

EXTERNAL IRRADIATION

In patients with thyroid cancers which do not take up radio-iodine, and particularly those which are locally unresectable (including almost all cases of anaplastic carcinoma and a high proportion of medullary carcinomas), external irradiation has an important role. A radical dose is required, typically of the order of 50–65 Gy (5000–6500 rad) in 5–7 weeks [12]. Such treatment is valuable both to delay local recurrence and also to treat or prevent troublesome symptoms from local obstruction. It can be curative, though rarely in patients with anaplastic carcinoma. In patients with thyroid lymphomas and small cell tumours, both of which are highly radiosensitive, external beam irradiation is the definitive treatment [13]. For these tumours a lower dose is adequate, of the order of 40 Gy (4000 rad) in 4 weeks. Since the total volume treated can be very substantial and at a site where spinal cord damage is a real threat, radical irradiation of the thyroid is technically difficult, especially if homogeneity of dosage is considered important. For this reason

several groups have developed sophisticated techniques using wedged field arrangements or arc rotation planning. Others prefer a more straightforward approach with a single anterior direct field, shaped by lead blocks in order to protect the larynx and, if necessary, the lungs. The radiation fields should cover the whole thyroid gland, and it is conventional to include the first-stage supraclavicular or cervical lymph nodes. The field may have to be extended inferiorly to include the upper mediastinal area if there is evidence of disease at this level. Intratracheal deposits, for example, are well described and can lead to haemoptysis.

RESULTS OF TREATMENT
FOR THYROID CANCER

For well-differentiated tumours the results of treatment are remarkably good. One substantial subgroup of patients, i.e. those below the age of 40 years with well-differentiated papillary carcinoma, have a normal survival pattern equal to that of a comparable population. The prognosis is affected by the age at diagnosis (the lower the better) and by the sex of the patient. In one large European co-operative study, 5-year survival rates were 60% for men and 75% for women [14]. Histological type also correlates with survival and, in general, the more well-differentiated the tumour the better the prognosis. Both papillary and non-invasive follicular carcinomas have a 10-year survival rate of the order of 75%. For papillary carcinoma, evidence of extrathyroid disease reduces the 10-year survival to about 50%. For medullary carcinomas the survival is only about 40% [12,15], a reflection of its early metastatic potential and the ineffectiveness of ^{131}I therapy, itself a reflection of its different histogenesis. Worst of all, anaplastic carcinoma has a very poor prognosis with about 5% of patients surviving 5 years and essentially no 10-year survivors. It is important to distinguish small cell carcinomas and thyroid lymphomas from the truly anaplastic group, since their prognosis is undoubtedly better, and thyroid lymphoma, though uncommon, has an extremely good prognosis. For anaplastic carcinoma even highly aggressive treatment including surgery, external irradiation (and sometimes chemotherapy) has failed to improve the outlook [16].

It is difficult to assess the separate contributions of surgery and radiation therapy since they tend to be used in a complementary fashion, and radiotherapy is usually offered only to patients in whom surgery has not been complete, i.e. those with a higher than usual risk of local recurrence and poorer ultimate survival. None the less, Tubiana's group [10] achieved a 10-year survival rate of over 70% in patients with papillary carcinoma who had undergone incomplete surgery. In follicular and medullary carcinoma the 10-year survival was 51% and 60% respectively. For patients presenting with metastases, treatment with radio-iodine (sometimes in combination with external irradiation to the primary tumour) may be very successful and gives an overall survival rate of about 22% at 12 years. This reflects not only the effectiveness of ^{131}I therapy but also the indolent nature of this tumour, even when metastatic.

Chemotherapy for recurrent or metastatic thyroid cancer has so far been disappointing. The most active single agent is doxorubicin, with a response rate of about 30%, and with proven activity in all cell types. In addition, bleomycin has produced well documented responses, and combinations of these and other agents have now been employed by several groups, reportedly with better response rates than with single agents alone. The difficulty with this approach is that the durations of response are on the whole very short, quite apart from the fact that many of these patients are elderly and have rapidly advancing disease. Chemotherapy has only a limited role in the management of metastatic carcinoma of the thyroid and treatment with external irradiation, radio-iodine and exogenous thyroxine should all be considered first.

CANCER OF THE ADRENAL GLAND

These rare tumours arise either from the adrenal cortex or the medulla, and in adults the ratio of adrenocortical carcinoma to malignant medullary tumours (malignant phaeochromocytoma) is approximately 2:1. Neuroblastoma, a common childhood tumour chiefly arising from the medulla, is discussed in Chapter 24.

Adrenocortical carcinoma

About a quarter of patients with adult Cushing's syndrome who have no obvious source of ectopic hormone production have an adrenal tumour, of which less than half are malignant [17]. Fewer than thirty cases are diagnosed in Britain per annum, and most of these are hormonally active, presenting with the features of Cushing's syndrome. In some patients, virilization, feminization or hyperaldosteronism (Conn's syndrome) are more obvious clinical features, although 30% of cases of adrenocortical carcinoma are non-functional. The mean age at presentation is 45 years, the female:male ratio is 2.5:1 and symptoms are usually present for 6−12 months before diagnosis. The endocrine symptoms are of glucocorticoid excess (45%), androgen excess (15%), both glucorticoids and androgens (35%), mineralocorticoids or oestrogens (5%). Benign adrenocortical tumours are typically yellowish in appearance and are adenomas often with large cell or giant cell patterns. Malignant tumours are usually more obviously necrotic or haemorrhagic, sometimes with pleomorphic morphology and frequent mitoses. Vascular invasion and distant dissemination (chiefly to bone, lung and liver) can occur. At presentation 70% have loco-regional disease and 30% have metastases. The diagnosis is usually made by biochemical measurement (persistent hypercortisolaemia with no suppression in response to dexamethasone, and a low plasma ACTH), CT scan confirmation of an adrenal tumour (Fig. 20.5) and, ultimately, tissue diagnosis fol-

Fig. 20.5 CT scan of abdomen showing adrenal tumour (arrowed). Normal anatomy of other structures is also clearly shown.

lowing laparotomy or CT-guided needle biopsy. Adrenal hyperplasia is usually bilateral, so unilateral adrenal enlargement is strongly suspicious of a benign or malignant tumour. Other imaging techniques include ultrasound and selective angiography with venous sampling. Non-functional tumours are more difficult to diagnose pre-operatively; clinical features are of a palpable abdominal mass (often a substantial size because of the 'silent' nature of the tumour), weight loss or fever. These patients are generally below the age of 20 years.

Treatment is primarily surgical, with wide resection which may necessitate a substantial thoraco-abdominal incision. A short course of pre-operative steroid therapy is often advocated. If there is evidence of metastatic disease, systemic treatment with o,p'-DDD (a derivative of the insecticide DDT) can be beneficial. In the majority of patients both a reduction in corticosteroid production and tumour regression can occur. Mitotane can often be given with little adverse effect but the full dosage of 8–10 g/day may produce side-effects of anorexia, nausea, diarrhoea, confusion and lethargy, limiting the acceptability of the treatment. Steroid replace-

ment is usually necessary. Where there is failure of response to o,p'-DDD, or if treatment has to be discontinued because of side-effects, palliation may be achieved by agents which interfere with steroid synthesis such as metyrapone or aminoglutethimide. Cushing's syndrome can be treated with aminoglutethimide. Chemotherapy using cisplatin and etoposide occasionally produces responses. Surgical resection or embolization of bulk disease should also be considered, as well as palliative radiotherapy for patients with painful bone metastases. Overall, the prognosis is not good. The median survival is 15 months, and only 20% of patients are alive at 5 years. Poor prognostic factors include age over 40 and metastases at presentation.

Adrenal medulla [18]

The cells of the adrenal medulla have a different derivation from those of the cortex, developing from neuroectodermal tissue and giving rise to both benign and malignant tumours. In adult life these include *phaeochromocytoma* (benign in 90% of cases), *ganglioneuroma* or *neuroblastoma*. In childhood, neuroblastoma is much the commonest of the adrenal medullary tumours and is discussed in Chapter 24.

Phaeochromocytomas can arise from the adrenal medulla (90%), organ of Zuckerkandl or adrenal medullary cell rests in the pelvis. They can occur sporadically or as part of a familial syndrome of multiple endocrine neoplasia (see Chapter 15). Other associated diseases are neurofibromatosis, von Hippel–Lindau and Sturge–Weber syndromes, cerebellar ataxia, and tuberous sclerosis/astrocytoma. About 10% are histologically malignant although the light-microscopical appearances are an unreliable guide to their clinical behaviour.

Phaeochromocytoma can occur at any age but patients are usually aged 40–60 years. Most patients are diagnosed as a result of investigation for hypertension, but the secretion of catecholamines by the tumour also causes

Table 20.2 Symptoms caused by phaeochromocytoma

Skin
Attacks of sweating, flushing, blanching

Cardiovascular
Hypertension, tachycardia, paroxysmal rhythm change,
   slow forceful beating chest pain, postural hypotension

Central nervous system
Headache, tremor, irritability, mood change, psychosis,
   anorexia

Metabolic
Weight loss, increased metabolic rate, glycosuria

symptoms (Table 20.2) which are the same for both benign and malignant tumours and include intermittent or paroxysmal headache, severe sweating attacks, postural hypotension, dys-rhythmias and chest pain. Some patients present primarily with an abdominal or pelvic mass.

Confirmation of the diagnosis is made by demonstration of excess catecholamines (adrenaline, noradrenaline and metabolites) in both urine and blood. The paroxysmal nature of the disorder may lead to false-negative plasma catecholamine measurement, and 24-hour urine collections are essential. Measurement of vanillyl mandelic acid (VMA) in the urine will provide the diagnosis in 85% of patients. In the others it may be necessary to resort to provocative tests using pharmacological agents. Phentolamine in *very small doses* (0.5–1.0 mg) will produce a fall in blood pressure of 25 mmHg lasting from 5 minutes to 4 hours. Histamine and tyramine provoke hypertension in these patients by liberating the excess catecholamines stored in nerve endings (but not in the tumour). The use of these drugs requires extremely careful monitoring.

Selective angiography and venous sampling may be necessary to localize the tumour though CT scanning generally gives excellent visualization of the adrenal. In most cases the diagnosis of malignancy can be made only when the resected specimen is examined histologi-cally, but occasionally a patient may have clinically obvious metastases.

Treatment of malignant phaeochromocytoma is by surgical resection with careful dissection and microscopical inspection of excision margins to ensure adequate surgical clearance. Surgical excision of single metastatic deposits has also been recommended. Pre-operatively the blood pressure is controlled by gradually increasing doses of phenoxybenzamine (to produce α receptor blockade). In patients with arrhythmia, a β blocking agent is added after the blood pressure is brought under control. (Fig. 20.6) Used alone they can precipitate severe hypertension. After good blood pressure control has been achieved for 10 days the resection is performed. During operation it is advisable to have continuous intra-arterial blood pressure monitoring with treatment of hypertension with phentolamine and arrhythmias with a β blocking agent. A fall in blood pressure following removal can usually be controlled by blood transfusions.

The use of chemotherapy for metastatic disease is purely anecdotal but alkylating agents and doxorubicin have been reported to be effective. In patients with symptomatic inoperable phaeochromocytoma both α and β blockers are valuable in controlling symptoms and may have

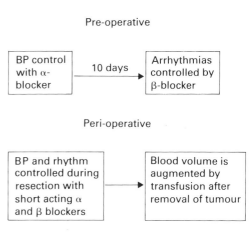

Fig. 20.6 Pre- and peri-operative management of phaeochromocytoma.

to be maintained for several years in patients with slow-growing tumours. Although long-term survival has been recorded, the majority of patients with malignant phaeochromocytoma die of the disease; extra-adrenal primary sites are said to have a particularly poor prognosis.

CANCER OF THE PARATHYROID GLANDS

This tumour is very rare with fewer than 100 cases in the world literature. Under 5% of all parathyroid tumours are malignant. The disease has been reported following irradiation of the neck. Most parathyroid carcinomas secrete PTH, causing hyperparathyroidism sometimes with a florid form of osteitis fibrosa cystica. The tumour tends to be slow-growing, and long-term survival frequently occurs if complete surgical removal is performed. Local recurrence can lead to severe pressure symptoms in the neck, but can be surgically resectable. Distant metastases occasionally occur, chiefly to lung and liver.

REFERENCES

1 Simpson W.J., McKinney S.E., Carruthers J.S., *et al.* Papillary and follicular thyroid cancer: prognostic factors in 1,578 patients. *American Journal of Medicine* 1987; **83**: 479–88.

2 Saad M.F., Ordonez M.G., Rashid R.K. *et al.* Medullary carcinoma of the thyroid: A study of the clinical features and prognostic factors in 161 patients. *Medicine* 1984; **63**: 319–42.

3 Mathew C.G.P., Easton D.F., Nakamura Y. *et al.* Presymptomatic screening for multiple endocrine neoplasia type 2A with linked DNA markers. *Lancet* 1991; **337**: 7–11.

4 Calmettes C., Ponder B.A.J., Fischer J.A. *et al.* Early diagnosis of the multiple endocrine neoplasia type 2 syndrome: consensus statement. *European Journal of Clinical Investigation* 1992; **22**: 755–60.

5 Lips C.J.M., Landsvater R.M., Höppener J.W.M. *et al.* Clinical screening as compared with DNA analysis in families with multiple endocrine neoplasia type 2A. *New England Journal of Medicine* 1994; **331**: 828–35.

6 Clark L., Ibanez M.L., White E.C. What operation for carcinoma of the thyroid? *Archives of Surgery* 1966; **92**: 23–26.

7 Leading article Thyroid cancer. *British Medical Journal* 1976; **1**: 113–14.

8 Sisson J.C. Applying the radioactive eraser: I-131 to ablate normal thyroid tissue in patients from whom thyroid cancer has been resected. *Journal of Nuclear Medicine* 1983; **24**: 743–45.

9 Mazzaferri E.L., Young R.L., Oertel J.E. *et al.* Papillary thyroid carcinoma: the impact of therapy on 576 patients. *Medicine (Baltimore)* 1977; **56**: 171–96.

10 Tubiana M., Schlumberger M., Rougier P. *et al.* Long term results and prognostic factors in patients with differentiated thyroid carcinoma. *Cancer* 1985; **55**: 794–804.

11 Ashcraft M.W., Van Herle A.J. Comparative value of serum thyroglobulin measurements and ^{131}I total body scans in follow-up study of patients with treated differentiated thyroid cancer. *American Journal of Medicine* 71: 806–14.

12 Moss W.T., Brand W.N., Battifora H. The thyroid. In *Radiation Oncology — Rationale, Technique, Results*, 5th edn. St Louis: Mosby, 1979: pp. 233–42.

13 Souhami L., Simpson W.J., Carruthers J.S. Malignant lymphoma of the thyroid gland. *International Journal of Radiation Oncology, Biology and Physics* 1980; **6**: 1143–8.

14 Byar D.P., Green S.B., Dor P.R., Williams D., Colon J. *et al.* A prognostic index for thyroid carcinoma — an EORTC study. *European Journal of Cancer* 1979; **15**: 1033–42.

15 Brooks J.R., Starnes J.F., Brooks D.C. *et al.* Surgical therapy for thyroid carcinoma: a review of 1249 solitary nodules. *Surgery* 1988; **104**: 940–46.

16 Leeper R.D. Symposium on thyroid cancer. *Medical Clinics of North America* 1985; **69**: 1079–96.

17 Luton J.-P., Cerdas S., Billaud L. *et al.* Clinical features of adrenocortical carcinoma, prognostic factors, and the effect of mitotane therapy. *New England Journal of Medicine* 1990; **322**: 1195–201.

18 Modlin I.M., Farndon J.R., Shepherd A. *et al.* Phaeochromocytomas in 72 patients: Clinical and diagnostic features, treatment and long-term results. *British Journal of Surgery* 1979; **66**: 456–65.

Chapter 21
Metastases from an Unknown Primary Site

In the majority of patients who present with symptoms from metastases, routine examination and investigation quickly disclose the underlying primary. However, 1–5% of all patients with cancer present with symptoms and signs due to metastases and, after initial investigation, the primary site remains undetected. In these cases the primary tumour is too small to be clinically apparent and simple investigations such as chest X-ray, full blood count and liver function tests fail to give the diagnosis. Usually the histological diagnosis, obtained from the metastasis, is of an adeno-carcinoma or poorly differentiated carcinoma.

There are few situations in medicine which are a greater test of clinical judgement. Faced with this situation, many physicians resort to a battery of investigations designed to disclose the primary site, but at the same time are aware that, if and when they find the primary tumour, it will make little or no difference to the management of the patient. Investigation is undertaken, almost as a ritual, to reassure both the physician and the patient that something is being done.

SITE OF PRESENTATION [1]

For the purposes of this chapter cases will be considered in which, despite full and appropriate examination, no primary site has been disclosed. The extent and nature of this preliminary investigation will depend on the site of the metastasis. The common metastatic sites include lymph nodes, bone, brain, liver and skin. Table 21.1 shows the most frequent primary tumours presenting at these sites. With each metastatic site, investigation will have a different emphasis. For example, a squamous carcinoma in a cervical node will lead to a strong suspicion that the nasopharynx or lung is the likely primary site and full examination including the larynx, pharynx and postnasal space will often give the diagnosis. Similarly an inguinal node or malignant ascites will lead to careful gynaecological examination. Management will then be as for the underlying malignancy. When initial investigation has failed to give any clue to the primary cancer, the physician must ask himself the question 'If I find the primary, will there be any treatment which offers a reasonable chance of palliation or cure?'

A particularly important group of tumours are germ cell tumours which, it is increasingly recognized, may present as a poorly differentiated carcinoma but are highly responsive to chemotherapy.

THE SITES OF ORIGIN OF METASTASIS FROM AN UNKNOWN PRIMARY

Curiously, the distribution of cancers which present as metastases from an occult primary is not the same as the overall distribution of cancer. In Table 21.2 the frequency of presentation of metastasis from an unknown primary is shown compared with the frequency of cancers in general. It is clear that the commonest tumours to present in this way are pancreas, lung, liver, stomach and colo-rectal cancer. Common cancers such as breast and prostate are much less frequent causes of metastasis from an unknown primary. This is probably

Table 21.1 Sites of metastases from an unknown primary

Site of metastasis	Likely primary site
High cervical nodes	Head and neck sites Thyroid Lung
Lower cervical nodes	Head and neck Lung, Breast Gut (especially L. supraclavicular node)
Axillary nodes	Lung Breast
Skin	Breast Lung Melanoma
Bone	Myeloma Breast Kidney Prostate Lung
Brain	Lung Breast Prostate Melanoma
Inguinal nodes	Vulva Anorectal Prostate Ovary
Disseminated intra-abdominal adenocarcinoma (including liver metastasis)	Ovary Stomach Pancreas Gut

Table 21.2 Sites of origin of carcinomas presenting as metastases from unknown site

	All unknown primary cases (%)	All cancers (%)
Pancreas	20	2
Lung	20	10
Unknown	15	—
Liver	10	2
Stomach	10	5
Colo-rectal	8	15
Breast	3	26
Thyroid	3	1
Renal	3	2
Prostate	3	18
Ovary	2	5
Other	3	14

Table 21.3 Treatable cancers which may present as metastases from an unknown primary

Curable tumours which must not be missed
Germ cell and trophoblastic tumours
Lymphomas
Well-differentiated thyroid cancer

Tumours which can be palliated by chemotherapy
Breast
Ovary
Small cell carcinoma of the bronchus

Tumours which can be palliated by hormone therapy
Breast
Prostate
Endometrial

because primary tumours in the breast are relatively easily detected clinically, while prostatic cancer is not infrequently associated with an elevation of the acid phosphatase or PSA which is a straightforward investigation often giving the diagnosis.

PROGNOSIS OF METASTASIS FROM AN UNKNOWN PRIMARY [2]

Several studies have shown that the survival of patients who present in this way is extremely poor. The median survival is usually only 3–5 months and only 10% of patients are alive at 2 years. This poor prognosis is probably related to the malignant potential of these tumours since at autopsy the primary is sometimes only very small. The tumour is presumably rapidly growing, with a tendency to early metastasis. The tumours which are associated with a less catastrophic prognosis are shown in Table 21.3 and it is these tumours in particular which one must not miss. Investigation must therefore be directed towards the confident exclusion of these tumours and, this having been done, there is probably no point in further investigation.

Several studies have shown that the yield of investigation is low when applied routinely to all patients in this situation. In one report the primary site was identified in only 10% of cases and in only 14 out of 266 cases was a treatable cancer detected [1]. In none of these was cure possible but palliation might have been considered. In most cases, therefore, a primary will not be found at presentation and even if it is, it is extremely unusual for a treatable disease to be discovered. A further problem in adopting an attitude of intensive investigation for all these patients is that the clinical studies frequently give false-positive and false-negative results, and the patient is then subjected to a number of further investigations, often invasive and invariably expensive, the end result usually being failure.

INVESTIGATION AND MANAGEMENT [3]

The following is a guide to management of this difficult problem. It must be emphasized that the degree to which investigation will be pursued will vary greatly with individual patients. The patient's age, fitness and degree of anxiety will all influence the decision as well as the possibility of finding a treatable tumour.

Review of histology

The most important first step is to discuss the biopsy with an experienced pathologist. Sometimes the pathologist may have a shrewd idea where the primary site might be, but because of lack of clinical information, has left the diagnosis open. Special stains may be useful in providing further information, for example, immunocytochemical staining for large cell lymphomas. These tumours are often difficult to distinguish from anaplastic carcinoma, but are very responsive to chemotherapy. Mucin stains may demonstrate intracellular mucin and point to an origin from the gut, pancreas or stomach. In recent years a large number of

Table 21.4 Useful immuno-histopathological investigation in diagnosis in metastasis from an unknown primary site

Cellular structure	Investigation or reagent	Tumour types identified
Cytokeratins	Cam 5.2	Carcinomas
Epithelial membrane antigen (EMA)	Antibodies to EMA	Carcinomas (especially breast, gut, ovary, pancreas)
Common leucocyte antigen (CLA)	Anti-CLA	Lymphomas (98% positive)
Desmin ⎫ intermediate Vimentin ⎭ filaments	Antibodies	Some sarcomas
S100 proteins	S100 antibodies	Melanoma
Thyroglobulin	Anti-thyroglobulin	Thyroid carcinoma
HCG	Anti-HCG	⎫
AFP	Anti-AFP	⎬ Germ cell tumours
PLAP	Anti-PLAP	⎭
Premelanosomes	EM*	Melanoma
Dense core granules	EM	Neuroendocrine tumours (small cell lung cancer)
Intermediate filaments	EM	Carcinoma

* EM, electron microscopy

monoclonal antibodies have been prepared which are reactive with membrane and cytoplasmic proteins and which may help to determine the cell of origin. It is extremely important not to miss a large cell lymphoma as a cause of an undifferentiated tumour, and antibodies to the common leucocyte antigen (see Chapter 26 and Fig. 3.12, p. 45) and to epithelial antigens such as cytokeratins can usually make this distinction.

Table 21.4 lists some of the more frequently used reagents. Many of these will work on paraffin sections, but some require frozen tissue. This is another reason why biopsy material should not be placed entirely in formalin when cancer is a possible diagnosis. Antisera to epithelial membrane antigens are available which help to define epithelial tumours such as breast cancer or other poorly differentiated adenocarcinomas. Antibodies to pre-keratin may be helpful in determining whether or not the tumour is of squamous origin; others react with melanoma associated antigens. If the node is taken from an axillary or a supraclavicular site, examination for oestrogen receptor positivity may be helpful in proving a breast origin of the tumour. Occasionally electron microscopy may help, for example in showing premelanosomes in malignant melanoma, or intercellular bridges in poorly differentiated squamous carcinoma. Undifferentiated germ cell tumours are curable cancers of young people which are easily overlooked. They may contain HCG and AFP and can be stained for the intracellular presence of these peptides by immunocytochemical techniques.

Biochemical and haematological investigation

Certain tests should be carried out as a routine. These include an acid phosphatase and/or PSA measurement in men over 40 years old to detect carcinoma of the prostate; HCG and AFP determinations in young patients in case the tumour is of germ cell type, and immunoelectrophoresis and examination of the urine for Bence Jones protein if myeloma is a possi-

bility. The blood film may show evidence of leucoerythroblastic anaemia and this is most commonly seen with breast cancer, occasionally in carcinoma of the lung and much less commonly in any other tumour. Polycythaemia and thrombocytosis may occur with renal carcinoma and hepatoma. Hepatomas also produce AFP (see Chapter 15).

Other investigations

The urine should always be examined. A fresh sample should be taken to look for red cells, which may indicate an underlying renal carcinoma. A chest X-ray is of course an essential examination and may disclose a carcinoma of the bronchus or enlarged mediastinal lymph nodes suggestive of a lymphoma.

Other more invasive investigations are of much more doubtful benefit. Although there is a temptation to go further and perform contrast radiology of the gut and kidneys, and CT scans of the chest and abdomen, these are seldom valuable or useful contributions to management since, by definition, the disease is disseminated at the time of presentation. There is a place for mammography if carcinoma of the breast is a serious differential diagnosis since the presence of a supraclavicular or axillary node does not rule out effective treatment of the tumour. In the final analysis the decision is one which requires judgement and skill. In the main, the less experienced the physician, the greater the number of investigations performed. It requires considerable clinical authority and careful explanation to help the patient understand that further investigation is not needed (or likely to be helpful) after the metastasis has been discovered and treatable causes excluded.

TREATMENT

The diagnosis of cancer presenting as metastasis poses a considerable burden on the patient and the doctor. The element of uncertainty in the situation and the serious nature and poor prognosis of the complaint make management difficult. Symptomatic treatments are always available and include local radiotherapy, analgesics and steroids, as used in metastatic cancer of known origin when it recurs. If the diagnosis has been established as a germ cell tumour or other treatable condition as outlined in Table 21.3, then of course treatment is along the appropriate lines. Approximately 80% of patients will have histological appearances of poorly differentiated adenocarcinoma or poorly differentiated carcinoma. Some of these patients may have a germ cell tumour and be curable by chemotherapy [4]. These patients often have tumour located in the midline (in the mediastinum or para-aortic region), are usually below 50 years old, and sometimes have a rapidly growing tumour which may have responded well to previous radiotherapy. In these cases, if the histology is poorly differentiated *adeno-carcinoma*, the response rate to germ cell chemotherapy is low (about 30%) and usually short-lived. If the histology is poorly differentiated *carcinoma* the response rate approaches 80% in some series and some patients are cured [5]. These findings indicate that younger patients with poorly differentiated carcinomas should receive platinum-based germ cell chemotherapy.

Some tumours may show neuroendocrine features (such as neurosecretory granules) on electron microscopy and these patients should receive chemotherapy as for small cell lung cancer (p. 238) since the response rate is high.

In many cases, however, no diagnosis will be reached, and the issue will then be to decide if chemotherapy should be used in an attempt to delay the progress of the disease. This depends very much on the clinical state of the patient and on the intensity of the patient's anxiety for treatment. Undoubtedly regressions can be induced with the use of drugs such as doxorubicin and mitomycin in combination, or combinations such as cyclophosphamide, methotrexate and 5-FU. Such regressions are usually short-lived and it is by no means clear whether the overall prognosis of patients will be improved even though it is likely

that responders will live longer than non-responders. The single most useful agent is doxorubicin, but this of course has the unwanted effects of nausea and alopecia. Our practice is to use a combination including doxorubicin in those patients who are young, relatively fit, and who have a strong desire for treatment [6]. All too often, however, there is a failure of response or only a short-lived response, and palliative treatment is all that can be offered.

In women in whom the histological diagnosis is adenocarcinoma, a trial of endocrine therapy with tamoxifen, aminoglutethimide or a progestogen is often worthwhile, even if there is no clinical or radiological evidence that the breast is the primary site.

Exceptionally an isolated cerebral metastasis can be removed surgically. Removal of solitary brain secondaries (even when the primary site is known) is associated with less likelihood of recurrence in the brain and better quality of life than control with radiation alone [7].

REFERENCES

1 Altman E., Cadman E. An analysis of 1539 patients with cancer of unknown primary site. *Cancer* 1986; **57**: 120−24.
2 Abbruzzese J.L., Abbruzzese M.C. Primary carcinoma: Natural history and prognostic factors in 657 consecutive patients. *Journal of Clinical Oncology* 1994; **12**: 1272−80.
3 Nystrom J.S., Weiner J.M., Wolf R.M. Identifying the primary site in metastatic cancer of unknown origin. Inadequacy of roentgenographic procedures. *Journal of the American Medical Association* 1979; **241**: 381−83.
4 Greco F.A., Vaughn W.K., Hainsworth J.D. Advanced poorly differentiated carcinoma of unknown primary site: recognition of a treatable syndrome. *Annals of Internal Medicine* 1986; **104**: 547−53.
5 van der Gaast A., Verweig J., Henzen-Logmans S.C., Rodenburg C.J., Stoger G. Carcinoma of unknown primary: Identification of a treatable subset? *Annals of Oncology* 1990; **1**: 119−22.
6 Woods R.L., Fox R.M., Tattersall M.H.N., Levi J.A., Brodie E.N. Metastatic adenocarcinomas of unknown primary site. A randomised study of two combination chemotherapy regimens. *New England Journal of Medicine* 1980; **303**: 87−89.
7 Posner J.B. Surgery for metastases to the brain. *New England Journal of Medicine* 1990; **322**: 544−45.

Chapter 22
Skin Cancer

AETIOLOGY AND PATHOGENESIS

It should not be surprising that skin cancers are the commonest of all malignancies, since the skin is the largest and most accessible organ of the body, directly exposed to whatever carcinogens are in our environment. It has been recognized for over 200 years that skin cancers can develop as a result of directly applied carcinogens, and the earliest described and perhaps best known example, noted by Percivall Pott in 1775, is the carcinoma of scrotal skin which affected chimney sweeps who came into direct contact with soot in the chimney flue. In the 19th century, an increase in the incidence of skin cancers was reported in patients who had been treated with medicines containing arsenic, and arsenical fumes had already been implicated as a contributing factor in the scrotal cancers of copper miners and smelters. Towards the end of the century, it was suggested that strong sunlight might be a promoter of skin cancer, and shortly after the discovery of radium, Becquerel proposed that ionizing radiation might be the component of sunlight responsible for malignant change. More recently, the carcinogenic roles of ultraviolet radiation, X-rays and chemicals has been confirmed; most important of all was the work of Yamagiwa and Ichikawa who were the first to demonstrate the carcinogenic properties of coal tar when applied directly to the skin of experimental animals [1], though it was Kennaway who isolated and identified the carcinogen as 3:4-benzpyrene. Over the past 40 years, the incidence of melanoma has doubled every decade, probably as a result of increased exposure to sunlight and perhaps also resulting from loss in our ozone layer [2].

Sunlight

Epidemiological studies have provided important clues to the aetiology of skin cancer. In general, its incidence varies directly in proportion to the intensity of sunlight, with the result that skin cancers are much more common in Australia (with the world's highest incidence rates) and South Africa, than in more temperate areas. The importance of sunlight is further suggested by the high proportion of skin cancers (particularly basal cell carcinomas) which occur in exposed areas of the body. In addition, certain races such as the fair-skinned Celts are particularly prone to developing skin cancer, probably due to a relative lack of protection by melanin pigment; in contrast, skin cancers are relatively uncommon in black races, presumably as a result of effective shielding by pigment in the superficial skin layers. In the past, large solar keratoses were often thought to transform into squamous carcinomas but that view is no longer widely held though these keratoses undoubtedly reflect cumulative solar damage. Most public information programmes about skin cancer emphasize the importance of avoiding over-exposure to sunlight [3]. In black people, the distribution of skin cancers is much less determined by sunlight exposure than in Caucasians, and is almost as common in unexposed areas such as the trunk and lower limbs. The use of psoralens and ultraviolet light 'A' (pUVA) in psoriasis is associated with a risk of cutaneous malignancy, particularly on the

413

male genitalia, and not only in cases where other carcinogens (such as X-rays) had been given in the past.

Occupational factors

Occupational carcinogens have in the past been an important cause of skin cancers, though increasing awareness of the hazards has substantially reduced these risks. However, industrial carcinogens such as petroleum derivatives, arsenicals, and coal tar are still in common use, and protective clothing is still important in prevention. Even more critical is the need to keep radiation exposure to an absolute minimum, particularly for those working with X-rays, including medical, nursing and radiographic personnel who require regular monitoring of radiation exposure throughout their working lives.

Immune suppression and viral causes

Recipients of renal allografts have an increased risk of cancer — possibly as great as 100 times that of the general population. The most common malignancies are those of the skin including squamous carcinoma, melanoma, basal cell carcinoma and Bowen's disease. The squamous carcinomas are more frequent than basal cell (a reverse of the usual pattern) and occur 20 times more often than in normal people. Sometimes the disease is severe and multifocal running an aggressive course.

Considerable interest has been aroused in the role of the wart viruses, *human papilloma virus* (HPV), in the aetiology of cancers of the skin and genital tract. A pattern is now emerging in which HPV appears to be associated with the appearance of cancer in particular clinical settings. The genome of HPV type 5 has been found in squamous carcinoma of the skin in a renal allograft recipient and also in the squamous cancers which occur in the rare inherited skin disorder *epidermodysplasia verruciformis* in which patients develop multiple warts. Although HPV is now less widely regarded as

the key aetiological agent, it seems extremely likely that it does indeed have carcinogenic properties.

Premalignant lesions

A group of premalignant skin lesions has been recognized in which malignant change, though not inevitable, is sufficiently common to justify very close surveillance. These lesions include:

INHERITED DISORDERS

Xeroderma pigmentosum

This autosomal recessive disease is characterized by greatly increased sensitivity to ultraviolet light leading to multiple solar keratoses, premalignant and ultimately frankly malignant skin lesions on exposed surfaces. The cancer can be squamous or basal cell carcinoma, or malignant melanoma. The defect appears to be due to UV-induced DNA damage causing a deficiency in the excision—repair mechanism for DNA.

Naevoid basal cell carcinoma syndrome (Gorlin's syndrome)

This syndrome is characterized by multiple basal cell carcinomas particularly on the face and trunk, associated with cleft lip and skeletal abnormalities which include frontal bossing, mandibular cysts and bifid ribs. It is inherited through a single autosomal dominant gene which has complete penetrance but variable expression. About 40% of patients do not appear to have an affected parent.

The syndrome is associated with an increased tendency to other neoplastic changes, notably ameloblastoma and squamous cell carcinoma of or around the jaw, meningioma, melanoma and many other sites [4]. Management may be particularly difficult in view of the hundreds of naevi or frank tumours these patients may develop. The skin tumours often develop in young adult life.

Albinism

This group of congenital diseases is associated with defective skin pigmentation and an increased tendency to solar keratosis and squamous carcinoma *in situ*.

Epidermodysplasia verruciformis

This is an autosomal recessive disease characterized by multiple flat warts. These and even non-affected skin may evolve into squamous carcinoma (see above).

CARCINOGEN-INDUCED DISORDERS

Arsenical keratoses

After exposure to inorganic arsenicals, keratotic lesions may develop 10 years or more later on the palms and soles. These lesions are premalignant although overt cancer is uncommon. The patients often have Bowen's disease and superficial basal cell carcinomas at other sites.

Solar keratoses

Although histologically similar to arsenical keratoses, the incidence of frank malignant change is much greater. The distribution is also different, since these lesions chiefly occur on the face and dorsal surfaces of the hands. Other changes of prolonged exposure to sunlight are present: furrowed elastic leathery skin, with wrinkling, atrophy and hyper- or depigmented patches.

Radiation dermatitis

Following exposure to modest doses of superficial radiation (often given many years before, for benign conditions, e.g. ringworm, acne or hirsutism), the skin may assume a characteristic appearance, with depigmentation, atrophy of the skin, hair and sweat glands, and telangiectasia. These areas are more susceptible to malignant change. Basal cell carcinomas on the scalp are usually related to previous irradiation and may arise in skin which shows no evidence of radiation change.

MISCELLANEOUS DISORDERS

Bowen's disease

Often considered with the premalignant skin disorders, this disease is more properly considered as a squamous cell carcinoma *in situ*, and is a superficial intra-epidermal carcinoma usually found on the trunk or limbs. Characteristically, this lesion spreads laterally within the cutis, commonly arising at several sites, and evolving slowly from a small erythematous papule to a crusting lesion. Histologically, the basal layer is intact but the epidermis shows premature keratinization and is disrupted with homogeneous cells with basophilic cytoplasm, small nuclei and frequent mitoses. There is an important association with internal malignancies, and as many as a quarter of all patients with Bowen's disease may develop a deep-seated carcinoma during the 10 years following diagnosis.

Leucoplakia

These are indurated whitish plaques, often fissured and with sharply defined borders, found on mucous membranes of the mouth. They may result from local irritation — ill-fitting dentures and smoking are frequently associated. The histology shows hyperplasia, hyperkeratosis and dyskeratosis; carcinoma *in situ* may arise, sometimes progressing to squamous cell carcinoma.

Genital carcinoma in situ

This disorder is now often regarded as a form of intraepithelial neoplasia. It presents as a persistent red papule or plaque on the penis. The relationship with HPV remains contentious. Pathologically there is an abnormal epidermis with an absent granular layer and small densely packed cells similar to those found in Bowen's disease. The lesion used to be called erythroplasia of Queyrat. Intraepithelial neoplasia may also be found on the vulva (see also Chapter 17).

BASAL CELL CARCINOMA

Basal cell carcinoma (rodent ulcer) accounts for over 75% of all cases of skin malignancy in the Western world. The age-specific incidence is shown in Fig. 22.1. They are epithelial tumours without any histological evidence of maturation or tendency to keratinization, and almost certainly arise from the undifferentiated basal cells of the skin, which normally differentiate into mature structures such as hair or sweat glands. Microscopically, these tumours are characterized by uniform cells with darkly stained nuclei

and little cytoplasm. The cells form a characteristic palisade (Fig. 22.2). The tumour generally arises on exposed areas, particularly the skin of the face and most characteristically around the nose, forehead, cheeks and lower eyelid although they may sometimes occur on the limbs. Macroscopically, these lesions are often described as being either nodular, pigmented, sclerosing (morphoeic), cicatrizing, infiltrating or ulcerative. The most typical appearance is that of a firm pink papule with a distinct raised edge, often serpiginous, with a pearly and telangiectatic appearance and with a slightly depressed or frankly ulcerated centre with or without a central crust. Although non-inflammatory and typically painless, they may irritate and will often bleed repeatedly if scratched.

Untreated, these tumours invade laterally with local destruction of cartilage or even bone; less commonly, such destruction may also result from deep extension. In the sclerosing variety, the typical features may be absent and the margin indistinct — making diagnosis more difficult. Superficial basal cell carcinomas, often multiple, also have an unusual appearance and

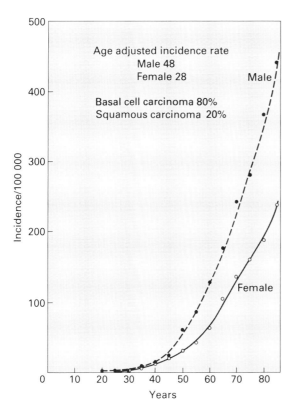

Fig. 22.1 Age-specific incidence of basal cell carcinoma and squamous carcinoma of the skin.

Fig. 22.2 Basal cell carcinoma of the skin, showing small nests of invading basal cells (×20).

are more commonly encountered on the trunk with, characteristically, a more plaque-like configuration, often with reddish scaling patches and a typical fine pearly edge. Very occasionally, cystic degeneration occurs in a basal cell carcinoma.

Despite the characteristically highly malignant microscopic appearance of basal cell carcinomas, metastasis to local lymph nodes or distant sites is exceptionally rare, a remarkable fact in view of the large size that many of these cancers can achieve, and an important contrast from the behaviour of squamous cell carcinomas. Multiple primary tumours, however, are not uncommon. In one American prospective study of 1000 patients with a basal cell carcinoma, 36% developed a second within a 5-year period. About 9% of Australian cases have multiple primary lesions at presentation [5].

Fig. 22.3 Squamous cell carcinoma of skin, showing invading masses of squamous epithelium forming keratin pearls (×20).

SQUAMOUS CELL CARCINOMA

Squamous cell carcinomas of the skin are less common than basal cell carcinomas (Fig. 22.1) though they share many characteristics of aetiology and site. Sunlight exposure, arsenic ingestion, and occupational carcinogens are all known to be important, as well as direct exposure to X-rays. Multiple squamous cell carcinomas of the hand were common among radiation scientists in the early years of this century until these hazards were recognized and methods of dosimetry improved. Histologically, these are typical keratinizing squamous lesions (Fig. 22.3) quite unlike the basal cell carcinoma, though diagnostic difficulties can occasionally occur with basal cell carcinoma and other lesions such as melanoma since more invasive and aggressive tumours may lack this characteristic feature. To some extent, the likelihood of local lymph node metastases can be predicted from the histological appearance, being more common with less well-differentiated tumours.

As with basal cell carcinomas, the commonest sites include the exposed areas of the head and neck, particularly the nose, temples, rim of the ear and lip, as well as the side and back of the neck, and the dorsal surfaces of the hand and forearm. The appearance of these lesions tends to resemble either a crusted scaly ulcer or a more nodular exophytic type of lesion, which can fungate if untreated. Small lesions may be impossible to distinguish macroscopically from basal cell carcinomas but the site of the tumour may be diagnostically helpful since squamous cell carcinomas, though commonest on the face, have a much more widespread distribution than basal cell carcinomas and a shorter history. A skin tumour of the hand or forearm is much more likely to be of squamous cell origin. Squamous cell carcinoma may also be difficult to distinguish macroscopically from the usually benign condition of keratoacanthoma, characterized by a locally rapidly advancing, discrete and often bulky papule, usually occurring on the face or neck, and typically with a central plug of keratin filling the ulcerated central part of the lesion.

Squamous cell carcinomas arising in an area of radiation dermatitis are both clinically and histologically more aggressive than other varieties, though the mean latent interval is about 20 years. In one large series of nearly 400 patients, the mortality was 10%. These tumours are now less frequent because of higher energy radiotherapy equipment, and the infrequent use of radiotherapy for benign skin disorders and arthritic conditions. This is also true of squamous carcinomas arising from chronic burn ulcers, *Marjolin's ulcer*, though this used to be a common problem, typically with a lengthy period of quiescence terminated by a highly aggressive phase with metastases to the lungs and other sites. A similar type of squamous cell carcinoma occasionally develops in chronic sinus tracts of osteomyelitis or other chronic infections. Squamous carcinomas can also develop in dysplastic or scar areas resulting from chronic skin diseases such as lupus vulgaris or lupus erythematosus, and are also reportedly more common in areas of vitiligo, particularly in black people.

Squamous carcinomas arising at mucocutaneous junctions such as the anus and vulva tend to be aggressive, as do those developing in areas of radiation-damaged skin, patches of Bowen's disease, or against a background of carcinoma *in situ*. In many cases, deep invasion and early metastasis takes place even though the primary lesion may appear unchanged. Sweat gland carcinoma, an uncommon condition, may also behave unpredictably. These tumours most commonly arise in the axilla and anogenital regions, and should be distinguished from the rare sebaceous gland cancers.

Treatment of basal cell and squamous cell carcinoma

Because of the frequency and characteristic appearance of these tumours, treatment without firm histological diagnosis is sometimes advocated. In general this is an unwise policy and has been shown to be dangerous since the lesions most likely to metastasize are those least likely to have been correctly clinically diagnosed [5]. Elderly patients may, however, be too unwell to withstand even the mild trauma of a surgical or drill biopsy under local anaesthetic. In all other cases, a biopsy should first be obtained. Benign conditions such as papillomas, sclerosing haemangiomas and keratoacanthomas can all be macroscopically confused with a basal or squamous cell carcinoma, and occasionally these two major types of skin cancer can themselves be difficult to distinguish from each other.

There are several effective methods of treatment, including electrocautery and curettage, cryosurgery, excisional surgery, chemosurgery, radiotherapy and topical chemotherapy. Since all of these methods have their strong adherents and each method yields a very high success rate, formal comparisons are difficult. In addition, approaches such as electrocautery and cryosurgery are in general confined to such small lesions (usually under 5 mm diameter) that the very high success rate of over 95% is not representative of an unselected group of patients.

Electrocautery is not usually used for tumours at difficult sites such as the margin of the eyelid or nasolabial fold, or for deeply infiltrating tumours. Cryosurgery, usually using liquid nitrogen, is also effective for small lesions, particularly for superficial tumours such as Bowen's disease and the most superficial of basal cell carcinomas. It can be extremely useful in elderly or immobile patients [6]. Chemosurgery, an interesting technique first described by Mohs [7], employs a zinc chloride paste fixative which is applied to the tumour, partly destroying it and allowing easy removal from the underlying skin whilst preserving its histological pattern. Further zinc chloride paste is then applied to any area of the residual tumour, and the whole process can be repeated. Currently the zinc fixative is often omitted. This method can be useful even for fairly large tumours and at sites where radiotherapy may be hazardous (see below), though the technique is time-consuming and laborious, and demands great expertise and care particularly in the histological assessment. Despite these potential drawbacks, the use of this technique, often referred to as micrographically controlled surgery, is now used far more frequently [6].

For basal cell and squamous cell carcinomas too large to be treated by electrocautery, most dermatologists would agree that the real choice in therapy lies between excisional surgery and radiotherapy. Each has its advantages. Excisional surgery is quick, does not require multiple visits to hospital, and is the only method producing a complete specimen for the pathologist to ensure that total microscopic excision has been achieved. On the other hand, for tumours of large size a general anaesthetic is usually required, and for still larger lesions, skin grafting or flap rotation may well be necessary, contributing to a less acceptable final cosmetic result as well as the risk of a higher postoperative complication rate than with simple excision alone. With tumours at difficult sites such as the inner canthus of the eye, surgery is probably best avoided since there is a risk of damage to the nasolachrymal duct, and surgical reconstruction can be very difficult. In general, however, the results of surgery are very good and an excellent cosmetic result can be achieved. This is true for both basal cell and squamous cell carcinomas, though a wider excision of squamous cell carcinomas is usually recommended because of the possibility of local lymphatic spread. Despite the known tendency of squamous cell carcinomas to metastasize to local lymph nodes, there is no place for routine lymph node dissection, although surgical excision is undoubtedly the treatment of choice for clinically involved regional lymph nodes.

Radiotherapy is also highly effective, with a cure rate of over 90%. It is especially useful for tumours on the face, particularly around the eye, nose and nasolabial fold where tumours may infiltrate deeply and prove difficult to excise surgically, without in some cases an unacceptable deformity. Both the columella of the nose and the ala nasae are difficult surgical sites, and radiotherapy is usually curative and gives excellent cosmetic results. One advantage

enjoyed by radiotherapists is the versatility of modern radiotherapy equipment, offering an energy and effective depth-dose of the irradiation beam which can be chosen to suit the individual tumour. Simple lead cut-outs can be tailor-made so that irregularly shaped tumours may be adequately treated without unnecessary treatment of large volumes of normal skin (Fig. 22.4). For tumours of the lower eyelid and other sites where shielding of deeper structures is desirable (e.g. gums, teeth and tongue in treatment of cancer of the lip), simple shielding can be repeatedly introduced, for each treatment session. Figure 22.5 shows a lead shield inserted under local anaesthetic into the lower conjunctival sac, to protect the eye whilst a tumour of the lower lid is treated. For tumours overlying bone or cartilage where low to moderate energy X-ray beams carry a risk of radionecrosis (see Chapter 5) direct electron beams can be employed with equally good results and far less risk of damage. There is some evidence that radiotherapy is particularly effective for basal cell carcinomas overlying bone or cartilage [8]. The major disadvantage of radiotherapy is that in order to produce the best cosmetic result, most radiotherapists feel that it is necessary to employ fractionated regimes of treatment over 2 weeks or more. Most patients are able to attend the radiotherapy department for several treatment sessions during this period, but for the elderly or infirm, the travelling may be tiring and a quick operation or treatment by a single large fraction of radiotherapy may be preferable.

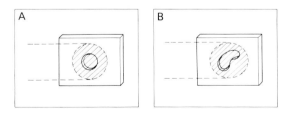

Fig. 22.4 Typical lead cut-outs for treatment of basal or squamous carcinoma. (A) Regularly shaped; (B) irregularly shaped.

Fig. 22.5 Treatment of skin cancer on lower eyelid.
(A) Typical position of tumour; (B) lead spatula inserted
into lower lid before each treatment, shielding cornea
and lens; (C) lead cut-out in position; (D) lateral view.

Table 22.1 Fractionation regimens in basal and
squamous cell carcinoma. Single fraction or 2-fraction
policies are generally adopted in elderly patients for
whom repeated visits may be difficult. In general,
however, better cosmetic results are achieved with more
prolonged fractionation.

$20-22\,\text{Gy} \times 1$
$14\,\text{Gy} \times 2$ (6 week gap)
$7.5\,\text{Gy} \times 5$ (7–10 days)
$6.75\,\text{Gy} \times 6$ (alternate days)
$6\,\text{Gy} \times 9$ (over 3 weeks)
$4.5\,\text{Gy} \times 10$ (over 3 weeks)

Treatment with a less highly fractionated
course of radiotherapy (such as the Sambrook
split course, in which two fractions of radiation
are given some 6 weeks apart), has a very
good cure rate but an undoubtedly higher incidence of late skin changes such as telangiectasia, atrophy and depigmentation. The aim of
longer courses of radiotherapy is to decrease
these late effects to a minimum, particularly
important for facial skin cancers where a very
high cure rate, coupled with a perfect cosmetic
result, should be the aim of every radiotherapist. Acute skin changes are much less
important (although sometimes irritating and
occasionally painful to the patient), and usually
consist of intense local erythema and inflammation, leading to early crusting, and finally,
resolution with healing which may take several
months to complete, particularly with larger
lesions. Common fractionation regimens are
shown in Table 22.1; they often reflect the
capacity of the radiotherapy department to treat
these common tumours, as much as the
individual preference of the radiotherapist.
Expressed in terms of the nominal standard

dose (see Chapter 5), these treatments aim for a
total of 1500–1900 ret. It is generally accepted
that squamous cell carcinomas require a wider
treatment field than basal cell carcinomas,
though most radiotherapists treat both lesions
to the same doses and their radiocurability is
probably identical [5]. Radiotherapy is not
indicated in the naevoid-basal cell carcinoma
syndrome in which it gives poor results with
marked skin damage.

Topical chemotherapy, usually using 5-FU,
has been increasingly employed in recent years,
particularly for recurrent lesions where surgery
and/or radiation therapy have already been
used. Although its precise role has not yet been
determined, the advantages of topical cytotoxic
therapy include the possibility of repeated use
where necessary, as well as its value in premalignant lesions and large areas of carcinoma
in situ where other methods of treatment might
be difficult. It is also valuable in treatment of
multiple lesions, particularly of the superficial
basal cell carcinoma type, but is not usually
recommended for thick or infiltrating lesions.
Topical cytotoxic therapy produces inflammation which is a disadvantage, although
steroids are helpful in alleviating this.

Overall results of treatment of both basal cell
and squamous cell carcinoma are excellent. Cure
rates of 90–95% are regularly achieved by surgery or radiotherapy; for smaller tumours
treated by curettage, cryosurgery or electrocautery the figures are claimed to be higher
still. Sadly, the occasional tumour is encoun-

tered (particularly with basal cell carcinoma) which proves resistant to all methods of treatment, usually with multiple recurrences of tumour, often at the margins of the treated area and sometimes over a period of 10 years or more. These cases are characterized by relentless local invasion and destruction both laterally and deeply. Distant metastases to bone, lung or elsewhere, are occasionally seen.

MALIGNANT MELANOMA

Epidemiology and pathogenesis

Malignant melanoma is a far less common skin tumour than the true carcinomas discussed above, but has a much worse prognosis. At present, it accounts for less than 2% of all skin cancers, with an annual incidence in Britain of about 3 per 100 000 population (Fig. 22.6). Its incidence appears to have risen sharply during the last four decades [2]. For this reason, if the incidence continues to accelerate at the present rate, 1 in 100 Americans will develop this disorder by the year 2000. There is a wide international variation and the disease is almost ten

times as common in Australia and New Zealand as it is in Europe. It occurs most frequently in patients between 40 and 70 years old, and is slightly more common in females than males. This is in contrast to basal cell and squamous carcinoma (Fig. 22.1) and implies that there is a difference in the relative importance of external factors, such as sunlight, in aetiology in these types of skin cancer.

Like other skin cancers, melanoma is more common in the white population than in the black, possibly as a result of the effectiveness of pigmented skin in screening out solar UV which has long been thought to be the most important factor in its aetiology [9]. The degree of sunburn, rather than sun exposure *per se*, may be an important aetiological feature. About 75% of all malignant melanomas occur on an exposed site, chiefly affecting pale complexioned white people especially those with red hair and freckles. Families have been described in which the disease occurs with unusual frequency [10]. The number of naevi on an individual's skin does seem to correlate quite closely with risk of developing melanoma [11]. In Australia, epidemiological studies have shown that the amount of received sunlight, as measured by distance from the equator, correlates well with the incidence of the disease. The importance of the earth's ozone layer probably lies in its protective effect, filtering out carcinogenic ultraviolet light.

Although trauma to superficial skin naevi has frequently been implicated as a cause of malignant change, there is little evidence to support this view. The most common skin sites of melanoma in white people are the head and neck, trunk and limbs. In black people the bodily distribution is different, with a greater likelihood of a primary site on the palms of the hands, soles of the feet and mucous membranes.

Much can be done to inform the public of the dangers of over-exposure to the sun, and information about the value of early diagnosis is clearly worthwhile since the outcome is so dependent on stage (see below). Forceful advertising campaigns through public media

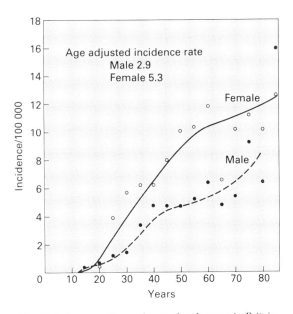

Fig. 22.6 Age-specific incidence of melanoma in Britain.

and in medical waiting areas have become commonplace.

Clinical and pathological features

Although more than half of all melanotic lesions arise from a pre-existing benign naevus, some undoubtedly develop at sites of previously normal skin; in many cases the primary site is never discovered, the patient presenting either with lymphadenopathy or with more wide-spread involvement. Post mortem studies have shown that most of the organs of the body are capable of harbouring a primary melanotic focus: larynx, oesophagus, trachea, bronchus, gastro-intestinal tract, and leptomeninges have all been implicated. Certainly all these organs (and many more) contain clusters of melanocytes, but why these should undergo malignant change remains completely unknown.

Diagnosis of malignant melanoma is not always straightforward. Almost all of us have pigmented melanocytic naevi (approximately twelve in the average white person), and many innocent pigmented naevi appear to enlarge slowly over the years. They are maximal in number in the third decade of life and then slowly disappear. Those undergoing any form of rapid change, particularly with ulceration or bleeding, must be regarded with great suspicion, and most dermatologists will advise excision biopsy. Other important skin conditions may be difficult to distinguish from malignant melanoma unless a biopsy is obtained; these include the pigmented basal cell carcinomas, solar keratoses, blue naevi, juvenile melanomas, pyogenic granulomas, sclerosing angiomas and benign pigmented melanocytic naevi.

The benign melanocytic naevi are derived from the intra-epidermal melanocyte whose origin is from the neural crest. There are important differences between the various types of naevus, which may have a bearing on the pathogenesis of malignant melanoma. *Junctional naevi* are well circumscribed, small, flat, pigmented lesions arising from clumps of pigmented cells at the junction of dermis and epidermis. The normal skin lines are not distorted. Their proliferation and penetration into the true dermis results in a *compound naevus*. These lesions are larger than junctional naevi and may be raised. Coarse hair may arise from these naevi and although the junctional activity may then abate, the pigmented cells deep in the dermis may then continue to multiply, resulting in an *intradermal naevus*. Here the melanocytes are no longer in contact with the epidermis. Clinically the lesion has very little pigmentation. It is usually a raised papule and is commoner in the older age groups. Although junctional naevi are certainly capable of malignant change, this happens only rarely. It is not clear how frequently melanoma arises in a common melanocytic naevus.

In the past decade there has been greater understanding of the importance of the *dysplastic naevus syndrome*, a skin condition originally recognized in familial melanoma but now regarded as more common in sporadic cases. These lesions tend to be larger than truly benign naevi, often irregular in outline and with more variable colour. The gene for familial dysplastic naevi has now been identified [12] and is located on chromosome 1. It is possible, though still far from proven, that the *ras* oncogene may be important in pathogenesis. It now seems clear that ultraviolet light can induce point mutations in the *ras* genes of basal melanocytes and keratinocytes. Despite the probable importance of the dysplastic naevus in the aetiology of malignant melanoma it should be recognized that the majority of these lesions appear stable or may even regress.

A history of enlargement of a pre-existing naevus can be obtained in 10–40% of patients with melanoma although this is not a reliable guide. A more definite precursor, though numerically far less frequently encountered, is the *lentigo maligna*, or Hutchinson's melanotic freckle. This is an epidermal lesion resulting from the maturation of atypical melanocytes, thought embryologically to result from neural crest tissue. It is one of three well recognized macroscopic varieties of malignant melanoma, accounting for up to 10% of all cases and, if suspected, demanding immediate surgical excision. The lesion is found in sun-exposed areas in elderly patients. At first there is a flat pigmented area on the skin which appears to represent a radial growth phase of the tumour. This expands slowly over many years. Later an invasive vertical growth develops, visible as nodules within the lesion. Surgical excision in the radial growth phase is often curative. *Superficial spreading melanomas* are usually larger lesions, often 2–3 cm in diameter, and chiefly occurring in middle-aged people. They have an irregular edge often with a pale central area. After 1–2 years the lesion may itch or ulcerate and may become nodular. The superficial growth phase has then given way to a deeper vertical penetration of the lesion. In general these melanomas evolve gradually in the first instance, though more rapidly than in lentigo maligna. In superficial spreading melanoma, about one-third of patients appear to have evidence of pre-existing dysplastic naevi. *Nodular melanomas* develop more rapidly still, and are almost always characterized by deep dermal invasion by the time of diagnosis. There is no histologically recognizable radial growth phase. The patients are usually middle-aged (Fig. 22.6) and areas of skin not exposed to light are often affected. Typically there is a raised nodule on the skin surface and the normal skin markings are disturbed. Ulceration occurs after 2–3 months and deep penetration occurs early. The association with a pre-existing naevus is less strong than in superficial spreading melanoma.

These three major types of melanoma account for almost 90% of all cases, the remainder arising from other types of naevus (congenital, blue, compound or intradermal), or from mucous membranes, meninges or other internal sites.

Stage of melanoma

The most important prognostic characteristics in malignant melanoma are the level of invasion (or microstage) and the clinical stage of the tumour.

MICROSTAGE

Clark and colleagues [13] described five separate levels of invasiveness (Fig. 4.1A), and demonstrated that prognosis correlated well with the depth of invasion, although subsequent work by Breslow suggests that vertical tumour thickness in millimetres may be an even better guide [14] and this method of pathological staging is now generally preferred. Tumours less than 0.75 mm in thickness very rarely metastasize. In addition, the *type* of primary melanotic lesion may also influence the prognosis, and nodular primary lesions in general have a worse prognosis stage for stage than the more common superficial spreading variety, which may well reflect the increased probability of nodal involvement with nodular lesions [15]. Thinner lesions can usually be diagnosed on simple histological criteria including nuclear atypia, asymmetry of the lesion, and the presence of single atypical melanocytes in the upper epidermis [16].

CLINICAL STAGE

No single clinical staging system has been universally accepted, although patients with obvious lymphadenopathy undoubtedly do less well than patients with cutaneous disease only. A simple scheme is shown in Table 22.2. Involvement of regional nodes is usually judged clinically, but patients with palpable and histologically positive regional lymph nodes have a 5-year survival of less than 20%, whereas those with impalpable local lymph nodes but microscopically confirmed lymph node invasion have

Table 22.2 Clinical stage of malignant melanoma

Stage I	Disease confined to local site
Stage II	Involvement of regional lymph nodes
Stage III	Distant metastases

a 5-year survival of over 50% [15]. Figures from Scotland confirm a survival rate of over 90% in patients with melanomas up to 1.49 mm in depth, a survival of 67% with tumours of 1.5 mm to 3.49 mm and only 38% where the tumour is thicker still [2].

In reality, the problem of classification and case-comparison is even more complex, since a surprising number of features are thought to have prognostic significance even in clinical Stage I disease (Table 22.3). The clinical diagnosis of regional lymphadenopathy or disseminated disease is undoubtedly of overriding prognostic significance. Important metastatic sites include liver, lung, spleen, heart and central nervous system (particularly brain but also meningeal involvement). Malignant melanoma can also metastasize to bone, and solitary bony metastases, in the absence of any other sign of dissemination, are well described.

STAGING INVESTIGATIONS

Once the diagnosis of melanoma has been established, clinical staging should naturally take account of these routes of spread, and simple investigations such as full blood count, chest X-ray and liver function tests should be undertaken in all patients.

Table 22.3 Prognostic factors in clinical Stage I malignant melanoma

Low risk
Radial (lateral) growth phase
Thickness <0.76 mm or Clark's level 2

Intermediate risk
Level 3 invasion
Up to 1.5 mm thickness

High risk
Level 4 or 5
1.5–4.0 mm invasion
High mitotic rate
Satellite lesions
Ulceration
Axial location or hands or feet

In patients with small, thin Stage I lesions, further investigation is not generally regarded as justifiable [2]. A fuller assessment including liver and brain scanning, will undoubtedly reveal an occasional case of unsuspected occult disease. Lymphography, abdominal CT scanning and/or abdominal ultrasonography may demonstrate unsuspected local or para-aortic lymphadenopathy. Although these investigations are difficult to justify as a routine, their increasing availability should allow for better prognostic detail. In particular, ultrasonography in skilled hands is a very valuable, simple and non-invasive technique in melanoma since it provides reliable information regarding both the liver and abdominopelvic lymph nodes. Recently the use of radiolabelled monoclonal antibodies (generally using ^{111}In or ^{123}I) for whole-body scanning has given additional information in some cases, identifying previously unrecognized metastatic sites.

Treatment of malignant melanoma

SURGERY

Local excision

For localized (Stage I) malignant melanoma, confined to the primary site, surgical excision is unquestionably the cornerstone of management. Because of the propensity of local lymphatic invasion, most surgeons recommend *wide* excision of the primary lesion, with a particularly generous clearance proximally. Although it can be difficult to confirm the need for this in every case, at least one study has demonstrated an increase of melanocytes in clinically and histologically normal epidermis surrounding a significant proportion of primary malignant melanomas, supporting the view that wide excision may be essential [15]. Wide excision usually requires split-skin graft coverage, and some authorities feel that for relatively good prognoses (i.e. Clark's level 1 or 2 (Fig. 4.1A) and lentigo maligna lesions), a less generous surgical excision, with primary closure, is adequate. Indeed, a well-controlled study from the WHO Melanoma Group has now shown that with tumours 1 mm or less in depth, more conservative surgical excision appears safe. The present view is that for each millimetre depth of tumour, a 1 cm margin is required, thus removing the need for surgical grafting in every case.

Depth of excision is also contentious, and will depend not only on the type of primary lesion but also on the site. Nodular lesions almost always invade deeply and demand deeper excision than primary lentigo maligna melanomas. Lesions of the hands and feet, for example subungual melanomas, are generally best dealt with by partial amputation of the digit. Nodular melanomas present a particular problem in view of their early deep invasiveness, and have usually invaded as far as the papillary-reticular junction (Clark's level 3) or more by the time of diagnosis. These lesions should therefore always be excised with wide clearance, and deeply down to at least as far as deep fascia. Skin grafting will almost always be required.

Regional lymph node dissection

Apart from primary surgical excision of the cutaneous lesion, the question of elective regional lymph node dissection frequently arises. Is it wise to undertake local lymphadenectomy in all cases of malignant melanoma? In patients with Stage I disease where no clinical lymphadenopathy is present, lymphadenectomy undoubtedly gives useful *prognostic* information. The presence of microscopic disease worsens the prognosis; 70% of cases with true Stage I (node-negative) lesions are alive at 5 years while only 50% of patients with occult regional lymph node involvement (proven only by surgery) survive this long.

Whether or not regional lymphadenectomy makes any therapeutic contribution to prognosis also remains uncertain. In general, there is agreement that for patients with good risk melanoma, i.e. a small lesion of a limb, not nodular in character and of Clark's level 1, there is nothing to be gained by lymphadenectomy. For deeper lesions, for example, nodular and spreading melanomas of Clark's level 3, 4 or 5, lymphadenectomy is often recommended.

Certainly most surgeons would favour dissection if there are clinically involved lymph nodes in the primary nodal drainage area, though it is doubtful whether such dissection genuinely adds to survival. Only 10% of patients with clinically detectable lymphadenopathy, confirmed at lymphadenectomy, are alive 5 years later [16]. This unhappy situation is closely analogous to what we know from breast cancer studies, in that local lymph node involvement undoubtedly implies disseminated (though often clinically undetectable) disease. In both of these illnesses, this prognostic information is gained by a procedure which is itself of doubtful benefit. Despite this dispiriting state of affairs, radical lymph node dissection for clinical Stage II melanoma is the only practical means of therapy with any serious chance of success at present. For the highly selected group of patients with high-risk clinical Stage II lesions of the distal portion of a limb, amputation may give the best chance of cure.

In Britain, few surgeons favour prophylactic lymph node dissection even in patients with high-risk lesions even though it provides useful prognostic information. This view is borne out by careful analysis of a large group of Australian patients [17]. The extremely high incidence of this disease in Australia and New Zealand has led to a special experience in the larger Australian centres, and the 5-year survival rates from Queensland appear better than for anywhere else in the world (Queensland 81%; England 61%; United States 37%). Although this might suggest particular expertise, it is also true that a higher proportion of Australian patients have primary melanotic lesions confined to the epidermis, and therefore likely to have a relatively good prognosis. Further results from Australia do suggest a possible benefit of prophylactic lymph node dissection in a small

group of patients with melanomas of intermediate thickness though the majority suffer
side-effects from this surgical procedure, without any obvious advantage.

RADIOTHERAPY

There are few reports of the use of radiotherapy
as an alternative to surgery for primary melanomas, though it is known that melanoma cells
in vitro are not completely radioresistant [18],
contrary to a long-held clinical belief that radiation therapy is of no value. Several reports
have demonstrated the clinical usefulness of
radiotherapy, which has in general been employed for patients in whom surgery is unsuitable, often because the lesion is too advanced.
Radiotherapy may be especially valuable in
lentigo maligna melanoma.

Since many lesions are on the extremities,
a high dose can usually be reached without
danger to internal structures. Further evidence
for the potential value of radiotherapy for surgically unsuitable lesions comes from assessment of radiation treatment for recurrent
or disseminated melanoma (see below). In
treating melanoma large infrequent fractions of
treatment (greater than 5 Gy) are used in an
attempt to overcome the shoulder effect which
is thought to be largely responsible for resistance (see Chapter 5).

CHEMOTHERAPY

Management of disseminated disease represents at present an almost insoluble problem.
The median survival for all patients with disease
beyond the regional lymph nodes is of the
order of 5 months, though patients with predominantly skin involvement have a median
survival of almost a year. Although malignant
melanoma is frequently cited as a tumour in
which spontaneous regression has been documented, the actual incidence of the phenomenon is no more than 1%, and lengthy survival
is exceptionally rare. None the less, with the
demonstration in the early 1970s of some degree

of sensitivity to cytotoxic chemotherapy, the
use of anticancer drugs for disseminated
malignant melanoma became widely adopted
although objective responses have been low
(Table 22.4), and the overwhelming majority of
these responses are less than complete. Furthermore responses are usually seen in skin, but are
very uncommon in liver, brain, bone and lung —
sites which are the main cause of death.

At present, the more active agents are thought
to be DTIC (dacarbazine) and vindesine, with
response rates of 20–30%. It is not clear whether
the use of drugs in combination offers genuinely superior results to treatment with single
agents alone, although improved results have
been claimed in some series. In addition to
dacarbazine, more recently evaluated agents
include nitrosoureas (notably BCNU and
fotemustine) and cisplatin. Use of these agents,
and also dacarbazine, may become more common with the advent of new generation 5HT$_3$
antagonists such as ondansetron, which clearly

Table 22.4 Chemotherapy in melanoma

Drug	Response rate* (%)
Single agents	
DTIC	22
Alkylating agents	10
Methotrexate	7
Cytosine arabinoside	10
Actinomycin D	13
Vindesine	15
Vincristine	10
Mitomycin C	14
Hydroxyurea	10
Nitrosoureas	14
Combination chemotherapy†	
DTIC + vinca	17
DTIC + nitrosourea	17
DTIC + vinca + nitrosourea	24
Vinca + nitrosourea	24
Vinca + nitrosourea + procarbazine	30

* Complete and partial response together. Most response
rates refer to cutaneous lesions. Responses are
uncommon in visceral lesions.
† Typical regimens.

offer superior control of nausea and vomiting than was previously possible. However, combinations such as BOLD (bleomycin, lomustine, vincristine and dacarbazine) have mostly failed to live up to their early promise when tested in larger groups of patients. Another experimental approach has been the use of high-dose chemotherapy (generally using melphalan, ifosfamide or dacarbazine) supplemented by autologous marrow transplantation. Such treatment has not as yet proven more beneficial than conventional chemotherapy and should not be used outside controlled clinical trials.

There is also some evidence of response to tamoxifen though reports are still scanty. Interestingly, there are well documented historic cases of remission (or, alternatively, sudden unexpected relapse) in melanoma patients who have become pregnant. In a small number, hormone-related tumour behaviour seems to have been clearly demonstrated.

REGIONAL LIMB PERFUSION

An alternative approach, for patients with primary melanoma of an extremity and with loco-regional or recurrent disease, is to consider the use of regional perfusion with cytotoxic drugs. This was first described by Creech in 1959, and proved an effective method of palliation [19]. Although this led to enthusiastic work in the 1960s and 1970s employing this technique as an adjuvant to primary surgical treatment, there is no convincing evidence that it reduces the likelihood of metastatic disease. The agents most commonly used are melphalan and cisplatin, the latter particularly in hepatic metastases. Responses are relatively common (up to 40%) though generally partial and short-lived. Regional perfusion has mostly been used for unresectable limb lesions with recurrent disease, or for widespread skin metastases confined to a single limb.

IMMUNOTHERAPY

Reports of occasional spontaneous regression of disease in melanoma, coupled with the demonstration of antigen and antimelanoma antibodies in the sera of a few patients with the disease [20], have led a number of groups to consider the use of 'active immunotherapy' in this disease. Non-randomized clinical trials using immunization with allogeneic melanoma cells or transfusions of allogeneic or autologous 'sensitized' leucocytes have been inconclusive and generally suggestive of, at best, only transient benefit. More recently, non-specific intralesional treatment with BCG has undoubtedly produced local responses in patients with recurrent cutaneous or nodal disease where direct injection of BCG is feasible. Unfortunately, most of these responses are short-lived, and of little or no value for patients with recurrent visceral or bone metastases.

Other forms of 'immunotherapy' including the use of levamisole and *Corynebacterium parvum*, are also currently under study. In addition, combined treatment of disseminated disease, using simultaneous administration of both chemotherapy and immunotherapy, are in progress at several centres, though the results have so far been discouraging. It seems that immunotherapy has at present little to offer. Claims for effectiveness have been from uncontrolled studies and randomized studies have failed to confirm any value.

BIOLOGICAL RESPONSE MODIFIERS AND HYPERTHERMIA

Following the interest in immunotherapy of melanoma in the 1970s, attention has more recently turned to the use of interferon, a biological response modifier of established value in other neoplasms, notably B cell lymphoid tumours (see Chapter 6). The interferons α, β and γ have all been shown to have activity though in most studies limited to about 10−20% of patients. Most responses are short-lived, though there are occasional exceptions, and generally confined to patients with a relatively small tumour burden. α-Interferon is also sometimes used for intralesional therapy and may occasionally result in complete disappearance of the injected lesion. Recent studies have attempted to assess α-interferon in combination with chemotherapy.

Interleukin-2 has also been used over the past 5 years, either as a single agent or given together with cultured autologous lymphocytes which appear to become cytolytic for the autologous tumour cells. These lymphokine-activated killer (LAK) cells may possibly then elicit a beneficial effect, reportedly up to 25% with a few unmaintained long-term responses. Unfortunately interleukin/LAK cell therapy has numerous dose-related side-effects making it difficult to use (see Chapter 6).

Hyperthermia, the use of heat treatment for cancer, has also been used with some success in melanoma, especially when combined with limb perfusion using melphalan chemotherapy. Although cell kill appears better at temperatures above 41–45°C, toxic reactions at this level can be severe and milder hyperthermia (39–40°C) is more commonly used. Studies of this approach continue, under the supervision of the EORTC and WHO.

PALLIATIVE RADIOTHERAPY

Palliative irradiation is undoubtedly useful in some patients with troublesome deposits, particularly for those with brain or osseous metastases. Although melanoma is not amongst the more radiosensitive of malignant diseases, it has been claimed that resistance can partly be overcome by the use of large infrequent fractions of treatment. When surgical treatment of the primary site is considered unsuitable, radiation therapy is the only possible alternative, and long-term control, both of primary and metastatic lesions, is achieved in about 25% of these cases. Newer approaches, including neutron and charged particle therapy, radiosensitizers and hyperthermia, are all being investigated. A further interesting type of regional treatment using novel irradiation is the concept of boron neutron capture therapy [21]. This approach exploits the uptake of phenylalanine (a molecule important in melanogenesis) into melanin-producing melanoma cells. The phenylalanine is coupled to boron to produce the boron-labelled melanin substrate analogue $^{10}B_1$-*p*-boronophenylalanine. If these cells are irradiated with non-toxic thermal neutrons, the ^{10}B nuclide 'captures' the neutrons and then disintegrates to produce a high-energy lithium atomic nucleus together with an α-particle. The energy is deposited locally, selectively destroying the melanin-synthesizing melanoma cells. This technique has been used in patients with melanoma with encouraging early results [21].

Prognosis

Prognosis in melanoma is always difficult to determine, a reflection of the multitude of potentially important features (Table 22.2). For patients with Stage I, about 50% will survive 5 years free of recurrence (Fig. 22.7), though it is important to recognize that late relapses occur, so that 5-year survival figures are not definitive. About one-quarter of patients with clinical Stage I disease have lymph node involvement at diagnosis (pathological Stage II), as shown by surgical series in which elective lymphadenectomy has been undertaken. Seventy-five per cent of these lymph node positive patients will later develop evidence of dissemination, and a further 20% of patients with true Stage I disease will develop distant metastases without ever having had local lymph node enlargement. About 20% of all patients destined to develop recurrent disease will remain disease-free during the first 5 years from diagnosis. For this reason a 5-year survival rate of 60% for Stage I melanoma signifies an overall cure rate of about 50%, i.e. only half of all patients presenting with the earliest stage of melanoma. There may also be a difference dependent on the primary site of the lesion. Analysis of over 12 000 cases from the Swedish Cancer Registry [22] demonstrated a worse prognosis for scalp and neck lesions, followed by those on the lower limbs and trunk. These data might have important

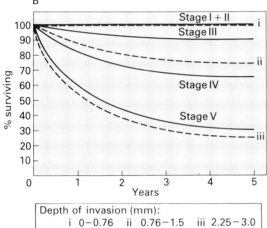

C	5-year survival
Trunk	40%
Arm	60%
Leg	60%
Head and neck	50%
Male	40%
Female	50%

Depth of invasion (mm):
i 0−0.76   ii 0.76−1.5   iii 2.25−3.0

Fig. 22.7 Prognosis in melanoma. (A) Prognosis related to stage grouping; (B) prognosis related to microstage; (I−V) and depth of invasion (dashed lines); (C) prognosis related to site and sex.

future implications, for example in determining the extensiveness of the initial surgery.

For patients with regional lymphadenopathy (Stage II) at diagnosis, the true cure rate is probably no more than 15% whilst those with disseminated disease at presentation have a median survival of less than 6 months. These dreadful figures will only improve with increased public and professional awareness resulting in earlier diagnosis and treatment. Although both chemotherapy and 'immuno-therapy' are at present relatively ineffective, it is at least now widely accepted that dissemi-nated melanoma is not totally resistant to treat-ment. One possible approach for the future is the further use of more intensive chemotherapy, in conjunction with haemopoietic growth fac-tors such as granulocyte-colony stimulating fac-tor (G-CSF) to allow higher doses to be given more effectively.

SKIN LYMPHOMAS

These are discussed in Chapter 26.

MISCELLANEOUS RARE TUMOURS

Dermatofibrosarcoma protuberans

This is a soft tissue sarcoma arising in the skin. It develops as firm nodules which grow slowly and may become large and be locally invasive. In general it does not metastasize but may recur after simple excision. Wide excision is the treat-ment of choice. Radiotherapy may be useful if major surgery (e.g. amputation) would other-wise be required.

Kaposi's sarcoma

Originally described by Kaposi in 1872, this sarcoma was a rarity in Europe until recently. Kaposi initially described the tumour in elderly Ashkenazi Jewish men and its incidence in Europe remained low at about 0.3 per million before the AIDS epidemic. In Africa, however, it is common and may account for 10% of all cancers in Kenya and Uganda. Curiously, there is some evidence that the disorder was increas-ing in frequency even before the AIDS epidemic.

There is a much higher frequency in renal allograft recipients and in patients with AIDS. In both these situations the tumour appears to be sustained by the immune suppression which if discontinued may allow regression of the neoplasm.

Pathologically the tumour is a proliferation of endothelial vascular channels with numerous spindle cells which are thought to be proliferating endothelial cells. There is often an infiltrate of lymphocytes and macrophages and if the spindle cell predominates, differentiation from a fibrosarcoma may be difficult. In the classic form of the disease a pigmented nodule appears on the leg or foot and grows very slowly. It may ulcerate but lymph node spread is unusual until multiple new lesions have appeared and the disease is more advanced. A form of the disease results in a brawny infiltration with diffuse swelling of the thigh or lower leg. This is a very indolent, unresponsive type of tumour.

The nodular form may become locally aggressive with invasion of deep tissues and formation of large masses. Another form occurs in children, which affects lymph nodes early with a clinical picture similar to lymphoma. In AIDS the disease occurs as a mixture of the nodular and lymphadenopathic forms and lesions may also appear on the mucous membranes. Some cases progress very rapidly indeed; others have a slow tempo. The presentation is often atypical in comparison to 'classical' Kaposi's sarcoma, with lesions at mucosal or inconspicuous sites. This form of disease seems particularly prevalent in homosexual males by contrast to other groups with HIV positivity.

Nodular localized disease is treated with radiotherapy. It is a sensitive tumour and single fractions of 8 Gy (800 rad) using electrons are effective, with a complete response rate of 60–90%. In cases of 'classic' non-AIDS related Kaposi's sarcoma, there is some evidence that radiotherapy doses should be higher in order to achieve adequate control. The tumour is also sensitive to chemotherapy. The most effective agents (with response rates) are actinomycin D (90%), DTIC (60%) and bleomycin (60%). Com-

bination chemotherapy gives a high proportion of complete responders. The usual combinations are actinomycin D and vinblastine, or actinomycin, vincristine and DTIC. α-Interferon produces tumour responses in about 40% of patients who have AIDS.

In the classic form of the disease patients live for many years. In AIDS related cases the prognosis is much worse, patients dying of opportunistic infections in addition to the sarcoma.

Merkel cell (primary cutaneous neuroendocrine) tumours

These curious and unusual tumours, often presenting as a discrete nodular mass, have attracted increasing attention in recent years. Histologically they are round cell tumours containing neurosecretory granules, and resemble small cell carcinoma. They can be surprisingly radiosensitive, and response rates of over 90% have been documented suggesting that the traditional therapeutic approach with surgery may be unnecessary. None the less 40% are locally recurrent (usually after surgery) and 55% give rise to regional node metastases. The overall 2-year survival rate is 72% (slightly better in women). So far about 450 cases have been reported in the world literature.

Extra-mammary Paget's disease

These lesions are located near apocrine sweat glands, in the ano-genital region, breast areola and axillae. They are probably a form of carcinoma *in situ*, and present as red, scaly plaques, slowly increasing in size. They are usually removed surgically.

Metastatic carcinoma

Nodules of secondary carcinoma are not infrequently found in the skin, especially with cancer of the breast and melanoma. If the diagnosis is in doubt excision biopsy may be necessary. If any treatment is required this will be of the underlying disease if possible. Radiotherapy is useful for ulcerating or painful deposits.

REFERENCES

1 Yamagiwa K., Ichikawa K. Experimental study of the pathogenesis of carcinoma. *Cancer Research* 1918; **3**: 1–29.

2 Mackie R.M. Diagnosis, detection and staging of cutaneous malignant melanoma. *Current Opinion in Oncology* 1990; **2**: 394–96.

3 Wakefield M., Bonett A. Preventing skin cancer in Australia. *Medical Journal of Australia* 1990; **152**: 60–61.

4 Gorlin R.J. Nevoid basal cell carcinoma syndrome. *Medicine (Baltimore)* 1987; **66**: 98–113.

5 Ashby M.A., Smith J., Ainslie J. *et al.* Treatment of non-melanoma skin cancer at a large Australian centre. *Cancer* 1989; **63**: 1863–71.

6 Walker N.P.J., Bailin P.L. Dermatological surgery. In R.H. Champion, ed. *Recent Advances in Dermatology*. Edinburgh: Churchill Livingstone, 1986. Chapter 11, p. 211.

7 Mohs F.E. *Chemosurgery in Cancer, Gangrene and Infections*. Illinois: C. Thomas, 1956.

8 Petrovitch Z., Kuisk H., Langholz B. *et al.* Treatment of carcinoma of the skin with bone and/or cartilage involvement. *American Journal of Clinical Oncology* 1988; **11**: 110–13.

9 Lancaster H.O., Nelson J.L. Sunlight as a cause of melanoma: A clinical survey. *Medical Journal of Australia* 1957; **1**: 452–56.

10 Anderson D.E., Smith J., McBride C.M. Hereditary aspects of malignant melanoma. *Journal of American Medical Association* 1967; **200**: 741–46.

11 Green A., Swerdlow A.J. Epidemiology of melanocytic naevi. *Epidemiological Review* 1989; **11**: 204–21.

12 Bale S.J., Dracopoli N.C., Tucker M.A. *et al.* Mapping the gene for hereditary cutaneous malignant melanoma-dysplastic nevus to chromosome 1p. *New England Journal of Medicine* 1989; **320**: 1367–72.

13 Clark W.H., From L., Bernadino E.A., Mihn N.C. The histogenesis and biologic behaviour of primary human malignant melanomas of the skin. *Cancer Research* 1969; **29**: 705–27.

14 Breslow A. Tumour thickness level of invasion and node dissection in stage I cutaneous melanoma. *Annals of Surgery* 1975; **182**: 572–75.

15 De Vita V.T., Fisher R.I. Natural history of malignant melanoma as related to therapy. *Cancer Treatment Reports* 1976; **60**: 153–57.

16 Stolz W., Schmoeckel C., Welkovich B. *et al.* Semi-quantitative analysis of histologic criteria in thin malignant melanomas. *Journal of American Academic Dermatology* 1989; **20**: 1115–20.

17 Davis N.C., McLeod R., Beardmore G., Little J., Quinn R., Holt J. Melanoma is a word not a sentence. *Australia and New Zealand Journal of Surgery* 1976; **46**: 188.

18 Barranco S.C., Romsdahl M.M., Humphrey R.M. Radiation response of human melanoma cells grown *in vitro*. *Cancer Research* 1971; **31**: 830–33.

19 Creech O., Ryan R.F., Krementz E.T. Treatment of melanoma by isolated perfusion technique. *Journal of the American Medical Association* 1959; **169**: 339–43.

20 Morton D.L., Eilber F.R., Joseph W.L. *et al.* Immuno-logical factors in human sarcomas and melanomas: A rational basis for immunotherapy. *Annals of Surgery* 1970; **172**: 740–49.

21 Mishima Y., Honda C., Ichihashi M. *et al.* Treatment of malignant melanoma by single thermal neutron capture therapy with melanoma-seeking [10]B-compound. *Lancet* 1989; **ii**: 388–89.

22 Thörn M., Adami H.O., Ringborg U. *et al.* The association between anatomic site and survival in malignant melanoma: an analysis of 12 353 from the Swedish Cancer Registry. *European Journal of Cancer* 1989; **25**: 483–91.

Chapter 23
Bone and Soft Tissue Sarcomas

INCIDENCE AND AETIOLOGY

Sarcomas are cancers of mesenchymal tissues. Although they are uncommon there is a great variety and a working classification is given in Tables 23.1 and 23.2. They occur in both children and adults and some types, such as osteosarcoma and Ewing's sarcoma, are most frequent in adolescence. There is a slight male preponderance. The age-specific incidence is shown in Fig. 23.1.

Table 23.1 Primary malignant bone tumours

Osteosarcoma
Variable malignancy, most benign form is parosteal osteosarcoma. Usually metaphyseal. Can be in flat bones. Age 10−20

Ewing's sarcoma
High-grade malignancy. Diaphyseal in long bones, often in flat bones. Age 10−20

Chondrosarcoma
Variable malignancy. Usually metaphyseal. Age 40−60

Other spindle cell tumours
Malignant fibrous histiocytoma ⎫
Fibrosarcoma ⎬ Age 30−50. Long bones. Metaphyseal usually, similar distribution to osteosarcoma
Haemangiopericytoma
Haemangioendothelioma ⎭

Other round cell tumours
Primary lymphoma of bone
Mesenchymal chondrosarcoma
Angiosarcoma

Giant cell tumour
Occasionally malignant. Epiphyseal. Age 30−40

BONE SARCOMAS

The best understood aetiological factor in bone sarcoma is ionizing irradiation [1]. From 1917 to 1926 many factories were established in the United States and Canada in which there was large-scale production of watches and instruments painted with paint which was made luminous by the action of radium on zinc sulphide. The deplorable factory conditions and the habit of the young female employees of pointing their brushes in their mouths led to radium poisoning with radionecrosis of the jaw, aplastic anaemia and, later, osteosarcoma at sites remote from the skull, and cancers of the skull air-spaces. The cumulative risk of developing osteosarcoma was as high as 70% over the ensuing 40 years.

Later, external beam irradiation was shown to be able to induce bone sarcoma. The latent period is usually about 10 years. Radiation-induced bone sarcoma is especially likely to occur in children and is one of the commonest second cancers complicating cancer treatment. Its occurrence is a major reason for avoiding bone radiotherapy in treatment of childhood cancer (Chapter 24).

Osteosarcoma occurs with a 500-fold increased incidence in patients who are cured of the familial form of retinoblastoma (see Chapter 24, p. 473). In this disease there is loss of both alleles at 13q14. Allele loss at this site has been found in sporadic cases of osteosarcoma. The retinoblastoma gene is described in Chapter 24, p. 470. Loss of heterozygosity and mutation of the p53 tumour suppressor gene on chromosome 17p is a frequent finding in sporadic

Table 23.2 Soft tissue sarcoma: a simplified classification

Tissue of origin	Benign neoplasm	Sarcoma
Fibrous tissue	Fibroma (single or multiple, as in fibromatosis)	Fibrosarcoma (including dermatofibrosarcoma protruberans)
Muscle		

Striated	Rhabdomyoma	Rhabdomyosarcoma
		  Embryonal
		  Alveolar
		  Pleomorphic
		  Botryoidal

Smooth	Leiomyoma (including uterine 'fibroids')	Leiomyosarcoma
Mixed origin		Malignant fibrous histiocytoma (possibly a mixture of other pathologies)
Fat	Lipoma	Liposarcoma
Blood vessels	Angioma, haemangioma	Haemangiosarcoma, Kaposi's sarcoma, lymphangiosarcoma, haemangiopericytoma
Peripheral nerves	Neuroma, neurofibroma neurilemmoma (including Schwannoma)	Neurofibrosarcoma, malignant neurilemmoma (including malignant Schwannoma and neuroepithelioma)
Pleura and peritoneum		Mesothelioma
Unknown		Synovial cell sarcoma Alveolar soft part sarcoma (malignant non-chromaffin paraganglioma)

osteosarcoma. A cancer familial syndrome was defined by Li and Fraumeni in 1969 and 1974. The Li—Fraumeni syndrome, in which sarcomas in childhood are associated with an increased incidence of cancer at an early age in close relatives, is now known to be related to a germ-line mutation in p53. The function of p53 is described in Chapter 3, p. 38.

In Ewing's sarcoma a characteristic translocation t(11:22) has been found both in cell lines and in primary tumours. The same translocation has been shown in neuroepithelioma and Askin's tumour suggesting that all three round cell tumours arise from a common lineage.

Although rare, primary malignant bone tumours are very important and their management is changing. Until the late 1960s the treatment was usually by amputation or radiotherapy alone, and the results were poor, with osteosarcoma and Ewing's tumour cured in only 10—20% of patients.

In recent years the management of malignant bone tumours has changed considerably. Local control of disease can often now be achieved without amputation by the use of internal prosthetic replacement. The use of intensive chemotherapy pre- and post-operatively has prolonged survival in both Ewing's tumour and osteosarcoma.

These changes have meant that the management of these uncommon tumours has become highly specialized. There is, therefore, a great deal to be said for treating these cases in centres with special experience in the complex surgery and chemotherapy (and sometimes radiotherapy) which is increasingly employed.

Osteosarcoma

This is the commonest malignant tumour of bone (31%) and accounts for 3—4% of all childhood malignancies. In Britain there are approxi-

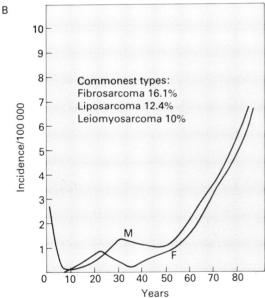

Fig. 23.1 Age-specific incidence of bone (A) and soft tissue (B) sarcomas.

mately 150 new cases each year. The term *osteosarcoma* is now preferred to osteogenic sarcoma which is a confusing term because so many different bone tumours make bone within their substance.

PATHOLOGY

The tumour usually arises in the epiphyseal region and consists of malignant osteoblasts which make osteoid. Within the tumour there may be areas of chrondroblastic or fibroblastic differentiation so that small biopsies may not be representative. The tumour cells produce alkaline phosphatase which is a useful cyto-chemical marker. Typically the tumour contains mixed fibroblastic, osteoblastic and chondro-blastic elements, but other forms are the telangiectatic type, in which there are blood-filled spaces in the tumour, and the small cell variant which may be difficult to distinguish from Ewing's sarcoma. The histological differential diagnosis includes other forms of primary malignant bone tumour or soft tissue sarcoma, especially malignant fibrous histiocytoma of bone. Histological grading of the degree of malignancy gives a rough guide to prognosis and is a prognostic variable which is taken into account in assessing comparisons between treatments.

Local invasion occurs when the tumour breaks through the bone and the periosteal surroundings (Fig. 23.2) and invades the soft tissue including the nerves and blood vessels around the joint. A staging system has been proposed, based on grade and compartmental extension (Table 23.3).

Juxtacortical (parosteal) osteosarcoma is an unusual variant in which new bone formation is especially dense and which presents as a large exostosis. The pathology and clinical behaviour is less malignant [1]. A further

Table 23.3 Staging system for bone sarcomas

Stage	Histological grade	Site
IA	Low	Intra-compartmental
IB	Low	Extra-compartmental
IIA	High	Intra-compartmental
IIB	High	Extra-compartmental
III	Regional or distant metastases	
	Any grade or local extent	

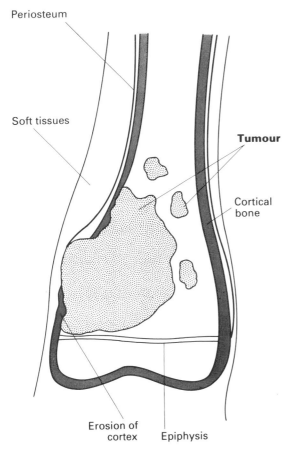

Periosteum

Soft tissues

Tumour

Cortical
bone

Erosion of
cortex   Epiphysis

Fig. 23.2 In this central osteosarcoma the tumour has
arisen next to the epiphysis. It has eroded the cortical
bone, broken through the periosteal barrier and spread
into the soft tissues. The 'islands' of the central tumour
are actually connected to the main tumour mass when
seen in three dimensions.

variant, *periosteal osteosarcoma*, has an intermediate degree of malignancy. Osteosarcoma
arising in Paget's disease occurs in an older age
group and often develops in flat bones. The
tumours are usually aggressive and metastases
occur early.

CLINICAL FEATURES

The disease mostly affects adolescents, the peak
incidence being in the age range 10–20 years
during the adolescent growth spurt. Boys are
affected more often [1.5 : 1]. Most of the tumours

occur round the knee and the lower femur and
upper tibia account for 60% of all cases. The
presentation is with pain and swelling, often
brought to attention by minor trauma. On
examination there is usually a firm swelling
which may be warm and tender with limitation
of movement of the joint [2].

RADIOLOGICAL APPEARANCES

Generally there is a destructive lesion in the
metaphyseal region, usually but not always
with new bone formation in spicules. There
may be a Codman's triangle caused by elevation
of the periosteum (Fig. 23.3). The parosteal
variety is associated with slow growth, exostosis and dense new bone, and the telangiectatic
type with rapidly progressive destruction. The
way in which the radiological appearances are
produced by the tumour extension is clearly

Fig. 23.3 Osteosarcoma of the lower left femur. There is
extensive bone destruction with elevation of the
periosteum (Codman's triangle) and new bone
formation.

Fig. 23.4 Fine detail X-rays of sagittal longitudinal slabs of resection specimens of osteosarcoma. (A) Classical osteosarcoma of distal femur in a boy aged 14 years. The lesion stops at the unfused epiphysis. It is destroying the cortex and extends subperiosteally, lifting the periosteum and forming a Codman's triangle. There are spicules of new bone formation. This is the commonest site for osteosarcoma. (B) Parosteal osteosarcoma in an 18-year-old male, arising from the posterior aspect of the distal femur (the typical site of this tumour). The tumour is confined to the outer aspect of the cortex and contains trabecular bone which is covered with fibrous tissue on the outer surface. The bone cortex is intact and the medulla is not involved. The fused epiphysis is visible. (C) Periosteal osteosarcoma of the mid femur in a woman aged 50 years. The tumour is made up of radiolucent tumour cartilage and shows patchy calcification. In a few places there is a trabecular pattern with mineralized tumour osteoid. There is involvement of the subadjacent medulla. (We are indebted to Dr Jean Pringle of the Royal National Orthopaedic Hospital, for these preparations.)

shown in X-rays of thin sections taken through the whole specimen (Fig. 23.4).

INVESTIGATION

Routine investigation should include chest X-ray, isotope bone scan which may show skeletal metastases and a CT scan of the thorax. This should be performed before surgery. CT scanning is the most sensitive method of detecting pulmonary metastases and these will be present in about 30% of cases. If local resection is contemplated (see below) a CT and MRI scan of the affected limb is essential to delineate tumour extent (Fig. 23.5). The serum alkaline phosphatase is frequently elevated and can be used as an approximate guide to disease activity. MRI scanning (Fig. 23.6) is now frequently used to determine the extent of the soft tissue component and the intramedullary extension. In interpreting these scans care must be taken not to confuse oedema with soft tissue infiltration.

Fig. 23.5 CT scan of osteosarcoma of the left femur. At this level the bone X-ray was only slightly abnormal. The scan shows erosion of the cortex, periosteal reaction and considerable soft tissue swelling.

TREATMENT

Surgery

Until recently, amputation was the main surgical treatment. For tumours around the knee the amputation is at mid-thigh level. To be of value the stump must extend at least 10 cm from the ischial tuberosity. Higher tumours, or those which extend high up the femoral shaft, are treated by disarticulation.

There is increasing use of conservative surgery in which a massive internal prosthesis is inserted after removal of the tumour (Fig. 23.7). The functional results are excellent for the lower femur and upper tibia, but somewhat less satisfactory in the upper humerus. Pathological fractures and/or extensive infiltration along the bone shaft or into soft tissue make prosthetic replacement less feasible. Increasingly, conservative limb-preserving surgery is now performed for pelvic tumours, either with removal of part of the pelvic ring without reconstruction (for tumours of the pubis and ischium not involving the hip joint) or with insertion of a metallic prosthesis. Local recurrence of the tumour is becoming less common with skilful surgery and with the use of pre-operative chemotherapy. Local recurrences can usually still be successfully treated by amputation.

Fig. 23.6 MR scan of the lower femur in a 16-year-old girl with osteosarcoma. A large soft tissue mass surrounds the lower femur, extending into the soft tissues.

Chemotherapy

Early experience with alkylating agents indicated that metastatic osteosarcoma was seldom responsive to chemotherapy. In the early 1970s very high-dose methotrexate (vHDMTX) with folinic acid rescue was shown to produce regression in 40% of patients with pulmonary metastases from osteosarcoma, although these responses were usually short-lived. Methotrexate was then used as adjuvant therapy after amputation. Although the results seemed initially encouraging, it later became apparent that metastasis with this regimen was delayed but not prevented.

The use of complex and intensive adjuvant chemotherapy appeared to be associated with an increase in survival from 20–25% without chemotherapy to 45–80% with treatment. The numerous early series had too few patients and did not include a randomized comparison with no chemotherapy. This led to controversy over the contribution of chemotherapy to survival. This issue was resolved by the publication of two controlled trials which showed a significant advantage for immediate chemotherapy [2,3] (Fig. 23.8).

Modern adjuvant programmes typically use cisplatin, doxorubicin and HDMTX. Ifosfamide is also active. Although other agents such as cyclophosphamide, bleomycin and actinomycin are sometimes used there is little evidence to suggest they are effective. In large-scale studies about 60% of patients are cured [4].

It is now usual to employ chemotherapy before surgery (induction or neo-adjuvant chemotherapy) as well as postoperatively [5] (Fig. 23.9). This has the advantages of starting systemic treatment early, of allowing time for the

Fig. 23.7 Endoprosthetic replacement of osteosarcoma of the distal femur. Following chemotherapy the tumour was resected and the lower femur and knee replaced by the prosthesis. Chemotherapy was then continued for 3 months. This patient walks normally, can run and climb stairs.

Fig. 23.8 Relapse-free survival in a randomized trial of adjuvant chemotherapy in operable osteosarcoma. The control group received chemotherapy only on relapse. The vertical bars are 95% confidence intervals. Patients randomized and refusing randomization have been amalgamated in this graph. Data from Link *et al.* [2] with permission.

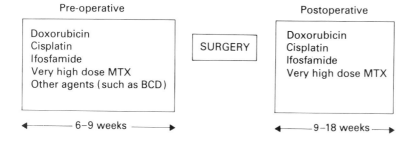

Pre-operative

Doxorubicin
Cisplatin
Ifosfamide
Very high dose MTX
Other agents (such as BCD)

← —— 6–9 weeks —— →

SURGERY

Postoperative

Doxorubicin
Cisplatin
Ifosfamide
Very high dose MTX

← —— 9–18 weeks —— →

Fig. 23.9 Schematic representation of a typical chemotherapy programme for osteosarcoma. BCD is a combination of bleomycin, cisplatin and actinomycin D. MTX is methotrexate. Limb preservation surgery is increasingly employed.

manufacture of an endoprosthesis, of facilitating surgery if the tumour reduces in size, and of allowing histological assessment of response when the tumour is resected. The hope that non-responding tumours would have a better prognosis if the chemotherapy was changed postoperatively, has not been fulfilled. A better strategy appears to be to give all the most active drugs initially.

The role of intra-arterial administration of cytotoxic drugs is still being assessed in osteosarcoma. Both HDMTX and cisplatin can be used in this way. Although high response rates are claimed it is not clear if these are better than with the same doses and schedules given intravenously.

Treatment of pulmonary metastases

Patients who develop pulmonary metastases may still be curable by surgery [6]. If a patient develops pulmonary metastases, CT scanning should be used to determine if he or she is operable. Adjuvant chemotherapy after amputation may not only delay or prevent pulmonary metastases but also benefits patients by reducing the number of pulmonary metastases when they do occur, sometimes allowing a potentially curative resection. The prognosis after metastasectomy is better if the lesions are unilateral, if there are less than six, if they appear late after chemotherapy has stopped, and if they are entirely resected. When a metastasis is detected chemotherapy is often started using agents which have not previously been given, and if no new metastases have appeared within 2–3 months, thoracotomy is undertaken. This approach helps to prevent needless thoracotomies in patients destined to develop further pulmonary metastases early and to die quickly of their disease.

Radiotherapy

In the days before chemotherapy, high-dose radiotherapy to the primary tumour was employed in order to avoid amputation in those destined to die of metastases. If these did not occur within 6–12 months a delayed amputation was performed. Unfortunately, local radiotherapy seldom provides long-lasting control of the primary and local recurrence and fractures often occur. Radiotherapy is still of great value in palliation of an advanced tumour and in treatment of painful bone metastases.

There was considerable interest in the use of low-dose whole lung irradiation in the 'prevention' of pulmonary metastases [7]. In reality the radiotherapy is to treat established but invisible metastases. Doses around 17.5 Gy in 20 fractions are usually used — which does not result in radiation pneumonitis. Some studies have shown prevention, or delay in onset, of pulmonary metastases, others have not and the value of this treatment remains uncertain. Its use has been superseded by chemotherapy.

Parosteal and periosteal osteosarcoma

Parosteal osteosarcoma is a rare slow-growing variant which arises from the surface of the bone, usually the distal posterior femur (Fig. 23.4B). It metastasizes late and adjuvant chemotherapy is not indicated. Treatment is by wide local excision. Periosteal osteosarcoma (Fig. 23.4C) is rare and is of a higher grade than parosteal lesions. There are usually areas of chondroblastic differentiation. Although less likely to metastasize than classical central tumours, chemotherapy may be indicated.

Chondrosarcoma

This is the second commonest bone tumour but occurs later in life than osteosarcoma, with a peak incidence at 40–60 years. It may arise *de novo* as a sarcomatous transformation of benign enchondromata, in multiple enchondromatosis (Ollier's disease) and, rarely, in Paget's disease.

PRESENTATION

These tumours are usually slow growing. The commonest site is the pelvis, followed by the femur, humerus, scapula and ribs. The most usual symptom is of a painful swelling, but in slow-growing lesions pain may not be a symptom at first. The disease tends to grow more rapidly in younger patients.

The X-ray typically shows a destructive bone lesion with areas of calcification normally as flecks (rather than spicules as in osteosarcoma) (Fig. 23.10).

PATHOLOGY [8]

The low-grade tumour resembles cartilage but without tumour osteoid being formed and with a greater degree of cellular pleomorphism. Low-grade tumours tend to be locally invasive and not to metastasize but pulmonary metastases are frequent in high-grade tumours. Sometimes low-grade tumours change to a more malignant variety after repeated local recurrence. At this stage a spindle cell component may dominate the histological appearance.

TREATMENT

The mainstay of treatment is surgery with

Fig. 23.10 Chondosarcoma of the ilium. The ilium is eroded by the tumour which shows patchy calcification. The tumour extends into the soft tissues laterally.

complete removal of the tumour with associated soft tissues. In a long bone this can sometimes be accomplished, without amputation, by *en bloc* resection and insertion of an endo-prosthesis. In the pelvis a surgical approach is often impossible. Radiotherapy is used as a palliative treatment but the tumour is radio-resistant and local control is usually short-lived [9]. From the little evidence available the tumour also appears to be resistant to cytotoxic drugs unless the tumour is dedifferentiated when responses may occur to drugs such as cisplatin, doxorubicin and ifosfamide.

Mesenchymal chondrosarcoma

This rare variant occurs in teenage children and

young adults. The axial skeleton and skull bones are often affected. The tumour contains small cell components which may make distinction from a round cell sarcoma difficult. It responds to chemotherapy but radical excision is essential for survival. Radiation may be used if the resection margins are not clear at operation. Chemotherapy regimens are usually based on cisplatin, doxorubicin and ifosfamide.

Ewing's sarcoma

This is a malignant round cell tumour of bone whose aetiology is unknown. The characteristic chromosomal translocation is discussed on p. 434. The peak incidence is 10–20 years and like osteosarcoma it is slightly more common in males (1.5:1). It is very rare in Africans and African-Americans.

PRESENTATION

Pain and swelling are the usual symptoms and may be present for many months before diagnosis. Pulmonary symptoms, due to metastases, may first bring the patient to the doctor. The flat bones of the pelvis are the commonest site of involvement although the femur is the commonest single bone to be involved, and the tibia and humerus less frequently. The tumour can also arise in the vertebrae, skull and ribs (Fig. 23.11). Fever and weight loss are not infrequent especially with large and metastatic tumours.

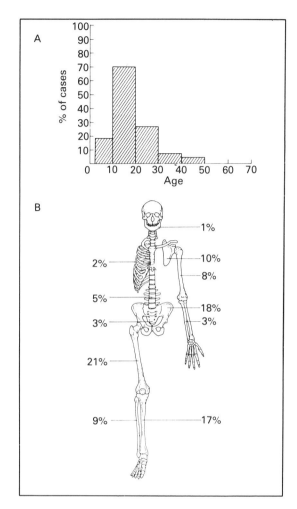

Fig. 23.11 Ewing's sarcoma. (A) Age at onset; (B) site of primary tumour.

PATHOLOGY

The tumour usually arises in the diaphysis and occasionally in the metaphysis. Epiphyseal involvement is unusual. Histologically it consists of small round cells. It resembles and must be distinguished from non-Hodgkin's lymphoma, metastatic neuroblastoma and some types of rhabdomyosarcoma. On conventional histology it may be impossible to distinguish Ewing's sarcoma from primitive neuroectodermal tumours (PNETs) of other types (such as

Askin's tumour). Indeed, it seems likely that classical Ewing's sarcoma and PNET are part of a spectrum of round cell tumours showing varying degrees of neural differentiation. Immunohistochemical techniques will show neural markers in PNETs (such as neurone-specific enolase, and the neural cell adhesion molecule). When PNET presents in bone it is not clear if the prognosis is substantially different from Ewing's sarcoma. Differentiation from lymphoma can be made by use of antibodies to the common leucocyte antigen (which stain lymphoma) and by the lack of surface immuno-globulin in Ewing's sarcoma.

The tumour typically permeates the medullary and cortical bone and for this reason, wide margins are needed in planning radiotherapy or surgery. Glycogen can often be demonstrated in the cytoplasm by the periodic acid-Schiff (PAS) stain and the distinction from these other tumours can usually be made on clinical, radiological and biochemical grounds. Metastases to lung and to the bones occur frequently.

INVESTIGATION

Diagnosis is by biopsy and expert opinion on the histology. The X-ray usually shows a diffuse erosion in a flat bone (Fig. 23.12) or in the diaphyseal region of a long bone (Fig. 23.13). There is a marked periosteal reaction sometimes with an 'onion skin' appearance, usually with evidence of a soft tissue mass which is often extensive.

Further investigation should include a full blood count which may show anaemia and leucocytosis in advanced or rapidly progressive cases; chest X-ray, CT scan of the primary site and of the thorax which may show single or multiple metastases; isotope bone scan to detect bone metastases which are common; plasma LDH and liver function tests; and urine VMA if there is a possibility that the diagnosis is neuro-

Fig. 23.13 X-ray of Ewing's tumour of the femur. Note the diaphyseal position, the periosteal elevation, and the new bone formation.

blastoma. MR scanning is invaluable in indicating the degree of intramedullary and soft tissue extension of the tumour.

TREATMENT

This must be both local and systemic. Local treatment alone is associated with cure in only 10–20% of cases and the prognosis has been improved considerably by the addition of adjuvant chemotherapy.

Local treatment [10]

Unlike most primary bone sarcomas Ewing's sarcoma is highly radiosensitive. For this reason the mainstay of local treatment has been radical megavoltage radiotherapy. Doses of 55–65 Gy are given to the primary site in 2 Gy fractions, over 6–7 weeks. Care must be taken not to irradiate all the soft tissues of a limb to this dose, or troublesome oedema will occur below the irradiated site. In practice this involves careful avoidance of a strip of soft tissue the

Fig. 23.12 Ewing's sarcoma of the right ilium. The bone is diffusely expanded by a large radiolucent tumour.

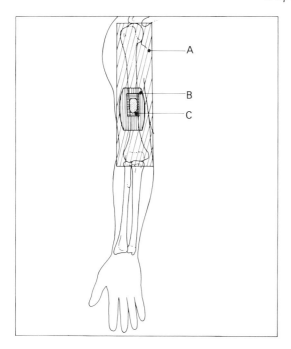

Fig. 23.14 Radiation fields in Ewing's sarcoma. (A) The whole bone is irradiated to a modest dose (30 Gy); (B) the field is shrunk down to the tumour and adjacent bone to 45 Gy; (C) the tumour itself is boosted to 60–70 Gy. If the tumour is well clear of the epiphyses these may not be included in the radiation field.

whole length of the treatment field (Fig. 23.14). Additionally the last 15–20 Gy are given to a smaller field around the residual tumour, i.e. using a 'shrinking field' technique.

In recent years troublesome late local recurrences have been seen in some patients after treatment with radiotherapy and chemotherapy. For this reason there is increasing use of surgical excision and endoprosthetic replacement of bone as an adjuvant to chemotherapy and radiotherapy. Surgery alone may sometimes be sufficient to gain control, but because of the permeating nature of the tumour, a combination of surgery and radiation is sometimes necessary. Another reason for wishing to avoid radiation is the risk of later development of radiation sarcoma. The problem is that surgery for large tumours often proves to be histologically intralesional so that follow-up

radiation cannot be avoided. The decisions between surgery and radiation are therefore highly complex. Malignant round cell bone tumours should be managed by those who are very familiar with these problems and not in hospitals with limited experience.

Chemotherapy

Adjuvant chemotherapy is an essential part of management and has been responsible for the improved prognosis in recent years [11]. The most useful agents are doxorubicin, cyclophosphamide, vincristine, actinomycin D and ifosfamide. Responses are also seen with etoposide, methotrexate and nitrosoureas. A variety of different combinations is in use, with none showing a clear superiority. It is probable that all first-line agents should be used and that the dose of drugs should be kept as high as possible. In recent years the tendency has been to use chemotherapy very intensively over a period of 9–12 months rather than to use lower doses for 1–2 years. A typical regimen begins with ifosfamide, doxorubicin and vincristine for 12 weeks followed by local treatment (with surgery and radiotherapy). Chemotherapy is continued postoperatively with actinomycin substituted for doxorubicin when the maximum dose of doxorubicin has been reached. The patient must be kept under regular review during this time with regular blood counts and chest X-rays, with bone scans when clinically indicated.

PROGNOSIS

In localized disease, the use of radical local treatment with the most intensive chemotherapy regimens [11] has led to 50–60% 5-year survival. Most of these children have probably been cured. Although many factors have contributed to this improved survival there is little doubt that chemotherapy has been the major influence.

Pelvic lesions have a worse prognosis than limb tumours. Very small tumours (for example, in the jaw, and small bones of the hand and feet) have an excellent prognosis and it is not clear how much chemotherapy is necessary in these cases. The main determinants of prognosis are tumour volume and the presence of metastases. Large tumours are both more likely to recur locally and to metastasize.

Patients presenting with metastatic disease may frequently obtain a complete response of the tumour followed by later relapse. These very high risk patients are increasingly considered for very high dose chemotherapy with autologous bone marrow or peripheral blood stem cell support. Preliminary results suggest that a minority of these patients may be cured by this procedure.

Giant cell tumour of bone (osteoclastoma)

This tumour occurs at the age of 20–40 years and typically involves the epiphysis of a long bone. It causes a well defined lytic lesion which eventually erodes the cortex of the bone, giving rise to soft tissue extension. The presentation is with pain and swelling typically around the knee, the tumour occurring with equal frequency on the lower femur and upper tibia. X-ray shows a lytic lesion. Similar cystic changes can be caused by aneurysmal bone cysts or the cystic lesion of osteitis fibrosa cystica (primary hyperparathyroidism).

Pathologically the tumour consists of giant cells and spindle cells. Occasionally the appearances are frankly malignant and the tumour is then more locally invasive and metastases may occur. The tumours can be graded (I–III) according to the appearance of the stromal cells. There is some dispute about whether radiation treatment encourages malignant transformation. This is an uncommon development in the tumour and usually it is the more aggressive (Grade III) tumours which are irradiated, so the issue is not clear.

The treatment is usually by thorough curettage of the entire cavity of a localized lesion. The cavity can be obliterated by bone chips. More extensive lesions can be treated by excision and endoprosthetic replacement of bone. Some tumours are not amenable to surgery, for example those in vertebrae. In these cases, radiotherapy at modest dose (40–50 Gy) over 4–5 weeks is the mainstay of treatment. There is no known effective chemotherapy although drugs used in osteosarcoma treatment have been used. Solitary pulmonary metastases can be excised, sometimes without recurrence.

Other malignant spindle cell tumours
of bone (Malignant fibrous histiocytoma, fibrosarcoma, haemangiopericytoma, haemangioendothelioma)

These tumours have a similar anatomical distribution to osteosarcoma but occur in the age range 30–50 years, and in the diaphysis a little more commonly. The fibrosarcomas are often of low grade. Many of the tumours are associated with a long history of pain before the diagnosis is established by X-ray followed by biopsy. Haemangioendothelioma has a propensity to occur in many bones at presentation, or with patchy involvement at several sites in the same bone. Treatment is by excision. High-grade tumours including malignant fibrous histiocytoma are often treated with chemotherapy as well. Malignant fibrous histiocytoma is sensitive to HDMTX, ifosfamide and doxorubicin [12]. The prognosis is poor with surgery alone (30% overall survival at 3–4 years) but it seems that chemotherapy will improve this. Like osteosarcoma these tumours tend to be resistant to radiotherapy, although radiotherapy may be helpful as an adjuvant to surgery, or for local recurrence.

Other round cell tumours of the bone
(Primary lymphoma of bone, mesenchymal chondrosarcoma (see p. 441), angiosarcoma)

This heterogeneous group of tumours is usually of high-grade malignancy with a propensity for metastasis.

NON-HODGKIN'S LYMPHOMA
OF BONE

Non-Hodgkin's lymphoma may occur in bone and be completely localized with no evidence of disease elsewhere. Nevertheless, the risk of spread is great. The tumours are lytic and destructive, typically having ill-defined margins. Both high-grade and low-grade tumours are described. In Europe they are usually B cell disorders, but T cell lymphomas are possibly more common in Japan. An associated soft tissue mass is often present. Full staging is essential (see Chapter 26) to determine if there is systemic spread and to ensure that the bone lesion is not a metastasis from a nodal lymphoma. Radiotherapy (30–40 Gy) controls the local disease, and systemic chemotherapy is now usually given especially if there is any doubt about whether the tumour is localized (Chapter 26), and in all high-grade tumours. In elderly patients with clinically localized disease it is permissible to follow an expectant policy and treat with cytotoxic agents only if metastasis occurs. Very rarely, the tumour may arise at a number of bone sites in a multifocal distribution.

ANGIOSARCOMA

This is an exceedingly rare undifferentiated tumour. Treatment is normally with radiation and chemotherapy, using similar agents to those effective against Ewing's tumour.

SOFT TISSUE SARCOMAS

Progress in the management of adult sarcomas has been hampered by the relative rarity and heterogeneity of these tumours, which makes it difficult for any single clinic or co-operative group to develop a large experience. In addition, they are relatively unresponsive to radiotherapy and chemotherapy and many of these tumours have a high incidence of local recurrence after surgery. Recently, characteristic chromosomal translocations have been identified in many of the tumours. Although few advances have been made in adults the clinical behaviour of these

tumours is at least becoming clearer, and one or two important points in management have begun to emerge over the past few years. In childhood sarcomas the picture is different, with some degree of responsiveness to chemotherapy proving the rule, leading in many instances to an improvement in survival rate (Chapter 24). This difference is chiefly due to important differences in histological subtypes between typical childhood and adult sarcomas, of which the childhood preponderance of embryonal rhabdomyosarcoma is perhaps the best example.

Aetiology

Most cases of soft tissue sarcoma are sporadic although a few families have been reported where two siblings have developed a soft tissue sarcoma. Patients with von Recklinghausen's disease have a tendency towards malignant change in fibromatous or neurofibromatous lesions (neurofibrosarcoma is the typical tumour type). Angiosarcoma of the liver occurs more frequently in workers who are chronically exposed to PVC. Patients with gross lymphoedema may rarely develop a lymphangiosarcoma of the oedematous limb (Stewart–Treves syndrome), most typically in the upper arm, following radiotherapy for breast carcinoma. Soft tissue sarcoma is one of the tumours which occurs in the Li–Fraumeni syndrome (p. 434). Soft tissue sarcoma may also arise in a previously irradiated area.

Pathology and clinical features [13]

Soft tissue sarcomas can arise wherever mesenchymal tissue is present (Table 23.2). The commonest varieties in adults result from malignant transformation of fibrous tissue (fibrosarcomas); striated muscle (rhabdomyosarcoma); smooth muscle (leiomyosarcoma); fat (liposarcoma) and blood vessels (haemangiopericytoma, angiosarcoma and Kaposi's sarcoma). Tumours of peripheral nerves (Schwannoma, neurofibrosarcoma, etc.) are discussed in Chapter 11 and mesothelioma in

Chapter 12. Other rarer tumours occur and are discussed below.

FIBROSARCOMA

These tumours are composed of fusiform fibroblasts which form collagen strands and reticulin. The histological definition of malignancy may be difficult and well-differentiated tumours such as dermatofibrosarcoma protruberans seldom metastasize but may be locally invasive. Anaplastic tumours invade locally and also spread rapidly to the lungs.

These tumours usually arise on the limbs or trunk but may occur in any soft tissue. Typically, the patient notices a painless firm lump. In dermatofibrosarcoma protruberans, the history is of a slowly enlarging skin nodule becoming violaceous and later ulcerating.

'MALIGNANT FIBROUS HISTIOCYTOMA'

In the last 10 years this term has become more widely used as a pathological entity. It is not a new disease and cases previously diagnosed as poorly differentiated fibrosarcoma or pleomorphic rhabdomyosarcomas are now often included in this category. It is probable that the term does not describe a specific tumour but an appearance which can be found in sarcomas of many types. The typical histological pattern is one of malignant spindle cells often arranged in a 'storiform' or herring-bone fashion. As with fibrosarcomas the presentation is usually with a painless lump or nodule though this tumour can also occur as a primary bone tumour (p. 445).

LIPOSARCOMA

These tumours arise in fat. The well-differentiated neoplasm has areas of mature fat and myxoid cells and may remain localized for several years. Poorly differentiated tumours are pleomorphic, contain numerous giant cells and metastasize to the lungs and liver. Clinically, these tumours present in middle age and occur in subcutaneous fat and in retroperitoneal tissues. They do not arise from pre-existing lipomas.

RHABDOMYOSARCOMA

This is a complex group of tumours with several distinct subtypes:

Embryonal rhabdomyosarcoma

These tumours occur in early childhood and young adult life. They consist of malignant spindle and round cells, and usually occur in the head and neck and orbit (Chapter 24).

Alveolar rhabdomyosarcoma

This tumour is composed of large, round and polygonal cells. It occurs in adolescents and young adults and has a wider, anatomical distribution, often presenting in the trunk. These are highly malignant tumours and metastasize early.

Pleomorphic rhabdomyosarcoma

In these tumours the cells vary greatly in size and shape and giant cells are often present. Many are now classified as malignant fibrous histiocytoma. They occur in adult life (over the age of 30 years), usually on the limbs, arising from deep muscle groups.

Botryoidal rhabdomyosarcoma ('sarcoma botryoides')

These tumours consist of polypoid growths in the urinary and genital tracts, usually in young children. Histologically the tumour consists of an area of cells with high mitotic activity surrounded by acellular oedematous tissue.

LEIOMYOSARCOMA

The uterus is much the commonest site of origin, and it is thought that the tumours usually occur as a result of malignant change in a uterine fibroid (leiomyoma). The histological diagnosis is usually made after hysterectomy for fibroids. Other leiomyosarcomas arise from smooth muscle at other sites such as subcutaneous tissue, stomach, bowel and retroperitoneum.

SYNOVIAL SARCOMA [14]

These tumours arise around joints, bursae and tendon sheaths. The cell of origin is not known but is not the synovial lining cell. A consistent chromosomal translocation is present, t (X;18) (p11.2; q11.2). Pathologically the monophasic form consists of sheets of spindle cells and in the biphasic form there are 'glandular' spaces lined by cuboidal epithelial cells. The tumours may contain calcified areas. Tumours with few mitoses and a large 'glandular' component have a better survival. Synovial sarcomas occur in young adults, especially in the hands, feet and knees but do not involve the joint lining. They present as hard lumps near a joint. Local spread and metastasis occur and local recurrence after excision is frequent. They are chemosensitive tumours.

ANGIOSARCOMA, LYMPHANGIOSARCOMA AND HAEMANGIOPERICYTOMA

Angiosarcomas are rare, highly malignant neoplasms arising from the vascular endothelium itself. Rarely, they arise in the liver (Chapter 15). Angiosarcomas usually arise in the skin, subcutaneous tissues and glandular sites such as breast and thyroid. Lymphangiosarcomas may arise in areas of chronic oedema (e.g. in the arm after mastectomy). Haemangiopericytoma (glomus tumour) is thought to arise from the contractile cells (pericytes) in small blood vessels. It usually occurs in the extremities and retroperitoneal spaces but is also found in the head and neck. Benign and malignant variants exist.

KAPOSI'S SARCOMA

This important tumour is dealt with in Chapter 22. It arises from endothelial cells and presents as pigmented skin lesions which grow slowly. Formerly, the tumour was commonest in Jewish and Italian men, and was much more frequent in West Africa than in Europe or the United States. This has changed with the recognition of AIDS, in which Kaposi's sarcoma occurs much more frequently, and with a much more aggressive course.

ALVEOLAR SOFT PART SARCOMA

This rare neoplasm occurs in young adults, usually women. It is usually a slow-growing tumour, occurring typically in the extremities, and typically arising in the thigh in adults and in the head and neck in children. Although lung metastases usually occur, they grow slowly and may be compatible with long survival.

EPITHELIOID SARCOMA

This is a rare tumour, recently described, occurring on the extremities and with a tendency to spread to skin, bone and draining nodes. The cell of origin is unknown, but the histological appearances can be similar to a carcinoma or chronic inflammatory lesion.

CLEAR CELL SARCOMA

This tumour typically arises in the extremity, usually around the knee in a young adult. Ultrastructurally the tumour contains premelanosomes and it may be a form of undifferentiated melanoma.

Investigation and staging

Clinical staging in soft tissue sarcoma is important for management and also offers a guide to prognosis. Chest X-ray is the most important investigation since many of these tumours metastasize to the lungs. Lymph node metastases are frequent, particularly in alveolar rhabdomyosarcoma and Ewing's sarcoma. Other important distant sites include the liver, bone marrow and brain.

Staging investigation should therefore include chest X-ray and CT scan of the thorax if possible, since the latter is the most sensitive means of detecting pulmonary metastases. Lymphangiography is occasionally indicated. MR scanning is essential to determine the extent of the tumour and infiltration into local structures. Operability is better assessed by this means than by any other.

Although there is no generally accepted staging system the classification originally proposed by Russell *et al.* [15] is useful prognostically (Table 23.4).

Management of the primary tumour

Biopsy is always required for an accurate diagnosis. The most satisfactory procedure is a needle biopsy followed by a planned approach to local and systemic treatment in collaboration with medical and radiation oncologists and surgeons. Sadly, the patient with a lump on a limb is often operated upon by an inexperienced surgeon who has no prior knowledge of the diagnosis. Where a sarcoma is suspected preoperatively and confirmed by frozen section, it is unwise to attempt an excision biopsy at the same procedure since such surgery is inadequate and definitive surgery must be undertaken at a second operation. This is also true when excision biopsy of a 'benign' mass has been attempted, and the diagnosis of malignancy was not suspected even at operation.

Table 23.4 Staging of soft tissue sarcomas [15]

Stage I	Low-grade (1) tumour No nodal or distant spread
Stage II	Intermediate grade (2) tumour No nodal or distant spread
Stage III	High-grade (3) tumour No nodal or distant spread
Stage IV	A Tumour of any grade with lymph node metastases only B Distant metastases

T_1 tumours are less than 5 cm diameter
T_2 tumours are more than 5 cm diameter
Grade is based on necrosis, pleomorphism and mitotic activity

Examples are leiomyosarcoma of the uterus which is usually diagnosed after hysterectomy for fibroids, and soft tissue sarcomas of the head and neck region, which frequently present with cervical lymphadenopathy rather than with the primary tumour itself.

Traditionally, radical surgery has usually been recommended for soft tissue sarcomas arising in the extremities, and amputation has been widely used. For high lesions of the thigh, this may require disarticulation or even hemipelvectomy in an attempt to control the tumour. These radical operations were introduced because of the risk of local recurrence.

Removal of the tumour without a margin of normal tissue (so-called marginal excision) carries an average local failure rate of 80%. Wide local excisions are accompanied by failure rates of 45% with surgery alone. Radical excisions, such as compartmentectomy (see below) or amputation have local failure rates of 10–20%. These figures led to the adoption of radical surgery as the mainstay of treatment.

The common problem of distant metastases, coupled with the realization that radiotherapy can play a useful part in local control, has led over the past 10 years to a modification of this view. Wide surgical excision, coupled with high-dose irradiation, may sometimes be accepted as a satisfactory alternative with of course a far happier outcome than can be achieved by amputation. The radiation dose must be high (at least 60 Gy in 6 weeks) to minimize the risk of local recurrence. For tumours of the limbs the dose can often be taken to 70 Gy. The affected compartment should be considered at risk and uniformly irradiated to this high dose. A strip of skin and subcutaneous tissue should be left unirradiated to allow adequate lymphatic drainage from the distal limb. A proportion of these patients develop local recurrence which may well require amputation, but wide local excision plus radical radiotherapy offers a satisfactory method of local control in the large majority (80–90%) of all patients with soft tissue sarcomas of the extremities. Surgical removal of the whole of the affected compartment (compartmentectomy) is usually recommended. These are often technically more difficult operations than amputation, in view of the important structures which have to be preserved, as well as the need to resect a large volume of tissue with primary closure wherever possible (Fig. 23.15). Radiotherapy is not always recommended for grade 1 (very low grade) tumours treated with wide local excision since the risk of recurrence is low. The dose and timing of radiation and the use of pre-operative radiotherapy, are issues requiring further study.

Radiotherapy treatment is particularly valuable in soft tissue sarcomas with multiple or extensive primary sites, such as soft tissue angiosarcomas or Kaposi's sarcoma. Recent reports in both of these tumours confirm a high degree of local control using wide field

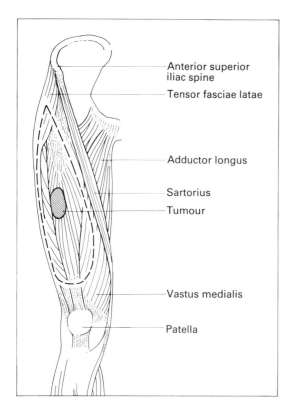

Fig. 23.15 Compartmentectomy. The diagram illustrates the wide surgical excision of soft tissue, situated, in this case, in the rectus femoris.

irradiation, sometimes in combination with surgery, with durable remissions (possibly cures) lasting 10 years and more, even in patients with multifocal sites of primary disease, for example on the scalp.

The management of soft tissue sarcomas of childhood is further discussed in Chapter 24.

CHEMOTHERAPY FOR SOFT TISSUE SARCOMAS

The past 10 years have seen a renewed interest in the chemotherapy of soft tissue sarcomas. A number of agents are effective in producing partial (or occasionally complete) remissions in patients with local recurrence and/or metastatic disease. A wide variety of agents has been shown to have activity, although in general the response rates to single agents are low and of brief duration. In the occasional patient a complete and durable response to chemotherapy is obtained. Responses of metastatic tumour lasting several years have been observed. Many classes of drug have activity (Table 23.5) including vinca alkaloids (vincristine), alkylating agents (cyclophosphamide and particularly ifosfamide), antimetabolites (particularly methotrexate) and antitumour antibiotics (including actinomycin D and doxorubicin).

Undoubtedly, the most responsive of these tumours are the embryonal rhabdomyosarcomas, in which the success of combination regimens (particularly employing vincristine, actinomycin D, doxorubicin and cyclophosphamide) for metastatic disease has led to their routine use as adjuvant treatment immediately following local radiotherapy and/or surgery. At least 60% of patients with embryonal rhabdomyosarcomas can be cured with modern adjuvant chemotherapy and cure is even possible in patients with evidence of residual disease postoperatively and in a proportion of patients with metastatic disease. The majority of these patients will be children or young adults, sadly these encouraging results have not so far been seen with other forms of soft tissue sarcoma.

Table 23.5 Chemotherapy in soft tissue sarcoma

Drug regimen	Approximate response rate (%)
Single agents	
Ifosfamide	30
Doxorubicin	25
DTIC	15
Cyclophosphamide	10
Vincristine	10
Methotrexate	10
Cisplatin	10
Actinomycin	10
Combination chemotherapy	
Doxorubicin, DTIC (AD) ifosfamide, doxorubicin	25–35
Vincristine, actinomycin, cyclosphosphamide (VAC)	20
Vincristine, doxorubicin, DTIC (VADIC)	35
Doxorubicin, cyclophosphamide methotrexate (ACM)	30
Cyclophosphamide, vincristine, doxorubicin, DTIC (CYVADIC)	40
Cyclophosphamide, vincristine, doxorubicin, actinomycin (CYVADACT)	35

A wide variety of single agents and combination regimens has been used in soft tissue sarcomas (Table 23.5). Although some groups have claimed a 42% response rate with doxorubicin and dacarbazine (DTIC), a careful review of over 350 patients has indicated that the response rate is approximately 25% of patients. A much smaller proportion of patients will achieve complete response but the addition of cyclophosphamide and vincristine to these two drugs has increased the complete response rate only to about 40%, at the cost of considerable toxicity. Nonetheless it is worth reiterating that complete responses may last for years. Responses occur more frequently in women.

New agents under active study include ifosfamide, with a reported response rate of 30%, making it one of the most active of all single agents yet encountered. Epirubicin is also active with similar response rates. Attempts at improving these figures have centred on the use of these drugs in combination. The combination of ifosfamide and epirubicin may be the most effective yet tested.

The use of chemotherapy as an adjuvant to surgery with or without radiotherapy remains very controversial. The single most important reason for this is that the trial sizes are far too small to detect differences of less than 20% in survival, and improvements of this size are clearly implausible with present drugs. A list of the results is given in Table 23.6 from which it can be seen that both positive and negative results have been obtained.

Further very large-scale studies, with longer follow-up are needed, but the differences in survival are likely to be small. The problem is made more difficult by the heterogeneity of histology, grade, stage and site. At present adjuvant chemotherapy is best offered in the setting of a trial, or in younger adults with high-grade tumours where the risk of metastasis is very high. Synovial sarcoma appears unequivocally more chemosensitive than other sarcomas, and in view of the age of the patients, chemotherapy should probably always be incorporated into treatment for this condition.

For advanced, metastatic disease other studies will be necessary to elucidate small but possibly important differences in chemotherapy effectiveness and also to monitor toxicity. If the initial promising results with ifosfamide can be confirmed, it may be possible to increase the cure rate by including this drug in adjuvant programmes. These possibilities, together with a more humane approach to the management of the primary lesion, may allow us to view the next 10 years with guarded optimism.

Survival

The survival correlates with stage and site: 5-year survival for Stage I is 80%; Stage II, 60%; Stage III, 30%; Stage IV, 10%. The more distal the tumour the better the prognosis. Lymph node spread is important prognostically and is commoner in rhabdomyosarcoma and synovial sarcoma. The prognosis for retroperitoneal

Table 23.6 Adjuvant chemotherapy in soft tissue sarcoma

Trial	Number of patients	Drug	5-year survival (months)	
			No chemotherapy	Chemotherapy
No benefit				
EORTC	326	CyVADIC	74	79
ECOG	75	DOX	66	68
NCI*	72	DOX, Cy, MTX	58	60
UCLA*	114	DOX	74†	78†
Mayo	61	CyVADIC + ACT	71	71
Some benefit				
NCI‡		DOX, Cy	60	82
Rizzoli Institute, Italy		DOX	67	87

* Trunk, retroperitoneal, head and neck. † Disease-free survival. ‡ Extremity. DOX, doxorubicin; Cy, cyclophosphamide; MTX, methotrexate; ACT, actinomycin; IC, imidazole, carboxamide; V, vincristine; AD, adnamycin (doxorubicin)

tumours is poor with 5-year survival of 15–35%. This figure is worse for higher grade lesions and those where no surgical removal is possible.

REFERENCES

1 Souhami R.L. The aetiology of bone sarcomas. In Souhami R.L., ed. *Clinics in Oncology Bone Tumours*, vol. 1. London: Ballière, 1987.

2 Link M.P., Goorin A.M., Miser A.W. *et al.* The effect of adjuvant chemotherapy on relapse free survival in patients with osteosarcoma of the extremity. *New England Journal of Medicine* 1986; **314**: 1600–06.

3 Eilber F., Guiliano A., Eckardt J. *et al.* Adjuvant chemotherapy for osteosarcoma: A randomized prospective trial. *Journal of Clinical Oncology* 1987; **5**: 21–26.

4 Winkler K., Beron G., Kotz R. *et al.* Neoadjuvant chemotherapy for osteosarcoma: Results of a cooperative German/Austrian study. *Journal of Clinical Oncology* 1984; **2**: 617–24.

5 Rosen G., Marlowe R.C., Caparros B. Primary osteogenic sarcoma. The rationale for pre-operative chemotherapy and delayed surgery. *Cancer* 1979; **43**: 2163–77.

6 Goorin A.M., Delorey M.J., Lack E.E. *et al.* Prognostic significance of complete surgical resection of pulmonary metastases in patients with osteogenic sarcoma: analysis of 32 patients. *Journal of Clinical Oncology* 1984; **2**: 425–31.

7 Van der Scheuren E., Breur K. Role of lung irradiation in the adjuvant treatment of osteosarcoma. *Recent Results in Cancer Research* 1982; **80**: 98–100.

8 Mankin H.J., Cantlay K.D., Lipielo L. *et al.* The biology of human chondrosarcoma. 1. Description of the case, grading and biochemical analyses. *Journal of Bone and Joint Surgery: American Volume* 1980; **62**: 160–76.

9 McNaney D., Lindbery R.D., Ayala R.G. *et al.* Fifteen year radiotherapy experience with chondrosarcoma of bone. *International Journal of Radiation Oncology, Biology and Physics* 1982; **8**: 181–90.

10 Razek A., Perez C.A., Tefft M. *et al.* Intergroup Ewing's sarcoma study: local control related to radiation dose volume and site of primary lesion in Ewing's sarcoma. *Cancer* 1980; **46**: 516–21.

11 Rosen G., Caparnos B., Nirenberg A. *et al.* Ewing's sarcoma. Ten year experience with adjuvant chemotherapy. *Cancer* 1981; **47**: 2204–13.

12 Bacci G., Springfield D., Picci P. Adjuvant chemotherapy in the treatment of malignant fibrous histiocytoma in the tibia and femur. *Journal of Bone and Joint Surgery: American Volume* 1985; **67**: 620–25.

13 Marsden H.B. The pathology of soft-tissue sarcomas with emphasis on childhood tumours. In D'Angio G.J., Evans A.E., eds. *Bone and Soft-tissue Sarcomas*. London: Edward Arnold, 1985, pp. 14–46.

14 Cagle L.A., Mirra J.M., Storm F.K. *et al.* Histologic features relating to prognosis in synovial sarcoma. *Cancer* 1987; **59**: 1810–14.

15 Russell W.O., Cohen J., Enzinger F. *et al.* A clinical and pathological staging system for soft-tissue sarcomas. *Cancer* 1977; **40**: 1562–70.

Chapter 24
Paediatric Malignancies

INTRODUCTION: AN APPROACH TO CANCER IN CHILDREN

The diagnosis of cancer in a child is an exceptional and painful test of the strength of family life. Happy families usually cope better with the shock, grief and disruption. When the diagnosis has been made, the physician must take time to be alone with the parents explaining the diagnosis, prognosis and approach to investigation and treatment. Over half of all children with cancer are cured: with many diseases a cautiously optimistic account can be given. The parents will sometimes feel angry about the diagnosis and may direct this towards the doctor. Often they feel that they have been responsible in some way, in that there is a genetic factor to which they have contributed, or that the cancer has arisen as a result of avoidable physical or mental trauma or faulty diet. They need to express these feelings and must be reassured that they are not to blame.

Talking to children and their parents requires tact, humanity, patience and a clear head. Every new case will prove an additional test of these qualities, and the doctor will have to deal with the guilt, anguish and anger of the parents as well as the physical and emotional suffering of the child. All children, except for the very youngest, need some account of why they are in hospital and what is likely to happen, and with older children and adolescents these explanations will need to be accurate and complete. It is impossible to make any generalization about how much to tell. Children of 6—8 years will understand that they are ill, and grasp the elements of treatment. At 10—11 years

they will know more, and teenagers will know about cancer and leukaemia. The physician must talk to the child and try to gauge his or her feelings and understanding. For children of about 11 years or more, a personal and private relationship with the doctor is important. They often want to ask questions directly and are anxious to avoid upsetting their parents. At other times they may feel that the truth is being filtered by their parents. The doctor should try to encourage the family to be open with each other with respect to the illness. Honesty and frankness are important in gaining the parents' trust and in helping them to participate, whereas glossing over of the facts will leave them with insufficient detail to help them understand the implications of the diagnosis and treatment.

The complexity of treatment makes it difficult for any doctor to provide detailed answers to all the questions which a parent or the child might ask, but it is essential that a single experienced clinician should be seen to be in charge, so that both the patient and the parents can identify with an individual rather than a committee — always a danger whenever a large number of doctors are involved in a single patient's care.

With most childhood cancers, the disease is brought under control and the child feels and looks well, except for the side-effects of treatment. These side-effects come to dominate the illness, since the acute anxiety about the diagnosis fades with time and with the induction of a remission or disappearance of the tumour. The nausea, vomiting and hair loss, and the disruption of school and family life because of frequent hospital trips all place a great strain on the child and family who will need support and reassurance from the medical team. A skilled multidisciplinary team is an essential part of management. Case discussion with nursing staff, counsellors, psychologists and medical staff is a useful way of ensuring that treatment and support is made as effective as possible. In teenagers the disruption to school work, the blow to body-image and development, and the possible loss of contact with friends, mean that family and school will need to act in harmony with the hospital staff to try and minimize the stress of the illness and the disruption to the child's education.

After successful treatment the long-term sequelae of treatment may bring problems — intellectual and neurological impairment following brain tumours such as medulloblastoma (see Chapter 11), growth defects after extensive radiation (see Chapter 5) and infertility after chemotherapy.

If the disease recurs the implications for prognosis are usually grave. If there is still a chance of cure, intensive treatment may be needed again and the depression of morale in the child and family will make extra support necessary. If the chance of cure is slim, or non-existent, the parents must of course be told and the aims of palliative treatment explained. Many parents still hope that a cure will be found, yet they must at the same time begin to accept the likelihood of the child's death. The conflict may be great and there must be an opportunity for the family to express their feelings.

Parents may be angry that relapse has occurred and feel that they had been wrong to allow aggressive treatment with its attendant side-effects and all to no avail. This anger may be directed to the medical and nursing staff. Even at this difficult stage, gentle explanations remain important and the clinician in charge of the child will also need to remember that less experienced staff may themselves need to be reassured and supported. It is important for parents to know that freedom from pain or discomfort is usually possible, and that the child's survival will not be uselessly prolonged.

Very young children do not have a clear idea of death but may express their fears of separation in play or in conversation. Adolescents will usually have an adult perception of death. In dealing with a dying child the doctors should allow the patient and family to indicate how far and fast they wish to go in discussion and should not force unpalatable facts upon them. Many families need to retain some hope of recovery in dealing with the situation. At the same time 'anticipatory mourning' may begin and the doctor must be prepared to listen to expressions of anger and grief as part of the process of acceptance that the child will die.

TUMOURS OF CHILDHOOD

Although all childhood tumours are uncommon, cancer is the commonest natural cause of death in childhood, and of all causes, second only to accidents. Despite this chilling statistic, extraordinary advances have been made in the management of almost all of the common childhood tumours. Whereas 30 years ago it was unusual even to see the slightest response to treatment, nowadays with a better understanding of the diseases and far more effective treatments, some degree of responsiveness is the rule, and cure is frequently achieved (Table 24.1). As treatment policies become more sophisticated, paediatric oncology has become a specialized branch of cancer treatment. The purpose of this chapter will therefore be to outline general treatment principles and to emphasize the multimodal and team approach. There is little doubt that childhood cancer is best treated in a specialized paediatric oncology centre. With some tumours, the chances of survival are possibly improved by 10–15% [1]. Conversely in cancers such as Wilms' tumour, where results may be equal in survival to those in non-specialist centres, this is often at the expense of over-treatment in the non-specialist hospitals [2].

Aetiology and incidence

Little is known of the aetiology of childhood

Table 24.1 Relative frequency and survival in childhood cancer [1]

Tumour	Incidence/ million/year	Total cases (%)	5-year survival rate (%)
Leukaemia	30	31	
Acute lymphoblastic	25		70
Acute myeloblastic	5		26
Brain tumours	20	19	50
Lymphoma	17	13	
Hodgkin's disease	8		88
Non-Hodgkin's	9		70
Neuroblastoma	8	7	43
Wilms' tumour	7	6	79
Soft tissue sarcoma	5	7	61
Osteosarcoma	3	2	54
Ewing's sarcoma	2	2	42
Retinoblastoma	3	3	91
Germ cell tumour	0.5	2	84

tumours. Ionizing radiation may be a predisposing cause, either when given during pregnancy or as a result of deliberate irradiation, for example to the thymus for thymic hyperplasia which has been responsible for an increased risk of thyroid carcinoma. Transplacental carcinogens have long been thought to be a possible cause of childhood cancer, but have been difficult to identify until the recent demonstration of the association of adenocarcinoma of the vagina in teenage girls with treatment of the mother 20 years previously with diethylstilboestrol for early threatened abortion [3].

Genetic factors are occasionally involved. Several tumours of childhood are now known to be associated with chromosomal abnormalities. Some of these are acquired and are discussed in the sections on the tumours concerned. Others are heritable (constitutive) abnormalities and these are listed in Table 3.4, p. 36. Some congenital malformations appear to be associated with paediatric tumours. There is an increased risk of tumours (usually neurogenic sarcomas) developing in children with von Recklinghausen's disease. The rare syndrome of hemihypertrophy may be associated both with Wilms' tumour and hepatoblastoma. Wilms' tumour can be associated with aniridia and a wide variety of congenital abnormalities.

In addition to the inherited diseases (Table 3.4, p. 36) in which there is an increased risk of cancer, there are inherited gene mutations which give rise to a high risk of cancer without any other manifestations. One of the best known examples is retinoblastoma, which has a marked familial incidence particularly in the bilateral form of the disease, where half the offspring of affected children will themselves develop the disease. The Li–Fraumeni syndrome is another example of a high risk of cancer in families of children with sarcoma (see p. 434). If a child with an identical twin develops acute leukaemia, then the risk of the twin also developing this disease is high. The overall risk of cancer in childhood is 1 : 600, but in siblings 1 : 300.

Geographical and racial variations also exist, which may eventually throw further light on aetiology. Liver cancer is commoner in the Far East, retinoblastoma in India, intestinal lymphoma in Israel and Burkitt's lymphoma in Uganda. In Britain and the United States the proportion of various groups of tumours is reasonably constant; 20–25% consist of tumours of the CNS and eye, 33% are leukaemias, and 35% are solid tumours (chiefly Wilms' tumour and neuroblastoma). Most of these tumours have their maximal incidence at ages 0–4 years, although some, such as bone tumours and lymphomas have a later peak, between 6 and 14 years. In general, younger children appear to have a better survival than older groups, particularly with neuroblastoma and retinoblastoma. With the relative improvement in treatments of other paediatric illnesses, cancer has assumed an increased importance as a cause of death despite the many advances in management.

Childhood tumours of the CNS are common, and are discussed with adult brain tumours in Chapter 11; leukaemia in Chapter 28, and paediatric lymphomas in Chapter 26.

Neuroblastoma

After brain tumours, leukaemia and lymphoma, neuroblastoma is the commonest of paediatric tumours, accounting for some 7% of the total. Over 80% of cases occur below 4 years of age. Most cases are sporadic but there are reports of twins with both affected, as well as families with two or more affected siblings. Most neuroblastomas show monosomy for the short arm of chromosome 1 (1p−) and the karyotype of chromosome 17 is often abnormal. There may be amplification of one of the *myc* family of oncogenes (N-*myc*). This is present in 30% of cases and the more invasive tumours show greater degrees of amplification.

PATHOLOGY

Neuroblastomas arise from neural crest tissue, which normally develops into the adrenal medulla and sympathetic ganglia. The common primary sites are therefore the adrenal medulla and the sympathetic nervous tissue in the retroperitoneum. However, tumours may also arise in the posterior mediastinum and spine, predominantly extradurally from paravertebral ganglia (Fig. 24.1). Because of their derivation from the adrenal medulla, elaboration and secretion of adrenal medullary hormones or metabolites are characteristic of these tumours (see below).

The tumour is composed of small cells with scanty cytoplasm, often in lobules with inter-

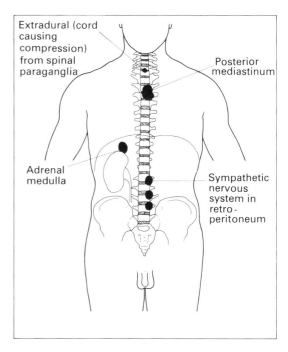

Fig. 24.1 Common primary sites of neuroblastoma.

vening fibrous or fibrovascular septa and with evidence of neurofibrillary tissue, often arranged as rosettes. Wide variations in degree of differentiation are seen, sometimes in a single specimen. Neuroblastomas are almost always PAS−ve, unlike Ewing's sarcoma, rhabdomyosarcoma or ganglion cell tumours. Immunocytochemical techniques, using monoclonal antibodies to neuroblastoma-associated antigens, have proved helpful in diagnosis of difficult cases. Neuroblastoma expresses NCAM on its surface. Monoclonal antibodies have been made to this and other surface antigens. The tumours also express the intermediate filament vimentin. Electron microscopically, the tumour cells contain electron-dense granules and in this respect are similar to tumours of the APUD system (see Chapter 15).

Neuroblastomas tend to spread very widely (Fig. 24.2), by local, lymphatic and haematogenous routes, and important sites of blood-borne dissemination include bone marrow (often forming clusters of large, poorly differ-

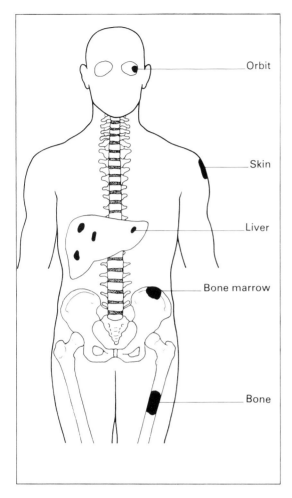

Fig. 24.2 Common sites of distant metastasis in neuroblastoma.

CLINICAL FEATURES

Clinical presentation is unusually varied, due to the variety of primary sites, the early wide dissemination and the secretion of pharmacologically active metabolites (Table 24.2). The commonest presentation is of an abdominal mass, sometimes painless but often accompanied by mild or recurrent abdominal pain. Other common syndromes include irritability, fever, lethargy, anaemia or bone pain from a metastasis. Occasionally, lymph node or skin metastases, hepatomegaly or proptosis are the first clinical signs. Subcutaneous metastases often have a blue/black colour. Liver metastases may be painful. Other primary sites of presentation include presacral neuroblastoma causing urinary frequency or obstruction, posterior mediastinal tumours causing dyspnoea; intraspinal tumours causing spinal cord compression; cervical sympathetic tumours causing Horner's syndrome and olfactory bulb tumours

Table 24.2 Presenting symptoms of neuroblastoma

Constitutional
Fever, malaise, weight loss, anaemia

Primary site
Adrenal: pain and abdominal mass
Presacral: loss of bladder control, frequency of micturition
Paravertebral: spinal cord compression
Cervical sympathetic: Horner's syndrome
Olfactory bulb: unilateral nasal block and epistaxis

Metastases
Liver: pain, weight loss, fever
Bone: pain (preceding X-ray change), anaemia, pathological fractures
Orbit: proptosis
CNS: malignant meningitis

Remote effects
Diarrhoea: ?due to secretion of vasoactive intestinal polypeptide
Myoclonus or opsoclonus
Hypertension

entiated cells), the liver (sometimes resulting in enormous hepatomegaly) and bone (often with a single destructive lesion as the typical neuroblastoma deposit). Unlike other paediatric soft tissue tumours, the lungs are seldom the site of metastases. Skin and periorbital metastases are common. An unusual characteristic is the ability of this tumour to undergo spontaneous remission and cure, even when disseminated. Although frequently described, this phenomenon is in fact a rarity with an incidence of about 3% and almost exclusively confined to infants under the age of 12 months.

(aesthesioneuroblastoma) causing nasal obstruction and epistaxis. There is an association between neuroblastoma and myoclonic or opsoclonic movements, though the mechanism is unclear.

DIAGNOSIS AND INVESTIGATION

The definitive diagnosis is by biopsy of the affected site but a confident diagnosis may already have been made biochemically. Catecholamine metabolites are produced in about 90% of all children with neuroblastomas and screening for urinary metabolites should be undertaken if the diagnosis is suspected. Homovanillic acid (HVA) or vanillyl mandelic acid (VMA) are the most reliable and widely used measurements. The diagnosis can often be made on a random urine sample. The random sample is reliable as long as HVA and VMA excretion are related to urine creatinine. Both HVA and VMA should be measured since either metabolite may be increased. Total catecholamine excretion can also be estimated. This will summate the output of metabolites of adrenaline, noradrenaline, metanephrine, normetanephrine, dopa and dopamine as well as HVA and VMA.

Radiological investigations are often extremely valuable. Plain X-ray of the abdomen will frequently demonstrate calcification in the primary tumour, typically with a diffuse pattern. Liver metastases may also calcify. The chest X-ray is often normal, though abnormal mediastinal shadowing often occurs with primary intrathoracic tumours (typically in the posterior mediastinum). Parenchymal lung metastases are very unusual. Skeletal survey and isotope bone scanning are useful in detecting osseous metastases. Bone marrow aspiration is mandatory in all cases of neuroblastoma. Over 40% of children have marrow involvement even when bone X-rays are normal. Marrow examination often yields the only evidence of secondary spread. Intravenous urography may show renal displacement often without intrinsic distortion of the renal calyces, though hydro-nephrosis or non-functioning kidneys may also occur with large obstructing tumours. Before the advent of CT scanning, aortography was abnormal in more than 80% of cases with an obvious mass, and abnormal tumour circulation could often be demonstrated. CT and/or MRI scanning and abdominal ultrasonography are now more frequently performed, giving excellent delineation of tumour as well as providing accurate imaging of the liver.

Meta-iodo-benzylguanidine (MIBG) is taken up by adrenergic nervous tissue and can be used to identify both primary and metastatic neuroblastoma. Using a higher radiation dose it is also undergoing study as a therapeutic agent.

Early diagnosis by screening urine of all 6-month-old babies has been attempted in Japan where it is now routinely offered. The effectiveness in saving life has not been proved and trials in Europe have not confirmed its value.

DIFFERENTIAL DIAGNOSIS

The clinical diagnosis of neuroblastoma is not always straightforward, particularly if the child presents with failure to thrive and without other obvious abnormalities to suggest a diagnosis of malignancy. The most important distinction in children presenting with an obvious abdominal mass lies between neuroblastoma and Wilms' tumour. Although the urinary and radiological investigations usually give a firm answer, it can be difficult to distinguish between the two, especially where urinary catecholamines are normal and where CT scanning fails to confirm that the mass is unequivocally renal or adrenal. Other abdominal tumours which may cause diagnostic difficulty include hepatoblastoma and intestinal lymphoma. If the child presents with bone metastases, these may be difficult to distinguish radiologically from a primary Ewing's tumour, bone lymphoma or even a non-malignant cause such as osteomyelitis or tuberculosis.

Difficulty may also occur when the child

presents with spinal cord compression when a variety of malignant and non-malignant causes must be considered. These include intraspinal cysts, neurofibroma, spinal tuberculosis, primary intraspinal tumours, medulloblastoma and other CNS tumours which seed within the CNS (see Chapter 11), or other rare causes of extradural compression, such as Hodgkin's disease.

CLINICAL STAGING

Clinical staging of neuroblastoma is important both prognostically and also as a means of selecting the most appropriate treatment. Although several classification schemes have been suggested, all are based on an accurate assessment of the detailed extent of spread. Although it is known that the degree of histo-logical differentiation (i.e. tumour grade) may influence prognosis, this information, though potentially useful, is difficult to fit into a simple staging classification. The same can be said for catecholamine excretion and age, though age at diagnosis is probably the single most important prognostic factor [5]. The most widely used classification [6] is based on extent of disease so as to produce a system that is practical for clinical use (Table 24.3).

Up to 70% of children have disseminated tumour at diagnosis, often in the bone marrow. The prognosis worsens with increasing stage. However, the IV-S category has been defined because these children have a surprisingly good prognosis with a survival rate similar to patients with stage I tumours. This might suggest a difference in sensitivity to treatment, depen-dent on the site of dissemination. However, it is also important to realize that most IV-S patients are under the age of 1 year, and patients of this age have a much better prognosis and a higher incidence of spontaneous regression.

In addition to age and disease extent, the primary site is also prognostically important. Tumours arising in the mediastinum and the neck have a better prognosis than those in the abdomen, probably since more are localized at

Table 24.3 International staging system for neuroblastoma

Stage I	Localized tumour confined to the area of origin; complete gross excision, with or without microscopic residual disease; identifiable ipsilateral and contralateral lymph nodes negative microscopically
Stage IIA	Unilateral tumour with incomplete gross excision; identifiable ipsilateral and contralateral lymph nodes negative microscopically
Stage IIB	Unilateral tumour with complete or incomplete gross excision; with positive ipsilateral regional lymph nodes; identifiable contralateral lymph nodes negative microscopically
State III	Tumour infiltrating across the midline with or without regional lymph node involvement; or, unilateral tumour with contralateral regional lymph node involvement; or, midline tumour with bilateral regional lymph node involvement
Stage IV	Dissemination of tumour to distant lymph nodes, bone marrow, liver, and/or other organs (except as defined in Stage IV-S)
Stage IV-S	Localized primary tumour as defined for Stage I or II with dissemination limited to liver, skin, and/or bone marrow

the time of diagnosis. This is particularly true with thoracospinal lesions which produce early spinal cord compression (so-called dumb-bell tumours). Oddly enough, pelvic tumours also appear to have a better prognosis, and more frequently undergo differentiation to ganglio-neuroma or even a spontaneous remission; again this may relate to the fact that most of these children are under the age of 15 months.

Other, biological, factors have recently been identified which correlate with prognosis [7]. These include N-*myc* amplification, hypo-diploidy and karyotypic abnormalities of chromosome 1 which are all associated with a poor prognosis. Hyperdiploidy and normal N-*myc* are associated with better outcome. Serum neurone specific enolase and serum ferritin, if elevated, have also been reported as associated with a worse prognosis.

CLINICAL MANAGEMENT

Current clinical management of neuroblastoma is unsatisfactory and refinements in treatment are continuously being suggested. Unlike many of the paediatric malignancies, chemotherapy has not yet made a significant improvement in the survival of these children, though the chemosensitivity of this tumour is not in doubt.

Local treatments with surgery, and/or radiation therapy are therefore critically important, and may be curative in children with localized disease. In one surgical series, a 2-year survival rate of 84% was achieved by the use of surgery alone in apparently localized cases. Radiotherapy is usually recommended after incomplete excision, but probably best avoided where surgery appears complete. Long-term survivors have certainly been documented where surgery was incomplete, but supplemented by postoperative radiotherapy, though the contribution of radiotherapy is difficult to quantify since almost all patients will have had at least a partial or subtotal surgical excision. Most children with clinical Stage II and III disease will be in this category. Even in children with Stage IV disease, in whom chemotherapy may be the most important part of treatment, attention must be paid to controlling the primary disease.

In Stage IV cases chemotherapy is usually the first treatment but radiotherapy and surgery will often be required at a later stage in order to achieve control of the bulky primary tumour. Some surgeons feel that in this situation, preoperative irradiation makes surgery technically easier. In these more advanced cases, the local treatment is usually withheld until at least 2 cycles of chemotherapy have been given. Low-dose hepatic irradiation has been given for Stage IV-S tumours but is not now widely used.

Guidelines for treatment of neuroblastoma are given in Table 24.4. Combinations of vincristine, cyclophosphamide, actinomycin D

Table 24.4 Guidelines for treatment of neuroblastoma

Stage I	Surgery alone
Stage II	Surgery with postoperative irradiation if surgery incomplete. Chemotherapy sometimes used
Stage III	Chemotherapy followed by 'debulking' surgery with local irradiation and further chemotherapy
Stage IV	As for Stage III, but intensive chemotherapy is the mainstay of treatment
Stage IV-S	If possible no treatment is given. If the child has symptoms because of tumour size, surgery ± minimal chemotherapy is justified

and doxorubicin are usually used. Newer agents such as cisplatin, etoposide and ifosfamide are increasingly used in combination therapy. All of these drugs have been shown to be active as single agents in neuroblastoma. Most drug combinations contain vincristine, actinomycin D and cyclophosphamide (Table 24.5) often with other agents. These are generally well tolerated and yield higher response rates than treatment either with single agents or with pairs of drugs, though the overall cure rate of only 10−20% is disappointing. Recent attempts to intensify treatment, either by the use of more agents (such as cisplatin and etoposide) or by increasing the drug dosage are of interest. The use of high-dose chemotherapy and autologous bone marrow transplantation in high-risk cases may improve survival, but results are difficult to interpret [8].

Although overall results remain disappointing, survival has improved in recent years as a result of better diagnosis, treatment strategy, biochemical monitoring and possibly chemotherapy. Survival is clearly related to age and stage (Fig. 24.3), and children living beyond 3 years from diagnosis are usually considered cured.

Table 24.5 Chemotherapy for neuroblastoma

Single agents Vincristine Actinomycin D Doxorubicin Cyclophosphamide High-dose melphalan Cisplatin Etoposide	}	Response rates are not well characterized for any of these agents but are in the range of 30% with few sustained complete responses

Combination chemotherapy
VAC I   Vincristine, actinomycin
        and cyclophosphamide
VAC II   Vincristine, doxorubicin
        and cyclophosphamide
	}	With both regimens response rates appear to be approximately 60% with 10– 20% sustained complete responses

OPEC   Vincristine
        Cisplatin
        Etoposide
        Cyclophosphamide
		60–70% complete and partial remission with 20–30% sustained

Wilms' tumour

INCIDENCE AND AETIOLOGY

Wilms' tumour (nephroblastoma) accounts for about 6% of all paediatric tumours, and has been recognized as a distinct clinical entity since the end of the last century. With neuroblastoma it forms much the largest group of intra-abdominal malignancies of childhood.

None the less there are pronounced differences between the behaviour of these two tumours, particularly in their response to treatment.

Although most cases are sporadic, a familial predisposition has been noted. Aniridia, hemihypertrophy, hamartoma, genito-urinary and musculoskeletal malformation are other well known associations.

The most consistent abnormality is deletion at the level of band 13 of the short arm of

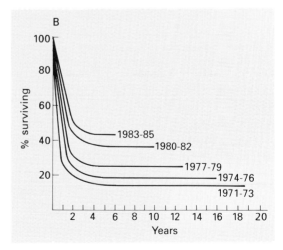

Fig. 24.3 (A) Survival related to stage in neuroblastoma and (B) neuroblastoma survival in the United Kingdom in the period 1971–85.

chromosome 11 (p13). In the case of aniridia–Wilms' tumour this deletion may be visible karyotypically (Fig. 24.4). Other described abnormalities are XX/XY mosaicism and trisomy 8 or 18. The peak age of incidence is 3–5 years, though rarely it has been discovered at birth. There is a slight male preponderance.

PATHOLOGY

Almost the whole kidney can be replaced either by a centrally or peripherally placed tumour, often exhibiting areas of patchy haemorrhage or degeneration, and sometimes with a lobulated appearance. Necrosis and cystic change are both common and although a very large size may be attained without obvious extra-renal involvement, extension of solid cores of tumour cells along the renal vein and inferior vena cava are common. Other direct sites of spread may include the perinephric fat, colon, adrenal gland or liver as well as the renal pelvis

itself, and the local draining lymph nodes. Occasionally the tumour may be extra-renal in origin, presumably arising in ectopic cell rests from mesonephric crest migration. Bilateral presentation occurs in 5–10% of cases which are usually regarded as being bilateral primary tumours rather than secondary spread. Bilateral Wilms' tumour can also be metachronous. Children with bilateral tumours are younger and have 10 times the incidence of associated congenital anomalies.

Histologically, the tumours contain both mesenchymal and epithelial elements, often admixed and with differing stages of maturity. Within the epithelial element, there is usually evidence of a renal origin with embryonic tubular or glomerular structures sometimes lined by recognizable epithelium and occasionally arranged in rosettes. Undifferentiated stroma may form a large proportion of the tumour though this too may show areas of differentiation to form smooth muscle, bone or cartilage. A variety of histological types has been described, which probably represent differing degrees of differentiation. Some tumours are so undifferentiated as to defy unequivocal histological diagnosis. About 5% of tumours are anaplastic. Nuclear enlargement and hyperploidy are associated adverse features. Typically, such tumours have a great propensity to metastasis. More highly differentiated forms also occur, and a specific group of 'mesoblastic nephromas', with only minimal nuclear pleomorphism and mitotic activity, a very low metastatic potential, and often surgically curable [9].

CLINICAL FEATURES

As with neuroblastoma, the common presentation is with a symptomless, painless abdominal mass more commonly on the left and often discovered by the parent or during a routine examination. There may be recurrent abdominal pain of moderate severity. Abdominal distension is common, though unlike neuroblastoma these tumours tend not to cross the

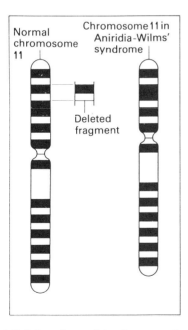

Fig. 24.4 Deletion of part of the short arm of chromosome 11 in aniridia–Wilms' syndrome.

midline. Haematuria occurs in 30% of cases. Hypertension is unusual but is occasionally severe and sometimes accompanied by complications such as retinopathy or encephalopathy. It is thought to be due to excess renin production by the tumour or to renal ischaemia from renal artery stenosis. Fever, anorexia and lethargy are also common presenting symptoms.

About one-fifth of children with Wilms' tumour have evidence of distant metastases at presentation, though figures from central referral hospitals suggest a much higher incidence (up to 60–70%), representing a preponderance of advanced and complicated cases. Direct spread to extra-renal fat and other local organs is common, and local nodal spread occurs predominantly to the para-aortic and other intra-abdominal lymph node groups. Haematogenous spread occurs typically to the lung parenchyma, brain and bone, though liver, mediastinum, vagina and testis are well known secondary sites (Fig. 24.5). Bilateral renal involvement in the absence of evidence of metastatic spread is well recognized.

INVESTIGATION AND STAGING

Plain chest and abdominal X-rays will help to define the extent of the primary tumour and demonstrate obvious pulmonary metastases. CT scanning of the chest is advisable since it is more sensitive in detecting pulmonary spread. Intravenous urography, abdomino-pelvic ultrasonography and in selected cases renal angiography, will give accurate pre-operative information as to the size and extent of disease. Visualization of the inferior vena cava (IVC) is important prior to surgery and can be achieved with ultrasound or contrast veno-graphy. CT or MRI scanning of the abdomen gives the most precise definition of the tumour size.

Routine urine examination often reveals microscopic haematuria, and measurement of catecholamine excretion may be necessary in cases which are difficult to distinguish clinically

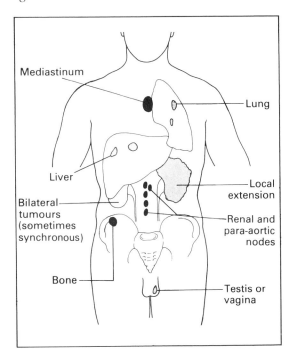

Fig. 24.5 Common sites of metastasis in Wilms' tumour.

from neuroblastoma. Isotope bone scanning is usually recommended since symptomless bone secondaries may be present. These investigations should help distinguish the true Wilms' tumour from a variety of malignant and non-malignant conditions which it may clinically resemble.

Although neuroblastoma is the most important differential diagnosis, other intra-abdominal childhood tumours may cause difficulty, such as retroperitoneal sarcoma and hepatoblastoma. Important non-malignant causes of childhood abdominal masses include renal haematomas, hydronephrosis, multilocular cystic kidney, horseshoe kidney, perirenal haematoma and splenomegaly, almost all of which are uncommon though frequent enough as a group of disorders to cause diagnostic problems.

Staging systems have become more logical with increased understanding of the natural history of these tumours and of the importance of complete surgical removal. At present, the

National Wilms' Tumour Study Staging System (Table 24.6) is most widely used [10].

This staging system has now been successfully used for 10 years, and data are accumulating to suggest that extent of disease at operation and the presence of lymph node involvement are the most influential prognostic factors. Large referral centres which treat a substantial number of children undoubtedly have better results than smaller hospitals where the occasional case is treated, a finding with the unavoidable implication that non-specialist clinicians should be strongly dissuaded from treating the occasional child with a curable cancer.

MANAGEMENT

There should be close co-operation between paediatric surgeon, radiotherapist, paediatric oncologist and pathologist to ensure that all clinicians will have the opportunity to assess each child before surgery is performed. There has been some controversy over the use of pre-operative biopsy. If this is done it should be a fine-needle biopsy to minimize the risk of intra-abdominal dissemination. Even in the presence of obvious metastatic disease, careful assessment of operability should be made since control of the primary tumour without surgery is always difficult. The advent of effective irradiation and chemotherapy has allowed surgeons to reconsider operating on children whose tumours were inoperable at first presentation.

Guidelines for the management of Wilms' tumour are set out in Table 24.6. Surgical removal should be performed in order both to remove the tumour in its entirety, without biopsy or other disturbance of the capsule, and to assess the extent of intra-abdominal disease with careful delineation of any area of residual tumour. Enlarged lymph nodes should generally be resected or at least biopsied.

Postoperative chemotherapy with combinations of vincristine, actinomycin D and/or doxorubicin should be used (Table 24.7). How-

Table 24.6 Staging and guidelines for the management of Wilms' tumour

Stage I	Tumour limited to the kidney, and completely resected. Renal capsule intact, tumour removed without rupture, no residual disease	Surgery and vincristine
Stage II	Tumour extends beyond kidney but is completely resected. Penetration is into the perirenal soft tissue or fat; infiltration of renal vessels outside the kidney, or para-aortic lymph node involvement. No residual tumour	Surgery; adjuvant combination chemotherapy using vincristine and actinomycin D
Stage III	Residual tumour confined to the abdomen, or tumour biopsied or ruptured before or during surgery. Involved lymph nodes beyond para-aortic chains; tumour not completely resected	As for Stage II but whole abdominal irradiation for diffuse spread and chemotherapy includes doxorubicin
Stage IV	Distant blood-borne metastases (usually to lung, liver, bone and/or brain). Lymph node metastases beyond the abdomen	Surgery and more intensive combination chemotherapy
Stage V	Bilateral tumours at presentation	Individual treatment often including bilateral renal surgery with low-dose postoperative radiotherapy and adjuvant combination chemotherapy

Table 24.7 Chemotherapy in Wilms' tumour

	Response rate (complete and partial) (%)
Single agents	
Vincristine	70
Doxorubicin	60
Actinomycin D	40
Cyclophosphamide	35
Etoposide	30
Cisplatin	30
*Combination therapy**	
Actinomycin D and vincristine	95
Vincristine, doxorubicin	90
Vincristine, doxorubicin, cyclophosphamide	90

* Response rates are approximate as these combinations have not been thoroughly tested in metastatic disease, and different combinations are used in different stages of the disease.

ever, the possible roles of pre-operative chemotherapy and routine postoperative irradiation of the tumour bed remain controversial. There is a growing evidence that pre-operative chemotherapy is valuable in the management of doubtfully resectable tumours.

Although for 30 years or more, postoperative radiotherapy has been employed routinely as an adjuvant to surgery, the development of effective chemotherapeutic regimens has led to a reappraisal of the role of radiotherapy.

In Stage I disease, postoperative radiotherapy confers no benefit in children under the age of 2 years treated by 'adjuvant' actinomycin D; this is possibly true for older children as well.

Children with Stages II and III should be treated postoperatively with combination chemotherapy and most of these children also receive postoperative radiotherapy including treatment to the whole abdomen in those with diffuse spread. There is some evidence that combination chemotherapy using vincristine, actinomycin D and doxorubicin gives a better

survival rate than the use of two drugs alone.

Stage IV disease should be treated with intensive combination chemotherapy. The successful treatment of disseminated Wilms' tumour demands an aggressive approach, often requiring surgical resection of both pulmonary and hepatic metastases with multiple courses of both radiotherapy and chemotherapy. The more widespread use of chemotherapy has also led to discontinuation of total lung irradiation which in the past was a common method of treatment for mediastinal or pulmonary metastases.

In patients with bilateral (Stage V) disease, treatment is usually with surgical removal of the tumour where possible, often by total nephrectomy on the more affected side and partial nephrectomy on the other. Low-dose postoperative radiotherapy and chemotherapy are usually given.

Unlike neuroblastoma the routine use of chemotherapy has radically altered the outlook in this disease, which was the first of the solid tumours in which adjuvant chemotherapy was established as an important part of the initial management. Most patients tolerate this treatment without too much difficulty. Avoidance of radiotherapy wherever possible has undoubtedly reduced the long-term complications such as growth retardation within the irradiated area, scoliosis, and radiation-induced second tumours — often an unresectable and rapidly fatal sarcoma. Trials are in progress to further clarify the details of postoperative treatment. At present, important chemotherapy-induced complications include nausea and vomiting, peripheral neuropathy, alopecia, and skin reactions (including recall phenomena in previously irradiated areas, following actinomycin D treatment).

Treatment of recurrent disease is always difficult because of the previous administration of chemotherapy and radiotherapy. The same agents may again be effective, particularly in cases where recurrence is late, well after discontinuation of the initial adjuvant chemotherapy. Other drugs such as cisplatin, vinblastine, bleomycin and etoposide may be of value in children resistant to first-line treatment. Palliative irradiation (sometimes in combination with surgery) may also be useful for brain, lung, extradural, bony and hepatic metastases.

PROGNOSIS

The prognosis in Wilms' tumour has improved greatly as a result of routine adjuvant chemotherapy, though a better understanding of the role of surgery, radiotherapy and supportive care have also contributed. At present, the prognosis in this disease is better than for any other childhood malignancy and the overall survival rate is now 80–90% (Fig. 24.6). Several prognostic factors are known to be important including age at diagnosis (the younger the better), histological findings such as degree of differentiation (with a better prognosis in well-differentiated tumours) and tumour stage. Prognosis for Stage I disease is excellent with 5-year survival rates of at least 90%; with Stage IV disease this falls to 54% [10].

Soft tissue sarcoma

INCIDENCE, AETIOLOGY AND CLASSIFICATION

Soft tissue sarcomas account for 7% of childhood tumours with an incidence of 0.8 per 100 000 children. Little is known of their cause although genetic factors are important in the Li–Fraumeni syndrome.

The histological types of soft tissue sarcoma in children are similar to those found in adults (see Chapter 23), but the relative frequency is different with rhabdomyosarcoma and fibrosarcoma predominating (Table 24.8).

Rhabdomyosarcoma

This tumour is much the commonest soft tissue sarcoma of childhood. *Embryonal rhabdomyosarcoma* is the most frequent histological type

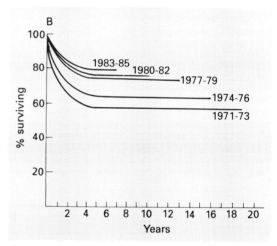

Fig. 24.6 (A) Survival related to stage in Wilms' tumour and (B) results of treatment in the United Kingdom, 1971–85.

Table 24.8 Childhood soft tissue sarcoma

	Relative frequency (%)
Rhabdomyosarcoma	52
Fibrosarcoma (including histiocytoma)	10
Mesenchymoma	6
Synovial sarcoma	6
Liposarcoma	4
Leiomyosarcoma	2
Vascular sarcomas	5
Others	15

with a peak incidence at 2–5 years. *Alveolar rhabdomyosarcoma* is commoner in adolescence. The tumours can arise at a variety of sites: in the head and neck (chiefly the orbit, nasopharynx, oropharynx or palate), the pelvis (particularly bladder, uterus and vagina) or less commonly, the extremities or trunk.

PATHOLOGY

There are four main histological subtypes of rhabdomyosarcoma: embryonal, alveolar, pleomorphic and mixed types. The first two account for more than 90% of all cases. Macroscopically, the tumours are usually nodular, often with a surrounding inflammatory and oedematous reaction. Although they may appear to be circumscribed, true encapsulation is very uncommon. Sarcoma botryoides has a characteristic macroscopic appearance, described as resembling bunches of grapes, which consist of mucinous polyps of tumour.

Microscopically, these tumours are highly malignant. Pathological diagnosis can be difficult, particularly if cross-striation is regarded as an essential part of the histological diagnosis. Electron microscopy should always be performed if possible, since the appearances are characteristic (Fig. 24.7).

Embryonal rhabdomyosarcoma

This is often poorly differentiated, with long slender spindle-shaped cells with a single central nucleolus and eosinophilic cytoplasm, often without obvious cross-striations. The cells usually have an irregular pattern without the cellular arrangements which are characteristic of alveolar rhabdomyosarcoma. Sarcoma botryoides is a polypoid form of embryonal rhabdomyosarcoma. The embryonal group is the commonest form of paediatric rhabdomyosarcoma and accounts for the majority of head and neck and genito-urinary cases.

Fig. 24.7 Electron micrograph of a portion of rhabdomyoblast. Thick and thin filaments are shown, and there is formation of Z bands (arrowed) (×26 600).

Alveolar rhabdomyosarcoma

This arises more commonly on the limbs and trunk. Microscopically these tumours have a more organized pattern and the cells tend to be separated by connective tissue bands. The typical cell is round with scanty eosinophilic cytoplasm which is sometimes vacuolated and may contain glycogen. Cross-striations are often seen, and giant multinucleate cells are common. Pleomorphic rhabdomyosarcomas are rare in childhood, and almost always arise in skeletal muscle.

All varieties are highly malignant and exhibit rapid growth with early dissemination, though embryonal rhabdomyosarcoma often presents greater problems of local recurrence. Early lymph node involvement is common, producing obvious lymphadenopathy which may be the initial presenting feature, particularly in head and neck tumours. Blood-borne metastases are also frequent, particularly to lung and marrow, though other sites such as brain, liver and other soft tissue sites may also be involved.

Clinically, the commonest presentation is with a painless mass either clearly visible in the case of extremity and trunk lesions, or causing displacement as with the characteristic proptosis of orbital rhabdomyosarcoma which accounts for 30% of all head and neck cases.

In the pelvis, the commonest primary sites are the genito-urinary tract and perianal area. Deep-seated tumours may cause indirect symptoms such as facial palsy and discharge from the ear with tumours in the middle ear; airway obstruction and nasal discharge from nasopharyngeal primaries; and dysphagia from tumours in the oropharynx. Lymph node metastasis is common with testicular and genito-urinary sites and may be the presenting sign, but is very unusual with head and neck (particularly orbital) primaries.

INVESTIGATION AND STAGING

Important investigations include a chest X-ray (with whole lung tomography or CT scanning if possible); isotope, liver and bone scanning; ultrasonography; CT and/or MRI scanning of the abdomen (in patients with abdominopelvic primary tumours). In head, neck and orbital cases, detailed plain radiographs, tomography, CT and/or MRI scanning are essential to determine the local extent of the primary site. Bone marrow examination is probably worthwhile. The most widely used staging notation is shown in Table 24.9, together with the relationship between initial stage and prognosis.

MANAGEMENT

As with most paediatric tumours, current management is complex and, for the majority of patients, includes surgery, radiotherapy and chemotherapy since none of these modalities alone gives satisfactory results. This integrated multimodal approach to treatment has led to a substantial improvement in prognosis during the past 20 years [11]. Until recently, radical

Table 24.9 Stage and prognosis in rhabdomyosarcoma in childhood

		Prognosis (3-year survival)
Group 1	Localized disease completely resected	82%
Group 2	Localized and/or regional disease with residual microscopic tumour following local therapy	60–70%
Group 3	Regional disease with gross residual tumour after local treatment	55%
Group 4	Distant metastatic disease	30%

surgical removal of the primary was always felt to be mandatory, a view which has undergone revision in recent years. Combination chemotherapy should now be used as the initial treatment, followed by local treatment with surgery and radiotherapy. Although surgery should be as complete as possible, careful judgement is required in order to avoid the risk of long-term mutilation. This has led, for example, to an increasing preference for wide excision (including compartmentectomy) rather than amputation for children with tumours of the extremities. When coupled with radical postoperative irradiation and early (adjuvant) chemotherapy this approach gives acceptably low local recurrence rates and allows for later amputation in the small number of cases where local recurrence occurs in the absence of more generalized disease.

With more deeply situated primary tumours such as nasopharynx, primary surgery plays no part other than to establish the histological diagnosis. In some of the deeply situated but more accessible abdominopelvic primaries, the role of surgery is more uncertain, though it is increasingly accepted that major procedures such as total cystectomy or exenteration should not be performed in the first instance since effective irradiation and chemotherapy may result in cure with far less long-term damage. Combinations of chemotherapy and irradiation are increasingly used to achieve local control in orbital rhabdomyosarcoma, and it is sometimes possible to save the eye. Embryonal and alveolar rhabdomyosarcoma are relatively sensitive to irradiation (particularly embryonal rhabdomyosarcoma), though high doses are required for effective control (50−60 Gy, 5000−6000 rad, over 5−6 weeks).

Chemotherapy has now been established as an important part of treatment both in metastatic and recurrent cases, and also as an adjuvant to local treatment. Many agents are known to produce objective responses in significant numbers of patients, including vinca alkaloids, alkylating agents, actinomycin D, doxorubicin, methotrexate, ifosfamide, cisplatin, carboplatin and etoposide (Table 24.10). Chemotherapy of metastatic disease usually produces only temporary remission. Treatment with combination chemotherapy is preferable using, for example, vincristine, actinomycin D and cyclophosphamide, though actinomycin D

Table 24.10 Chemotherapy in rhabdomyosarcoma in childhood

	Response rate (complete and partial) (%)
Single agents	
Vincristine	30
Actinomycin D	35
Doxorubicin	30
Cyclophosphamide	40
Mitomycin C	35
Cisplatin	33
Ifosfamide	30
Etoposide	20

Combination chemotherapy regimens
Vincristine, actinomycin D, cyclophosphamide
Vincristine, actinomycin D, cyclophosphamide, doxorubicin
Other regimens including cisplatin, ifosfamide and etoposide as part of study protocols especially in poor prognosis disease

should not be given synchronously with radiation because of dangerous recall phenomena, and cyclophosphamide is usually deferred until after radiotherapy because of the danger of myelosuppression. Adjuvant chemotherapy is usually continued for 9−12 months. Localized tumours only require 6 months therapy. Tumours in special sites may require particular treatment strategies; for example, in parameningeal tumours prophylactic treatment with intrathecal chemotherapy and cranial irradiation may be needed.

At present, multicentre studies in both Europe and the United States are attempting to provide answers to several unresolved issues such as the need for radiotherapy, the most acceptable and effective form of adjuvant chemotherapy, and the duration of adjuvant treatment.

PROGNOSIS

With adjuvant chemotherapy, the overall survival rate has improved, and in patients with loco-regional disease (Groups 1−3), 2-year survival rates of up 80% have been reported, compared with a 2-year survival of perhaps 25% before the era of effective chemotherapy. Recurrence tends to occur early, usually (90%) within the first 2 years. The stage of disease is the most important prognostic factor; both the extensiveness of the primary lesion (which will govern the likelihood of resectability) and the presence of metastases affect survival. As with other paediatric tumours, age at presentation also affects prognosis; in one study the median survival for children under 7 years was 78 months, compared with 18 months for older children [12], though the younger children had less extensive disease at the time of diagnosis, and in general a more favourable tumour type (predominantly embryonal rhabdomyosarcoma) than older children. Site may also be important, and orbital tumours in general have a better prognosis although other head and neck tumours, particularly nasopharynx, have a poor prognosis presumably due to their inaccessibility, late presentation and unsuitability for surgical resection as well as propensity for spread to CNS.

Retinoblastoma

INCIDENCE AND INHERITANCE

Retinoblastoma is a rare but important tumour with a familial incidence. The rate appears to have doubled over the past 40 years and it now has a frequency of one case per 15000 live births, accounting for about 3% of all childhood malignancies. Its increasing incidence is due in part to the fact that it is an inherited disease in which survival is increasing, which in turn leads to an increase in the number of children born to previously affected parents.

Most children with retinoblastoma have a normal karyotype. In those with associated mental retardation (see below) a deletion on the long arm of chromosome 13 is present (13q14). Recombinant DNA probes have shown chromosome loss, and loss of heterozygosity at this site in all patients. Tumour formation only occurs when both genes are lost.

The Rb gene codes for a nuclear phosphoprotein which is DNA-binding and which binds to oncoproteins from DNA tumour viruses. The introduction of the normal Rb gene product suppresses tumorogenicity. The Rb gene may be inactivated in other tumours, for example small cell carcinoma of the lung and breast cancer. The gene product appears to have a general cell cycle suppressor function.

Patients with retinoblastoma have a greatly increased likelihood of developing a second tumour. Those with bilateral (inherited) disease have a 20% risk of a non-ocular cancer of which the commonest is osteosarcoma, and occasionally Ewing's sarcoma, Wilms' tumour and soft tissue sarcoma.

Although most cases of retinoblastoma are sporadic (non-familial), retinoblastoma is an important example of a congenital malignancy. It is inherited by an autosomal dominant gene, though some individuals can apparently carry this defective gene without developing the tumour. Sporadic non-familial cases are mostly unilateral, with only a small risk that the offspring of these patients will subsequently develop the disease (Fig. 24.8). However, in the occasional sporadic bilateral case, there is a 50% chance of the offspring developing the disease. In retinoblastoma families, most affected children will themselves develop bilateral disease so that in apparently unilateral familial cases, a close watch must be kept on the contralateral eye. In genetic counselling (Table 24.11) it is also important to recognize that about 4% of normal parents of an affected child produce more than one child with the disease. Retinoblastoma can rarely be associated with mental retardation, microcephaly; and skeletal deformity; a deletion at 13q14 may be observed. A group of patients has been reported in which bilateral retinoblastoma was associated with pinealoblastoma.

PATHOLOGY

Retinoblastoma is typically multifocal. This is presumably due to spread of tumour within the retinal layers, as well as to synchronous tumour development within different parts of the retina in cases of bilateral disease, since spread via

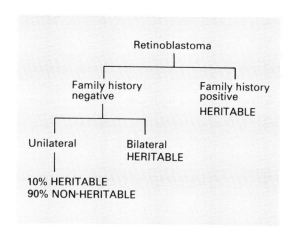

Fig. 24.8 Inheritance of retinoblastoma.

Table 24.11 Genetic counselling in retinoblastoma

Bilateral disease is almost always familial

Offspring of survivors of hereditary retinoblastoma, or of bilateral sporadic cases, will have a 50% chance of developing the tumour

Unaffected parents with a child with unilateral disease have a 1–4% chance of having another affected child

Survivors of unilateral sporadic disease have a 7–10% chance of having an affected child, and are therefore presumed to be silent carriers

If two or more siblings are affected there is a 50% chance that subsequent siblings will have the tumour

Unaffected children from retinoblastoma families may occasionally (5%) carry the gene but if they have an affected child the risk in subsequent children is 50% since the parent is then identified as a silent carrier

the optic nerves and chiasm does not generally occur. The commonest route of spread, particularly of the endophytic type of tumour, is forward into the vitreous humour, and this growth within the globe tends to occur before other involvement of periglobal structures or backwards spread to the intracranial space. Retinal detachment may occur during this process, but extension of growth into the choroid does not usually occur other than with very large tumours. Invasion of the sclera may also occur, carrying a poor prognosis; the optic nerve itself may be directly invaded by the tumour via the lamina cribrosa and thence to the subarachnoid space with dissemination of tumour cells into the CSF and consequent seeding along the base of the brain.

Microscopically, retinoblastoma typically consists of an admixture of undifferentiated and small cells with deeply staining nuclei and scant cytoplasm, though larger cells are often found, sometimes with a tendency to rosette formation around the central cavity. Traditionally this was considered to be a gliomatous tumour, from glial elements derived from spongioblasts though electron microscopy has more recently suggested an origin in the photo-receptor cells.

Blood-borne metastases occur, most commonly to the bone marrow, liver, lymph nodes and lungs.

CLINICAL FEATURES

Most children present under the age of 2 years, usually with a white pupil ('cat's eye reflex'), or less commonly, with strabismus, glaucoma, defects in visual fixation, or inflammatory changes within the eye. Any family history of retinoblastoma should immediately raise suspicion, and the most important investigation is a careful ophthalmological examination by an experienced ophthalmic surgeon. This gives an assessment of tumour site, extent, involvement of the contralateral eye and evidence of multicentricity. Only the ophthalmologist can reliably exclude important non-malignant diseases such as toxocara or retinal dysplasia, though biopsy is accepted as unwise since this may provide a pathway for tumour dissemination.

INVESTIGATION

Tumour calcification may also be present, although this may only be visible radiologically. Chest X-ray, full blood count and isotope bone scanning should be performed in all cases, with CSF examination whenever there is a suspicion of CNS involvement. Orbital CT or MRI scanning and ultrasound may be useful as a means of assessing extensiveness of disease.

STAGING

Size, site and multicentricity of tumour has led to the widely accepted clinical staging system which has now been in clinical use for over 25 years (Table 24.12).

This simple system depends on ophthalmoscopic examination with accurate diagrammatic representation of the retinal lesion in relation to standard reference landmarks such as the optic nerve head, ora serrata (junction of the retina and ciliary body), etc.

Table 24.12 Staging and prognosis (percentage of 3-year survival) in retinoblastoma

Stage I	Single or multiple tumours of size less than 4 disc diameters at or behind the equator (90–100%)
Stage II	Single or multiple tumours of size 4–10 disc diameters at or behind the equator (90–100%)
Stage III	Tumours anterior to the equator or a single tumour larger than 10 disc diameters at or behind the equator (70–85%)
Stage IV	Multiple lesions, some greater than 10 disc diameters. This group includes any lesion extending anteriorly to the ora serrata (70–75%)
Stage V	Massive tumours involving over half the retina, or tumours with vitreous seeding (33–70%)
Stage VI	Residual orbital disease. Extension into the optic nerve and through the sclera (30%)

TREATMENT

Treatment depends on the presenting stage. In recent years treatment philosophy has sharply altered away from immediate or early enucleation of the more severely affected eye, to a more conservative policy with a much greater reliance on radiotherapy as the preferred local technique. The excellent results of this approach (see below) are highly dependent on careful ophthalmological assessment in every case. Eradication of tumour with preservation of vision has in most cases become a realistic aim.

With very small tumours, cryosurgery or photocoagulation are both effective, though with tumours near the optic disc or macula, external beam irradiation is preferable because light coagulation close to these critical parts of the eye carries a risk of permanent visual damage. For these tumours, external irradiation using a single lateral field is both simple and effective.

For larger tumours (3–10 mm) brachytherapy (see Chapter 5) with radioactive cobalt plaques is frequently used, but smaller tumours near the optic disc or macula are better treated with external beam irradiation. With single tumours above 10 mm, external beam irradiation of the whole eye is the treatment of choice, and usually requires multifield treatment to ensure homogeneous irradiation of the whole globe, particularly where there is a risk of vitreous seeding. Use of an anterior field allows for more adequate sparing of the contralateral eye even though the lens and cornea are unavoidably treated. This technique is also suitable where there are multiple tumours confined to one eye. A dose of 35 Gy (3500 rad) in 3–4 weeks is sufficient to control most intra-ocular retinoblastomas.

With obvious infiltration of the optic nerve, enucleation is preferable, though many large but non-invasive tumours have been successfully treated by external irradiation alone.

With bilateral tumours, preservation of sight is more difficult, and it is best to treat each eye individually on its own merits rather than assuming that enucleation of the worse eye will invariably be required. Where there is residual tumour in the orbit, postoperative irradiation should certainly be given to include the whole orbit and optic foramen, and in some cases, where there is a risk of CNS dissemination, whole brain or even craniospinal irradiation should also be considered. A dose of 50 Gy (5000 rad) in 5 weeks is both effective and well tolerated in children requiring postoperative irradiation of the orbit, in whom the radiation tolerance of the eye is no longer a consideration. Particular care is required to ensure immobilization either by means of a head cast, or with sand bags.

In all cases of retinoblastoma, treatment planning must be precise, aiming to cover all areas of disease without unnecessarily jeopardizing the lens of both the affected and the contralateral eye. Fortunately, with the radiation dose required to control most retinoblastomas (35–40 Gy (3500–4000 rad) in 3½–4 weeks), significant complications are now uncommon, though in the early years of radiotherapy, radiation complications were frequent, often producing irreversible loss of vision. The commonest complication, cataract formation, is unavoidable when anterior beams are used, though of course not all cataracts are clinically significant and, if necessary, lens extraction is fairly simple and effective. Vascular injury from irradiation, though easily visible to the ophthalmologist, rarely impairs vision, though occasionally retinal haemorrhage may result in secondary glaucoma which can be troublesome. This is particularly well recognized where a second course of irradiation has been given for recurrent disease. Irreversible damage to the orbital bones may prevent normal growth, a particular problem in infants. Finally, radiation-induced second tumours have been reported in several series, though some retinoblastoma families have a known tendency to develop second malignancies, particularly osteogenic sarcomas at any site within or distant from the irradiated volume. In one large series of nearly 400 patients, the incidence of radiation-induced tumours was over 11%, though many of these patients had received repeated courses of treatment, resulting in enormous doses of irradiation.

PROGNOSIS

The results of treatment are very good (Table 24.12), particularly in early cases and where specialized facilities and experienced clinicians are available. Ninety-percent cure rates are widely achieved and for one large series, children with Stages I and II disease had a cure rate of 100%, and even those with Stages IV and V disease had a cure rate of 75%. When conservative measures have failed, enucleation of the eye can be curative, though there is still a 10–15% overall mortality rate, due to intracranial spread or distant metastases. A few children, successfully treated, will later die from a second radiation-induced tumour (usually osteosarcoma). Limitation of total radiation dose will probably reduce the incidence of this tragic complication of treatment.

For patients with high-risk tumours (including those with extra-ocular metastases at presentation), cytotoxic chemotherapy has been used, either with single agents or with combinations of drugs. Vincristine, actinomycin D, doxorubicin, methotrexate and cyclophosphamide are the drugs most usually employed in combination chemotherapy. The results of treatment for advanced and extra-ocular retinoblastoma are poor and a well-designed study of adjuvant chemotherapy for these high-risk tumours is desirable. Surgical or radiation cure is rare in patients with massive orbital disease or extensive optic nerve involvement at presentation. In these very advanced cases, death is equally likely to result from intracranial involvement as from distant metastases, and although combination chemotherapy, whole brain irradiation and/or intrathecal chemotherapy have undoubtedly produced worthwhile responses, no cures have yet been reported.

Histiocytoses [13]

This is a group of disorders comprising 3–4% of paediatric tumours, whose origin is considered to be from the macrophage/monocyte series of cells. These cells arise in the bone marrow, circulate briefly as blood monocytes and then migrate to tissues where they form fixed macrophages in the liver (Kupffer cells), spleen, lung, bone marrow and tissues (histiocytes). In some ways they behave like cancers since they are often multifocal, sensitive to cytotoxic agents and irradiation, and can be fatal.

The classification of histiocytoses has recently been altered and is now based on the nature of the histiocytic infiltrate.

1 Class 1 histiocytosis is characterized by the presence of the Langerhans' cell. These cells may not be genuinely malignant and may respond to immunological mediators. Under electron microscopy the cells show typical Birbeck granules. Opinion is still divided as to whether this is a malignant disease. In some cases, however, monoclonality of cells has been demonstrated.

2 Class 2 lesions are characterized by a reactive macrophage infiltrate (the normal nodal architecture being preserved).

3 Class 3 is a malignant histiocytic tumour, including monocytic leukaemia. These are discussed in Chapter 28.

LANGERHANS' CELL HISTIOCYTOSIS (LCH, CLASS 1 HISTIOCYTOSIS)

This used to be called histiocytosis X, which included the spectrum of syndromes of Letterer−Siwe disease, eosinophilic granuloma and Hand−Schüller−Christian disease. Letterer−Siwe disease, an acute disease with its onset in infancy, is characterized by hepatosplenomegaly, lymph node enlargement, thrombocytopenia and skin rash. A greasy, scaly, scalp or nappy (diaper) rash is usually the presenting feature. Widespread infiltration of the skin, liver, lungs, spleen and bone marrow gives rise to hepatic dysfunction, dyspnoea and marrow failure. Lytic lesions in bone are common. The form of the disease previously called eosinophilic granuloma forms a spectrum ranging from a single, isolated bone lesion, typically in older children, to multiple punched-out bone lesions. The prognosis is worse below the age of 3 years. Presentation is usually with bone pain or lymphadenopathy. The disease may regress spontaneously. Other patients present with multiple eosinophilic granulomas. Occasionally, diabetes insipidus may occur, due to pituitary involvement as well as exophthalmos from orbital deposits (Hand−Schüller−Christian disease). Enlargement of liver and spleen occurs, as does skin infiltration, but the disease is less aggressive than Letterer−Siwe disease. As with eosinophilic granuloma, the disease may become quiescent and does not usually relapse if the activity ceases for 3−4 years. Diabetes insipidus is permanent, and chronic neurological disability may occur as may cirrhosis with portal hypertension.

Mortality is highest in infants and in children with organ infiltration (lung, liver, bone marrow). Single bone lesions can be treated by curettage and local steroid injection. Radiation in low dosage is often dramatically effective but carries the risk of bone sarcoma in later life. More generalized disease can be treated with cytotoxic drugs of which the most useful are prednisolone, vinblastine, etoposide, chlorambucil and methotrexate. However, the disease may follow a very indolent course and may even remit completely even without treatment and it is important to avoid toxicity. In many cases (especially those where the disease is confined to the bone or skin) treatment can be withheld for long periods of time.

Rare paediatric tumours

The tumours described above, the intracranial tumours of childhood, and the leukaemias and lymphomas, constitute 92% of all childhood malignancies; the remaining 8% are made up of a variety of uncommon diseases seen only sporadically even in large paediatric centres. Some, such as hepatoblastoma and orchioblastoma are rare but 'genuine' paediatric tumours whereas others, such as adenocarcinoma of the kidney or transitional cell carcinoma of the bladder are essentially adult tumours seen very rarely in the paediatric age group. The principles of management of these rare paediatric malignancies are not yet clearly established. The importance of a joint approach with full pretreatment assessment by paediatric surgeon, radiotherapist and paediatric oncologist (working closely with a histopathologist with special experience in these tumours), cannot be emphasized too strongly.

Germ cell tumours

All of the adult germ cell tumours (see Chapters

17 & 19) are occasionally seen in childhood. In addition, specific childhood forms occur though none is common.

SACROCOCCYGEAL GERM CELL TUMOURS

These are the most common germ cell tumours of childhood and the commonest tumour of the newborn. The female : male ratio is 4 : 1. Clinically, there is a large swelling between the coccyx and rectum, and the tumour arises on the inner margin of the distal part of the coccyx. Approximately 10% of tumours in the newborn are malignant, but above 3 months of age 50% are malignant. The tumour should be surgically excised, but if there are malignant elements (embryonal carcinoma, choriocarcinoma), chemotherapy should be given despite its toxicity in infants.

HEAD AND NECK GERM CELL TUMOURS

Ten per cent of childhood teratomas arise in the head and neck. The sites are very variable (orbit, soft tissue, nasopharynx), and they may cause respiratory obstruction. Treatment is with surgery and chemotherapy (if malignant). Pineal teratomas are discussed in Chapter 11.

TESTICULAR GERM CELL TUMOURS

The main histological variants are the yolk sac tumour (endodermal sinus tumour, Teilum tumour, orchioblastoma), embryonal carcinoma and differentiated tumour. Below the age of 2 years, yolk sac tumours are probably less likely to metastasize than in older children. The differentiated tumours are benign. Before effective chemotherapy was available, 9% of children under 2 years old were alive 2 years after treatment, while only 25% of older children survived. This difference may be less marked since the advent of platinum-based chemotherapy. The management follows the guidelines outlined for adult testicular tumours (see Chapter 19).

SEX CORD AND STROMAL TUMOURS OF THE TESTIS

Leydig cell tumours and Sertoli cell tumours occur rarely, the Leydig cell tumour at age 4–5 years and the Sertoli cell tumour below the age of 2 years. Leydig cell tumours which may be accompanied by testicular virilization, are slow growing and cured by orchidectomy. Sertoli cell tumours may cause feminization, and orchidectomy is adequate treatment.

Gonadoblastomas are very rare tumours, chiefly found in patients with testicular feminization (XY or XY/XO karyotype with dysgenetic gonads and feminine phenotypes).

The tumour develops in an abnormal gonad which is frequently indeterminate or no more than a rudimentary streak. The testes may be maldescended, in which case they are present in the inguinal canals or abdomen.

OVARIAN GERM CELL TUMOURS

The classification of these tumours is discussed in Chapter 17. Dysgerminomas, embryonal carcinoma and teratoma are managed as outlined in Chapter 17; as in adults, surgery and combination chemotherapy are the major modalities though radiotherapy is important in dysgerminoma.

Hepatoblastoma

This tumour is discussed on p. 292.

LATE SEQUELAE OF TREATMENT OF CANCER IN CHILDHOOD

As more children and adolescents survive cancer, we are becoming increasingly aware of late effects of treatment. The importance of these problems has, in turn, led to a re-examination of the primary treatment in some stages of some tumours, if the same survival can be achieved at less long-term cost. There are three areas of particular concern: effects on growth, gonadal function and the occurrence of second cancers.

Growth [13]

Studies in acute lymphoblastic leukaemia (ALL) where both chemotherapy and prophylactic cranial irradiation were administered have shown significant decreases in height during treatment, which is regained to a varying degree when treatment stops. The site of damage is not definitely known but growth hormone (GH) deficiency and a lack of responsiveness of the epiphysis to GH, induced by chemotherapy, certainly plays a part. In children treated with radiation for brain tumours, growth retardation is greater in those who are also given chemotherapy. It is not known which cytotoxic agents are most likely to produce growth impairment.

Radiation of a growing epiphysis results in an arrest of bone growth at that site. The dose required to produce a permanent closure of the epiphysis is not known with certainty but most schedules of treatment for cancer will do so. In a young child this may lead to a gross disparity in limb length, failure of development of the spine (after mantle treatment for Hodgkin's disease, for example) or asymmetry of the chest wall.

Gonadal function [14]

Children treated with nitrosoureas and procarbazine for brain tumours have a high incidence of gonadal dysfunction. Although puberty progresses normally, follicle stimulating hormone (FSH) levels are high (and LH to a lesser degree). In later life the boys have small testes and severe oligospermia. In girls ovarian function appears to return to normal and prospects for fertility are good. It is not known if their menopause will be premature. In some ALL protocols spinal irradiation may affect either the ovaries or the testes.

In boys who do not receive alkylating agents there is much less germinal epithelial damage. If MOPP therapy has been given for Hodgkin's

Table 24.13 Relative risk of bone cancer according to primary diagnosis [14]

Diagnosis	Relative risk
Retinoblastoma	1000 ×
Ewing's sarcoma	650 ×
Rhabdomyosarcoma	300 ×
Wilms' tumour	125 ×
Hodgkin's disease	100 ×

disease severe oligospermia and high FSH levels are the rule. Damage appears to be less long lasting if treatment is given prepubertally.

Second cancers

The possibility of inducing a second cancer by treatment is particularly important in childhood cancers because of the long period of risk. One of the commonest types of second cancer is bone sarcoma [15], and the relative risk depends on the primary diagnosis (Table 24.13). The secondary cancer is usually osteosarcoma and it typically develops in the radiation field (though this is not the case in the inherited form of retinoblastoma (Fig. 24.8)).

Acute non-lymphoblastic leukaemia may develop after treatment with chemotherapy — alkylating agents and nitrosoureas appear to be the drugs most likely to be associated. The risk seems higher after treatment for Hodgkin's disease (where radiation is often also given). Leukaemia is also more common after brain tumour treatment. Overall the relative risk of leukaemia determined by the Late Effects Study Group was 14-fold [16].

REFERENCES

1 Stiller C.A. Centralisation of treatment and survival rates for cancer. *Archives of Diseases in Childhood* 1988; **6**: 3−23.
2 Pritchard F., Stiller C.A., Lennox E.L. Overtreatment of children with Wilms' tumour outside paediatric oncology centres. *British Medical Journal* 1989; **299**: 835−36.
3 Herbst A.L., Robboy S.J., Scully R.E., Poskanzer D.C.

Clear cell adeno-carcinoma of the vagina and cervix in girls: Analysis of 170 registry cases. *American Journal of Obstetrics and Gynecology* 1974; **119**: 713−24.

4 Li F.P., Tucker M.A., Fraumeni J.F. Childhood cancer in siblings. *Journal of Pediatrics* 1976; **88**: 419−23.

5 Breslow N., McCann B. Statistical estimation of prognosis for children with neuroblastoma. *Cancer Research* 1971; **31**: 2098−2103.

6 Brodeur G.M., Seeger R.C., Barrett A. *et al*. International criteria for diagnosis, staging and response to treatment in patients with neuroblastoma. *Journal of Clinical Oncology* 1988; **6**: 1874−81.

7 Evans A.E., D'Angio G.H. Prognostic factors in neuroblastoma. *Cancer* 1987; **59**: 1853−59.

8 Dini G., Philip T., Hartmann O. *et al*. Bone marrow transplantation for neuroblastoma: a review of 509 cases. *Bone Marrow Transplantation* 1989; **4** (suppl. 4): 42−46.

9 Bolane R.P. Congenital and infantile neoplasia of the kidney. *Lancet* 1974; **ii**: 1497−99.

10 Wolff J.A. Advances in the treatment of Wilms' tumor.

Cancer 1975; **35**: 901−4.

11 D'Angio G.J., Breslow N., Beckwith J.B. *et al*. Treatment of Wilms' tumour: Results of the third National Wilms' Tumour Study. *Cancer* 1989; **64**: 349−60.

12 Maurer H.M., Beltangady M., Gehan E.A. *et al*. The Intergroup Rhabdomyosarcoma Study 1. A final report. *Cancer* 1988; **61**: 209−20.

13 Clayton P.E., Shalet S.M., Morris-Jones P. *et al*. Growth in children treated for acute lymphoblastic leukaemia. *Lancet* 1988; **i**: 460−62.

14 Livesey E.A., Brook C.G.D. Gonadal dysfunction after treatment of intracranial tumours. *Archives of Diseases in Childhood* 1988; **63**: 495−500.

15 Tucker M.A., D'Angio G.J., Boice J.D. *et al*. Bone sarcoma linked to chemotherapy and radiotherapy in children. *New England Journal of Medicine* 1987; **317**: 588−93.

16 Meadows A.T., Baum E., Bellani-Fossati F. *et al*. Second malignant neoplasms in children: An update from the Late Effects Study Group. *Journal of Clinical Oncology* 1985; **3**: 532−38.

Chapter 25
Hodgkin's Disease

In the last 25 years the prognosis of Hodgkin's disease has greatly improved, both for patients with localized disease who are often curable by radiotherapy, and for those with disseminated disease treated with cytotoxic drugs. Success has not only been achieved because of the introduction of entirely new methods of treatment, but also because it has become increasingly apparent how radiotherapy and chemotherapy can be employed to best advantage. There have also been improvements in staging techniques and a better understanding of the patterns of spread which have led to more rational treatment. In this respect Hodgkin's disease has been a model which has led to improvements in management of other malignant tumours.

INCIDENCE AND EPIDEMIOLOGY

The incidence of Hodgkin's disease rises steeply from the age of 10–20 years. There is a slight fall in middle age, followed by a rise after 50 years to reach a maximum at age 70 years and over (Fig. 25.1). The male:female ratio in Western countries is about 1.5:1. Although the incidence varies in different parts of the world the male predominance usually holds (Table 25.1).

While the reliability of cancer statistics differs from country to country, the reported variation in incidence appears to reflect genuine differences in the frequency of the disease rather than in the accuracy of diagnosis [1]. In some countries such as Colombia and Nigeria the incidence in childhood (age 5–14) is five times that in Britain, but in adult life it is four times

Table 25.1 Hodgkin's disease. Annual incidence rates (per 100 000) in various countries

	Male	Female
England	2.2	1.3
USA		
Whites	2.3	1.4
African-Americans	1.3	0.7
Japan	0.6	0.3
Ceylon	0.1	0.1

less common. In these countries the history also tends to be less favourable compared with Western Europe and North America. In Japan and possibly other Far East countries, the incidence appears to be substantially lower than in the West.

AETIOLOGY

Genetic, family and social factors

There have been several studies on the association of Hodgkin's disease with histocompatibility antigens, but the results have been conflicting. In part this is due to technical problems with typing reagents and in selection of cases for analysis. In prospective studies of unselected cases, HLA-A1 has been shown to occur with a marginally increased frequency compared with controls, and HLA-A12 in younger patients with good histology.

There have been many reports of families where two or more members have developed Hodgkin's disease, sometimes with presen-

Fig. 25.1 Hodgkin's disease. Age-specific incidence.

tation is very close in time. In the family of a patient the risk of siblings having the disease is greater than normal, possibly about six times that of the normal population, with siblings of the same sex are most likely to be affected [2]. The meaning of rare but dramatic clusters of cases is unknown but suggests an environmental rather than a genetic cause. There is no definite relationship with social class although there have been suggestions that it may be commoner in classes.

Some studies have suggested an increased incidence of Hodgkin's disease among woodworkers in the United States, but this is not the case in Britain. Schoolmates and health care personnel have been stated to be at higher risk of exposure to a hypothetical, transmissible, causative agent. Carefully designed and controlled studies have not confirmed this [3].

Infections

The infectious agent which has the strongest claim to an association with Hodgkin's disease

is the Epstein–Barr virus (EBV). Infectious mononucleosis (which is caused by EBV) has often been reported as occurring immediately before the presentation of Hodgkin's disease. Cells similar to Reed–Sternberg (RS) cells have been found in lymph node biopsies from patients with infectious mononucleosis. However, case–control studies (see Chapter 2) have failed to show an association, but cohort studies have usually done so although the increased risk appears marginal and such studies do not constitute proof of a causal connection. EBV genome can be detected by southern hybridization in 40% of all cases. The positive cases are the European form of EBV. RS cells also express EBV latent membrane protein. The proportion of cases expressing EBV is lowest in nodular sclerosing disease and in the 15–35 age range. The role of EBV remains open. It is possible that it is one of several causative or contributing agents. It is also possible that abnormal immune responses may make an individual more susceptible both to EBV infection and Hodgkin's disease.

There have been many attempts to find evidence that retroviruses (e.g. RNA tumour viruses, see Chapter 3) are involved in the aetiology of Hodgkin's disease. Sequences of DNA homologous with murine leukaemia virus RNA have been reported in extracts of spleen from patients with Hodgkin's disease, but not in normal spleen. The interpretation of this finding is open to question, however, since neoplastic cells constitute only a small proportion of the cells in spleens involved with Hodgkin's disease.

PATHOLOGY

The Reed–Sternberg (RS) cell

Lymph nodes from patients with Hodgkin's disease contain two categories of cells. The first is the cell which is the hallmark of the disease and which is thought to be the malignant component — the RS cell or its mononuclear counterpart (Fig. 25.2). The second category

Fig. 25.2 Section of a lymph node in Hodgkin's disease, showing typical binucleate Reed−Sternberg cell and mononuclear Hodgkin's cell (×400 original magnification).

consists of a pleomorphic cellular infiltrate, the composition of which varies considerably in different patients.

The malignant cells are large, often with slightly basophilic cytoplasm. The nuclei are usually lobulated and there may be two or more in a single cell. The classical RS cell has two or more nuclei usually with large nucleoli which are acidophilic. The mononuclear variety of cell is sometimes seen in reactive inflammatory nodes, and cells with a similar appearance to RS cells may occasionally be found in infective lesions (infectious mononucleosis) and a variety of other lymphoproliferative disorders such as phenytoin-induced lymph node enlargement and non-Hodgkin's lymphoma. The RS cells have some of the cytological characteristics of the dendritic cells which are found in the paracortical region of normal lymph nodes. In spite of intensive investigation the origin of the malignant cell in Hodgkin's disease has not yet been elucidated. The reason for, and significance of, the infiltrate of normal cells which make up the bulk of the nodal enlargement in the disorder is similarly obscure.

The techniques of immunohistochemistry and molecular genetics have been used in Hodgkin's disease in an attempt to characterize the RS cell. Immunophenotyping using a variety of B-cell reacting monoclonal antibodies frequently shows B cell characteristics in RS cells. CD20 and CD15 are usually expressed. Light chain restricted immunoglobulin expression has now been shown in the Hodgkin's cells in nodular lymphocyte predominant Hodgkin's disease (an unusual variant which may terminate in a B cell lymphoma after many years). CD30, an activation antigen on lymphoid cells, is strongly expressed on RS cells (and on other lymphomas and so-called Ki-1 positive lymphomas). Soluble ED30 is found in the serum of untreated patients.

T cell markers and T cell receptor gene rearrangement may also be found on RS cells. It is not clear if this implies that RS cells can be cells of different lineages since T cell receptor gene rearrangement can be detected in some of the B cell neoplasms.

To date no consistent karyotypic abnormality has been found in Hodgkin's disease although a variety of chromosomal translocations have been detected.

Classification

The histological classification which is now widely used is based on the Lukes−Butler scheme [4] which divides the microscopic appearance into four categories.

1 *Lymphocyte predominant.* The appearances are of small lymphocytes with scarce RS cells and their mononuclear variants. Some cases of lymphocyte predominant disease (the 'nodular' forms) are possibly a variety of B cell lymphoma, as described above, relapsing late as a high-grade B cell lymphoma.

2 *Nodular sclerosis.* There are broad bands of collagen (not simply fibrosis) separating cellular nodules of Hodgkin's disease. Nodular sclerosing disease has been subcategorized into two groups (1 and 2) where 1 has a lymphocyte predominant infiltrate in the nodules and 2 has

a more pleomorphic appearance with numerous RS cells. In one report patients in group 1 had a better prognosis [5], although this is not fully confirmed.

3 *Mixed cellularity.* The infiltrate is pleomorphic with lymphocytes, macrophages, eosinophils and polymorphs.

4 *Lymphocyte depleted.* There is either diffuse fibrosis with fewer RS cells, or a reticular type with numerous RS cells or their mononuclear variant.

The nodular sclerosing and mixed cellularity categories make up 80–90% of all cases. Prognostically, lymphocyte predominant histology is most favourable and lymphocyte depleted least so. Mixed cellularity is generally considered to be a histological appearance with less favourable prognosis than nodular sclerosis, but this is not the case in patients with advanced disease treated with chemotherapy.

Sometimes the pathologist has great difficulty in deciding if the patient has Hodgkin's disease or not and mistakes can occur. The clinician should be very careful in cases which have atypical histology obtained from non-nodal sites, and with clinically odd presentations such as isolated disease presenting in the gut or skin. The differential histological diagnosis includes:

• reactive nodes with immunoblasts which may be seen in infectious mononucleosis, other herpes virus infections, or toxoplasmosis;
• hypersensitivity to drugs such as phenytoin;
• angio-immunoblastic lymphadenopathy (see Chapter 26);
• T cell lymphoma (see Chapter 26);
• metastatic melanoma; and
• non-Hodgkin's lymphoma, particularly the distinction from sclerosing B cell mediastinal lymphoma and Ki-1 lymphoma (Chapter 26, p. 519).

In patients with proven Hodgkin's disease, other histological abnormalities may be found. For example at staging laparotomy, the spleen or liver may show granulomatous infiltration of unknown cause. A further example may occur after intensive chemotherapy when the lymph nodes may show an unusual appearance, with vascular invasion and atypical, lymphocyte-depleted histology with few inflammatory elements — appearances similar to a non-Hodgkin's lymphoma.

ABNORMAL IMMUNITY IN HODGKIN'S DISEASE

It has long been recognized that host defence against infection is abnormal in advanced Hodgkin's disease even before treatment. Radiotherapy and chemotherapy can impair these defence mechanisms still further. An increased susceptibility to tuberculosis was noted in 1932 and subsequently it was confirmed that the tuberculin skin test was frequently negative in Hodgkin's disease. These observations have been extended and it is now clear that depressed delayed-hypersensitivity reactions to a variety of antigens including candida, mumps and histoplasmin are frequently found. These impaired responses are more common in patients with advanced disease and with constitutional symptoms. When attempts are made to induce delayed hypersensitivity to artificial antigens such as dinitrochlorobenzene (DNCB), it is frequently found that there is anergy to the antigen, particularly in patients with more advanced disease. *In vitro* tests have not yet elucidated the nature of the defective cell-mediated immunity.

The cause of these abnormalities remains obscure but there is little doubt that patients with Hodgkin's disease are especially susceptible to opportunistic infections. These include infections with bacteria such as pseudomonas and tuberculosis, fungi such as candida and aspergillus, and viruses such as herpes zoster and herpes simplex. In all of these diseases, susceptibility is probably due to depressed cell-mediated immunity.

The more advanced the disease, the greater the likelihood of anergy, but there is little clinical value in tests of immune competence as part of the routine investigation of a newly diagnosed case. The degree of spread of the disease is better assessed by more straightforward investigations.

The treatment of patients with advanced disease with cytotoxic drugs is hazardous for many reasons; one of the most important is the profound additional depression of immunity which may lead to fatal infection.

THE CLINICAL FEATURES

In the vast majority of cases the clinical presentation is straightforward [6]. The patient has accidentally noticed an enlarged, painless lymph node in the neck or elsewhere, and a biopsy gives the diagnosis. The initial site of presentation (Fig. 25.3) includes cervical nodes (70% of all cases), axilla (25%) and inguinal area (10%). The lymph nodes usually grow slowly and are sometimes visible on photographs months or years before being noticed by a patient. Occasionally the nodes are

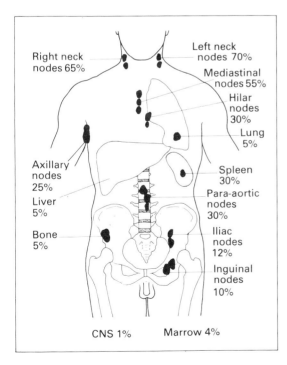

Fig. 25.3 Frequency of sites of involvement at presentation in patients with Hodgkin's disease.

Right neck nodes 65%
Left neck nodes 70%
Mediastinal nodes 55%
Hilar nodes 30%
Lung 5%
Axillary nodes 25%
Spleen 30%
Para-aortic nodes 30%
Liver 5%
Bone 5%
Iliac nodes 12%
Inguinal nodes 10%
CNS 1%   Marrow 4%

described as growing very rapidly and sometimes they are tender if there has been a recent upper respiratory infection. The nodes may fluctuate in size with such infections and may mislead the physician into believing that the node enlargement is only inflammatory.

Twenty-five per cent of all patients have constitutional symptoms at presentation. Fever is the commonest of these and is generally of low grade but may occasionally be hectic, up to 40°C, which usually occurs in the evening and falls to normal in the morning. In advanced disease, bouts of fever lasting 1 or 2 weeks may occur (Pel−Ebstein fever) but this is unusual and not specific for Hodgkin's disease. Drenching sweats may occur at night, waking the patient from sleep. Lesser degrees of sweating occur in many normal individuals and are hard to evaluate. Weight loss occurs, as in any other malignancy, but is especially associated with advanced or bulky disease. The triad of constitutional symptoms (fever, sweats and more than 10% loss of body weight), is of very great importance since cases with one or more of these have a much poorer prognosis.

Generalized pruritus occurs in 5−10% of patients at the time of presentation, but many patients will develop this symptom during the course of the disease when it relapses. If severe, it can be a most disabling symptom, the skin becoming excoriated from scratching, especially at night. The cause is unclear although release of histamine by the tumour has been postulated. The symptom abates with successful treatment. Alcohol-induced pain is felt in involved lymph nodes in a very small number of patients (2−5%). It is aching or stabbing in nature, comes on within minutes of drinking and lasts from a few minutes to an hour [7]. It is chiefly associated with mediastinal disease of nodular sclerosing histology.

Other rare systemic features of Hodgkin's disease include autoimmune haemolytic anaemia (although a positive antiglobulin test in the absence of haemolysis is more common) and immune thrombocytopenia. A variety of erythematous skin rashes may occur, including erythroderma, erythema multiforme, psoriasiform lesions and bullous eruptions.

Enlarged nodes may produce symptoms due to compression. Examples include limb oedema and pain due to nerve entrapment; cough, stridor or superior vena caval obstruction from mediastinal disease; obstruction of the inferior vena cava or the ureters by para-aortic nodes; obstructive jaundice due to nodes in the porta hepatis. Internal mammary node enlargement may give rise to a chest wall mass in the para-sternal region. In contrast to non-Hodgkin's lymphoma the tonsil and Waldeyer's ring are rarely involved, and when this does occur it is usually associated with upper cervical node involvement.

Hodgkin's disease occasionally presents as a pulmonary lesion and then must be distinguished from infection or other bronchial neoplasms by sputum cytology, culture and biopsy. Endobronchial Hodgkin's disease is very rare — the clinical features being wheezing and haemoptysis. Much more commonly, pulmonary infiltration occurs from direct spread from enlarged hilar or mediastinal nodes. Pulmonary nodules of Hodgkin's disease are easily missed on conventional chest X-rays, and whole-lung tomograms or CT scans are very useful when the diagnosis is in doubt. Pleural infiltration usually presents as an effusion, and is nearly always associated with mediastinal and pulmonary disease. If the mediastinal disease is massive, the pleural effusion may be due to lymphatic obstruction rather than direct invasion by tumour. The same is true for chylous effusions. A diagnosis of pleural infiltration can only be made reliably by biopsy or by a CT scan showing nodules of tumour in the pleura or subpleural lung. Cytological examination is usually unrewarding since RS cells are rarely found.

Bone marrow involvement occurs at presentation in approximately 5% of patients and is nearly always associated with widespread disease elsewhere, and with constitutional symptoms. The diagnosis is by marrow trephine biopsy. The number of positive routine marrow biopsies in patients with early stage disease is very small, but a normal blood count does not preclude involvement in those with advanced disease. Marrow involvement is, however, more likely if there is anaemia, thrombocytopenia or leucopenia. The disease is focal within the marrow so false-negative biopsies are frequent.

Occasionally the bones are involved in a more localized way by Hodgkin's disease, either by direct spread from adjacent nodes, or by metastatic spread (in which case there is usually widespread disease elsewhere). The commonest histology is nodular sclerosis. The presentation is with pain, the serum alkaline phosphatase is elevated, X-rays may show either osteoblastic or osteolytic lesions, and an isotope bone scan is positive. A solitary bone deposit does not necessarily indicate Stage IV disease (i.e. diffuse involvement of an extranodal tissue, see Table 25.2) and may respond to local treatment, with a good prognosis.

Skin and subcutaneous infiltration are uncommon as presenting features but may occur in the context of aggressive disease over lymph node masses or in their drainage areas. The nodules of tumour are often painless but may ulcerate. Subcutaneous lesions may occur in the breasts. Primary cutaneous Hodgkin's disease is a great rarity.

When Hodgkin's disease involves the central nervous system it is usually spinal rather than cerebral. This is a rare presentation and usually occurs by extension through the intervertebral foramina from adjacent lymph nodes to cause epidural compression. The clinical features are of root pain, paraesthesiae or spinal cord compression. All are medical emergencies because there is a serious risk of paraplegia (see Chapter 8). Laminectomy and radiotherapy are the normal methods of diagnosis and treatment. If the diagnosis is known, prompt treatment with radiotherapy alone is usually adequate. Compression of the spinal cord may be localized and does not necessarily constitute an indication for chemotherapy. Rarely, Hodgkin's disease may present with leptomeningeal spread, with a clinical syndrome of basal malignant meningitis causing cranial nerve palsies, or symptoms and signs of raised intracranial pressure.

The gut is rarely the primary site of Hodgkin's disease and the diagnosis should be viewed with suspicion, since gastro-intestinal non-Hodgkin's lymphomas are so much more common. Nevertheless, there are isolated cases of the disease arising in the oesophagus, stomach, small and large bowel. The presentation is usually indistinguishable from other tumours at these sites. When the disease occurs in the small bowel it usually affects the terminal ileum and may cause malabsorption syndrome.

The urinary tract is seldom clinically involved, and the commonest manifestation is ureteric compression with hydronephrosis. It is very unusual for direct renal infiltration to be clinically apparent. Rarely, cases of nephrotic syndrome occur, which are due to immune complex glomerulonephritis or to compression of the renal veins by tumour masses.

Hodgkin's disease may be accompanied by paraneoplastic syndromes. In the central nervous system, patients may rarely develop progressive multifocal leucoencephalopathy. This is a relentless, fatal, demyelinating disorder, now known to be caused by a papovavirus and characterized by dementia, disorientation and focal signs leading to coma and death. Subacute cerebellar degeneration has also been recorded, with progressive ataxia, especially truncal ataxia, due to degeneration of Purkinje cells in the vermis. The Guillain−Barré syndrome occurs in the disease more commonly than would be expected by chance. There are a few cases of segmental, granulomatous angiitis in the brain, which may respond to treatment of Hodgkin's disease and which are possibly related to varicella-zoster infection. These paraneoplastic syndromes are discussed further in Chapter 9.

PATTERNS OF SPREAD

In early Hodgkin's disease some lymph node groups are much more commonly involved than others (Fig. 25.3). By far the commonest site of presentation is the neck, while involvement of mesenteric nodes is rare. Following localized treatment, adjacent lymph nodes are the most frequent sites of relapse, a finding which led to the introduction of extended field radiotherapy. In more detailed analyses, certain patterns of spread have been found (bilateral cervical node enlargement is unusual unless there is also mediastinal disease; mediastinal disease is itself frequently associated with involved neck nodes). Nodular sclerosing Hodgkin's disease in the mediastinum is more frequently found in women and is not usually associated with subdiaphragmatic disease. Splenic involvement is uncommon when the presentation is with isolated inguinal node enlargement. In the abdomen the coeliac plexus is the commonest site of node involvement [8].

When the disease involves the liver or bone marrow, splenic disease is nearly always present; involvement of the liver with sparing of the spleen is so unusual that the pathological findings should be questioned. It is not clear if splenic involvement is a source of dissemination although vascular invasion in splenic Hodgkin's disease may signify a worse prognosis.

STAGING CLASSIFICATION

As with many cancers, the adoption of a generally agreed staging notation has been of immense value for a number of reasons. First, because it has encouraged clinicians to compare like with like in trials of treatment; second, because stage correlates closely with prognosis; and finally because it focuses attention, in individual cases of the disease, on the importance of knowing the degree of spread of the disorder before considering the treatment options. Nevertheless, it is surprising how commonly the process of 'staging the patient' is regarded as an end in itself without regard to the value of the information gained by what are often expensive, uncomfortable and sometimes dangerous investigations. Understanding the full extent of the disease is only important if it will influence treatment. In Hodgkin's disease this is often, but not always, the case. The Ann Arbor classification [9] is widely used as a description of clinical or pathological stage and is outlined in Table 25.2. This staging notation (with explanatory notes) is used throughout this chapter.

There is a distinction to be made between the anatomical description of the extent of the disease on the basis of clinical examination, routine chest X-ray, lymphangiography and isotope scans (clinical stage) and the description based on information obtained by biopsy and laparotomy (pathological stage). The former is obviously likely to underestimate the extent of the disease, especially in patients with more aggressive disease and those with constitutional symptoms.

When comparison is made between the results of clinical and pathological staging (based on laparotomy) it is generally found that for each clinical stage there is a 25–30% chance of error as judged by pathological stage (Table 25.3). While most of these errors are the result of underestimation of the extent of disease using clinical criteria, some patients in whom disease is judged to be widespread are shown to have less extensive disease on pathological staging. An example of this 'down-staging' of disease is seen in patients who have a palpable spleen but no evidence of histological involvement at laparotomy.

INVESTIGATION

Haematology and biochemistry

Full blood counts are normal in most patients with localized nodal disease without constitutional symptoms (Stages IA and IIA). Mild anaemia, polymorphonuclear leucocytosis and a high erythrocyte sedimentation rate (ESR) are more common with advanced disease. The anaemia is usually normochromic or slightly hypochromic and is typical of the anaemia of chronic disease. Rarely, autoimmune haemo-

Table 25.2 Ann Arbor staging classification for Hodgkin's disease

Staging classification

Stage I	Involvement of a single lymph node region or of a single extralymphatic site or organ
Stage II	Involvement of two or more node regions on the same side of the diaphragm, or of a localized extranodal involvement and one or more lymph node regions on the same side of the diaphragm (IIE)
Stage III	Involvement of lymph nodes on both sides of the diaphragm which may include the spleen (IIIS) or a localized extranodal site (IIIE) or both (IIISE)
Stage IV	Diffuse involvement of one or more extralymphatic organs

Notes

1 Suffix A: no constitutional symptoms. Suffix B: constitutional symptoms present. These are fevers, night sweats and/or loss of 10% or more of body weight over 6 months. Pruritus is not included
2 Localized extranodal involvement can at times be difficult to distinguish from Stage IV disease. A good working rule is that localized spread means that the lesion in question could still be treated with radiotherapy
3 Stage III disease can be usefully subdivided according to the extent of intra-abdominal node involvement. Stage III_1 means involvement of spleen, splenic, coeliac or portal nodes or any combinations of these. Stage III_2 means involvement of para-aortic, iliac or mesenteric nodes with or without upper abdominal disease
4 In the case of the marrow or liver, diffuse involvement means the demonstration of any amount of unequivocal Hodgkin's disease since localized spread at these sites is not recognized and radiotherapy not regarded as a treatment option

lytic anaemia may occur at presentation. Lymphopenia usually signifies advanced disease but eosinophilia, which occurs in a few patients, has no prognostic significance. The ESR is a somewhat unreliable guide to extent and activity of disease but a high ESR (above 40) is usually associated with more widespread disease.

Liver enzymes and plasma bilirubin are often

Table 25.3 Clinical versus laparotomy (pathological) staging

	Positive at laparotomy	Negative at laparotomy
Spleen		
Clinically* + ve	50	50
Clinically − ve	24	76
Overall	28	72
Liver		
Clinically + ve	6	94
Clinically − ve	2	98
Overall	3	97
Abdominal nodes		
Clinically + ve	73	27
Clinically − ve	14	86
Overall	29	71

* Clinically positive means definitely abnormal lymphogram, hepatomegaly or splenomegaly.

abnormal with hepatic involvement, but isolated, modest elevation in aspartate transaminase or glutamyl transpeptidase sometimes occurs in the absence of proven involvement. The plasma alkaline phosphatase is often elevated, particularly in patients with advanced disease. Usually it is the liver isoenzyme which is responsible but bone phosphatase may sometimes be contributory. An elevated alkaline phosphatase is not conclusive evidence of extensive disease if it is an isolated finding.

Routine X-rays

CHEST X-RAY

The chest X-ray is an essential examination. Enlargement of mediastinal and bronchopulmonary lymph nodes is very common and the anatomical distribution of the lymph node groups is shown in Fig. 25.4. Mediastinal adenopathy is particularly common in women with nodular sclerosing disease. Massive mediastinal node enlargement may occur, leading to superior vena caval obstruction (Fig.

25.5). The thymus may be involved and often the mass projects laterally to the right and is seen anteriorly on lateral films. The bronchopulmonary lymph nodes may be enlarged with more subtle radiological changes. Usually there is associated mediastinal node enlargement.

The pulmonary changes may be due to compression of a bronchus, direct intrapulmonary extension from a lymph node mass or less commonly, to localized intrapulmonary Hodgkin's disease. Bronchial compression may cause atelectasis of a whole lobe with associated consolidation within the collapsed area. Direct extension from lymph nodes (Fig. 25.6) is not infrequent. In patients who have been treated with radiation to mediastinal nodes, extension of the disease into the lung may be very difficult to distinguish radiologically from radiation pneumonitis and fibrosis. Tuberculosis and other infections may produce similar radiological appearances. A chest X-ray may also

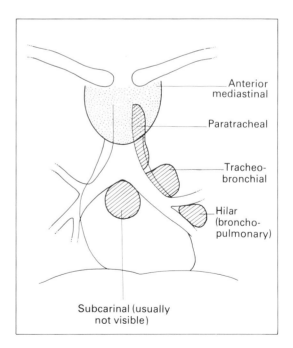

Fig. 25.4 Anatomical distribution of the major lymph node groups which may be involved in Hodgkin's disease.

Fig. 25.5 Chest X-ray showing a very large, well-defined mediastinal mass. The patient was a woman of 22, with nodular sclerosing Hodgkin's disease.

show enlargement of the cardiac shadow due to a pericardial effusion, or erosion of a rib or the sternum due to local extension from lymph nodes.

LYMPHOGRAPHY

In this technique lymphatic channels are can-

Fig. 25.6 CT scan of the abdomen in a patient with Stage III Hodgkin's disease. A large mass of lymph nodes is displacing the Barium-filled stomach to the left.

nulated, and low viscosity contrast material is injected slowly. X-rays of the pelvis and abdomen are taken at the time of injection and the next day. The hazards of the technique are that it is uncomfortable for the patient; sites of cannulation may become infected; local extravasation of contrast material may occur; and lymphocysts may develop, particularly at a site of previous inguinal node biopsy. In addition hypersensitivity reactions to the dye or contrast material can occur; and the contrast material embolizes in the lungs causing a transient reduction in diffusing capacity. This may be dangerous in patients with underlying lung disease.

The filling films show the lymphatic channels and nodes. There are usually anastomoses from each side at the level of the para-aortic nodes. The nodes are seldom shown clearly above L_1 but occasionally the thoracic duct can be seen and the left supraclavicular nodes are often outlined. Most information about the lymph nodes is obtained from the films at 48 hours. Normally the lymph nodes are 1–2.5 cm in size and homogeneous in texture. In the inguinal nodes there may be filling defects perhaps due to previous infections. There are several limitations of lymphography. First, some lymph groups are not normally outlined, such as the obturator, high para-aortic, splenic, renal hilar, mesenteric and porta hepatis nodes. Second, it gives no information about the spleen. Third, the technique and its interpretation depends on the skill and experience of the radiologist. Finally, lymphographic appearances cannot be fully evaluated without follow-up films. CT scanning has largely replaced lymphography.

Other imaging techniques

Ultrasound examination may demonstrate enlarged nodes and may be of value in the upper abdomen (see Chapter 4). The technique depends critically on the experience of the radiologist, so that assessment of its accuracy and value in routine use is difficult. In experienced hands the technique can be invaluable, particularly since it is entirely non-invasive and can be easily repeated. Thoracic CT scan will determine whether there is intrapulmonary spread of disease with greater accuracy than whole-lung tomograms, and in particular, will demonstrate small pulmonary and subpleural nodules of tumour.

Involvement of mediastinal nodes is delineated by the technique. Although, in practice, treatment decisions are not often altered by the routine application of thoracic CT scans, the additional information may lead to a change in treatment policy and the scans are of value in

Fig. 25.7 Involvement of hilar nodes with extension into the lung on the right.

the planning of involved field radiotherapy.

In the abdomen, CT scanning is probably less sensitive than lymphography in demonstrating abnormal pelvic, iliac and lower para-aortic nodes, but it can be useful in the upper abdomen, where lymphography is of limited value. Small foci of hepatic or splenic disease cannot be demonstrated. CT scanning of the abdomen is especially valuable if it shows widespread disease in asymptomatic patients, because the management will be altered.

Both ultrasound and CT scanning may alter treatment policy, but are not as accurate as laparotomy and give no information about microscopic splenic involvement. In asymptomatic patients with localized disease, liver scans seldom give useful information. Even in patients with constitutional symptoms and mildly abnormal liver function tests, the correlation between liver scans and laparotomy findings is poor. Occasionally a grossly abnormal scan will indicate the need for chemotherapy in a doubtful case, but such instances are rare.

Bone scanning may be useful in demonstrating isolated areas of involvement and is cheaper and more reliable than plain X-rays as a screening procedure. The information obtained from routine use is limited but if there is bone pain, it is an essential investigation, since a positive scan may change treatment policy if the cause of the abnormality is Hodgkin's disease. The areas shown up on scan must be examined radiologically since increased uptake on a bone scan has many causes including degenerative joint disease or previous trauma. The distinction between fibrosis and active disease can sometimes be made by MR or gallium scanning. These techniques do not add greatly to CT scanning at the time of first diagnosis, but are of value if the patient is being investigated for relapse after previous treatment. Higher dose gallium scanning is now usually used. Another indication is in determining whether a residual mediastinal abnormality, after chemotherapy, contains active tumour.

Barium studies of the stomach and bowel are unnecessary unless there are clear symptoms requiring investigation. In the stomach the usual radiological appearance of Hodgkin's disease is of a mass indenting the barium, occasionally with appearances suggesting ulceration. In the small and large bowel the typical appearance is of a long segment of infiltration with a coarse and distorted mucosal pattern and thickening of the bowel wall. The involvement may be patchy and discontinuous.

PERCUTANEOUS BIOPSY

Some of the indications for percutaneous biopsy have already been discussed. Marrow trephine is a worthwhile investigation in patients for whom treatment may be with radiotherapy alone, since an involved marrow will indicate the need for chemotherapy. However, in localized Hodgkin's disease without constitutional symptoms only 4% of patients will have a positive trephine biopsy. It may be difficult to decide whether the marrow is involved since typical RS cells may not be present. The mononuclear Hodgkin's cell may be found and may be sufficient for diagnosis. The involvement is usually focal so there are considerable sampling errors.

Percutaneous liver biopsy is not a reliable investigation since Hodgkin's disease may sometimes be focal within the liver. It can be useful in selected cases with abnormal liver function tests, constitutional symptoms or hepatomegaly, and if positive may remove the need for further staging procedures. There may be a considerable problem in interpreting liver biopsy material even if obtained at laparotomy. Focal mononuclear infiltrates are frequently found, and pathologists are usually reluctant to diagnose the disease on the basis of occasional malignant-looking mononuclear cells. In both liver and marrow, non-caseating granulomata may be found, the cause of which is unknown, and these should not be confused with Hodgkin's disease.

THE VALUE OF STAGING LAPAROTOMY AND SPLENECTOMY

The introduction of laparotomy and splenectomy by Kaplan, Rosenberg and co-workers at Stanford in the 1960s showed that even in patients with clinical, localized (Stages I or II) supradiaphragmatic disease, there was a significant chance of finding disease below the diaphragm. Since then there has been considerable debate about the necessity for this procedure in newly diagnosed Hodgkin's disease, and modern imaging techniques and the increased efficacy of chemotherapy have meant that the procedure is now used far less often.

The technical aspects of the laparotomy are very important. It is not a procedure for the non-specialist general surgeon because the information obtained may then be sub-optimal. The para-aortic lymph node chain is exposed and biopsies taken from as high and as low as possible. The spleen is removed, splenic hilar nodes are biopsied, as are iliac nodes if possible. The porta hepatis is carefully inspected. Wedge biopsies are taken from the lobes of the liver, and trephine biopsy from the iliac crest. One or both ovaries may be moved and repositioned, usually in a more central position (oophoropexy), in anticipation of possible pelvic node irradiation, since a central position allows shielding from irradiation without compromising the dose to iliac lymph nodes.

The diagnostic yield of laparotomy and splenectomy is shown in Table 25.3. Demonstration of occult disease is mainly in the spleen and para-aortic nodes. In most studies, about 40% of patients have been shown to have been 'under-staged' clinically, as judged by subsequent laparotomy and splenectomy. After an adequate staging procedure, the chances of subsequent relapse in the abdomen are 10%. The questions which therefore arise are:
• can we select the patients who should undergo the procedure?
• can we devise treatment strategies which make this operation unnecessary? and

• what are the immediate and long-term hazards of laparotomy and splenectomy?

There is no purpose to be served by a staging laparotomy and splenectomy if no change in the proposed treatment will follow. There is no known therapeutic benefit from removing a diseased spleen. For this reason patients who are known beyond doubt to have Stages IIIB, IVA and IVB disease on the basis of clinical evidence and preliminary investigations, should not be subjected to laparotomy since drug treatment will be used (see below). The aim of the laparotomy is to help in the planning of the areas to be irradiated and, in some cases, to decide whether chemotherapy should be used in place of, or in addition to, radiotherapy. In centres where it is routine practice to use chemotherapy for massive mediastinal disease and Stage IIIA disease (Table 25.2), a laparotomy is also unnecessary.

In clinically localized disease above the diaphragm, a laparotomy will disclose sub-diaphragmatic disease in 40% of patients. It is probable that in patients presenting in this way but not subjected to laparotomy, extended field radiation above and below the diaphragm, with irradiation of the spleen, produces as good relapse-free survival as radiation fields planned on the basis of laparotomy findings. Some centres have therefore employed these extensive radiation fields in preference to laparotomy. The disadvantage of this approach is that many patients will be overtreated with radiotherapy since only a minority will have intra-abdominal disease. High-dose radiation over an extended field has a considerable morbidity (see below) and this approach is not generally used. In other centres, it is still the practice, in disease localized to one side of the neck or to the mediastinum, to treat without laparotomy on the basis that in these patients the chances of finding disease are small and that if relapse occurs in the abdomen, effective salvage treatment is available. Many oncologists do not take this view, arguing that there is a risk of occult splenic involvement and that this may give rise to disseminated disease, putting the patient at risk. However, it seems that a policy of limited assessment followed by radiotherapy, with chemotherapy if relapse occurs, does not lead to reduced survival. The risks of laparotomy are small. The operative mortality in experienced hands is less than 1%. On the other hand, the procedure adds to the patient's discomfort and means that the treatment has been prolonged by a stay in hospital and convalescence. There is also a risk of morbidity associated with the procedure, such as subphrenic abscess, chest infection and venous thrombosis.

The long-term sequelae of splenectomy have been the subject of much investigation. In children below the age of 12 years, splenectomy seems unwise since the risk of bacterial infection, particularly with *Haemophilus influenzae* and *Streptococcus pneumoniae*, is increased. The problem is that patients with Hodgkin's disease are susceptible to infection by virtue of the immune suppression caused by the disease and its treatment. There seems little doubt that splenectomy adds to this susceptibility in children, and may also do so in adults although this is less well documented. For these reasons opinion has moved away from staging laparotomy. The result of this policy means that patients who have been treated for supradiaphragmatic disease with radiotherapy must be carefully watched for early symptoms of subdiaphragmatic relapse which will occur in a substantial minority. Prophylactic oral penicillin is of value in preventing late (sometimes fatal) bacterial infection.

The balance of advantages is therefore now against the use of staging laparotomy except in specific circumstances where a fundamental change in policy would result.

TREATMENT [10]

It is important that physicians treating patients with Hodgkin's disease realize that there is now a good chance of cure for all patients, even when they present with extensive disease. The mainstay of treatment of localized disease is radiotherapy, with chemotherapy for advanced disease, and combined modality treatment in particular clinical situations [11]. The best chance of cure is when the patient first presents. Careful assessment of the best treatment strategy is critical at this stage. While many patients can still be cured after relapse, recurrence of disease usually worsens the outlook.

In the past 15 years the methods of using radiotherapy and drugs have changed considerably. An understanding of the principles of these treatments in the disease is important in planning the correct approach in each patient.

Principles of radiotherapy

The development of megavoltage equipment has allowed greater doses to be given over a wider area without intolerable damage to normal intervening tissues (see Chapter 5). Like all lymphomas, Hodgkin's disease is highly sensitive to radiotherapy, so that modest doses are generally adequate. The probability of long-term control (Fig. 25.8) at the irradiated site is dependent on dose. The dose—response relationship is, however, less clear with doses above 30−35 Gy. It is uncertain whether the dose which is needed to eradicate clinically inapparent disease in adjacent nodes is the same or less than that required for enlarged nodes and bulky tumour masses. The usual practice at the present time is to treat both the involved and adjacent fields to the same dose level — usually in the region of 40 Gy in 25 daily fractions — though in some centres the uninvolved adjacent areas are treated to a lower dose, usually 35 Gy over 4 weeks.

There has been considerable debate over many years as to whether it is preferable to treat only the sites of clinical involvement (involved field, IF) or whether to extend the field to adjacent nodes (extended field, EF). The debate shifts its ground as new procedures such as staging laparotomy and combination chemotherapy are introduced and as 'salvage' treatment becomes more effective for relapse. For example, in patients with clinically localized cervical node disease, the possible advantage of EF radiotherapy such as the mantle field (Fig. 25.9) is less apparent if these patients do not have a staging laparotomy, since some of them will have undiagnosed (and therefore untreated) intra-abdominal disease and an even wider field would be necessary to treat such cases. Furthermore, now that chemotherapy for relapse after radiation failure is so much more successful than it was at the time when EF radiation was first introduced, the long-term survival advantage for EF rather than IF is not apparent. The radiation fields most commonly employed are the mantle field for treating disease in the neck, mediastinum and axillae, and the inverted Y field for nodes in the para-aortic and iliac regions (Fig. 25.9). The lungs, larynx and humeral heads are shielded. When large mediastinal masses are irradiated the field is often progressively contracted as resolution occurs, to avoid irradiating large volumes of lung (see Chapter 5).

Principles of chemotherapy

A wide variety of cytotoxic agents show activity against Hodgkin's disease. The approximate response rates obtained with the different drugs, when used as single agents in advanced disease, are shown in Table 25.4.

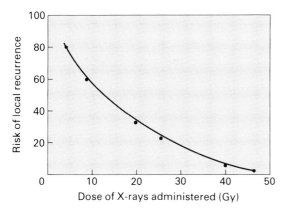

Fig. 25.8 The relationship between local recurrence rate and dose of radiation administered.

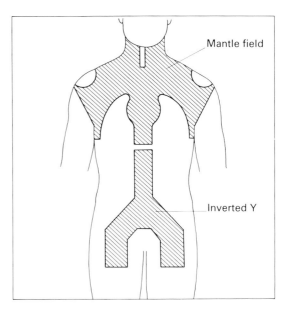

Fig. 25.9 Mantle and inverted Y fields. These are commonly employed fields. In this case the patient has been splenectomized.

When cytotoxic drugs are used as single agents the likelihood of a complete response is small and, if obtained, the response is not usually sustained for more than a few months even if the same drug or another is continued. Single-agent chemotherapy is therefore palliative and not curative. The use of a single cytotoxic drug impairs the subsequent response to other drugs either alone or in combination. For this reason the prior administration of single-agent chemotherapy is a grave mistake if there is a chance of cure with combination therapy.

The major step forward, therefore, was the evolution of modern combination chemotherapy in the 1960s. The drug regimen which has been most widely employed is the MOPP schedule introduced by DeVita and colleagues. The details of this and other commonly employed regimens are given in Table 25.5 with the approximate response rates. A total of six cycles of chemotherapy produces responses in a far higher proportion of cases than is seen with single-agent treatment, even when the latter is given in high dosage with curative

Table 25.4 Approximate % response rates to cytotoxic drugs

	Complete response	Partial response	Total
Alkylating agents			
Nitrogen mustard	10	50	60
Cyclophosphamide	10	45	55
Chlorambucil	15	45	60
Vinca alkaloids			
Vincristine	30	30	60
Vinblastine	30	30	60
Other agents			
Prednisolone	0	60	60
Procarbazine	20	35	65
Doxorubicin	10	45	50
Bleomycin	5	40	35
DTIC	5	40	45

intent. Equally important, most of the responses are complete and in most cases are sustained when chemotherapy is stopped. Mustine-containing combinations are no longer used in the United Kingdom because the chlorambucil-containing regimens are as effective and much less unpleasant without mustine. So-called 'hybrid' regimens have been developed in which seven or eight drugs, taken from two regimens which might be used in alternation, have been combined into a single cycle usually over 10–14 days. Response rates are high but there is no evidence that cure rate is increased. An example is the LOPP/EVAP hybrid regimen. Figure 25.10 shows the proportion of relapse-free patients after treatment with ChLVPP or MOPP. Previously untreated patients have a 40–50% chance of long-term relapse-free survival with these regimens and may be cured. The likelihood of achieving sustained complete response seems to be somewhat less in men, in patients over the age of 40 years and in those with marked constitutional symptoms. In these patients, alternating regimens of different drugs (e.g. MOPP and ABVD) may improve response and survival [12]. Response rate, duration, and survival are much worse if the patient has previously been treated

Table 25.5 Combination chemotherapy regimens and approximate response rates (%)

MOPP (28 day cycle)	
Mustine	6 mg/m^2 days 1,8 i.v.
Vincristine (Oncovin)	2 mg (max) or 1.4 mg/m^2 days 1,8 i.v.
Procarbazine	100 mg/m^2 days 1–19 p.o.
Prednisolone	40 mg/m^2 days 1–14 p.o.
EVAP (alternates with LOPP every 28 days)	
Etoposide	150 mg/m^2 days 1,2,3 (max 200 mg)
Vinblastine	6 mg/m^2 days 1,8 (max 10 mg)
Doxorubicin	25 mg/m^2 days 1,8
Prednisolone	25 mg/m^2 days 1–14 (max 60 mg)
ChLVPP (28 day cycle; for LOPP substitute vincristine for vinblastine)	
Chlorambucil	6 mg/m^2 days 1–14 p.o.
Vinblastine	6 mg/m^2 days 1,8 i.v.
Procarbazine	100 mg/m^2 days 1–14 p.o.
Prednisolone	40 mg days 1–14 p.o.
ABVD (28 day cycle)	
Doxorubcin (Adriamycin)	25 mg/m^2 days 1,15 i.v.
Bleomycin	10 mg/m^2 days 1,15 i.v.
Vinblastine	10 mg/m^2 days 1,15 i.v.
DTIC	375 mg/m^2 days 1,15 i.v.

with single or multiple drug therapy. Previous radiotherapy does not seem to jeopardize response although the toxicity may be greater (see below). The general principles of administration of the drugs are discussed in Chapter 6.

The response to chemotherapy is usually rapid, with disappearance of fever and reduction in tumour masses. Following six cycles of treatment there appears to be little advantage in maintenance chemotherapy although the use of a different regimen such as ABVD may prove to increase remission duration. If relapse occurs after ChLVPP or MOPP, temporary improvement may be obtained by further treatment with the same regimen. With the use of a different regimen (such as ABVD) prolonged survival is occasionally achieved, especially in those patients who relapse after having been treated and who obtain a complete remission.

TREATMENT ON RELAPSE INCLUDING HIGH-DOSE CHEMOTHERAPY [13]

Relapse after a standard chemotherapy regimen is a very adverse prognostic feature. Local relapse in a previously unirradiated nodal area can be treated by irradiation which, if the original disease was localized (e.g. to the mediastinum), should be with curative intent. Frequently the relapse will be more generalized and further chemotherapy will be the treatment of choice. If a single regimen has been previously used (e.g. ChLVPP) then a different regimen should be employed (e.g. ABVD).

Although durable remissions can be obtained with conventional chemotherapy, increasing interest is being shown in the results of high-dose chemotherapy with autologous bone marrow transplantation or peripheral blood stem cells as support [14]. These procedures are becoming less difficult. Depending on selection criteria about 30% of patients who receive high-dose chemotherapy in complete or partial second remission will have long-term freedom from progression. The cure rates are unknown. At present high-dose chemotherapy should be considered for patients with extensive (Stage III or IV) disease who are not in complete remission after initial chemotherapy; for patients who have relapsed quickly after remission; for patients who have relapsed after two different chemotherapy regimens, and for patients who are not responding completely to a salvage chemotherapy regimen.

Management as determined by stage

In the following discussion, guidelines are given as to the management of Hodgkin's disease at presentation according to clinical and pathological stage. Clinical practice varies considerably, so a consensus view is presented and difficult areas of management are considered separately.

CLINICAL STAGE IA, IIA;
PATHOLOGICAL STAGE IA, IIA OR
UNKNOWN

In this category patients have one or more groups of nodes involved on one side of the diaphragm, and investigation (possibly including laparotomy and splenectomy) has failed to show disease elsewhere. For this group of

Fig. 25.10 Relapse-free survival using MOPP chemotherapy. *Note*: later relapses do occur and approximately 50% of all patients are relapse-free at 10 years.

patients radiotherapy produces excellent results (Fig. 25.11). The usual practice for patients with cervical and mediastinal disease is to irradiate the mantle field (Fig. 25.9) to a dose of 40–44 Gy in 20–25 fractions. For those presenting with inguinal node disease the inverted Y field is generally used. The use of chemotherapy in localized disease and the treatment of massive mediastinal disease are discussed separately. The best method of management when laparotomy has not been performed is a matter of considerable controversy. Three treatment strategies have been advocated.

1 To treat with either mantle field or IF irradiation only, and to rely on salvage irradiation or chemotherapy on relapse. The advantage of this approach is that it avoids overtreatment of a large number of patients, especially those with good histology in whom the risk of occult intra-abdominal disease is small. However, the question of whether treatment on relapse is as effective as early treatment is as yet unanswered. Diminished survival with delayed treatment has been reported, but mostly from trials conducted in the days before combination chemotherapy.

2 To treat with total nodal irradiation (TNI) including the spleen. This is associated with good results but many patients will be overtreated by this approach, and if systemic relapse occurs soon after TNI, the toxicity of chemotherapy may be very considerable.

3 To treat with mantle radiotherapy followed by six cycles of ChLVPP or MOPP, or with chemotherapy followed by irradiation. Again many patients will be overtreated and long-term sequelae of radiotherapy and chemotherapy are worrying (see below). Excellent long-term disease-free survival is usually obtained and this approach may be safest if the histology and other prognostic factors (e.g. ESR) are adverse.

The policy for this group of patients will, therefore, vary in different institutions. Most centres do not perform laparotomies on clinical Stages IA and IIA patients. Some centres then treat all of them by **2** or **3** above. In the United Kingdom

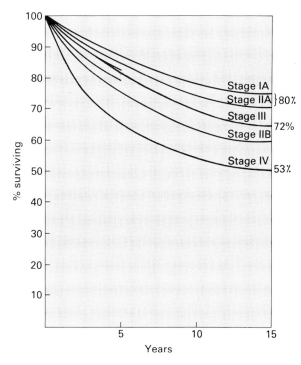

Fig. 25.11 Survival related to stage in Hodgkin's disease. Figures are approximate and incorporate results using different treatment strategies.

most major centres adopt strategy **1**, reserving chemotherapy for relapse.

CLINICAL STAGE IIIA; PATHOLOGICAL STAGE IIIA

In this category patients have presented with localized disease but scanning or laparotomy has demonstrated spread to lymph nodes in the abdomen or spleen. The distinction between $IIIA_1$ and $IIIA_2$ is useful in deciding on treatment within the IIIA category as a whole. Although Stage $IIIA_1$ patients (see Table 25.2) can be treated with TNI, reserving chemotherapy for relapse, Stage $IIIA_2$ patients do not do well with this approach and the prognosis is improved by adding chemotherapy to the TNI. However, a recent trial has indicated that chemotherapy alone may be as effective as TNI and chemotherapy in Stage IIIA and in most centres, current policy would be treatment with chemotherapy, reserving radiation for sites of residual or initially bulky disease, given at the completion of the chemotherapy programme.

CLINICAL STAGE IIB, IIIB, IVB

The patient presents with constitutional symptoms and widespread disease or more localized disease (IIB) and is either found to have extensive disease at laparotomy or, more commonly, the pathological stage is unknown. The mainstay of treatment is chemotherapy with ChLVPP, MOPP or a more complex chemotherapy regimen. In poor prognosis patients (see principles of chemotherapy, above) there may be an advantage in treatment with alternating regimens such as ABVD but this is uncertain. Although pathological Stage IIB disease (an unusual category) can be treated with EF radiotherapy alone, the risk of relapse is high and if IF radiotherapy is used the results are very poor, with early relapse very likely.

Clinical problems

There are a number of problems in management which occur frequently and which do not fall readily into any of the above categories.

MASSIVE MEDIASTINAL DISEASE

It is not uncommon to find a huge mediastinal mass in a relatively asymptomatic patient, in which the mass, on chest X-ray, occupies more than one-third of the transverse diameter of the chest or is greater than 10 cm across (Fig. 25.5). Several studies have suggested that it is difficult to control the disease by radiation alone and that early chemotherapy improves both relapse-free survival and overall survival. At present the data are somewhat conflicting, but many physicians would treat such patients with both radiotherapy and combination chemotherapy. The usual practice is to give chemotherapy first, allowing a smaller volume to be irradiated.

COMBINED MODALITY TREATMENT IN STAGES IA AND IIA

In early disease the use of chemotherapy in addition to radiotherapy has been the subject of considerable investigation but it is by no means standard practice. While relapse-free survival is better than with radiotherapy alone, overall survival is not improved because 'salvage' treatment is increasingly effective on relapse. Involved field radiotherapy and chemotherapy without laparotomy are probably the equivalent in terms of effectiveness of EF radiotherapy after full staging procedures. At present there is no definite indication for using chemotherapy early in IA and IIA disease although some centres do so if there are many groups of nodes involved.

HODGKIN'S DISEASE IN CHILDHOOD

Results of treatment of Hodgkin's disease in childhood are as good or better than in adults. The disease appears particularly sensitive to chemotherapy in children. There are, however, several problems in management of the disease in young children. First, high-dose radiation profoundly affects bone growth and, for example, in the case of vertebrae, the child's prospect of reaching a normal height is reduced (see Chapter 8). Second, in children, splenectomy is associated with an increased risk of bacterial infection, particularly with pneumococci. Third, the long-term consequences of treatment in childhood are not yet fully understood.

In children with clinical Stage I, with minimal disease, the yield of staging laparotomy is small. Such patients can be treated by IF irradiation without laparotomy, with good results. For children with clinical Stages II and III disease and with bulky Stage I disease, EF irradiation produces a relapse-free survival of about 50% at 5 years. However, there is a strong argument for treatment with low-dose (20–25 Gy) EF irradiation, to avoid radiation sequelae, with six cycles of MOPP or equivalent, often given as three cycles before and after radiotherapy. Relapse-free 5-year survival of about 80% is achieved by this means and staging laparotomy is avoided. Chemotherapy alone may be as effective as the combined modality treatment and it is clearly preferable to avoid EF radiation wherever possible. As in adults, chemotherapy is the mainstay of treatment of Stages IIIB and IV disease.

HODGKIN'S DISEASE DURING PREGNANCY (see also Chapter 8, p. 157)

Occasionally Hodgkin's disease is diagnosed for the first time during pregnancy. If this happens during the first 20 weeks, it is probably best to advise termination and then to proceed to the usual evaluation and treatment. During the last trimester, provided the patient is not ill, it is possible to wait until delivery before investigation and treatment. More difficult problems arise if the pregnancy is advanced (20 weeks or more) and the disease is progressing and/or the patient is constitutionally unwell, or if the pregnancy is early but termination is refused.

In a woman in advanced pregnancy in whom treatment cannot be delayed until delivery because the disease is advanced or growing rapidly, it is probably best to treat with combination chemotherapy. There are several reports of normal full-term children born to women who have received combination chemotherapy during pregnancy but clearly it is prudent to postpone such treatment for as long as possible. Single-agent chemotherapy was used in the past but this is not good practice since there is little to suggest that the adverse effects on the fetus are less and there is a grave problem of worsening the long-term prognosis by this treatment. If a woman refuses termination early in pregnancy and has progressive disease, chemotherapy should be delayed as long as possible to allow the early, crucial stages of fetal development to proceed. If the patient has apparently localized supradiaphragmatic disease but it is

felt inadvisable to wait until after delivery, localized radiotherapy is given and full investigation is deferred. In this situation, where a decision has to be made between chemotherapy and irradiation, abbreviated staging using ultrasound can be helpful.

If a woman with previously diagnosed, investigated and treated Hodgkin's disease relapses during pregnancy, then similar considerations apply. In women who have been successfully treated for Hodgkin's disease there is no evidence that pregnancy will provoke recurrence or adversely affect prognosis.

TOXICITY OF TREATMENT

The toxicity of radiotherapy and chemotherapy has been dealt with in general terms in Chapters 5 and 6. The following brief account specifically concerns Hodgkin's disease.

Acute toxicity of chemotherapy

Bone marrow depression is a common accompaniment of all standard chemotherapeutic regimens in Hodgkin's disease. Most centres make dosage reductions in response to depressed blood counts, rather than delay the cycle, although delay may be necessary on occasions. The toxicity tends to be cumulative and particular care should be taken as treatment progresses, especially in the elderly, in those who have received EF radiotherapy in the past and in ill patients with extensive disease. After TNI the problem is particularly severe since over 50% of the adult haemopoietic marrow is within the irradiation field. Recovery of the marrow after TNI takes years and is often incomplete, so chemotherapy should be introduced with caution in these patients.

Immunosuppression. Treatment adds to the depression of cell-mediated immunity (CMI) which is commonly present in advanced disease. Lymphopenia is an invariable consequence of EF irradiation and persists for several months after treatment. Depression of CMI is induced by most cytotoxic agents, especially alkylating agents and steroids. For this reason herpes zoster and herpes simplex are very common in heavily treated patients and may be life-threatening. Less common nowadays is reactivation of tuberculosis, but other opportunistic infections such as pneumocystis, cytomegalovirus and aspergillosis are occasionally seen.

Long-term complications of radiation

Radiation pneumonitis, leading to fibrosis, is a relatively common complication if the radiation dose is above 40 Gy. For this reason very large mediastinal masses require special consideration. Chemotherapy is often used to produce tumour shrinkage before irradiation, though it is not clear whether it is sufficient to irradiate the residual volume only. For smaller nodal areas complications are exceptionally rare.

Occasionally mediastinal irradiation may cause pericarditis with a pericardial effusion which usually resolves. This may cause pain but is usually asymptomatic. Constrictive pericarditis is an extremely uncommon complication of mediastinal irradiation using modern techniques. Radiation damage to coronary arteries seems to be very rare.

Clinical hypothyroidism is an infrequent (5%) complication of mantle field irradiation, although transiently elevated TSH levels are more frequent (30%). Radiation damage to the bowel following infradiaphragmatic irradiation may rarely occur giving rise to diarrhoea (sometimes bloody), steatorrhoea and intestinal obstruction. It is related to both the volume and the total dose administered and it is more likely to occur if the bowel has been tethered in one site by previous inflammation or surgery.

In the CNS the commonest symptom of radiation damage is Lhermitte's syndrome of tingling and paraesthesiae in the legs, often provoked by neck flexion. This usually passes off with no sequelae. Transverse myelitis should not occur with modern planning techniques. Very high repeated doses over peripheral

nerves can rarely lead to peripheral neuropathy, usually within 1–5 years.

Impaired spermatogenesis occurs with doses of irradiation to the testes as low as 50 cGy and is more rapid, complete and long-lasting with higher doses, being invariable and often permanent above 5 Gy (see Chapter 5). During pelvic irradiation, with effective shielding, the dose should be below 100 cGy. The dose which causes permanent cessation of ovarian function is higher than for the testis. Oophoropexy is sometimes carried out to take the ovaries outside a possible pelvic irradiation field (see above).

Long-term complications of chemotherapy (see Chapter 6)

Female fertility may be depressed after MOPP but the effect is inconsistent. Persistent amenorrhoea and the onset of the menopause are more likely to occur in older, premenopausal women. Amenorrhoea frequently occurs during treatment but normal menstruation usually returns and many patients have had children after treatment. There are anecdotes of fetal abnormalities as a result of such pregnancies but the risk is not clear. The hazard of teratogenicity during chemotherapy, on the other hand, is usually regarded as an indication for termination.

Azoospermia is almost inevitable after MOPP or its variants. Procarbazine and the alkylating agents appear to be responsible. Recovery from sterility is rare. Sperm storage prior to chemotherapy is strongly advised for men who are concerned about the effects of fertility. In advanced Hodgkin's disease oligospermia is common before treatment begins.

During the first 5 years after MOPP chemotherapy the cumulative risk of herpes zoster is approximately 15% and is 50% after MOPP with TNI. Disseminated zoster (9%) is more common in those receiving combined modality treatment than with chemotherapy or radiation alone (2%). Bacterial infections, especially pneumococcal, also occur more often, particularly in children, in patients over 50 years, and probably in those who have had splenectomy.

SECOND MALIGNANCIES [15,16]

In recent years it has become apparent that following chemotherapy for Hodgkin's disease, there is an increased risk of the patient developing a second malignancy. The association was first documented for acute non-lymphocytic leukaemia (ANL). At present, the risk of developing ANL in the 7 years after chemotherapy alone, or combined modality treatment, is approximately 2%. However, in patients over the age of 40 years, the risk of ANL may be higher. It is now apparent that the role of solid tumours is greater than that of leukaemia and occurs with a relative risk of 4 for lung cancer, 17 for non-Hodgkin's lymphoma and 2 for all other tumours. Lung cancers and breast cancer are especially likely to occur in the radiation field, as are bone sarcomas. However, the relative risk is greatest for combined modality treatment. The cumulative probability is shown in Fig. 25.12.

Both alkylating agents and procarbazine are potential carcinogens, but the cause of the increased incidence of ANL is not known. ANL may be less common after ABVD; however, this regimen has been introduced into clinical practice more recently than MOPP, and since the leukaemia risk is highest more than 5 years after chemotherapy, it is too soon to assume that ABVD is not as leukaemogenic. The risk of leukaemia relates to survivors rather than to those treated. It is important to appreciate that the risk of Hodgkin's disease is far greater than the hazard from a second malignancy.

Fig. 25.12 Second malignancies after treatment for Hodgkin's disease from [15] with permission.

REFERENCES

1 Correa P., O'Connor G.T. Epidemiologic patterns of Hodgkin's disease. *International Journal of Cancer* 1971; **8**: 192–201.

2 Grufferman S.G., Cole P., Smith P.G., Lukes R.J. Hodgkin's disease in siblings. *New England Journal of Medicine* 1977; **296**: 248–50.

3 Smith P.G., Pike M.C., Kinlen L.J., Jones A., Harris R. Contacts between young patients with Hodgkin's disease. A case-control study. *Lancet* 1977; **ii**: 59–62.

4 Lukes R.J., Butler J.J. The pathology and nomenclature of Hodgkin's disease. *Cancer Research* 1966; **26**: 1063–83.

5 MacLennan K.A., Bennett M.H., Tu A. *et al*. Relationship of histopathological features to survival and relapse in nodular sclerosing Hodgkin's disease: a study of 1659 patients. *Cancer* 1989; **64**: 1686–93.

6 Urba W.J., Longo D.L., Hodgkin's disease: review article. *New England Journal of Medicine* 1992; **326**: 678–87.

7 Atkinson K., Austin D.E., McElwain T.J., Peckham M.J. Alcohol pain in Hodgkin's disease. *Cancer* 1976; **37**: 895–99.

8 Irving M. The role of surgery in the management of Hodgkin's disease. *British Journal of Surgery* 1975; **62**: 853–62.

9 Lister T.A., Crowther D., Sutcliffe S.B. *et al*. Report of a committee convened to discuss the evaluation and staging of patients with Hodgkin's disease: Cotswolds Meeting. *Journal of Clinical Oncology* 1989; **7**: 1630–36.

10 Santos A., Valagussa P. Advances in the treatment of Hodgkin's disease. *Current Opinion in Oncology* 1992; **4**: 821–28.

11 Yelle L., Bergsagel D., Basco V. *et al*. Combined modality therapy of Hodgkin's disease: 10 year results of National Cancer Institute of Canada Clinical Trials Group multicenter clinical trial. *Journal of Clinical Oncology* 1991; **9**: 1983–93.

12 Canellos G.P., Anderson J.P., Propert K.J. *et al.* Chemotherapy of advanced Hodgkin's disease with MOPP, ABVD and MOPP alternating with ABVD. *New England Journal of Medicine* 1992; **327**: 1478–84.

13 Hoppe R.T. Development of effective salvage treatment programs for Hodgkin's disease: an ongoing clinical challenge. *Blood* 1991; **77**: 2093–95.

14 Armitage J.O., Bierman P.J., Vose J.M. *et al.* Autologous bone marrow transplantation for patients with relapsed Hodgkin's disease. *American Journal of Medicine* 1991; **91**: 605–11.

15 Swerdlow A.J., Douglas A.J., Vaughan-Hudson G. *et al.* Risk of second primary cancers after Hodgkin's disease by type of treatment: analysis of 2846 patients in the British National Lymphoma Investigation. *British Medical Journal* 1992; **304**: 1137–43.

16 Tucker M.A., Coleman C.N., Varghese A., Rosenberg S.A. Risk of second cancers after treatment for Hodgkin's disease. *New England Journal of Medicine* 1988; **318**: 76–81.

Chapter 26
Non-Hodgkin's Lymphomas

INCIDENCE AND AETIOLOGY [1]

Recent years have seen a considerable growth in our knowledge of the aetiology of non-Hodgkin's lymphomas (NHL). They are a heterogeneous group of neoplasms which, in Western countries, occur predominantly in the elderly. The overall age-specific incidence is shown in Fig. 26.1 but this obscures markedly different age incidences with some of rarer forms of NHL (which occur in childhood or early adult life). It seems clear that the incidence of NHL is rising quite rapidly but the causes are not known. The AIDS epidemic has contributed to the rising incidence of B cell lymphomas as shown by Fig. 26.2.

Geographical distribution

BURKITT'S LYMPHOMA

In 1958 Burkitt reported cases of a lymphoma occurring in the jaw and abdomen of Ugandan children. The jaw tumours occurred maximally at 3 years of age. Burkitt showed that the tumour appeared in regions of high humidity — the wet tropical areas. The tumour was then reported in Papua New Guinea in the same climatic regions and cases are now reported in the Western countries but with an incidence of only 1% of that in Africa. Western cases have few jaw tumours and in Middle Eastern cases the ileocaecal region is more usually involved. The Epstein–Barr virus (EBV) was identified in cultured tumour cells from African cases, and almost all African cases have high serum titres of anti-EBV. Since almost all the normal popu-

Fig. 26.1 Age-specific incidence of non-Hodgkin's lymphoma.

lation has been infected a co-factor has been postulated — possibly falciparum malaria. This is also suggested by the lower incidence of the tumour in cities and in regions where malaria has been controlled. The age of onset is higher in children who have migrated to areas of high malaria endemicity.

503

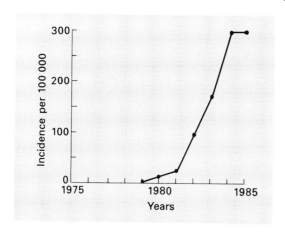

Fig. 26.2 Incidence of non-Hodgkin's lymphoma in never-married men aged 25–44 in San Francisco according to year.

LYMPHOMA OF THE MIDDLE EAST

Lymphoma is a common Middle Eastern cancer (10% of all cancer cases), but they differ from European cases in that many are intestinal, often arising in a background of diffuse small intestinal thickening generally termed immunoproliferative small intestine disease. Current hypotheses favour the view that this is an early stage of lymphoma.

ADULT T CELL LEUKAEMIA/LYMPHOMA

A lymphoma characterized by skin rash, hepatosplenomegaly and hypercalcaemia was reported in 1977 in patients from the southern Japanese island of Kyushu. Later, cases were described in the United Kingdom in patients from the Caribbean and in the United States. A T-lymphotrophic virus was isolated in Japan and in the United States and shown to be identical. This is now designated HTLV1. The virus is transmitted in breast milk and possibly in semen. There are recent suggestions that the HTLV1 lymphoma may also be endemic in eastern China. It is not clear what environmental stimulus causes activation of an infection acquired in infancy — the age of onset of the overt disease is 40–60 years. The overall

incidence in Japan is 5 per 100 000 and 3 per 100 000 in the Caribbean. HTLV1 also causes spastic paraplegia in Jamaica.

Viral causes

The role of HTLV1 in lymphoma has been discussed above. HTLV2 is a virus initially isolated from a case of hairy cell leukaemia (p. 561) and subsequently in another case. However, few patients or controls have been identified who have antibodies. Both are retroviruses which differ morphologically. They all have three genetic regions — *gag* (which codes for a structural protein), *pol* (which produces reverse transcriptase which allows transcription into DNA) and *env* which codes for an envelope protein. Like the AIDS virus (HIV used to be called HTLV3) they have a tropism for CD4 lymphocytes but the receptor on the lymphocyte is not known for either.

The Epstein–Barr virus is a herpes virus containing double-stranded DNA in the core surrounded by a capsid, and an envelope derived from the cell it has infected. The virus is B lymphotrophic, entering the cell by the C3d complement receptor. Infected cells producing the virus die, but in some cells a latent infection occurs without viral assembly. Epstein–Barr virus genome has been demonstrated in Burkitt's lymphoma cells, carcinomas of the nasopharynx, some B cell lymphomas in AIDS and the Wiskott–Aldrich and Chediak–Higashi syndromes (Table 26.1). The relationship between EBV infection and tumour development is still not well understood (see above). In X-linked lymphoproliferative syndrome (discussed below), 70% of patients develop severe, fatal infectious mononucleosis or B cell lymphoma. The tumour cells often contain EBV DNA but, unusually, the lymphoma cells are polyclonal. It seems likely that EBV-infected cells in these immune-suppressed individuals are able to proliferate and in some cases a true monoclonal B cell tumour supervenes.

Recently a new herpes virus has been isolated

Table 26.1 Disorders predisposing to development of lymphoma

Congenital
Chediak–Higashi syndrome
Ataxia telangiectasia
Wiskott–Aldrich syndrome
Swiss-type agammaglobulinaemia
Klinefelter's syndrome
Coeliac disease
Bloom's syndrome
X-linked lymphoproliferative disease

Acquired
Acquired immune deficiency syndrome (AIDS)
Chronic immune suppression (e.g. renal allograft recipients)
Sjögren's syndrome
Rheumatoid arthritis
Common variable hypogammaglobulinaemia

from a variety of patients with both B cell and T cell lymphomas and from lymphomas in AIDS patients. This has been designated human B cell lymphotrophic virus (HBLV) or human herpes virus 6 (HSV6). It is unrelated to EBV and in some areas of the United States and Europe 60% of individuals are seropositive. High serum levels have been found in Hodgkin's disease and in other lymphomas. The virus has also been found in glioblastoma cells. Its role in oncogenesis remains obscure.

HIV-related lymphomas

In 1984 a series of 90 patients with AIDS were described who had developed NHL [3]. The clinical features of these lymphomas are discussed on p. 517. Almost all are B cell tumours. B lymphocytes in HIV infected patients have a high level of spontaneous proliferation, but the stimulus is not known. Both EBV and cytomegalovirus have been proposed as possible causes, as has co-infection with HTLV1.

Lymphomas in other immune-deficiency states

Table 26.1 indicates the wide range of dis-

orders predisposing to NHL, with the majority clearly suggesting states of immune deficiency. In organ transplant recipients, lymphomas account for one-third of all the associated malignancies. The tumours are usually immunoblastic and often intracranial. If the immunosuppression has included cyclosporin A in high dose, the lymphomas are more frequent and often nodal or intestinal. With other immunosuppressive treatment, intracerebral lymphoma is more common. In ataxia telangiectasia and Wiskott–Aldrich syndrome there is a high incidence of lymphoma. In these cases, and in transplant recipients, there are well documented associations with EBV infections.

In the X-linked lymphoproliferative syndrome (discussed above) immune deficiency in young boys is associated with overwhelming EBV infection.

Coeliac disease

Patients with this disease have a 200-fold increase of lymphoma of the intestine. The tumours are T cell in origin and have distinct clinical features (p. 523).

MOLECULAR GENETICS OF LYMPHOMA [2]

A reciprocal translocation of chromosomal material between chromosome 8 and 14 (t(8;14) (q24;q32)) in tumour cells in Burkitt's lymphoma was the first consistent genetic abnormality discovered in lymphoma. More than 80% of tumours have this translocation. Translocations between 8 and 22 (t(8;22)) and from 2 to 8 (t(2;8)) were described later in the remaining tumours. Subsequently, the Ig heavy chain locus was mapped to 14q32 and the light chain was found at 2p11 and at 22q11. Each of these sites is the site of gene rearrangement in the normal B lymphocyte. The break on the 8 chromosome is always at band 8q24 which is the C-*myc* proto-oncogene site.

There is now known to be heterogeneity at the site of the Ig locus break. The C-*myc* is abnormally expressed for B cells, although it is at a level appropriate for proliferating cells. Interestingly, the endemic cases do not show c-*myc* rearrangement, but the sporadic cases do.

Follicle-centre cell lymphomas of the follicular type show a characteristic chromosomal translocation in 85% of cases. This is between 14q32 (the heavy chain locus) and 18q21. The breakpoint on chromosome 18 is rearranged in the majority of follicular lymphomas. The gene is referred to as *bcl*-2 (B cell leukaemia and lymphoma 2). Sensitive techniques such as the polymerase chain reaction (PCR) can detect low levels of cells containing the rearranged sequence.

T cell malignancies also show non-random chromosomal abnormalities. The most common site is at 14q11 which is the site of the T cell receptor gene (α and δ chains).

It is still not clear what role these lympho-specific translocations play in oncogenesis. They sometimes appear to develop earlier in the cell lineage than the phenotype of corresponding tumour would suggest (i.e. the tumour differentiates), and to be related to control of proliferation appropriate to that cell lineage.

The most important clinical application of molecular techniques has been the detection of rearrangement of antigen-receptor genes as a manifestation of clonality. These genes (T cell receptor genes and immunoglobulin genes) rearrange during normal development of the cells producing an antigen-specific clone. Neoplastic expansion of a clone is accompanied by a specific rearrangement which can be detected using molecular and immunological techniques. The most commonly employed technique is Southern blot hybridization after the DNA has been cut into fragments using a restriction enzyme. This technique can detect a clonal cell population when the population constitutes 2–5% of the cells tested.

PATHOLOGY [3]

There is a bewildering profusion of terminology to describe the pathological appearance of non-Hodgkin's lymphoma. This has come about because the enormous growth of knowledge in cellular immunology in the last decade has led to attempts to classify the tumour according to what is known about normal lymphocyte development. At the same time conventional pathological descriptions of the diseases have been developed and refined to accommodate the widely differing clinical features and prognosis. Attempts have also been made to combine both pathological and immunological descriptions, and immunocytochemical staining of fresh-frozen biopsy material is increasingly employed for accurate diagnosis. This has led to increasing difficulty for the clinician and general pathologist. What follows, therefore, is a brief guide to the basis of the immunological contribution to our understanding of these diseases, followed by a synopsis of how the diseases are described in pathological terms.

During fetal life precursors of T lymphocytes are formed and migrate to the thymus, and thence to the developing lymph nodes and spleen. Maturation into mature T cells takes place at various stages especially in the thymus. The sequence of maturation can be defined by their surface antigen structure. Monoclonal antibodies to T cell surface antigens have been especially helpful in this respect. The sequence of maturation is shown in Fig. 26.3. By the time the T cell leaves the thymus its function as a helper cell or cytotoxic/suppressor cell is established.

In the lymph nodes the T cells lodge in the paracortical region (Fig. 26.4) and around the central arterioles in the spleen. Some T cells recirculate from the lymphatic system to the blood and thence from the blood back to the lymph nodes where they enter the paracortical region through post-capillary venules.

Early B lymphocytes are formed in the fetal liver and subsequently in the bone marrow. From there they migrate to the lymph nodes. They are found in the follicles which consist of an outer mantle zone of small lymphocytes and a germinal centre composed of cells where the

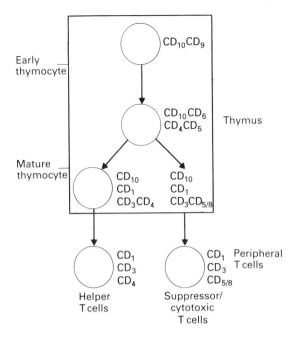

Fig. 26.3 T cell surface phenotype during maturation in the thymus. The T cell antigens are identified by monoclonal antibodies and are helpful in categorizing the various forms of T cell lymphoma and leukaemia.

nucleus is either irregular in shape or large and round. The cells with a nucleus of irregular outline are called cleaved cells or *centrocytes* and those with a large round nucleus, non-cleaved or *centroblasts*. Some B lymphocytes

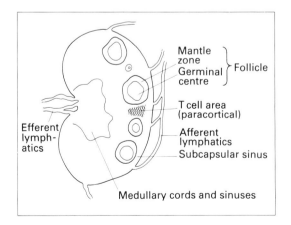

Fig. 26.4 Lymph node structure.

recirculate between nodes and blood. After contact with antigen, B cells transform into antibody-secreting plasma cells.

As B cells terminally differentiate, the genes which code for the enormous variety of potential immunoglobulin molecules rearrange to code for one Ig molecule only. At this point the 'clonal' nature of the cell is established. Similarly, rearrangement of the genes which code for the four components of the T cell antigen-receptor occurs during T cell clonal development in the thymus. This rearrangement can be detected relatively simply using molecular biological techniques. In a cell suspension which may contain lymphoma cells (which are clonal) clonal rearrangement can be detected if as few as 5% of the cells constitute the tumour population. Gene rearrangement is therefore a useful technique for determining, for example, marrow contamination. Detection of a chromosomal abnormality (such as the 14:18 translocation in follicular lymphoma) by PCR is even more sensitive but is not possible in tumours which do not have such abnormality.

Macrophages, or mononuclear phagocytes, are formed from pluripotent haemopoietic stem cells in the marrow. They are liberated into the bloodstream as monocytes and lodge in tissues at sites of inflammation (histiocytes). They also play a part in repopulating the 'fixed' tissue phagocytic cells — Kupffer cells, splenic, alveolar and peritoneal macrophages. The antigen-presenting cells (dendritic cells) in lymph nodes and spleen may also be part of the mononuclear phagocyte system. A simplified guide to the stage in differentiation of lymphocytes and macrophages to which various non-Hodgkin's lymphomas and leukaemias correspond is shown in Fig. 26.5 and a synopsis of the immunological classification of lymphoreticular neoplasms is shown in Table 26.2.

In the early 1970s it was realized that the majority of lymphomas were derived from cells of the follicular centre and consisted of either centrocytes (cleaved cells) or centroblasts (non-cleaved cells), or a mixture of the two. As immunological techniques developed, more

Table 26.2 Cell of origin of lymphomas

B cell tumours	T cell tumours
Follicular lymphomas of centrocytes and centroblasts	Cutaneous T cell lymphoma
Diffuse lymphomas centroblastic, centrocytic, immunoblastic	T cell lymphoma of mediastinum with convoluted nuclei
Lymphoplasmacytoid (Waldenström's)	Peripheral T cell lymphoma
Chronic lymphatic leukaemia	Other lymphoblastic and immunoblastic lymphomas usually of diffuse type
Burkitt's lymphoma	*Macrophage tumours*
Heavy chain disease	?Some diffuse large cell 'lymphomas'
	Histiocytic medullary reticulosis

Fig. 26.5 Simplified scheme of cell origin of non-Hodgkin's lymphomas. (A) Origin of B cell and T cell lymphomas; (B) origin of macrophage tumours.

individual cell types were identified within the lymphomas and classification developed accordingly. The following cell types have been identified: small lymphocytes (B and T), lymphoplasmacytic cells, plasma cells, centrocytes (small and large), centroblasts (small and large), immunoblasts (B and T), and lymphoblasts (B and T).

B cell neoplasms make up the majority of non-Hodgkin's lymphomas (Table 26.2). The most common are all the follicular lymphomas which are derived from the B cell of the follicle centre. However, these cells do not always form follicles and may also give rise to a diffuse lymphoma.

T cell lymphomas probably constitute about 10% of non-Hodgkin's lymphomas (Table 26.2). The T cell lymphomas can be divided into three broad categories:

- cutaneous lymphomas;
- thymic lymphomas; and
- peripheral T cell lymphoma.

Morphologically they are diffuse with a wide variety of cellular morphology.

It is not yet clear how many lymphomas are neoplasms of malignant macrophages. Those which are should not, strictly speaking, be called lymphomas. The term 'histiocytic lymphoma' is now regarded as erroneous since many of the tumours which were originally described are B cell neoplasms. There is still uncertainty about how frequently true macrophage (histiocytic) tumours occur. Histochemical evidence has suggested that they may account for 5% of diffuse large-cell lymphomas (Table 26.2).

Although the immunological classification of lymphoma is logical and in many respects superior, the pathological diagnosis in most departments rests on conventional light microscopical appearances (Fig. 26.6). Earlier classifi-

Fig. 26.6 Histological appearance in non-Hodgkin's lymphoma. (Original magnification × 400). (A) Follicle centre cell lymphoma predominantly containing centrocytes but with scattered centroblasts (arrowed); (B) follicle centre cell lymphoma composed principally of centroblasts; (C) peripheral T cell lymphoma showing proliferating high endothelial venules (arrowed) and a mixture of small and large lymphocytes, some with clear cytoplasm, others showing an irregular nuclear outline.

cations divided the lymphomas according to whether there was nodule formation or the node was diffusely replaced by tumour. The term 'nodular' is sometimes used synonymously with 'follicular'. In most instances the pattern is due to the formation of follicles by the neoplastic cells and the term follicular rather than nodular should be used to describe these tumours. These categories (follicular and diffuse) were then divided according to cell type: well-differentiated lymphocytic; poorly differentiated lymphocytic; mixed lymphocytic and histiocytic; histiocytic; and undifferentiated. The term 'histiocytic' was a misnomer (see above) but the classification emphasized the prognostic significance of the microscopic appearances. The follicular lymphomas had a good prognosis and lymphocytic lymphomas a better outlook than histiocytic or undifferentiated. This scheme is still widely used.

A panel of pathologists have devised a working formulation which allows some cross-reference between the classifications. It has been criticized for not being immunologically based but it is given here because it is used increasingly. This formulation was not intended to supplant existing classifications but to allow increasingly bewildered clinicians to steer their way through the maze of classifications and terms used in publications, text books and by their local pathologists. The formulation is given in Table 26.3.

One major difficulty with any classification is that within a single lymph node, or group of nodes, areas of follicular or diffuse change may both occur, and both small and large cells are often found. Furthermore, follicular lymphomas frequently evolve into diffuse large cell forms during the course of their natural history.

A rule of thumb with respect to prognosis is that the greater the degree of follicle formation

Table 26.3 Working formulation for clinical usage (with alternative terminology in italics)

Low-grade malignancy
A Diffuse small cell differentiated lymphocytes, consistent with chronic lymphatic leukaemia. Plasmacytoid features may be present
B Follicular. Small cleaved cells — *centrocytes*. Some diffuse areas
C Follicular mixed small and large cleaved cells. Some diffuse areas

Intermediate grade malignancy
D Follicular. Large centrocytes and centroblasts — *cleaved and non-cleaved*. Diffuse areas
E Diffuse. Small cleared cell — *centrocytic*
F Diffuse. Small and large cell — *small and large centrocytic and centroblastic*
G Diffuse. Large cleaved and non-cleaved cells — *large centrocytes and centroblasts*

High-grade malignancy
H Diffuse large cell, immunoblastic type
I Diffuse lymphoblastic cells sometimes convoluted
J Diffuse small non-cleaved cells — *centroblasts*

Other
Mycosis fungoides
Unclassifiable
Plasmacytomas — *extramedullary*

the better, and that small well-differentiated lymphocytes are associated with a better prognosis than lymphoblastic, immunoblastic or other large cell types.

CLINICAL FEATURES

Non-Hodgkin's lymphomas usually arise in peripheral lymph nodes, but may also develop at a wide variety of extra-nodal sites. The clinical features of extra-nodal lymphomas are described later (see pp. 521–528).

PRESENTATION OF NODAL DISEASE

Painless enlargement of a lymph node is the most frequent presentation of non-Hodgkin's lymphoma, and the commonest site is the neck. Sometimes the nodes fluctuate in size which can lead to delay in diagnosis. Non-Hodgkin's lymphomas tend to be more widespread at presentation than Hodgkin's disease and to be present at more unusual lymph node sites, for example, Waldeyer's ring. Although the presentation is usually straightforward the enlarging lymph node mass may cause initial symptoms due to compression, for example swelling of the arm or leg, simulating deep venous thrombosis or superior vena caval obstruction.

Retroperitoneal lymph node enlargement can result in backache and obstructive renal failure, and nodes in the porta hepatis may cause obstructive jaundice. Widespread infiltration of the liver is usually accompanied by weight loss, anorexia and fever.

Even without liver involvement, constitutional symptoms are not infrequent with weight loss, night sweats and fever. Intra-abdominal lymphoma may present with fever of unknown origin, especially if there is hepatic or bone marrow involvement.

Clinical examination must be meticulous. The neck should be carefully examined and it is often easier to determine the extent of disease in the neck if the examination is carried out from behind the patient. Node enlargement should be sought in the pre- and post-auricular regions, in the occipital, supra- and infraclavicular areas, and deep behind the sternomastoid. The axilla should be carefully examined both in the apex and the walls. Epitrochlear nodes are often missed. In the abdomen the size of the liver and spleen should be noted and an attempt made to examine abdominal and retroperitoneal nodes by deep palpation. The inguinal nodes are often slightly enlarged in normal individuals but pathological inguino-femoral nodes may extend downwards into the medial aspect of the thigh. Examination of the oro- and nasopharynx should be routine, as should rectal examination which may lead to detection of large masses of pelvic nodes.

Diagnosis and investigation of nodal lymphomas

The diagnosis is by node or tissue biopsy. Although there is usually little difficulty about the diagnosis, other conditions may simulate lymphoma (see Table 26.4) especially at extra-nodal sites, and precise immunological classification is becoming increasingly important in management. For these reasons a lymph node biopsy should be regarded as an important clinical investigation and not as a trivial affair.

Too often inexperienced surgeons biopsy a superficial node, which shows reactive hyperplasia, or a node in the neck or groin which may not be obviously abnormal. If there is a deeper clearly pathological node this should be removed. Immunohistochemistry helps a great deal in diagnosis, particularly in distinguishing large cell lymphomas from anaplastic carcinoma, and in the diagnosis of T cell tumours. Some of these investigations can only be done on fresh or frozen tissue so the biopsy should not be placed in formaldehyde and the pathologist will advise as required. If the node shows reactive hyperplasia or an equivocal result one should not hesitate to biopsy another node if the clinical suspicion is high. If the nodes are in an inaccessible site it may be necessary to proceed to laparotomy or mediastinotomy. It is often better to do this than to repeatedly biopsy equivocally enlarged peripheral nodes.

Table 26.4 Lymph node enlargement simulating lymphoma

Follicular histology
Reactive hyperplasia
Rheumatoid arthritis and related arthritides
Angiofollicular hyperplasia
Toxoplasmosis

Diffuse histology
Phenytoin sensitivity
Dermatopathic lymphadenopathy
Angioimmunoblastic lymphadenopathy with
    dysproteinaemia
Metastatic carcinoma and melanoma

Other histologies
Sinus histiocytosis with massive lymph node
    enlargement
Infectious mononucleosis
Cat scratch fever
Metastatic carcinoma (especially melanoma)

Staging notation

The staging notation is the same as that employed for Hodgkin's disease (see Table 25.2). Unlike Hodgkin's disease the great majority of patients will have Stages III and IV disease at presentation.

In the investigation of non-Hodgkin's lymphoma there are certain routine tests which are inexpensive, harmless, and sometimes rewarding and these should be performed. A chest X-ray may show hilar, mediastinal or paratracheal node enlargement. Parenchymal lung lesions are less common as are pleural effusions, but the latter occur not infrequently when there is massive mediastinal disease. Occasionally the effusion is chylous due to rupture of lymphatics in the mediastinum. Lung infiltrates and effusions which contain lymphoma cells usually occur when there is associated mediastinal or hilar disease.

The blood count may show anaemia, which

is usually normochromic and typical of the anaemia of chronic disease (with a low serum iron and iron-binding capacity). Occasionally it is due to autoimmune haemolysis and a Coombs test and reticulocyte count should be performed if this is suspected. The blood film may show circulating lymphoma cells. However, immunological methods may detect a malignant population which is not apparent on the blood smear, and the proportion of patients with blood involvement will certainly prove to be higher than the present 10% of cases identified by the blood film. Recent methods of demonstrating monoclonality in B cells have been applied to bone marrow and have suggested a high level (30−50%) of involvement in both follicular and diffuse lymphomas. An abnormal blood film implies marrow disease, but this may not always be detected on aspiration and biopsy. Conversely marrow involvement on biopsy is not always associated with an abnormal peripheral blood picture. The blood urea and electrolytes should be measured to exclude renal failure. The liver enzymes should also be measured since a rise in alkaline phosphatase and transaminases may indicate liver infiltration and the alkaline phosphatase and bilirubin may be elevated if there are nodes in the porta hepatis causing compression.

Other investigations include CT scanning of the abdomen or pelvis to demonstrate intra-abdominal or pelvic disease, an intravenous urogram if there is evidence of renal impairment, and X-rays and bone scan if there is bone pain or tenderness at a particular site. Before the advent of CT, lymphography was widely used to demonstrate pelvic and para-aortic nodes. Most patients (80%) with nodular lymphoma have abnormal lymphograms, and approximately 60% of those with diffuse lymphoma. CT scanning is a less troublesome alternative to lymphography and has about the same sensitivity. It has the advantage of being able to demonstrate nodal masses in the mesentery and in the upper abdomen — sites poorly demonstrated by lymphography.

How far should these tests be done as a routine and combined with more invasive tests such as liver or marrow biopsy? This depends on what the treatment strategy is to be. If there is a prospect that the disease is localized and the patient might be cured by radiotherapy, extensive investigation is needed to define the true extent of the disease. But if the treatment is to be with palliative local radiotherapy, for example in an elderly patient with clinically localized disease, then invasive investigations are meddlesome. If the histology and clinical features indicate widespread poor-prognosis disease then intensive chemotherapy will be used and it becomes irrelevant to persist with unpleasant investigations such as liver biopsy.

Most cases of non-Hodgkin's lymphoma presenting as a nodal disease should be regarded as widespread, irrespective of histology. In both nodular and diffuse lymphomas it is likely that there will be evidence on mediastinal and abdominal CT, and a not inconsiderable chance of detecting disease in the marrow or liver. While 30% of patients have *clinically* localized disease (Stages I and II) at presentation, after sequential investigation the proportion falls to about 15%. Laparotomy makes little contribution to assessment of spread.

THE MANAGEMENT OF NON-HODGKIN'S LYMPHOMA PRESENTING AS NODAL DISEASE

Follicular lymphomas [4]

These lymphomas constitute 30−40% of all cases. They are tumours of the follicle centre (B cell) and are a mixture of small cleaved centrocytes and large centroblasts. Depending on the proportion of these cells they are referred to as follicular small cleaved (centrocytic) mixed or large cell (centroblastic) lymphoma. The distinction from diffuse lymphomas of the follicular centre cell is occasionally arbitrary since a single node may show follicular and diffuse changes especially in the large cell (centroblastic)

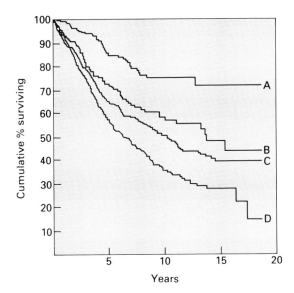

Fig. 26.7 Prognosis in follicular non-Hodgkin's lymphoma. The curves indicate the death from lymphoma according to stage at presentation. A, Stage I/IE (*n* = 244); B, Stage II/IIE (*n* = 186); C, Stage III/IIIE (*n* = 397); D, Stage IV/IVE (*n* = 423). The relationship between prognosis and clinical stage is clearly shown. Fifteen-year overall cause-specific survival is 37%. Data from the British National Lymphoma Investigation with grateful thanks to Dr Gillian Vaughan Hudson.

types. Spontaneous fluctuations in lymph node size and even regressions occur.

An unusual form of lymphoma with a nodular appearance is the *mantle-zone lymphoma* derived from small B cells surrounding the follicle. This has a different phenotype from the follicular centre cell.

The translocation from 18q21 to 14q32 at the site of the heavy chain enhancer has been previously discussed. The large cell variants appear to have the highest growth fraction and small cell the lowest and this may account for the greatest likelihood of cure of the large cell variant by chemotherapy.

The tumours occur in middle or old age with painless (often prolonged) enlargement of nodes. Marrow and blood involvement is fre-

quent, especially in the centrocytic types. Clinical Stages I and II disease occurs in 40% of cases but only 20% have Stages I and II after investigation.

STAGES I AND II FOLLICULAR SMALL CELL AND MIXED LYMPHOMA

In this group localized or extended field irradiation produces impressive results with 60–80% of patients free of the disease at 10 years. Recurrence is frequent at adjacent lymph node sites but further radiation can be given. The use of total nodal irradiation has been suggested but this may be overtreatment for many patients. The current data suggest that about 50% of patients will be cured by treatment of involved and adjacent lymph nodes. Additional chemotherapy has not yet been shown to be unequivocally beneficial when radiation is used. However, in Stage II disease in the elderly population, excellent symptomatic control can be obtained with the use of intermittent oral chlorambucil which is sometimes combined with prednisolone.

STAGES I AND II FOLLICULAR LARGE CELL (CENTROBLASTIC) LYMPHOMA

This is a much less common form and has a more rapid course. In true Stage I disease radiation therapy may cure some patients. Relapse-free survival is prolonged if chemotherapy (such as CHOP) is added [4]. Chemotherapy alone with CHOP or pro MACE-MOPP produces excellent results. At present the weight of evidence favours intensive chemotherapy as the mainstay of treatment and the role of radiation is less clear.

STAGES III AND IV FOLLICULAR 'CENTROCYTIC' LYMPHOMA

This disease is best described by the term 'mantle zone' lymphoma. It is indolent, but spreads to the bone marrow. Management is similar to that described for mixed follicular lymphoma (below).

Some of these patients with low-grade follicular lymphomas will live for several years without symptoms from their disease (Fig. 26.7). There has been considerable debate about how soon treatment (with chemotherapy) should begin. The median period before symptoms develop is 4 years. It seems that no advantage in survival is obtained with an immediate treatment policy versus a 'watch and wait' approach [5].

However, certain groups of patients clearly do not do well — poor prognostic features include B symptoms, anaemia and hepatosplenomegaly. There are therefore cogent reasons for considering a more aggressive treatment policy in these patients. A high proportion of complete remissions can be obtained with intensive chemotherapy, but the duration may be short. α-Interferon appears to prolong the time to relapse or progression. As with Stages I and II follicular mixed centrocytic/centroblastic disease this may matter less in elderly patients but seems unwise in patients below the age of 55. In these patients high-dose chemotherapy is being assessed in second and third relapse (see below).

With low-dose oral chemotherapy, symptoms can usually be brought under control. However, with this approach relapse will occur relatively quickly and the interval between treatments will shorten. A high response rate is obtained with more intensive regimens (CHOP-Bleo, M-BACOD, C-MOPP, ProMACE-CytaBOM) with 70% complete responses of whom 60% are still in remission at 4 years. In contrast a trial from the National Cancer Institute in the United States demonstrated no advantage to early intensive combination chemotherapy in Stages III and IV disease. Recent reports indicate that α-interferon can prolong the remissions induced by chlorambucil although benefit in survival has not yet been shown. Poor prognosis is

indicated by systemic symptoms, high serum LDH and poor performance status.

It is still not clear if intensive therapy will increase cure rate. The role of high dose chemotherapy (with bone marrow or blood stem cell support) is under evaluation in young patients. The large cell (centroblastic) form is more aggressive, resembling the more common diffuse centroblastic disease, and is treated accordingly.

Adult diffuse intermediate and high-grade lymphoma [5,6,7]

Included in this category are follicular large cell lymphoma and the diffuse tumours called centrocytic/centroblastic, large cell, immunoblastic, undifferentiated, and pleomorphic peripheral T cell lymphomas. The largest group is the diffuse large cell type. These are usually B cell tumours but T cell tumours can appear identical clinically and it is not clear if there is any prognostic significance to the cell type. Immunoblastic tumours are usually of B cell origin and lymphoblastic may be B or T cell. The justification for grouping them all therapeutically is that there is no clear reason for adopting different treatment strategies in each type. The major prognostic determinants are measures of bulk and symptoms, not of cell lineage.

The patients are usually middle-aged or older. Most cases are Stages III or IV but large cell types are localized (I or II) in 25% of cases. Stage IV disease, large tumour masses, high LDH and constitutional symptoms are poor prognostic features. Routine investigation includes chest and abdominal CT scanning and bone marrow aspiration and biopsy.

Treatment is with intensive combination chemotherapy. The CHOP regimen has been widely used (Table 26.5) but in the last 10 years more intensive combinations are becoming more favoured. These regimens have incorporated the following features: additional agents such as methotrexate, cytosine arabinoside and etoposide, treatment at closer intervals to avoid the problem of relapse between cycles,

Table 26.5 Combination chemotherapy regimens in advanced diffuse nodal non-Hodgkin's lymphoma

Regimen	Drug	Dose
CHOP (21 days)	Cyclophosphamide	$1\,g/m^2$ d1*
	H-doxorubicin	$70\,mg/m^2$ d1
	O-vincristine	$2\,mg$ IV d1
	Prednisolone	$100\,mg$ p.o. d1−5
M-BACOD (21 days)	Methotrexate	$200\,mg/m^2$ d18,15 (with folinic acid)
	Bleomycin	$15\,mg/m^2$ d1
	A-doxorubicin	$45\,mg/m^2$ d1
	Cyclophosphamide	$600\,mg/m^2$ d1
	O-vincristine	$2\,mg/m^2$ d1
	Dexamethasone	$6\,mg/m^2$ p.o. d1−5
Pro(M)ACE-CytaBOM (21 days)	Prednisolone	$60\,mg/m^2$ d1−14
	A-doxorubicin	$25\,mg/m^2$ d1
	Cyclophosphamide	$650\,mg/m^2$ d1
	Etoposide	$120\,mg/m^2$ d1
	Cytarabine	$300\,mg/m^2$ d1
	Bleomycin	$15\,mg/m^2$ d8
	O-vincristine	$2\,mg/m^2$ d8
	Methotrexate	$120\,mg/m^2$ d8 (with folinic acid)
MACOP-B (one cycle)	Methotrexate	$400\,mg/m^2$ d8,36,64
	A-doxorubicin	$50\,mg/m^2$ d1,15,29,43,57,71
	Cyclophosphamide	$350\,mg/m^2$ d1,15,29,43,57,71
	O-vincristine	$2\,mg/m^2$ d8,22,36,50,64,78
	Prednisolone	$75\,mg/m^2$ p.o. d1−84 (reducing)
	Bleomycin	$20\,mg/m^2$ d22,50,78

* dl etc. denotes which day of the cycle this chemotherapy should be given

and the use of multiple drug combinations (such as ProMACE-CytaBOM; Table 26.4) to overcome drug resistance. Typically treatment durations of 6−8 months are used, but the MACOP-B regimen lasts only 12 weeks with chemotherapy cycles being given weekly. The regimens are very myelosuppressive and mucositis is common especially with MACOP-B. The best results require the maximum dosage and the risks of toxicity are constantly present. The more intensive programmes are not suitable for elderly or infirm patients and considerable care is needed in all patients regardless of age.

With many of these regimens complete response rates (in single-institution, selected series) are 80% or greater. Relapse is uncommon after 3 years, and cure rates as high as 60−70%

may be achieved. If complete response is not attained the outlook is poor — most patients die within 2 years. Failure to attain early complete response may be an indication for autologous bone marrow transplantation (see below).

Adult lymphoblastic lymphoma [8]

These are diffuse high-grade lymphomas characterized by cells with scant cytoplasm, small nucleoli and nuclei which may be of a convoluted or non-convoluted form. The mitotic rate is high. There is often strong phosphatase activity. The immunophenotype is variable but many are T cell tumours. Both T cell and B cell forms express terminal deoxyribonucleotidyl transferase (tdt). The cells may show a variety of T cell markers (Fig. 26.3) and some have a clearly 'thymic' pattern of antigen expression. B cell types may show common acute lympho-blastic leukaemia antigen (CALLA). Chromo-somal breaks at the location of the T cell receptor α and δ chains are frequent (14q11).

The disease is most frequent in adolescence and in young adults and in males more than in females. A mediastinal mass and superior vena caval obstruction is frequent. There is wide-spread nodal involvement. Bone marrow in-volvement is frequent and the distinction between this and lymphoblastic leukaemia is sometimes a matter of definition. Many haema-tologists will call this leukaemia if there are more than 25% of lymphoblasts in the marrow. Although involvement of the CNS at diagnosis is unusual, it may occur during the course of the disease especially if there is marrow involvement.

Treatment has depended to some degree on whether these patients have been regarded as having leukaemia or lymphoma and on whether they are children or adults. There is no clear clinical basis for this. In children, haematology units have used either ALL protocols or those based on the LSA$_2$L$_2$ regimen (p. 520). Both these regimens are relatively successful but the LSA$_2$L$_2$ probably cures only half of the patients; other regimens such as COMP or A-COP appear to be at least as effective. All employ intrathecal treatment as prophylaxis for CNS disease. Established CNS disease is treated as described on p. 525. With the introduction of intensive chemotherapy regimens, the prognosis has im-proved with a 3-year relapse-free survival of 60%. Poor prognostic [6] features are age greater than 30, high initial white count and a failure to obtain complete response. The role of high-dose chemotherapy (and autologous marrow or blood stem cell support) is under investigation for these patients.

Small non-cleaved cell lymphomas
(SNCC lymphomas, Burkitt's lymphoma, lymphoblastic lymphoma — Burkitt's type)

These tumours are characterized by diffuse infiltration of lymph nodes with cells with a round nucleus with multiple nucleoli, scanty cytoplasm containing lipid, and macrophages. The distinction between Burkitt's and non-Burkitt's type is somewhat arbitrary. The cells are B cells with surface IgM. They express HLA-DR, CALLA, CD19, CD20 and CD21 — all B cell markers. The chromosomal translocations are described on p. 506.

In Western countries about 30% of childhood NHL and 1–2% of adult cases are of Burkitt type. In so-called 'endemic' areas (equatorial Africa, New Guinea) the incidence is 40 times higher than in the West where the incidence is 2 per million below the age of 20.

The presentation and management of Burkitt's lymphoma in childhood is discussed below (p. 521). In adults the patients have tra-ditionally been treated with one of the regimens outlined in Table 26.4. This may not be the correct policy, and in recent years there has been increasing evidence of improved results if protocols based on the childhood regimens are adopted. Recent results are comparable with those obtained in children. The regimen consisted of CHOP with intermediate dose MTX, and cytosine arabinoside and MTX given intrathecally.

Bone marrow transplantation in non-Hodgkin's lymphomas [9]

Although modern combination regimens will cure 50–60% of patients with high-grade NHL those who relapse are seldom, if ever, curable by conventional chemotherapy. High-dose chemotherapy with autologous bone marrow transplantation (ABMT) or peripheral blood stem cell (PBSC) support can achieve an increase in drug dosage of 5–7-fold. Whether this is adequate to cure a patient with a tumour resistant to lower doses is the essential question which surrounds the procedure. Above these doses non-haematological toxicity is likely to be fatal. Major improvements in supportive care, the use of ABMT or PBSC support and haemopoietic growth factors have all reduced the morbidity and mortality from the procedure.

Evidence from uncontrolled trials [9] shows that in relapsed patients about 30−40% of cases will live beyond 3 years after high-dose treatment and 60−75% of patients will have a major response. Prognostic factors include general health, tumour mass, the responsiveness of the tumour to previous chemotherapy and the number and variety of previous regimens. These encouraging results have led to the use of the procedure in first remission in high-risk patients, or in patients failing to achieve complete response (CR) with the first treatment. The problem here is that in those patients who have a CR the cure rate may be as high as 60%, and in the others a wide variety of prognostic factors means that randomized comparison of the new treatment is essential.

Such randomized trials have not been completed, so the value of the procedure is not yet firmly established. It should be considered in patients who fail to achieve CR with initial treatment, in selected patients with poor-prognosis tumours (such as high-grade T cell lymphomas, adult lymphoblastic lymphoma, poor-prognosis high-grade nodal lymphoma of follicular centre cells) even in first CR, and patients who, after first relapse, achieve a second CR.

One problem with ABMT is the potential contamination of the transfused marrow by tumour. A wide variety of 'purging' procedures has been adopted to eliminate residual tumour cells, but, as yet, there is no convincing evidence that these are necessary or effective. The problem therapeutically is the residual disease in the patient rather than in the marrow.

AIDS-related non-Hodgkin's lymphomas [10]

The occurrence of NHL in patients infected with HIV is now regarded as part of the defi-

nition of AIDS. These lymphomas are usually large cell immunoblastic or small non cleaved-cell lymphomas. Many arise in extra-nodal sites such as the CNS (see p. 525), a feature also apparent in the lymphomas arising in other immuno-deficiency states.

Typically the NHL occurs in a patient who has had AIDS for 1−2 years and whose CD4 cell count is very low. It is estimated that as more patients with AIDS live longer (due to antibiotic therapy) one-third or more will develop NHL. Coincident infection with HTLV1 is increasingly recognized especially in intravenous drug abusers.

Chemotherapy response rates are low (CR less than 50%) and often of short duration. Poor prognostic features are AIDS present before diagnosis of NHL, poor performance status, low CD4 count and extra-nodal disease. Opportunistic infections are frequent. Haematological toxicity, especially after long-term AZT treatment, often makes full dosage impossible. Treatment of CNS disease is discussed on p. 526.

NON-HODGKIN'S LYMPHOMA IN CHILDHOOD

Incidence and aetiology

Non-Hodgkin's lymphomas are rather more common in children than Hodgkin's disease (1.5:1) and are the third most frequent childhood cancer. Approximately 0.6 per 100 000 children below 15 years develop the disease each year with a peak onset age of 6−10 years (Fig. 26.1). A variety of inherited diseases predispose to childhood NHL (Table 26.1). The other aetiological factors are discussed on pp. 503−5.

Pathology

The distinction between childhood NHL and leukaemia is to some extent a semantic one. Many childhood lymphomas spread to the bone marrow and the frequency of diagnosis of marrow involvement is increasing as tech-

Table 26.6 Pathology of childhood non-Hodgkin's lymphoma

Diffuse lymphoblastic lymphoma: B cell, T cell
Diffuse large cell lymphoma
Burkitt's lymphoma

Table 26.7 Distribution of main primary site of disease in children with non-Hodgkin's lymphoma (%)

Intra-abdominal	30
Peripheral nodes	25
Mediastinal	22
Skeleton	7
Nasopharynx	10
Subcutaneous and skin	3.5
Epidural	1
Thyroid	0.5
Testis	0.5
Breast	0.5

niques for the demonstration of monoclonality of B cells (e.g. light-chain restriction) are improving. A convention is to regard more than 25% infiltration as compatible with lymphoma. The lymph nodes almost always show diffuse involvement and follicular patterns are very rare. The main types are shown in Table 26.6. Diffuse lymphoblastic lymphoma is the commonest type. Some of these tumours show a convoluted nuclear morphology, form rosettes with sheep red blood cells, and react with anti-T cell reagents, i.e. are T cell tumours. Others show surface Ig, i.e. are B cell tumours. Other tumours have neither T nor B markers.

Approximately 20% of cases are large cell lymphomas which are of diverse lineage. Some appear to be tumours of the follicle centre cell, others are B cell immunoblastic tumours, while yet others express T cell histiocytic markers. Many of these tumours express the CD30 antigen (ki-1, Ber-h2) which characterizes activated B and T cells. The majority of these appear to be peripheral T cell tumours.

Childhood NHL has a greater tendency to involve extra-nodal sites such as the gut, bone marrow and CNS. The lymph nodes of Waldeyer's ring and the mediastinum are frequently involved. A staging system is shown in Table 26.6; the distribution of the main mass of disease at presentation is shown in Table 26.7 and a staging system in Table 26.8. About 50% of the tumours arising in the mediastinum are of T cell origin.

Table 26.8 A simple staging system for childhood non-Hodgkin's lymphoma and Burkitt's lymphoma

Stage	Description
I	A single nodal area, or single extra-nodal site excluding the mediastinum
II	A single extra-nodal tumour with involved regional nodes Two or more nodal areas on one side of the diaphragm Primary gut lymphoma and mesenteric nodes
III	Two or more nodal sites above and below the diaphragm All primary intrathoracic tumours Extensive primary intra-abdominal disease All paraspinal or epidural tumours
IV	Involvement of CNS or marrow

Burkitt's lymphoma

I	Single extra-abdominal site
II	Multiple extra-abdominal sites
III	Intra-abdominal tumour
IV	Intra-abdominal tumour with extra-abdominal sites

Childhood B cell lymphomas

The majority of NHL in childhood are B cell tumours. These diffuse lymphomas are either of large cell type or consist of small non-cleaved

cells. The large cell lymphomas are usually found in boys and are often extra-nodal occurring in the nasopharynx, lung, mediastinum, bone, soft tissues and tonsils.

The small non-cleaved cell lymphomas are either Burkitt's lymphoma, or a form in which the cells are more pleomorphic. Burkitt's lymphoma occurs predominantly in Africa but is occasionally seen in Western countries. In Africa the presentation is usually with jaw or orbital tumours which grow rapidly. Other sites of involvement include the ovaries, retroperitoneal tissues, kidneys and glandular tissues such as breast and thyroid. Lymph node and marrow invasion is infrequent. Spread to the CNS is common and occurs early, often with paraplegia and cranial nerve palsy. A staging system which relates to prognosis is shown in Table 26.8. In Western countries Burkitt's lymphoma is more likely to present with an abdominal mass, or with enlarged cervical nodes. Marrow involvement is more frequent than in African cases.

Many childhood B cell lymphomas are generalized diseases with a risk of marrow and CNS involvement. However, some cases have a lower risk of meningeal spread. These cases include localized tumours of the gut, and patients with localized nodal disease. With localized gut lymphoma it is not clear if any treatment should be given after a complete resection, but it is the usual practice to treat with chemotherapy. Central nervous system prophylaxis does not appear to be necessary in these cases.

Childhood T cell lymphomas

These tumours often present with anterior mediastinal or cervical node enlargement. They disseminate rapidly to the bone marrow, the central nervous system, and to the testes. The cells may have convoluted nuclei and focal acid phosphatase activity in the cytoplasm. They usually exhibit T cell markers, reacting with T cell monoclonal antibodies and also show expression CD30 (see above). In childhood, Ki-1 (CD30 positive) lymphomas may be accompanied by a skin rash (lymphomatoid papulosis) which may be the presenting feature on which a rapidly evolving lymphoma develops [11].

Histologically the mediastinal tumours are described as lymphoblastic. The distinction between the childhood and adult forms of lymphoblastic lymphoma is arbitrary, and this and the treatment are more based on historical patterns of care rather than on clear evidence that such distinctions are important.

The patients are usually males and there may be superior vena cava obstruction at presentation which may need urgent treatment (usually with steroids and vincristine) before the diagnostic biopsy can be taken. This therapy can make subsequent diagnosis difficult, but the situation may be life-threatening and aggravated by biopsy under anaesthetic. Marrow failure from infiltration, or CNS symptoms, may be the presenting feature.

In many large treatment series these childhood tumours have not been characterized by modern methods. It now appears that many pleomorphic large cell lymphomas of childhood are T cell tumours even when there is no mediastinal mass present.

Diagnosis and investigation of childhood non-Hodgkin's lymphoma

Diagnosis is by lymph node or tissue biopsy. Initial staging investigations should be performed quickly since progress of the disease may be rapid. A marrow aspiration and biopsy should be performed and the CSF examined for cells. Biochemical tests of liver and kidney function are necessary with measurement of plasma calcium and urate since the tumour lysis syndrome (see Chapter 8) may occur when treatment starts.

Precise immunohistochemical definition of the tumour is now often possible. Although at present the relationship to prognosis is not clear, in the next few years the application of these techniques may allow a more precise definition of risk and therefore lead to greater precision in selecting treatment.

Treatment of large-cell non-Hodgkin's lymphoma in childhood

During the 1960s the prognosis of acute lymphoblastic leukaemia in childhood was improving rapidly with the use of more intensive drug regimens and prophylactic treatment of the CNS. Childhood lymphomas were, however, still rapidly fatal, 85% of children dying within 1 year and only 10–15% surviving 5 years.

In 1971, Wollner and her colleagues at the Memorial Sloan-Kettering Cancer Center in New York proposed a protocol of treatment for childhood lymphomas based on ideas derived from treatment of leukaemia. This protocol, known as LSA_2L_2, has greatly improved management and 5-year survival of 70–80% is now obtained with few children relapsing beyond this time. The LSA_2L_2 protocol has the following components.

• An intensive induction regimen using cyclophosphamide, vincristine, doxorubicin, prednisolone and intrathecal methotrexate.

• A consolidation phase using antimetabolites — cytosine arabinoside, thioguanine, asparaginase.

Fig. 26.8 Results of intensive chemotherapy of large cell non-Hodgkin's lymphoma in childhood.

• A maintenance phase lasting 1 year, using sequential alternating pairs of drugs.

The results of protocols of this type are shown in Fig. 26.8. Survival is better in Stages I and II disease.

In a randomized study [12] in paediatric non-Hodgkin's lymphoma of all stages comparing the LSA_2L_2 protocol with a slightly less aggressive regimen (COMP), the Children's Cancer Study Group in the United States found little difference between the two treatments, and better disease-free survival at 2 years for localized disease (81%) than for generalized disease (46%).

In non-localized disease the LSA_2L_2 protocol proved better than the COMP regimen for patients with lymphoblastic disease. Lymphoblastic lymphoma in childhood tends to present with mediastinal disease and includes many cases of T cell lymphoma. Non-lymphoblastic disease tends to be more localized and have an intra-abdominal presentation. In cases with a better prognosis (Stages I and II disease, Table 26.6) a recent trial has shown that radiotherapy can be omitted from the treatment and that treatment of moderate intensity combined with intrathecal methotrexate is associated with a 4-year survival of nearly 90%. There are considerable potential long-term advantages in reducing the amount of chemotherapy and radiation which these children receive. Failure of bone growth, bone cancers, leukaemia and sterility are sequelae of childhood treatment which may be avoided if less intensive treatment can be given without diminished survival.

The optimum treatment for the tumours expressing CD30 has not yet been defined but regimens based on COMP or the LSA_2L_2 programme have generally been employed.

Other regimens have been used, some of which include cranial irradiation as prophylactic CNS treatment. With the LSA_2L_2 protocol, using intrathecal methotrexate only, the incidence of CNS relapse is about 16%. The incidence is probably lower when cranial irradiation is used in addition. The risk of CNS disease appears to be low for those with

Stage I nodal disease, and those whose intra-abdominal lymphoma has been resected.

The agents usually employed in treating this disease are cyclophosphamide, vincristine, methotrexate and prednisolone (COMP). Almost all children will have a complete remission but 50% will relapse. Cure is still possible if CNS relapse occurs, but many regimens now include some form of CNS prophylaxis.

Children who survive 2 years will probably be cured. The 2-year disease-free survival figures for each stage (Table 26.8) are A and B 80%; C 65%; and D 40%. In Stage C it is advisable to remove as much bulk as possible before treatment. With 90% removed the results approach those for stage A. More aggressive regimens are being developed for Stage D cases including very high dose chemotherapy with autologous bone marrow transplantation.

EXTRA-NODAL PRESENTATION OF NON-HODGKIN'S LYMPHOMA

Non-Hodgkin's lymphomas may present at a variety of extra-nodal sites, and when they do there are particular problems in diagnosis and management. In addition to presentation at an extra-nodal site, there may be involvement of these sites at a time when the nodal lymphoma relapses and disseminates. In this latter circumstance, this is usually part of a generalized spread of the disease. Treatment will be palliative if there has been intensive previous chemotherapy.

The account which follows concerns the management of non-Hodgkin's lymphomas presenting at an extra-nodal site, in the absence of clinically overt disease elsewhere.

Gastro-intestinal lymphoma [13]

Lymphomas may occur at any site in the gastro-intestinal tract but the stomach and the small intestine are most frequently involved. The aetiology and pathogenesis are not well understood. The gut-associated lymphoid tissue in a normal individual shows a well-defined pattern of lymphocyte traffic. Immunoglobulin bearing cells in the follicle centre of small intestinal lymphoid nodules (Peyer's patches) migrate into the bloodstream and return to the lamina propria of the small bowel where they differentiate to plasma cells. A similar 'homing' mechanism may take place with gastric and large bowel lymphocytes and with lymphocytes bearing immunoglobulin of other classes.

NON-HODGKIN'S LYMPHOMA OF THE STOMACH

Pathology and clinical features

Lymphoma of the stomach is an uncommon tumour, comprising less than 0.5% of all gastric neoplasms. The patient is usually middle-aged or elderly but the disease can affect young adults. In many cases the tumour begins as a low-grade lesion in the mucosa with destruction of the glandular tissue — 'lymphoepithelial lesions'. This low-grade tumour may occur diffusely in the stomach and remain localized to the stomach wall for several years. Some tumours are of large cell type and spread early to adjacent lymph nodes. As with small intestinal lymphoma, it is possible that the lymphoid cells in the low-grade tumours are specific B lymphocytes, with the property of homing to gastric mucosa with little tendency to spread or lodge in other sites until late in the disease.

The two most widely used staging systems are given in Table 26.9. The TNM system is limited by the failure to give weight to the importance of the finding of nodal involvement not adjacent to the stomach (II_1 versus II_2 disease in the Ann Arbor system).

The presentation of gastric lymphoma is similar to that of adenocarcinoma of the stomach with nausea, anorexia and upper abdominal discomfort as the chief symptoms and occasionally haematemesis, or chronic iron deficiency anaemia being associated. Barium meal shows

Table 26.9 Staging systems for gastric lymphoma

	TNM	Ann Arbor
Limited to stomach wall	I	I
Mucosa alone	IA	
Submucosa	IB	
Serosal	IC	
Adjacent (perigastric) nodes	II	II$_1$
Non-adjacent intra-abdominal	III	II$_2$
Nodes outside abdomen	III	III
Disseminated, non-nodal disease	IV	IV

a large gastric ulcer or appearances similar to adenocarcinoma of the stomach. On endoscopy, a malignant ulcer is usually seen but occasionally, the appearances can simulate a benign gastric ulcer. Biopsy evidence can be misleading since the specimen may show small lymphocytes which are hard to distinguish from an inflammatory infiltrate. Recently it has been reported that there is a close association between the low-grade gastric lymphoma of mucosa-associated lymphoid tissue (MALT) and infection with *Helicobacter pylori* [14]. Treatment of *H. pylori* infection may lead to remission of lymphoma but it is not known for how long.

Treatment

Treatment of gastric lymphoma has usually been by surgical resection if possible [15]. The lack of randomized trials means that clear-cut guidance concerning non-surgical treatment is difficult. The following account represents an assessment of the present position.

For low-grade tumours confined to the stomach (Stage I) it is reasonable, if resection has been complete, to follow an expectant policy with repeat endoscopy (yearly) to ascertain if new lymphoepithelial lesions are developing. If they do then chemotherapy should be given. The 'correct' chemotherapy is not known but it seems reasonable to use combination therapy (e.g. CHOP or equivalent) in younger patients and chlorambucil in the elderly. If the diagnosis

of a low-grade lymphoma has been made on biopsy and *H. pylori* infection is present, it seems reasonable to assess the response to anti-Helicobacter treatment. It is not clear if this treatment with or without cytotoxic chemotherapy can avoid the need for surgery.

For localized high-grade tumours and all tumours of Stage II or worse there is a higher risk of relapse. These relapses may be outside the abdomen (in 50% of cases of Stages II$_2$ or III disease). Stage II$_1$ low-grade tumours may be treated by gastric and upper abdominal radiotherapy but increasingly the preference is to use chemotherapy. Stage II$_1$ high-grade tumours are usually treated with combination chemotherapy. For Stage II$_2$ or III chemotherapy seems the most appropriate treatment and is clearly indicated for Stage IV disease.

SMALL BOWEL LYMPHOMA [16]

Pathology

Lymphoma of the small intestine represents the most common gut tumour of children below the age of 10 years and there is a rise in incidence in adults above the age of 50 years. There is a slight male preponderance (M : F, 5 : 1) and there are two predisposing conditions. In long-standing untreated coeliac disease there is an increased incidence of intestinal lymphoma, and in this situation the lymphoma has now been shown to be of T cell type and the bowel is usually widely involved. In the Middle East, there is a high incidence of intestinal lymphoma which is usually preceded by a diffuse plasma cell and lymphocytic proliferation in the small bowel, known as immunoproliferative disease of the small intestine. During this early phase there is an excess production by the plasma cells of the heavy chain of IgA — the α chain (α chain disease). At this early stage, the disease may respond to treatment with antibiotics, but it subsequently progresses and a B cell lymphoma develops which may be rapidly evolving. The secretion of α heavy chains in the blood may disappear at this stage.

In the typical case of intestinal lymphoma in Europeans, no predisposing cause has been detected. The neoplasm arises in the lymphoid tissues of the mucosa of the bowel, invades and ulcerates the mucosa, and penetrates through the bowel wall to the serosal surface. The lymphoma may begin, as in the stomach, with a low-grade lymphoepithelial lesion which spreads to involve the full thickness of the bowel wall, often above the site of the neoplasm. Histologically, many small bowel lymphomas are of the diffuse large cell type, but in adults some of the lymphomas are of lower grade [14].

Clinical features

In small bowel lymphoma the presentation is usually with subacute or acute intestinal obstruction with colicky abdominal pain, vomiting and constipation. There may be diarrhoea or even malabsorption but this is unusual. Gastro-intestinal haemorrhage occurs, usually of a chronic type leading to iron deficiency anaemia. When perforation occurs the clinical picture is typical of perforation of the bowel at any site. Occasionally patients may present with ascites, usually chylous in nature, but sometimes it is due to widespread dissemination of intraperitoneal lymphoma. When the disease has become more extensive within the abdomen, there may be fever and anaemia, and intestinal lymphoma is a cause of pyrexia of unknown origin.

The diagnosis is usually made at laparotomy or by a barium follow-through examination which may show infiltration of the bowel wall with ulceration and segments of narrowing above which are areas of bowel dilatation.

The management of non-Hodgkin's lymphoma of the small intestine is often difficult. This is in part due to the fact that the disease often presents as an acute surgical emergency and may be operated on by an inexperienced surgeon and adequate resection not carried out. Nevertheless, the prognosis is dependent on an adequate surgical excision of the tumour. A

Table 26.10 Staging of intestinal lymphoma

IA	Single tumour confined to gut
IB	Two or more tumours confined to gut
IIA	Local node involvement
IIB	Local extension to adjacent structures
IIC	Local tumour with perforation and peritonitis
III	Widespread lymph node enlargement
IV	Disseminated tumour (to liver, spleen and elsewhere)

simple system of staging related to prognosis is shown in Table 26.10.

All cases should be further staged with chest X-ray and bone marrow aspiration. A liver biopsy should be performed during the laparotomy. Complete local excision of the tumour with the cut ends free of disease, and without involvement of mesenteric nodes, will frequently result in a cure, and the role of radiation therapy and adjuvant chemotherapy is still to be determined in this type of case. If the lymphoma is of low-grade histology and complete excision has been carried out, then it is probable that no further treatment is needed. If, as is more likely, there is local node involvement and the histology is of a diffuse large cell type, most oncologists would treat the patient further and in recent years the tendency has been to use combination chemotherapy rather than to attempt to control the disease by local radiation. There is a particular danger in the use of combination chemotherapy in patients in whom the tumour has not been resected completely, with perforation of the bowel wall a result of tumour lysis. This has a high mortality. In unresectable tumours it is therefore prudent to begin chemotherapy in lower dose both to allow healing of the bowel wall as the tumour regresses more slowly, and to avoid neutropenia which will add to mortality if perforation occurs. Without combination chemotherapy the 5-year survival of diffuse lymphomas of the gut is about 20%, and of follicular lymphomas about 50%, but this clearly depends on the stage.

The combination of drugs usually employed will include cyclophosphamide, vincristine, doxorubicin and prednisolone in various regimens as for diffuse non-Hodgkin's lymphomas at other sites (Table 26.4). In children, the likelihood of CNS involvement is small and it does not appear that prophylactic treatment of the CNS is an essential part of management.

The lymphoma complicating coeliac disease presents particular problems. The preferred designation is 'enteropathy-associated T cell lymphoma'. The mean time of onset is 7 years after the diagnosis of coeliac disease but may be many years later. The lymphoma does not regress on a gluten-free diet and typically the patients do not show anti-gliadin antibody in the blood. Cutaneous and pulmonary spread of the lymphoma is characteristic. The small bowel is frequently involved with an ulcerative lesion which may be the harbinger of the malignant change. Resection of the lymphoma is carried out where possible. Although chemotherapy is usually given postoperatively the prognosis is bad due to the poor nutritional state of the patient and the risks of perforation and haemorrhage.

α-Chain disease

The lymphoma which follows immune proliferative small intestine disease (IPSID) is characterized by a transformation of the nodular mucosal infiltrate into a high-grade B cell lymphoma where there is secretion of α heavy chain (subclass 1). Recent studies have suggested that IPSID is a neoplasm from the beginning. Although in the early stage IPSID may regress with antibiotics, when it transforms to a high-grade tumour treatment with chemotherapy is difficult and usually unsuccessful [17].

LYMPHOMATOUS POLYPOSIS [18]

This is a rare disease in which polyps occur in the ileocaecal region in patients over 50 years of age. The polyps consist of a nodular or diffuse lymphoid (centrocytic) tumour and the mesenteric nodes are usually involved. The tumour disseminates widely early on. Treatment with chemotherapy produces regression but the prognosis is poor.

NON-HODGKIN'S LYMPHOMA OF BONE (see also Chapter 23, p. 446) [19]

Non-Hodgkin's lymphoma frequently invades the marrow and may sometimes cause localized bone lesions with pain, vertebral collapse and pathological fractures. Occasionally non-Hodgkin's lymphoma presents as a bone lesion and most of these cases are of large cell lymphoma formerly called 'reticulum cell sarcoma of bone'. Sometimes the lesion is localized with no evidence of non-Hodgkin's lymphoma at other sites, even after extensive investigations. In children, isolated lymphoma of bone may be mistaken for Ewing's sarcoma. Immunohistochemical studies will usually resolve any diagnostic difficulty. In most cases of non-Hodgkin's lymphoma of bone the lesion is confined to one bone and a long bone is usually affected. The antecedent history is often very long and the lesions are often very large with extensive soft tissue infiltration.

The diagnosis is based on the finding of a bone lesion in the absence of widespread lymphoma at other sites including the bone marrow. Pretreatment staging therefore includes CT scan of the abdomen and mediastinum and a bone marrow examination.

Although radiotherapy (40–45 Gy) produces local control in over 90% of cases, and should encompass a generous margin of normal bone and soft tissue, dissemination to lymph nodes occurs in approximately 50% of cases. It is usual practice therefore to give combination chemotherapy before radiotherapy. It is not known whether, in the era of intensive chemotherapy, radiation treatment can be dropped and at present local treatment is given even if the chemotherapy response is excellent. In the very elderly it is reasonable to treat with radiation alone in the first instance.

CNS involvement with lymphoma

Primary lymphomas of the brain and spinal cord occur but are rare. Usually the CNS is involved as part of the pattern of spread of generalized disease and there is a particular tendency for the CNS to be involved in diffuse lymphomas especially of childhood, of T cell type and when there is marrow involvement.

PRIMARY LYMPHOMA OF THE BRAIN [20]

These uncommon tumours occur more frequently in AIDS, in renal allograft recipients and in those on long-term immunosuppressive therapy. Except in AIDS, the histological appearances are usually of a follicular centre cell lymphoma with both centrocytic and centroblastic forms. Lymphoplasmacytic types also occur. They arise in the cerebrum in 70% cases, cerebellum and brain stem (25% of cases), and rarely in the spinal cord. They tend to be multicentric, and perivascular infiltration is common. Presentation is with the signs and symptoms of a brain tumour (Chapter 11, p. 207). Although rare in the spinal cord, seeding into the CSF occasionally occurs late in the disease. An unusual complication is migration of lymphoma cells into the vitreous of the eyes causing visual loss. The patients do not usually show lymphoma elsewhere at presentation or later in the disease. Bone marrow and CSF examination are essential staging investigations.

In the non-AIDS-related cases treatment is with radiotherapy but the disease can be difficult to control, local relapse being common even after doses as high as 45–50 Gy. Spinal irradiation is usually recommended. There are as yet too few data to know whether systemic chemotherapy improves results, although this is increasingly employed before radiation. The prognosis is not good and, if CSF seeding has occurred it is very difficult to cure the disease even with chemotherapy, neuraxis radiation and intra-thecal treatment.

At the start of the AIDS epidemic CNS lymphoma was recognized as an associated tumour. The tumour is a high-grade B cell neoplasm, typically occuring in patients already gravely ill with AIDS (many cases being diagnosed at autopsy). The presentation is with focal neurological signs, cranial nerve palsies, fits and mental confusion. On CT scan the tumour mass may be difficult to delineate and ring-enhancing lesions may make distinction from toxoplasmosis difficult. Treatment is difficult and unsuccessful. The patients are ill and immunocompromised. Radiation may help localized disease. Chemotherapy is associated with a great likelihood of opportunistic infection.

SECONDARY LYMPHOMA OF THE CNS

Involvement of the CNS occurs in about 9% of all cases of non-Hodgkin's lymphoma [12]. The clinical presentation is either with lymphomatous meningitis (55%) or with extradural compression (45%), see Fig. 26.9. The great majority of patients have diffuse large cell (centroblastic) lymphoma or diffuse centrocytic lymphoma as the primary disease. Light microscopical evidence of involvement of the bone marrow at diagnosis is present in 70% of cases, probably an underestimate if more sensitive tests of involvement are undertaken. The patients usually have advanced nodal spread at diagnosis, and involvement of retroperitoneal nodes is common. Lymphomatous involvement of the CNS is particularly frequent in childhood lymphomas and in lymphomas of T cell type.

The clinical presentation of lymphomatous meningitis is with cranial nerve palsies, mental confusion and raised intracranial pressure. Root lesions frequently occur due to compression and perivascular infiltration. The most important diagnostic test is lumbar puncture. The CSF is examined cytologically and, if possible, surface markers (light chain restriction, T cell markers) should be identified in an attempt to distinguish the cells from reactive lymphocytes which might be found in tuberculous or fungal

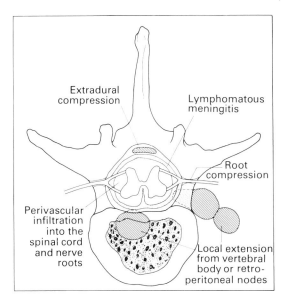

Fig. 26.9 Involvement of the spinal cord with lymphoma. Extradural compression may result from lymphomatous involvement of the vertebral body or by extension from para-aortic nodes. Leptomeningeal infiltration is probably haematogenous and is particularly common when bone marrow is involved.

meningitis and which may be part of the differential diagnosis.

Epidural compression usually occurs in the thoracic spine, but nerve roots may be compressed including the cauda equina. These patients usually have retroperitoneal lymphoma and sometimes intravertebral deposits. The clinical syndrome is with a paraparesis and is a medical emergency whose management is discussed in Chapter 8.

Lymphomatous meningitis is a serious complication and very few patients in whom it has developed will be cured. The management is with intra-thecal chemotherapy using methotrexate in combination with cytosine arabinoside and craniospinal irradiation. Patients at high risk (many childhood lymphomas and T cell lymphomas in childhood and adolescence) should receive prophylactic treatment of the CNS with intra-thecal methotrexate and craniospinal irradiation in an attempt to avoid this

complication. Although it has been argued that adult patients with large cell and undifferentiated lymphomas should receive CNS prophylaxis it does not in fact appear that the incidence of CNS disease in adults is rising as survival improves with chemotherapy (as it did in childhood leukaemia). Newer regimens for systemic treatment often include methotrexate and other drugs which penetrate the CSF and these may confer adequate protection. Alternatively, the risk of CNS disease in adults may be lower than had been predicted.

Non-Hodgkin's lymphoma of Waldeyer's ring

Non-Hodgkin's lymphoma may present in the lymphoid tissue of the oropharynx and nasopharynx, in the absence of clinical evidence of disease elsewhere. The histology may be follicular or diffuse, centroblastic or centrocytic. The presentation is with difficulty in swallowing and nasal congestion. There may be enlargement of cervical lymph nodes, or evidence of disease elsewhere.

Approximately 20% of patients have localized disease (Stage I) and 40% have involvement of cervical nodes (Stage II). Lymphangiography will demonstrate that half of the patients with Stage II disease have involved abdominal nodes (Stage III). Approximately 50% of patients have Stage III disease at presentation, and 10% of patients, Stage IV disease (in bone marrow or liver). Patients who present with Stage I disease do not usually prove to have more extensive disease on investigation.

The gastro-intestinal tract may be involved, and a barium meal and follow-through should be performed as part of the initial investigations.

For patients with disease localized to Waldeyer's ring and cervical nodes, treatment is usually with radiotherapy. Many patients (possibly 60%) will be free of disease at 5–10 years. For patients with Stages III and IV disease, treatment is with chemotherapy, but it is not clear if the prognosis has been greatly improved by modern regimens. In the past, most of these patients died before 5 years.

Ocular non-Hodgkin's lymphoma

Uncommonly the conjunctiva, the orbit and the globe of the eye can be the site of NHL. Orbital lymphomas present with unilateral proptosis, external ocular palsy and intra-ocular lymphoma with visual disturbance. Conjunctival lymphoma presents with swelling of the lid and visible tumour.

These tumours are uncommon, and their prognosis is not known with certainty. They must be distinguished from the more frequent benign lymphoid proliferations which affect the eye. They are usually treated with local radiotherapy, but systemic spread probably occurs in about half the cases.

Non-Hodgkin's lymphoma of the lung

Non-Hodgkin's lymphoma may spread to the lung either directly from mediastinal nodes or as part of a more widespread dissemination (usually in advanced and drug-resistant cases). Both Hodgkin's and non-Hodgkin's lymphoma may involve the lung and cause considerable diagnostic difficulty.

Lymphomatoid granulomatosis

This disease usually arises in the lung. It consists of a pleomorphic infiltrate, often involving vessel walls with areas of necrosis and atypical lymphoid cells. The disease is indolent often over many years. Malignant, invasive, lymphoma occurs in up to 50% of cases even if the disease is not considered malignant at the onset. In some cases T cell monoclonal proliferation has been demonstrated (by T cell receptor gene rearrangement). Cases have been described in AIDS. Spread to the skin and CNS occur. Local resection may be curative. More widespread disease has a worse prognosis but long-term remissions may be obtained by steroids and chemotherapy. Epstein–Barr virus genome has been demonstrated in one case.

Malignant angioendotheliomatosis [21]

This disorder is characterized by fever, dementia, neurological signs, organ failure and skin lesions. There is intravascular proliferation of atypical mononuclear cells within small blood vessels. Recent studies have shown this to be a lymphoid tumour with positive B cell markers and numerous karyotypic abnormalities.

Cutaneous non-Hodgkin's lymphoma

The skin is a frequent site of secondary spread of NHL of all types. It is usually involved in the context of disseminated and often drug-resistant disease. Clinically there are subcutaneous lumps or papular infiltrates in the dermis. The treatment is of the underlying disease where possible. Superficial X-rays are very helpful in controlling troublesome lesions and electron therapy is useful for widespread cutaneous infiltrates.

The skin may also be the site of a primary lymphoma and in recent years it has become apparent that these are often T cell in origin. The two major syndromes are *mycosis fungoides* and *Sézary's syndrome*.

MYCOSIS FUNGOIDES [22]

This rare disease is uncommon in black people and has an equal sex incidence. The onset is usually at 40–60 years of age, though many cases may have a long history with an origin much earlier in life. There are three well-recognized stages in the clinical evolution, although in individual cases they are often not easily separable.

In the *erythematous* or *pre-tumour* stage there is a rash which may resemble psoriasis with fine red scaly patches. There are often poikilodermatous changes which suggest the diagnosis. This phase may last for many years and the diagnosis can only be substantiated by biopsy. There is acanthosis, parakeratosis and clusters of histiocytes (Darier–Pautrier abscesses).

In the *infiltrative* or *plaque* stage there are indurated plaques. Microscopically there is infiltration of the upper dermis and epidermis with lymphoma cells which are helper T cells. In the cases seen in Britain there is usually no significant lymph node enlargement. If the nodes do enlarge, they may show 'dermatopathic lymphadenopathy' and, later, clear evidence of tumour infiltration.

In the *tumour* stage the lesions enlarge and ulcerate. Involvement of internal organs may occur.

The most important prognostic factor is extent of disease. A staging system is shown in Table 26.11 — 90% of Stage I patients are alive at 8 years, while median survival in Stage II disease is 5 years and Stage IV, 2 years.

Management [22]

Treatment in the first stage is symptomatic with antipruritic agents. Steroid creams and topical nitrogen mustard have also been used. More advanced lesions, if not too infiltrated, can be treated with PUVA. Wide-field irradiation is the treatment usually used in the mycotic stage. Whole-body electron therapy is increasingly preferred in order to avoid treatment of deeper structures. Visceral involvement is very difficult to treat effectively.

Table 26.11 A staging system for mycosis fungoides

Stage	Description
I	Plaque or eczematous lesions
II	Plaque lesions with clinically enlarged but pathologically negative nodes. Tumours present with or without clinically enlarged but pathologically negative nodes
III	Generalized erythroderma
IV	Any skin lesion with pathologically involved nodes or visceral involvement

Chemotherapy responses occur and the most active agents are alkylating agents, etoposide, cisplatin and methotrexate. Combination chemotherapy produces higher response rates which are of longer duration, but cures do not occur and survival may not be superior to single agents. Recombinant interferon produces responses but its role in therapy is not yet defined.

SÉZARY'S SYNDROME

The original description was of patients with generalized erythroderma and large atypical lymphocytes in the blood. The latter are now known to be T cells (of helper type). The skin shows infiltration with T cells. Lymph node enlargement and hepatomegaly may be present. The disorder can be regarded as a disseminated form of mycosis fungoides. The patient complains of intense itching, the skin becomes red and thickened and may be swollen. Hair is lost and palmar hyperkeratosis occurs with dystrophy and loss of nails. The circulating cells were called *cellules monstreuses* by Sézary. They do not infiltrate the marrow until late in the disease. Hepatosplenomegaly may occur and there may be lymph node enlargement.

Chemotherapy may produce remissions when the disease is widely disseminated, but the patient is not cured. Combination chemotherapy is usually employed. Responses to PUVA occur as in mycosis fungoides.

Non-Hodgkin's lymphoma of the thyroid

These tumours usually present as a rapidly enlarging thyroid mass in a middle-aged or elderly woman. They are associated with Hashimoto's thyroiditis, and areas of thyroiditis may be found in the gland on biopsy. Histologically they are usually diffuse large cell tumours which are generally of B cell type. Follicular and plasmacytoid forms are unusual, and T cell tumours are rare. The evolution of the disease in a gland affected by autoimmune disease is reminiscent of the development of lymphomas in Sjögren's syndrome. The mass does not take up radioactive iodine and cannot be distinguished clinically from other thyroid cancers. Diagnosis is made by biopsy or thyroidectomy. Radical surgery has little role in management, however, since the tumours are sensitive to radiotherapy.

Staging investigations are necessary since the prognosis is excellent with local treatment if the disease is confined to the gland. These investigations should include chest X-ray, abdominal CT scan and/or lymphogram, and marrow aspiration and biopsy. Relapse in the gut is relatively frequent and a small bowel barium examination may be useful.

If there is no local extension of the tumour from the gland and no evidence of involvement of adjacent nodes, radiotherapy (40 Gy in 4 weeks) to the gland and adjacent nodes will cure 90% of patients. Only 50% of patients with local and nodal extension will be cured, and the prognosis is also worse over the age of 65 years. Adjuvant chemotherapy should therefore be considered in these cases, and is clearly necessary for patients with more widespread disease. It seems likely that T cell tumours will also require chemotherapy. There are, as yet, few data to show whether chemotherapy will improve the prognosis.

Non-Hodgkin's lymphoma of the testis and ovary

Non-Hodgkin's lymphoma of the testis is usually a diffuse large cell (centroblastic) lymphoma. The patients are generally over the age of 50 years — an age when seminoma and teratoma are uncommon. The tumours are mostly unilateral but there is a considerable risk of contralateral involvement. Presentation is with a painless enlargement of the testis. After investigation most patients are found to have Stages I or II disease (Ann Arbor system, Table 25.2). The disease has a tendency to spread to abdominal nodes and to Waldeyer's ring. Occasionally CNS relapse occurs.

Staging investigations should include lym-

phangiogram and/or CT scan of the abdomen, and bone marrow examination. Localized disease (IE and IIE) can be adequately treated with radiotherapy to the pelvic and para-aortic lymph nodes. Bilateral or advanced (Stages III and IV) disease carries a poor prognosis and systemic chemotherapy is required.

TUMOUR LYSIS SYNDROME

This syndrome of hyperuricaemia and renal failure is particularly likely to occur in patients with Burkitt's lymphoma, those with large intra-abdominal tumours, and with T cell tumours with a large mediastinal mass. The cause, prevention and treatment of tumour lysis syndrome are discussed in Chapter 8.

REFERENCES

1 The emerging epidemic of non-Hodgkin's lymphoma. Current knowledge regarding aetiological factors. *Cancer Research* 1992; **52**. (This is a useful volume with several contributions on incidence, viral causes, immunosuppression and pathogenesis.)

2 McGrath I. *The Non-Hodgkin's Lymphomas.* London: Edward Arnold, 1990. This is a very useful general reference. The sections on molecular genetics are Chapter 6 (Haluska F.G. *et al.*) and Chapter 7 (Dalla-Favera *et al.*).

3 Isaacson P.G. Pathology of malignant lymphomas. *Current Opinion in Oncology* 1992; **4**: 811–820.

4 Rohatiner A., Lister T.A. Management of follicular lymphoma. *Current Opinion in Oncology* 1994; **6**: 473–79.

5 Coiffier B., Gisselbrecht C., Vose J.M. *et al.* Prognostic factors in aggressive malignant lymphomas: description and validation of an index that could identify patients requiring a more intensive therapy. *Journal of Clinical Oncology* 1991; **9**: 211–19.

6 Prestige B.R., Horning S.J., Hoppe R.T. Combined modality treatment for stage I–II large cell lymphoma. *International Journal of Radiation Oncology, Biology and Physics* 1988; **15**: 1633–40.

7 Fisher R.I., Gaynor E.R., Dahlberg S. *et al.* Comparison of a standard regimen (CHOP) with three intensive chemotherapy regimens for advanced non-Hodgkin's lymphoma. *New England Journal of Medicine* 1993; **328**: 1002–6.

8 Piccozi V.J., Coleman C.N. Lymphoblastic lymphoma. *Seminars in Oncology* 1990; **17**: 960–1104.

9 Goldstone A.H., Singer C.R.J., Gribben J.G. *et al*. Fifth report of EBMTG experience of ABMT in malignant lymphoma. *Bone Marrow Transplantation* 1988; **3** (suppl. 1): 33−36.

10 Levine A.M., Sullivan-Halley J., Pike M.C. *et al*. HIV-related lymphoma: Prognostic factors predictive of survival. *Cancer* 1991; **68**: 2466−72.

11 Kadin M.E., Sakko K., Berliner N. *et al*. Childhood ki-1 lymphoma presenting with skin lesions and peripheral lymphadenopathy. *Blood* 1986; **68**: 1042−49.

12 Anderson J.R., Wilson J.F., Jenkin D.T. *et al*. Childhood non-Hodgkin's lymphoma. The results of a randomized therapeutic trial comparing a 4-drug regimen (COMP) with a 10-drug regimen (LSA$_2$-L$_2$) *New England Journal of Medicine* 1983; **308**: 559−65.

13 Isaacson P.G., Spencer J. Malignant lymphoma of mucosa associated lymphoid tissue. *Histopathology* 1987; **11**: 445−62.

14 Wotherspoon A.C., Doglioni C., Diss T.C. *et al*. Regression of primary low grade B-cell gastric lymphoma of the mucosa-associated lymphoid tissue type after eradication of *Helicobacter pylori*. *Lancet* 1993; **342**: 575−77.

15 Gobbi P.G., Dionigi P., Barbieri F. *et al*. The role of surgery in the multi-modal treatment of primary gastric non-Hodgkin's lymphomas. *Cancer* 1990; **65**: 2528−36.

16 List A.F., Greer J.P., Cousa J.C. *et al*. Non-Hodgkin's lymphoma of the gastrointestinal tract. An analysis of clinical and pathological features affecting outcome. *Journal of Clinical Oncology* 1988; **6**: 1125−33.

17 Ben-Ayed F., Halphen M., Najjar T. *et al*. Treatment of alpha chain disease − results of a prospective study in 21 Tunisian patients by the Tunisian−French intestinal lymphoma study group. *Cancer* 1989; **63**: 1251−56.

18 O'Brian D.S., Kennedy M.J., Daly P.A. *et al*. Multiple lymphomatous polyposis of the gastrointestinal tract. A clinicopathologically distinctive form of non-Hodgkin's lymphoma of B cell centrocytic type. *American Journal of Surgical Pathology* 1989; **13**: 691−99.

19 Bacci G., Jaffe N., Emilani E. *et al*. Therapy for primary non-Hodgkin's lymphoma of bone and a comparison of results with Ewing's sarcoma. *Cancer* 1986; **57**: 1468−72.

20 Pollock I.F., Lunsford L.D., Flickinger J.C., Dameshek H.L. Prognostic factors in the diagnosis and treatment of primary central nervous system lymphoma. *Cancer* 1989; **63**: 939−47.

21 Molina A., Lombard C., Donlon T. *et al*. Immunohistochemical and cytogenetic studies indicate that malignant endotheliomatosis is a primary intravascular (angiotropic) lymphoma. *Cancer* 1990; **66**: 474−79.

22 Kuzel T.M., Springer E., Roenigk H.H., Rosen S.T. Mycosis Fungoides: time to define the best therapy. *Journal of the National Cancer Institute* 1990; **82**: 183−85.

Chapter 27
Myeloma and Other Paraproteinaemias

MYELOMA

Incidence and aetiology

Myeloma (multiple myeloma, myelomatosis, plasma cell myeloma) is chiefly a disease of the elderly. The incidence rises with age and is commonest in patients aged 65 and over (Fig. 27.1). It is almost twice as common in males. There is an annual incidence of approximately 3 per 100 000 and the disease is twice as frequent in the American black population as in the white. There is good evidence of a rising incidence over the past 25 years [1]. Family clusters have been reported, and there is an increased incidence in first degree relatives. Use of serum electrophoresis as a screening test reveals a far higher incidence of paraproteinaemia (a monoclonal immunoglobulin band), and up to 3% of an asymptomatic elderly population (70 years and older) have a monoclonal gammopathy detected by this means. Most of these patients will have a form of benign paraproteinaemia (see p. 533) but a minority subsequently develop symptomatic myeloma. As with other B cell neoplasms, there now appears to be an unequivocal relationship between radiation exposure and subsequent development of myeloma [2]. An increased incidence has been reported in a group of American radiologists, presumably due to life-long radiation exposure, and also in survivors of Nagasaki and Hiroshima with a delay of 20 years.

Pathogenesis

IMMUNOGLOBULIN ABNORMALITIES

Multiple myeloma is one of a group of B lymphocyte neoplasms which are characterized by continued synthesis and release of immunoglobulins (Table 27.1). In myeloma there is neoplastic proliferation of a clone of B lymphocytes resulting in the formation of large numbers of immature plasma cells which infiltrate the bone marrow and which can occasionally be found in the blood. The oncogenic event may, however, occur earlier in the B cell differentiation pathway but clonal expansion, giving rise to the clinical syndrome, occurs at the plasma cell stage (Fig. 27.2). Production of large amounts of a monoclonal immunoglobulin is, therefore, a finding characteristic of multiple myeloma. Calculations of growth rate in myel-

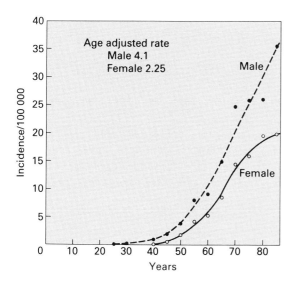

Fig. 27.1 Age-specific incidence of myeloma in Britain.

Table 27.1 Immunoglobulin-producing neoplasms

Benign
Monoclonal gammopathy of unknown significance
  (MGUS)
Cold agglutinin disease

Malignant
Myeloma
Waldenström's macroglobulinaemia
Primary amyloidosis
Non-Hodgkin's lymphomas
Heavy chain diseases (γ, α, or μ)

oma have indicated that the disease has usually been present for several years before the tumour has expanded sufficiently to cause symptoms [1].

The basic structure of normal immunoglobulins consists of two polypeptide light chains (with molecular weights of 22 000) and two heavy chains (molecular weights of 55 000−70 000). These are held together by covalent (disulphide) and non-covalent bonds (Fig. 27.3). There is variability in heavy chain structure, with five separate types of heavy

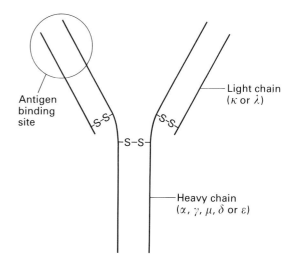

Fig. 27.3 Basic structure of immunoglobulin molecules. Two light chains are joined by disulphide bonds to two heavy chains. These are also joined by a variable number of disulphide bonds. The heavy chain varies in each immunoglobulin class, but light chains do not.

chain γ, α, μ, δ and ϵ. These differences form the basis of the five classes of immunoglobulin, IgG, IgA, IgM, IgD and IgE. Furthermore there are altogether 10 different heavy chain sequences, 4-γ, 2-α, 2-μ and only one each of δ and ϵ. Of the γ immunoglobulins, IgG$_3$ is particularly prone to polymerize, as is IgA and IgM. There are, however, only two types of light chain — kappa (κ) and lambda (λ). IgG, IgD and IgE are found in the plasma as single molecules with a molecular weight of 160 000−200 000. IgM is a macroglobulin (molecular weight 900 000) synthesized as a pentamer of IgG structure. IgA is formed by plasma cells in the gut and respiratory tract, and is therefore found in external secretions such as saliva, tears, bronchial and gastro-intestinal mucosa, as well as in the blood. It has an important role in primary defence against invading pathogens.

Normal immunoglobulins are diverse in their detailed structure since they are synthesized in response to a variety of antigenic stimuli. Each immunoglobulin molecule recognizes one antigenic structure only, and the portion of the molecule which confers this specificity is known

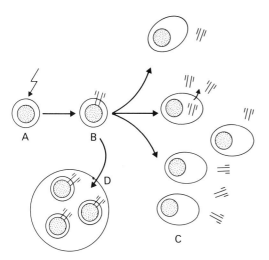

Fig. 27.2 Pathogenesis of myeloma. (A) Oncogenic event in a B cell; (B) expansion of a clone of malignant B cells; (C) proliferation of plasma cells leading to bone lesions and production of paraprotein; (D) suppression of normal B cells leads to hypogammaglobulinaemia.

as the idiotypic determinant. It is located at the highly variable antigen binding site (Fig. 27.3). By contrast, in myeloma the product of the neoplastic plasma cell clone is an immunoglobulin of a single homogeneous structure (i.e. a single idiotype). This tumour product is called myeloma protein or M-protein (not to be confused with IgM), or paraprotein. There is always light-chain restriction, that is, to either κ or λ type.

In most patients with myeloma, whole immunoglobulin molecules are often synthesized, but there may be a disproportionate production of one component so that free light chains may be produced. In approximately 1% of patients with multiple myeloma no monoclonal protein can be detected in the plasma or urine. In these patients (often termed nonsecretors) the myeloma cells can sometimes be shown to contain abnormal heavy or light chains in the cytoplasm which are not secreted. In about 25% of patients, only light chains are produced.

When free light chains are secreted into the blood, they cross the glomerular membrane and are therefore detectable in the urine. They have the unusual property of producing a cloudy precipitate when the urine is heated to 50–60°C, with dissociation of the precipitate as the temperature is raised near boiling point. Excretion of free light chains (sometimes called Bence-Jones protein (BJP) after Henry Bence-Jones who described it in 1850) occurs in 40–50% of all cases of myeloma, and may be the only detectable abnormal protein since about 25% of patients with myeloma do not synthesize complete immunoglobulin molecules. It is detected nowadays by immunoelectrophoresis of the urine.

The major classes of immunoglobulin have differing physical properties and when there is excess production these may be clinically relevant since many aspects of the disease are attributable to the physical characteristics or deposition of the immunoglobulin itself. For example, IgM has a high molecular weight and hyperviscosity syndrome is not uncommon (see below). IgA molecules polymerize in the plasma and will also cause hyperviscosity. Excess light chains may be deposited in the renal tubule and contribute to renal failure (see p. 536). Polymerization of light chains is one component of amyloid which also contributes to renal disease. The incidence of the different types of myeloma protein roughly parallels the concentrations of normal serum immunoglobulins (Table 27.2) and reflects the number of plasma cells normally found in each group. IgG myeloma is the commonest type, followed by IgA. IgM production is rarely due to a true myeloma but is usually part of Waldenström's macroglobulinaemia or NHL (see p. 543). IgD myeloma is very uncommon, and IgE exceedingly rare. More than 5×10^9 plasma cells must be present for the paraprotein to be detectable as a discrete immunoglobulin band.

In myeloma an assessment of tumour mass can be made using a formula which includes haemoglobin, calcium, presence of multiple bone lesions, paraprotein concentration and blood urea. Patients with a large tumour mass ($>0.5 \times 10^{12}$ cells) have a worse prognosis and respond less frequently to chemotherapy. Some of the important prognostic features are shown in Table 27.3. One of the more successful attempts to determine likely prognosis has used only serum β_2 microglobulin (s-β_2m) values and initial haemoglobin level, according to the formula: $1.156 \log (s-\beta_2 m[mg/l] - 0.007 Hb$

Table 27.2 Paraprotein frequency in myeloma

Immunoglobulin class	Frequency (%)
IgG	55
IgA	24
Bence-Jones only	25
IgM*	2
IgD	2
Biclonal	1
None detected	1

* Excluding Waldenström's macroglobulinaemia

Table 27.3 Prognostic features in myeloma

Good	Poor
Low serum β_2 microglobulin level <2 mg/l	High serum β_2 microglobulin level >2 mg/l
Haemoglobin >10 g/dl	Haemoglobin <8.5 g/dl
Serum calcium normal	Serum calcium >2.9 mmol/l
No lytic bone lesions	More than 3 bone lesions
Low paraprotein level	High paraprotein level
IgG < 50 g/l	IgG > 70 g/l
IgA < 30 g/l	IgA > 50 g/l
Urine light chains <2 g/24 hours	Light chains >5 gm/24 hours
Plasma urea <8 mmol/l	Urea >8 mmol/l

[g/l]). In this formula, larger values imply a worse prognosis [3].

Depression of production of normal immunoglobulin is a characteristic feature of the disease and one which helps to differentiate it from benign varieties of a monoclonal gammopathy (p. 542). It occurs most frequently and profoundly in IgG myeloma, and to a lesser extent in cases producing Bence-Jones protein only. The mechanism of suppression of normal Ig production is not clear. This depression affects all classes of normal immunoglobulin and contributes greatly to susceptibility to bacterial infection.

There are many other causes of monoclonal immunoglobulin production (Table 27.4). One disorder in particular, monoclonal gammopathy of unknown significance (MGUS), previously

Table 27.4 Causes of monoclonal gammaglobulinaemia other than myeloma

Monoclonal gammopathy of unknown significance (MGUS)

Non-lymphoid and lymphoid malignancy
Carcinoma of breast, gastro-intestinal tract, ovary, bladder, prostate and others
Soft tissue sarcomas
Melanoma
NHL
Waldenström's macroglobulinaemia

Autoimmune diseases
Rheumatoid arthritis
Polyarteritis nodosa

erroneously termed 'benign monoclonal gammopathy', is very common in the elderly and may cause diagnostic difficulty, particularly as it may later progress to myeloma. The current understanding of the MGUS–myeloma relationship is that a spectrum exists from the relatively benign disorder to the frankly malignant. Although MGUS shares certain features with myeloma, notably the excess immunoglobulin synthesis and occasional Bence-Jones proteinuria, the marrow plasma cell infiltrate is modest (<10%) and there are no bone lesions. Progression of MGUS to myeloma is well described and may occur slowly, with a period of 'smouldering' disease which can cause difficulty for the clinician.

This may be accompanied only by mild anaemia, appearance for the first time of BJP positivity and the emergence of moderate symptoms — and finally the need for treatment after as much as a decade of careful observation.

It is not yet clear which oncogenes or other DNA sequences are the most critical for myeloma development, either *de novo* or within an existing background of MGUS. Initial studies suggest that both the *myc* and *ras* oncogene series may be implicated. It is also known that of the cytokines, interleukin 6 (IL-6) is an important agent capable of stimulating plasma cell growth and differentiation, and lymphotoxin (TNFβ) is a known mediator of osteoclast activation and therefore of myeloma bone destruction.

PATHOLOGICAL FEATURES

In myeloma there is infiltration of both the bone and the bone marrow by malignant plasma cells (Fig. 27.4). Typically, these cells are round or oval, often with an eccentrically placed nucleus like their normal counterpart. The cytoplasm is densely basophilic, due to the RNA which produces the paraprotein, with a clear perinuclear zone where the Golgi apparatus is situated. Immunoglobulin is present in the rough endoplasmic reticulum. Abnormal forms are often present and these cells are large and may be bi- or tri-nucleate, sometimes with more than one nucleolus and the nucleus eccentrically placed. These abnormal forms may be diagnostically helpful when the degree of infiltration is small. The marrow infiltration is often patchy, unlike leukaemia — hence the name multiple myeloma — a focal tumour mass. The histological diagnosis is highly probable when the level of infiltration exceeds 20% of all nucleated marrow cells, but the diagnosis is not excluded by lesser degrees of involvement. The bone becomes destroyed by the tumour. Typically the lesions are lytic and fractures are common (Fig. 27.5). The mechanism of lysis is not fully

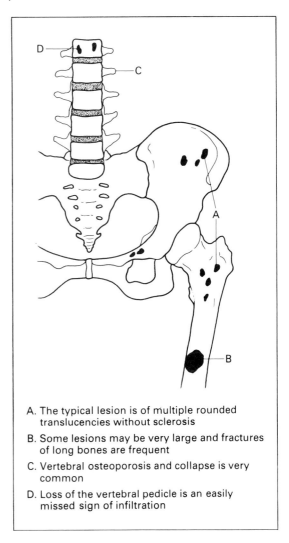

A. The typical lesion is of multiple rounded translucencies without sclerosis

B. Some lesions may be very large and fractures of long bones are frequent

C. Vertebral osteoporosis and collapse is very common

D. Loss of the vertebral pedicle is an easily missed sign of infiltration

Fig. 27.5 Diagrammatic representation of bone lesions in myeloma.

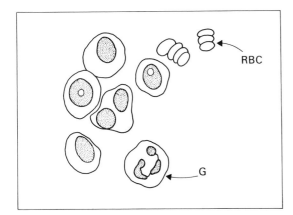

Fig. 27.4 A clump of myeloma cells in bone marrow. The cells are often large and sometimes contain more than one nucleus. The nucleus may be eccentrically placed or central. Red cells (RBC) are shown forming rouleaux due to the paraprotein; a granulocyte is also shown (G).

understood but osteoclastic activating factors produced by the myeloma or mature B cells have been described. Any bone can be affected and common sites include vertebrae, pelvis, skull, ribs and proximal long bones.

The kidney is affected in several ways (Fig. 27.6). First, light chains are taken up by distal renal tubular cells which are a major site of catabolism of normal light chains. The massive load of light chains results in tubular damage

A. Free light chains cross the glomerular basement membrane

B. Free light chains are deposited in cells of the distal tubule and collecting system and fill the collecting tubule causing obstruction

C. Amyloid is deposited in the glomerulus

D. Hypercalcaemia reduces glomerular filtration rate

E. Hyperuricaemia leads to distal tubular and interstitial urate deposition

Fig. 27.6 Renal damage in myeloma.

and large casts of light chains and albumin fill the tubule and obstruct the nephron, imposing a further load on the remaining nephrons. Specific defects in tubular reabsorption may occur, possibly due to the protein aggregation in renal tubule cells and leading to tubular reabsorptive defects with leakage of amino acids, glucose, potassium and phosphate (acquired Fanconi syndrome).

Second, amyloid deposition in the blood vessels of the glomerulus occurs in 10% of patients. It is especially common in those cases where light chains alone are produced. In myeloma (but not in all other circumstances), this protein consists in part of polymerized light chain fragments. λ Light chains are much more

likely to lead to amyloid formation. Other features of the disease which contribute to renal impairment include recurrent hypercalcaemia with dehydration, hypercalciuria and nephrocalcinosis, urate deposition and renal tubular leakage. Urinary tract infection is common and pyelonephritis may develop. Together, these processes constitute 'myeloma kidney'.

Occasionally there is deposition of malignant plasma cells in the kidney, or in other soft tissues producing localized swellings. This typically occurs late in the disease when there is a large tumour mass. Skin, lymph nodes, liver and spleen are the commonest sites.

Clinical features

Patients with multiple myeloma may be asymptomatic for many years before presenting with weakness, bone pain, anorexia and other symptoms due either to abnormal proliferation of the malignant plasma cells, to direct effects of the abnormal immunoglobulin, or to hypercalcaemia.

Diffuse bone pain is often the major complaint and skeletal abnormalities are present in about two-thirds of patients. The pain is typically dull or aching, and often felt in the spine, ribs or pelvis. Pathological fractures are common and acute back pain from a vertebral crush fracture is a frequent first presentation of myeloma. This may lead to acute cord compression (see Chapter 8). In its later stages, multiple myeloma may be among the most painful of all cancers with multiple sites of vertebral and long bone fracture from widespread malignant infiltration.

Typical radiological appearances include generalized osteopenia or osteoporosis (particularly evident in the dorsal and lumbar spine and sacroiliac area), and punched out osteolytic lesions, with little or no sclerosis (Fig. 27.5), although osteoblastic lesions are occasionally seen. Full radiological skeletal survey will often reveal unsuspected bone lesions and should always be performed at diagnosis. In addition to the ribs, vertebrae, and hips, these lesions are frequently and characteristically found in the skull, where they usually remain asymptomatic until they reach a large size. Biopsy of any of these sites reveals heavy infiltration with abnormal plasma cells.

Many patients present with fatigue and lassitude due to anaemia, and recurrent bacterial infection due to immune paresis. Nausea, anorexia and dehydration may be due to hypercalcaemia and lead to deteriorating renal function.

Hyperviscosity syndrome may develop in patients in whom the type and level of abnormal immunoglobulin contributes to an increase in plasma viscosity. This is most commonly seen in patients with Waldenström's macroglobulinaemia (see below) but also occurs in patients with myeloma especially with IgA, IgM and IgG$_3$ paraproteins. Clinically this syndrome consists of neurological symptoms, chiefly vertigo, confusion and transient ischaemic episodes; retinopathy with distended retinal veins, haemorrhages and papillo-edema; and hypervolaemia with increased vascular resistance. A bleeding tendency is frequently due to both thrombocytopenia and a clotting disturbance whose pathogenesis is not clearly understood, but is often due to interference of the coagulation system by the paraproteins. Although at presentation the platelet count is not usually below $50 \times 10^9/l$, coating of platelets by abnormal immunoglobulin may lead to reduced platelet aggregation. This may lead in turn to an abnormally prolonged bleeding time with purpura, epistaxis, mucosal bleeding and retinal haemorrhage. A positive Hess test, reduced thromboplastin generation time and defective clot retraction may all occur.

In addition to cord compression from direct involvement of the vertebrae by myeloma, patients often suffer other neurological complications. Direct extradural involvement may occur through involvement of nerve roots via the intervertebral foramina. Soft tissue deposits may occur in the orbit or base of skull, leading to proptosis or cranial nerve palsies. Carpal tunnel syndrome may develop, and is thought

to be due to amyloid infiltration. Patients may occasionally develop a mixed polyneuropathy and, rarely a multifocal leucoencephalopathy (Chapter 9).

Lymphadenopathy, hepatomegaly and splenomegaly are not usually present but may develop later in the course of the disease, particularly in IgD myeloma. Megaloblastic anaemia can occur, possibly due to defective folate metabolism, although many patients have some degree of macrocytosis with no megaloblastic change and of uncertain cause. Recurrent infection is also a common feature of the disease and is frequently one of the presenting complaints. Leucopenia predisposes to infection, as does the generalized depression of normal immunoglobulins. This immunoglobulin abnormality usually fails to become normal even with 'successful' treatment which may depress the monoclonal immunoglobulin band. Some patients also have impairment of phagocytosis and cellular immune responses.

The plasma volume may be high as a result of the increase in total plasma protein. This will contribute to the anaemia even when the total red cell mass is near normal. Congestive cardiac failure is occasionally encountered. The M-band is also responsible, by direct coating of erythrocytes, for the raised ESR and erythrocyte rouleaux formation which are so characteristic of multiple myeloma. Typically the ESR is more than 80 mm/hour. Bone marrow involvement is almost always demonstrable, although the distribution may be patchy, and for diagnostic purposes, direct biopsy of a tender area is more likely to be positive. Many haematologists advise against sternal marrow puncture in patients with myeloma, in view of the extreme fragility of bone and the danger of inadvertently entering the mediastinum. It is usually best to sample tender, or radiologically abnormal areas, wherever possible. Abnormal plasma cells can account for up to 95% of the nucleated cell population.

Hypercalcaemia is a common feature, chiefly attributable to the bone destruction from abnormal plasma cell proliferation, although other factors which activate osteoclasts have been described [4]. In many myeloma patients, a highly potent osteoclast activating factor (OAF) has been identified. Approximately one-third of patients have an abnormally elevated plasma calcium at diagnosis, and the majority develop hypercalcaemia during the course of the illness. Indeed myeloma is the diagnosis *par excellence* which may result in profound and treatment-resistant hypercalcaemia. Hyper-calciuria is even more frequent. In myeloma, the hypercalcaemia is often of sufficient severity to require emergency treatment (Chapter 8). The symptoms include polyuria, polydipsia, constipation, nausea, vomiting, dehydration and mental confusion.

Impaired renal function is common. Its pathogenesis has been described above. It is important to realize that once hypercalcaemia and renal impairment have developed, a vicious circle becomes established in which there is worsening renal function, increasing hyper-calcaemia, further dehydration with falling glomerular filtration rate, and increasing tubu-lar obstruction and dysfunction from light chain deposition. This is a medical emergency and its management is described below.

Diagnosis

In a typical case when there are bone lesions, anaemia, paraproteinaemia, hypercalcaemia and marrow involvement, there is no diagnostic difficulty. In less florid cases, the differential diagnosis can be difficult and may include:
1 other causes of anaemia, bone pain and hypercalcaemia such as metastatic cancer;
2 other causes of paraproteinaemia such as MGUS, occult primary tumours (Table 27.4), Waldenström's macroglobulinaemia or lym-phomas;
3 other causes of lytic lesions in bone such as breast, renal, thyroid or bronchial carcinoma;
4 other causes of spinal cord compression such as metastatic cancer;
5 other causes of anaemia and raised ESR such as connective tissue diseases, malignancy and

infection — especially where cold agglutinins are formed as in mycoplasma infections and infectious mononucleosis, although these patients are generally younger;
6 solitary plasmacytomas (see below); and
7 primary amyloidosis, which may be accom-panied by plamacytosis in the marrow and also by a proteinuria.

The diagnosis may sometimes be difficult es-pecially if there is minimal marrow involve-ment, no detectable paraprotein, or a solitary bone lesion on skeletal X-rays. In doubtful cases the marrow examination may have to be re-peated. However, if there is no pressing indi-cation for treatment, a period of observation may allow the diagnosis to be established more easily (Table 27.5). Occasionally, immunological testing using light and heavy chain antibodies to establish monoclonality may be necessary to exclude a 'reactive' plasmacytosis.

Treatment

When patients with myeloma present with dangerous manifestations such as dehydration, hypercalcaemia and/or spinal cord compres-sion, the first treatment should be to correct the

Table 27.5 Important investigations in myeloma

Haematological
Full blood count and erythrocyte sedimentation rate (ESR)
Marrow aspiration and biopsy
Serum viscosity

Biochemical
Urea and electrolytes, creatinine clearance
Serum calcium
Serum albumin
Quantitative immunoglobulins
Immunoelectrophoresis
Twenty-four hour urine for light chains and total protein and calcium excretion
β_2 microglobulins — plasma/urine

Radiological
Skeletal survey

metabolic disturbance or serious local problem (Chapter 8). Intravenous fluid replacement, correction of hypercalcaemia, local irradiation and occasionally decompressive laminectomy should, in these circumstances, take precedence. In the majority of patients, however, the presenting clinical syndrome is more slowly evolving and in contrast to these clinical emergencies there will be time to confirm the diagnosis before instituting treatment.

CHEMOTHERAPY

Chemotherapy with intermittent alkylating agent treatment (usually melphalan) has traditionally been the mainstay of treatment and has improved survival from a median of 6–12 months (untreated) to 2–3 years [5,6]. Usually given by mouth, doses vary from 6–10 mg/m^2 over 4–7 days every 4–6 weeks. Recent schedules have become more aggressive. The addition of oral prednisolone (often given in enteric-coated form as doses tend to be high) has slightly improved the remission rate. Typical doses range from 60–80 mg/m^2 with melphalan (4–7 days every 4–6 weeks) in divided doses and accompanied by an H$_2$ antagonist such as ranitidine 150 mg twice daily. More complex induction chemotherapy regimens are increasingly used (see below) although it is not entirely clear whether the more aggressive combinations provide a higher survival rate [7].

Combined melphalan–prednisolone oral therapy is generally well tolerated although some patients complain of nausea or steroid side-effects. In long survivors, there is undoubtedly a small risk of development of acute myeloblastic leukaemia related to chronic melphalan therapy [8]; this fatal complication has chiefly been noted in patients on long-term daily melphalan therapy rather than pulsed intermittent courses of treatment. Cyclophosphamide (75–150 mg daily by mouth) is sometimes used for patients who show no improvement with melphalan.

Most patients with myeloma (approximately 75%) will respond to oral chemotherapy, with improvement in symptoms, particularly pain, tenderness and hypercalcaemia. The paraprotein level generally falls within the first three cycles of chemotherapy, although the immune paresis of the unaffected immunoglobulins usually takes longer to recover, and may never do so. Other parameters such as haemoglobin, albumin and blood urea may return to normal limits and can be useful for monitoring progress. In patients who respond to chemotherapy, it is rarely necessary to continue the initial treatment beyond 6–9 courses, since little further is to be gained. By this time the patient will either have entered a 'plateau' phase, in which no further reduction of the paraprotein occurs, or the patient's immunoglobulin levels will be normal and treatment can reasonably be discontinued. In some cases the patient's paraprotein level will have risen throughout the early courses of melphalan–prednisolone therapy, in which case it is clearly necessary to consider alternative treatment.

In the past 10 years many more complex regimens have been tested, in an attempt to raise remission rates and duration, and ultimately to improve survival. Many agents show activity in myeloma and the newer regimens (Table 27.6) generally include a vinca alkaloid, multiple alkylating agents and doxorubicin together with high-dose prednisolone or dexamethasone. Immune modulators such as levamisole have sometimes been used (notably in the United States) and also α-interferon which clearly has activity in this disease, including use as maintenance therapy [9]. Although many have reported improved results with complex regimens, intensive (monthly) treatment with conventional melphalan and prednisolone may offer equally good results with fewer side-effects. In the United Kingdom, however, a recent prospectively randomized MRC myeloma study suggested that the ABCM regimen (Table 27.6) may be superior, although the melphalan in this trial was given without a steroid and at relatively modest dose [10]. Intensive regimens

Table 27.6 Chemotherapy trials in multiple myeloma [5–8,10]. Newer regimens compared with melphalan/prednisolone

Drug combination	Response rate (%)	Reported median survival (months)
All cases		
BCNU, cyclophosphamide and prednisolone (PCB)	49	36
Melphalan and prednisolone	52	36
MeCCNU, vincristine, melphalan and prednisolone	70	41
Melphalan and prednisolone	58	39
Vincristine, BCNU, melphalan, cyclophosphamide and prednisolone (VBMCP)	74	33
Melphalan and prednisolone	57	29
Early stage disease		
MeCCNU, vincristine, melphalan and prednisolone	85	48
Melphalan and prednisole	69	43
Vincristine, melphalan, cyclophosphamide and prednisolone alternating with vincristine, BCNU, doxorubicin and prednisolone (VMCP-VBAP)	54	44
Doxorubicin, BCNU, melphalan and cyclophosphamide (ABCM)	50	40

are clearly more toxic and may be difficult to apply in an elderly population. One well known combination of vincristine, infused doxorubicin and high-dose dexamethasone (VAD) requires insertion of a Hickman line, and considerable periods of in-patient care, also making it less widely acceptable. However, it seems reasonable to offer more intensive regimens such as ABCM, VAD or VMCP-VBAP to younger, fitter patients since it seems likely that this group may benefit. It is also in this group that the initial results of high-dose melphalan therapy (with or without autologous bone marrow transplantation) have appeared promising [11]. With this intensive but single-exposure treatment, complete remission is seen in about one-third of patients, with elimination of malignant plasma cells in the marrow, re-

duction of paraprotein to undetectable levels and return of normal marrow function. In many cases, the immune paresis has resolved as well, an impressive feature and unusual with conventional treatment. A further group, limited to young, fit patients, may possibly derive real benefit from allogeneic bone marrow transplantation if a donor is available [12]. However, this is a highly selected population and the technique is not yet widely applicable.

After discontinuation of oral first-line chemotherapy, patients should be carefully monitored since further treatment will always be required, although sometimes only after many months or years. If treatment with melphalan–prednisolone or other first-line chemotherapy is discontinued following a well-documented response, it is usually worth reinstituting the same therapy at the point of relapse since a second response is usually seen. Relapse is usually readily detectable by a rise in the monoclonal immunoglobulin band, although some patients become symptomatic again without such a rise. Further supportive therapy with blood transfusion, antibiotics or palliative radiotherapy is often required if the patient becomes anaemic, or develops infections or painful bony lesions.

Second-line chemotherapy in myeloma remains unsatisfactory, although successes have been claimed with combinations of doxorubicin, vincristine, nitrosoureas and other agents [8]. This also applies in the 25% of myeloma patients who do not appear to be conventionally responsive when first treated ('primary chemoresistance'). Responses to secondary chemotherapy are usually of short duration, and at the cost of inflicting more undesirable side-effects than are seen with melphalan/prednisolone. In an elderly population, careful judgement is always required before considering such treatment and it is important to establish that no further response can be obtained with first-line chemotherapy.

RADIOTHERAPY

Radiotherapy is of great value in multiple myeloma and is often required as part of the initial treatment, particularly for patients who present with painful bone deposits in the vertebrae or long bones especially if there is a likelihood of pathological fracture or cord compression. Radiotherapy is the most important modality in myelomatous spinal cord compression either alone or in combination with neurosurgical decompression. Myelography or MRI scanning should be performed if possible to define the full extent of the compression. Treatment should be started early at the onset of radicular pain. If delayed until signs of paraparesis have developed, the outcome is worse. For lytic deposits of long bones, radiotherapy is often combined with internal fixation, particularly where a weight-bearing long bone is af-fected. Since myeloma deposits are relatively radiosensitive, large doses are rarely required.

For spinal deposits, a total of 30 Gy (3000 rad) in 10 fractions over 2 weeks is commonly employed. Although shorter treatments, e.g. 5 Gy (500 rad) in 5 fractions over 1 week, are effective, many radiotherapists prefer to avoid the risks of short fractionation regimens where significant portions of the spinal cord are included in the volume (see Chapter 5 for a fuller discussion of radiation myelitis). In myeloma, lengthy portions of cord are often unavoidably treated. At other sites, treatment with shorter fractionation regimens is often used. Single fractions, 8–12 Gy (800–1200 rad) are effective and safe, which is of particular value in myeloma since patients often require frequent courses of treatment at multiple sites.

Success has recently been claimed with systemic or hemi-body irradiation in myeloma [13], and there is no doubt that treatment can be effective in patients with symptomatic relapse who are no longer responsive to standard chemotherapy treatment. Our practice is to offer treatment with low dose-rate super-voltage telecobalt to the upper half of the body to a dose of 7.5 Gy (750 rad), followed 6–8 weeks later by treatment to 10 Gy (1000 rad) to the lower half of the body (or vice versa). Toxicity includes nausea and vomiting, diarrhoea and alopecia. Pulmonary complications are unusual if the dose to the upper half of the body is kept below 8 Gy (800 rad). Overall median survival with this technique is 12 months in drug-resistant cases (with many survivors >2 years), comparable with second-line chemotherapy regimens but generally more acceptable. Hemi-body irradiation cannot, however, be recommended as first-line therapy to consolidate a chemotherapy remission.

Prognosis

Many patients with myeloma experience remissions and relapses requiring careful judgement for optimal choice and timing of therapy. Some patients survive for 5 years

or more, requiring little in the way of chemotherapy, but repeated courses of radiotherapy
and general support measures. Such patients
usually have a low tumour burden based on
simple criteria (Table 27.3). Large retrospective
analyses of patients with myeloma have shown
that tumour burden is a good predictor of response and survival [9]. Median survival in the
best prognostic categories is approximately
5 years, compared with only 6 months in the
worst groups (Fig. 27.7). Since many patients
with myeloma eventually develop renal failure,
it is not surprising that simple measures of
renal function are often regarded as the single
most important prognostic criterion at diagnosis, although in recent years, more weight
has been given to initial β_2 microglobulin level
and number of bone lesions. Apart from recurrence and increasingly severe renal dysfunction,
the other important group of myeloma complications results from progressive pancytopenia
both from crowding of normal elements by
abnormal plasma cells, and also from therapy.
Anaemia often requiring transfusion at an ever
decreasing interval, infection and thrombocytopenia with bleeding are all common and

contribute to ill-health and eventually to death.
Occasionally, hypercalcaemia may become
totally resistant to treatment.

SOLITARY PLASMACYTOMA

Solitary plasmacytoma is a single plasma cell
lesion, found either in bone or soft tissue (particularly nasal or oral cavity, bowel or bronchus)
with the typical histological finding of malignant plasma cell infiltration, as in multiple
myeloma. In many patients, no other evidence
of myeloma develops provided adequate local
treatment with radiotherapy is given. However,
solitary plasmacytomas can be the initial manifestation of myeloma and these patients should
be carefully investigated since a proportion
with apparently solitary lesions will prove to
have multiple myeloma at the outset. Patients
with true solitary plasmacytomas should be
followed up regularly since a proportion of
them will undoubtedly develop myeloma later,
although latent periods of several years are not
unusual. This progression is more common
in those who present with a plasmacytoma
in bone than in those where the site is extramedullary. There is no proven benefit in
aggressive treatment of solitary plasmacytomas
with chemotherapy in the expectation that this
will prevent the development of generalized
myeloma.

MONOCLONAL GAMMOPATHY OF UNKNOWN SIGNIFICANCE (MGUS)

There are many diseases in which a monoclonal
immunoglobulin band is found but without
evidence of a plasma cell neoplasm (Table 27.4).
The commonest cause, and the one which
creates greatest diagnostic confusion, is MGUS,
which is a disease of the elderly. It is common,
with a prevalence of 0.5% in adults over 40
years and 3% over 70 years; it accounts for 40%
of all paraproteinaemias. The concentration of
monoclonal immunoglobulin is usually less
than 30 g/l. A large majority (85%) have an IgG
paraprotein. There is no other abnormality of

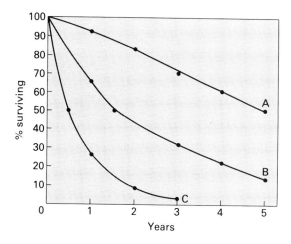

A. Low tumour mass (median survival 5 years)
B. Intermediate mass (median survival 2 years)
C. High tumour mass (median survival 6 months)

Fig. 27.7 Prognosis in myeloma related to tumour mass.

plasma proteins or symptoms of the kind found in patients with multiple myeloma. Bence-Jones protein is occasionally found. The ESR is usually raised. Monoclonal gammopathy of unknown significance requires no treatment although it clearly predisposes to myeloma.

MACROGLOBULINAEMIA

This group of conditions is characterized by the production of monoclonal IgM. The causes are given in Table 27.7.

Benign macroglobulinaemia follows a similar course to other forms of MGUS (see above).

Cold agglutinin disease is a disease of the elderly in which the patients suffer from vascular disturbances in the extremities due to intracapillary agglutination of red cells in parts of the body exposed to cold. A deep blue-violet discolouration may occur (acrocyanosis) which may lead to gangrene. In addition, a moderate haemolysis is usually present.

Physical examination reveals little in the way of abnormalities apart from the spleen being slightly enlarged. The disease is due to a monoclonal IgM which has the property of being a cold agglutinin. If simple measures — gloves or mittens and warm boots — are inadequate, treatment with alkylating agents can be helpful.

WALDENSTRÖM'S MACROGLOBULINAEMIA

This condition, which typically occurs in the elderly, is characterized by bone marrow infiltration with lymphoid cells which have the appearance of an 'intermediate' form between lymphocytes and plasma cells (lymphoplasmacytoid). Monoclonal lymphocytes are present in both blood and bone marrow, and the tumour morphology in this disease is suggestive of a differentiating B cell neoplasm. There is often an enlargement of lymph nodes, liver and spleen. Unlike IgM myeloma, bone lesions are very uncommon although diffuse osteoporosis may occur. There is production of a monoclonal IgM, often in very large amounts, sometimes producing hyperviscosity.

The patient typically presents with ill-health and weakness, sometimes with night sweats. The symptoms of hyperviscosity may predominate with headache, mental confusion, retinal haemorrhages and renal impairment. Renal disease is less common than in myeloma. The macroglobulin may produce haemolytic anaemia or act as a cold agglutinin. It may produce haemorrhage by interaction with platelets and clotting factors. Purpura and bleeding are not infrequent. Investigations reveal anaemia, variable thrombocytopenia, a raised serum IgM and occasionally immune paresis.

Treatment and prognosis

The disease is usually only slowly progressive and, in the absence of symptoms, treatment can be withheld. Chlorambucil or cyclophosphamide, given in a small daily dose, usually produce regression of lymphadenopathy and a fall in IgM levels. Steroids are of little value.

Since IgM is intravascular, plasmapheresis will produce reduction of viscosity and is essential if clinical hyperviscosity is present. It should be repeated until chemotherapy reduces IgM production. The prognosis is variable, but average survival is 3–4 years from diagnosis. In aggressive cases, combination chemotherapy as for myeloma may be valuable.

Table 27.7 Causes of macroglobulinaemia

Benign
Benign macroglobulinaemia
Cold agglutinin disease

Neoplasms
Waldenström's macroglobulinaemia
IgM myeloma
Non-Hodgkin's lymphomas
Chronic lymphatic leukaemia

HEAVY CHAIN DISEASES

These diseases are lymphocyte neoplasms in which there is production of incomplete heavy chains of immunoglobulin, without light chains. The first patient was described by Franklin in 1964 [14]. So far, only γ, α and μ heavy chain diseases have been described. Interestingly, each has distinct clinical features.

γ-Heavy chain disease

γ-Heavy chain disease usually affects elderly patients, producing lymphadenopathy, tonsillar enlargement, palatal oedema, and hepatosplenomegaly. Bone lesions are unusual. Occasionally there are associated autoimmune diseases such as systemic lupus erythematosus or Sjögren's syndrome. Anaemia is common but the bone marrow may not show any diagnostic features. The lymph nodes may be replaced with lymphoplasmacytoid cells, but may not be diagnostic. The γ-heavy chain fragment is found in serum or urine and there may also be immune paresis.

Chemotherapy is usually minimally effective. Although this disease may occasionally regress without treatment, survival time is usually not greater than 3 years.

α-Heavy chain disease (see also Chapter 26 p. 524)

This important disease is the commonest of the heavy chain diseases and is chiefly found in young Mediterranean adults and in the populations of the Middle East and South America. It is a disease of the small bowel although occasionally the stomach, large bowel and post-nasal space are affected. Typically, the disease occurs in adults aged 20−30 years. There is frequently a history of gastro-intestinal disturbance extending over many years, and some patients have been previously diagnosed as having immune proliferative disease of the small intestine. Because of massive lymphoid infiltration of the bowel, severe malabsorption

and diarrhoea develop and, although the histological appearances may initially not appear to be malignant, a true lymphoma usually develops.

α-Heavy chains are present in the blood but their detection is difficult. The marrow is not involved and liver, spleen and lymph nodes are not enlarged. The diagnosis is made by small bowel biopsy. Treatment with cytotoxic chemotherapy at the stage of frank lymphoma is only temporarily effective. Whole abdominal irradiation has sometimes been used. Before this stage, treatment with oral tetracycline may produce long remissions.

μ-Heavy chain disease

In this very rare disease, μ-heavy chains are found in the plasma. The clinical disease mimics long-standing chronic lymphatic leukaemia, or a non-Hodgkin's lymphoma, usually with marked visceral organomegaly, and treatment is similar to that used for these diseases.

REFERENCES

1 Velez R., Beral V., Cuzick J. Increasing trends of multiple myeloma mortality in England and Wales 1950−1979: are the changes real? *Journal of the National Cancer Institute* 1982; **69**: 387−92.

2 Cuzick J. Radiation-induced myelomatosis. *New England Journal of Medicine* 1981; **304**: 204−10.

3 Cuzick J., Cooper E.H., MacLennan I.C.M. The prognostic value of serum β_2 microglobulin compared with other presentation features in myelomatosis. *British Journal of Cancer* 1985; **52**: 1−6.

4 Mundy G.R., Raisz L.G., Cooper R.A., Schechter G.P., Salmon S.E. Evidence for the secretion of an osteoclast stimulating factor in myeloma. *New England Journal of Medicine* 1974; **291**: 1041−46.

5 Gregory W.M., Richards M.A., Malpas J.S. Combination chemotherapy versus melphalan and prednisolone in the treatment of multiple myeloma: an overview of published trials. *Journal of Clinical Oncology* 1992; **10**: 334−42.

6 Niesvisky R., Siegel D., Michaeli J. Biology and treatment of multiple myeloma. *Blood Reviews* 1993; **7**: 24−33.

7 Durie B.G.M., Dixon D.O., Carter S. *et al.* Improved survival duration with combination chemotherapy induction for multiple myeloma. *Journal of Clinical*

Oncology 1986; **4**: 1227−37.

8 Alexanian R., Dimopoulos M. Drug therapy: the treatment of multiple myeloma. *New England Journal of Medicine* 1994; **330**: 484−89.

9 Mandelli F., Avvisati G., Amadori S. *et al.* Maintenance treatment with recombinant interferon α-2b in patients with multiple myeloma responding to conventional induction chemotherapy. *New England Journal of Medicine* 1990; **322**: 1430−34.

10 MacLennan I.C.M., Drayson M., Dunn J. Current issues in cancer: Multiple myeloma. *British Medical Journal* 1994; **308**: 1033−36.

11 Selby P.J., McElwain T.J., Nandi A.C. *et al.* Multiple myeloma treated with high dose intravenous melphalan. *British Journal of Haematology* 1987; **66**: 55−62.

12 Barlogie B., Gahrton G. Bone marrow transplantation in multiple myeloma. *Bone Marrow Transplantation* 1991; **7**: 71−79.

13 McSweeny E.N., Tobias J.S., Blackman G. *et al.* Double hemibody irradiation in the management of relapsed and primary chemoresistant myeloma. *Clinical Oncology* 1993; **5**: 378−83.

14 Franklin E.C., Lowenstein J., Bigelow B., Meltzer M. Heavy chain disease. A new disorder of serum gammaglobulin. *American Journal of Medicine* 1964; **37**: 332−50.

Chapter 28
Leukaemia

Leukaemias are neoplastic proliferations of white blood cells. Although uncommon, they have been the subject of detailed investigation because of the insights they give into aetiology and pathogenesis of the malignant process. The intensive chemotherapy which has been responsible for the increasing cure rate in acute leukaemia has served as an example for the treatment of other malignancies. Allogeneic bone marrow transplantation was developed as a treatment for acute leukaemia. Autologous bone marrow transplantation (ABMT) has also been widely used in treatment of acute leukaemia and some of the findings have been of great importance in designing studies of ABMT in solid tumours. For these reasons, the principles of management are described in this chapter, but more detailed discussion and guidance is given in articles and books mentioned on pp. 565–6.

INCIDENCE AND AETIOLOGY [1]

In childhood (below 15 years of age), acute lymphoblastic leukaemia (ALL) accounts for 80% of all cases, acute myeloblastic leukaemia (AML) and its variants accounting for 17% of the remainder, and chronic granulocytic leukaemia (CGL) approximately 3%. The death rate from acute leukaemia in the population is approximately 7 per 100 000. The disease is slightly more common in males (3:2), and its incidence over the last decade appears to have been constant. Acute leukaemia is most common in the elderly (Fig. 28.1A & B), and over 15 years of age 85% of cases are AML. In adults, AML and ALL have a very similar

prognosis, but childhood ALL has different clinical features and a much better prognosis than adult ALL, or AML at any age.

A variety of aetiological factors have been implicated. Ionizing irradiation is leukaemogenic. Survivors of the Hiroshima and Nagasaki atom bombs have an increased risk of leukaemia and the risk is greater for those who were near the centre of the explosions. AML and CGL are the most frequent types. The increased incidence began 2 years after the explosion and then declined after 6 years (Fig. 28.1C).

There is controversy over the possible link between residence near nuclear establishments and childhood leukaemia. The reported increase in incidence has been disputed. If true it may be due to radiation effect but it is also compatible with a transmissible agent such as a virus or other community-based experience.

Exposure to certain chemicals increases the risk of leukaemia. Benzene and some of its derivatives predispose to the development of both leukaemia and aplastic anaemia. An excess of leukaemia (predominantly AML) has been reported in refinery workers. Other occupations with increased risk appear to be welders and workers in industries using DDT.

One of the most worrying causes of leukaemia is anticancer treatment itself. There is an increase in risk of leukaemia after treatment for Hodgkin's disease (see also Chapter 25, p. 500) and ovarian cancer [2]. The risk increases with time from treatment. There is a higher relative risk for young patients. In treatment-related leukaemia typical chromosomal abnormalities occur of which the most consistent is loss of the whole or long arm of chromosome 5 and/or 7.

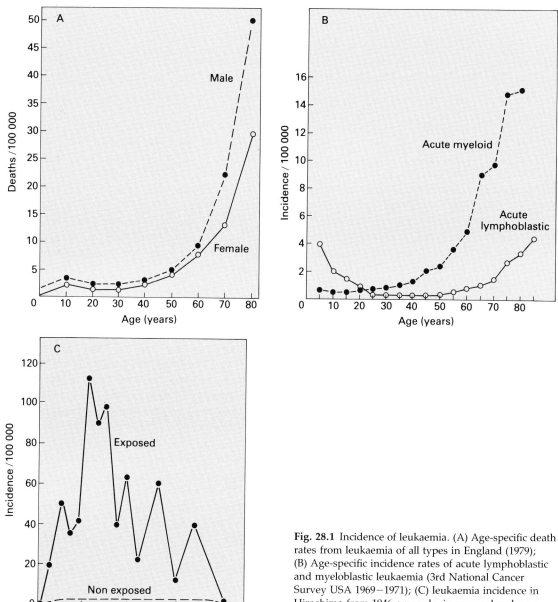

Fig. 28.1 Incidence of leukaemia. (A) Age-specific death rates from leukaemia of all types in England (1979); (B) Age-specific incidence rates of acute lymphoblastic and myeloblastic leukaemia (3rd National Cancer Survey USA 1969–1971); (C) leukaemia incidence in Hiroshima from 1946 onwards, in exposed and non-exposed individuals. (From Wintrobe M. *Blood Pure and Eloquent*. McGraw Hill, 1980, p. 528. With permission.)

This also occurs following benzene exposure. The region 5q band 23–32 appears to be consistently, and critically, deleted. This region contains genes which code for haemopoietic differentiation antigens, GM-CSF, IL-3 and IL-5. Both occupational exposure to petro-chemicals and cytotoxic drugs are associated with karyotypic abnormalities on chromosomes 5 and 7.

Smoking increases the risk of leukaemia by

50%. The risk is mainly for AML and acute myelomonocytic leukaemia (AMML) (see below). The risk of childhood leukaemia is also probably increased in children whose mothers smoked marijuana or who were exposed to benzene and other solvents in pregnancy.

Certain constitutive abnormalities predispose to leukaemia. In Down's syndrome (trisomy 21) there is an increased risk of acute leukaemia — usually ALL in younger patients. Bloom's syndrome, Fanconi's anaemia and ataxia telangiectasia are all autosomal recessive diseases characterized by chromosome breakage and an increased risk of leukaemia. A defective DNA repair mechanism may be responsible; AML is the usual leukaemia in Fanconi anaemia, and ALL in ataxia telangiectasia.

THE ACUTE LEUKAEMIAS

Pathology and classification

In recent years there has been a considerable growth of knowledge about the maturation of haemopoietic and lymphoid cells. Acute leukaemias often retain many of the cytoplasmic and membrane characteristics of their normal counterparts, so it is possible to relate the various types of acute leukaemia to a particular stage of myeloid or lymphoid maturation. A simplified scheme is shown in Fig. 28.2.

The diagnosis is made from blood and marrow films and careful staining and preparation are essential. In the typical case there are leukaemic blasts in the blood and the marrow is packed with uniform-looking blast cells. Cases of ALL almost always show these appearances but in adult AML the leukaemic process may be much more subtle with few blasts in the blood. The marrow must show over 30% of blasts for the diagnosis to be made with confidence. When there are less than 20% blasts the diagnosis of myelodysplastic state is usually made (see p. 558).

The acute leukaemias have been subdivided on morphological grounds using a scheme de-vised by a French–American–British study group [3]. An outline is given in Table 28.1. With the exception of acute promyelocytic leukaemia, the prognostic significance of this subdivision is doubtful.

In AML, the myeloblasts may contain Auer rods which are pink staining rod-like inclusions which are probably aberrant forms of the cytoplasmic granules found in normal granulocyte precursors. These granules are often prominent in the cytoplasm in AML and are particularly frequent and often large in the M_3 variety (hypergranular promyelocytic leukaemia). In monocytic leukaemia (M_5) the blasts are large with abundant cytoplasm and in erythroleukaemia (M_6) there are erythroblasts and myeloblasts in the marrow.

The commonest form of ALL (L_1) is characterized by scanty cytoplasm and fewer nucleoli. In the less common form (L_2) the blasts are larger, with a larger nucleolus. This form, which is more common in adults, is more easily mistaken for AML and may account for some cases designated as undifferentiated leukaemia.

Cytochemical stains help to determine the type of leukaemia if there is doubt. The commonly used stains are shown in Table 28.2. These stains may help to confirm the diagnosis in doubtful cases. In occasional instances of undifferentiated acute leukaemia, the cyto-

Table 28.1 A morphological classification of acute leukaemia [3]

AML
M_1 myeloblastic (no maturation, undifferentiated)
M_2 myeloblastic (some maturation)
M_3 hypergranular promyelocytic
M_4 myelomonocytic
M_5 monocytic
M_6 erythroleukaemia
M_7 megakaryoblastic

ALL
L_1 small monomorphic cells
L_2 large heterogeneous cells
L_3 Burkitt-like

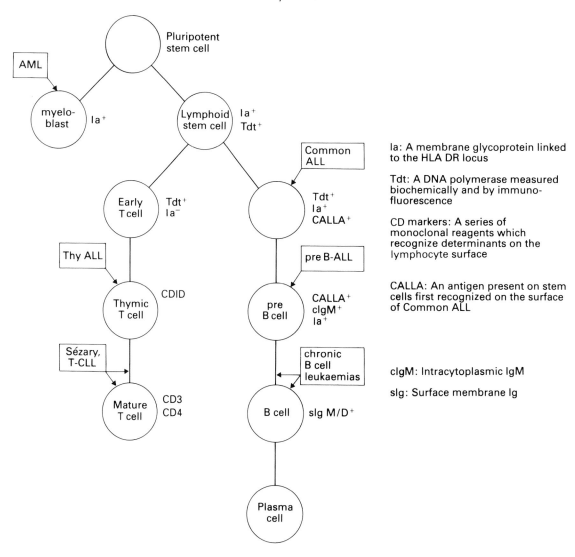

Fig. 28.2 Maturation of haemopoietic and lymphoid cells in relation to types of leukaemia.

chemical stains are unhelpful. Some further help in diagnosis may be obtained by using the membrane markers shown in Fig. 28.2. In ALL in particular, these markers may help to distinguish common ALL from T cell ALL and Burkitt's lymphoma (Table 28.3).

IMMUNOLOGICAL PHENOTYPE IN LEUKAEMIA [4]

The normal maturation sequence of lymphoid

and myeloid cells is accompanied by expression of cell surface and cytoplasmic proteins which can be detected by antibodies. In leukaemia this antigen expression can be used to 'phenotype' tumours which reflect different stages of maturation. Some of the subdivisions have little prognostic or therapeutic importance but they help in understanding the pathogenesis of leukaemia. An abbreviated summary is given in Table 28.3.

Table 28.2 Cytochemistry and lineage-characteristics of acute leukaemia

Phenotypic feature	Leukaemia
Sudan black	+AML −ALL
Myeloperoxidase	+AML −ALL
α-Naphthyl-butyrate esterase	+AML −ALL
Tdt expression*	ALL (T and B)
Ig gene heavy chain rearrangement	(B) ALL
TCR† gene arrangement	(T) ALL
Cytoplasmic or surface Ig	(B) ALL
TCR expression	(T) ALL

* Tdt: a DNA polymerase measured by fluorescence or biochemically

† TCR: T cell receptor

CHROMOSOMAL ABNORMALITIES IN LEUKAEMIA (Table 28.4)

A wide range of acquired karyotypic abnormalities have now been found in leukaemia and in recent years a more precise definition of the genes involved has become possible. Progress is being made in understanding how these genetic changes lead to the development of leukaemia. It seems likely that, as in other cancers, several sequential changes are necessary for the development of the full malignant characteristics.

In *chronic myelocytic leukaemia* (CML) the Philadelphia (Ph') chromosome is found which is a chromosome 22 with a reciprocal translocation from between 9q (band q 34.1) and 22q (band 11.2). This moves the *C-abl* (tyrosine-kinase) proto-oncogene from 9 to 22 and fuses it to a gene at the breakpoint cluster region (*bcr*). Production of fusion protein results in a 210 MW in CML (and another, 185 kDa, in ALL) [5]. The function of these proteins is not known. When CML undergoes blastic transformation (see below) further chromosomal abnormalities occur. It has been shown that cases of CML which are Ph' −ve sometimes have a more restricted *abl−bcr* translocation which is not detected cytogenetically. Other translocations have been described in CML but almost all involve a translocation with new chromosomal material next to the *bcr* gene.

In *AML* and *AMML* there are specific chromosomal abnormalities associated with the different categories (M_1–M_7) described in Table 28.1. These are outlined in Table 28.4. This represents

Table 28.3 Immunological phenotypes of leukaemia

Cluster designation*	Antigen	Leukaemia
CD2	Sheep erythrocyte rosette receptor	T cell
CD3	T lineage	T cell
CD4	T cell helper/inducer	T cell
—	T cell receptor	T cell
CD10	B cell lineage (CALLA)† (endopeptidase)	B cell
CD19	Pan B cell	B cell
CD20	B cell lineage	B cell
CD22	Myelin-associated glycoprotein	B cell
CD11b	C3 bi-receptor	AML, AMML
CD33	Myeloid lineage	AML, AMML
CD36	Myeloid	AML, AMML
CD41,42	Megakaryocytic glycoproteins	Megakaryoblastic
CD45	Common leucocyte antigen	All leukaemias
CD34	Progenitor cell antigen	Primitive leukaemias

* Refers to categories assigned at international workshops on classification of leucocytes

† CALLA: common acute lymphoblastic leukaemia antigen (formerly designated)

a very simplified summary of many different abnormalities in a rapidly changing field. In these leukaemias the leukaemic event occurs at the stem cell level and is followed by defective maturation. The connections between the chromosomal change and the maturation defect remain unknown as yet.

Acute lymphoblastic leukaemia (ALL). In T cell ALL breakpoints occur at 14q11 which is the site of the T cell receptor genes (α and β) and 7q33–36 (β T cell receptor). Translocation of oncogenes such as C-*myc* (t(8;14) (q24;q11)) to this site, similar to that found for Ig genes in Burkitt's lymphoma, may result in disordered cell growth. Another T cell specific translocation is t(11;14). Chromosome 9p is frequently deleted or translocated in ALL and is especially associated with lymphomatous clinical features.

ONCOGENE PRODUCTS IN LEUKAEMIA

As described in Chapter 3 a variety of 'oncogenes' code for proteins involved as receptors for growth-inducing ligands or enzymes which transmit the signal from the membrane to the cytoplasm leading to growth and differentiation. In leukaemia some of the gene translocations and deletions described above involve oncogenes, which may thereby be inappropriately activated or mutated leading to disordered growth. Thus, the receptor for colony stimulating factor (CSF-1) is the product of the C-*fms* gene and is expressed in acute non-lymphocyte leukaemia. The intracytoplasmic domain has protein tyrosine kinase activity. CD20 (Table 28.3) is a B-cell protein with signal transduction properties. Both of the fusion proteins resulting

Table 28.4 Common chromosomal abnormalities in leukaemia

Leukaemia	Abnormality
CML	t(9;22)(q34.1;q11.2) Demonstrable karyotypically in 80% of cases. More restricted translocation in many of the remainder. In ALL this translocation has a very poor prognosis
AML	
M_1	t(8;21). Good prognosis
M_2	t(8;21). Good prognosis
M_3	t(15;17)(q22;q11). Good prognosis
M_4	Various translocations involving 11q23 (poor prognosis), inversion of 16
M_5	t(9;11), other translocations of 11q23. Poor prognosis
T cell ALL	t11;14 (p13;q11). Poor prognosis
	Deletions and translocation of 9p
	t(10;14)(q24;q11). Poor prognosis
	t(7;19)
B cell ALL	t(8;14)(q11). Very poor prognosis
	t(11;14)
	t(1;19). Rather poor prognosis
Undifferentiated or ALL	t(4;11)(q21;q23). Very poor prognosis
CLL	Trisomy 12. Worst prognosis
	Deletion 13q14. Worst prognosis

CML: chronic myelogenous leukaemia; AML: acute myelogeneous leukaemia; ALL: acute lymphoblastic leukaemia; CLL: chronic lymphocytic leukaemia from the *abl—bcr* translocation in CML and ALL (above) have tyrosine kinase activity and are leukaemogenic in mice. p53 (Chapter 3, p. 38) is frequently mutated in CML and the resultant protein has defective function being unable to serve as a check to entry into cell cycle. These examples indicate that the result of the genetic instability is to give rise to proteins which may alter growth and differentiation in the cell.

Clinical features and management of acute leukaemias [6]

ACUTE LYMPHOBLASTIC LEUKAEMIA (ALL) IN CHILDHOOD

The disease usually presents at the age of 4–5 years, and the symptoms are due to marrow infiltration causing anaemia, thrombocytopenia, infection and bone pain, especially in long bones. As with other forms of acute leukaemia the history is of a few weeks of malaise, sometimes with fever even in the absence of obvious infection. Oral and pharyngeal ulceration may occur and bone pains are frequent. Although petechiae are often found on examination, presentation with other haemorrhagic phenomena is less common.

On examination the child is usually pale. There may be lymph node enlargement, splenomegaly and slight hepatic enlargement. The bones may be tender on pressure particularly over the sternum. Skin petechiae are common (and may also be seen on the palate) and as haemorrhages in the eye, either in the retina or as larger subhyaloid haemorrhages. Skin infiltration with leukaemia is uncommon and takes the form of plaques of tumour of purple colour.

Occasionally the patient has symptoms of meningeal involvement at presentation. This usually manifests itself as headache, vomiting and neck stiffness. Cranial nerve palsies may occur as in other forms of malignant meningitis. Investigation usually reveals anaemia, thrombocytopenia and an elevated total white cell count (WBC) with numerous lymphoblasts. In

40% of cases, the total WBC is not elevated but blasts are usually present. 'Aleukaemic leukaemia' is a term used to describe those cases where blasts are not present in the blood film (approximately 5% of cases). In all cases a bone marrow examination is essential, with cyto-chemical and immunological studies when possible (as outlined above). A chest X-ray is usually normal, but in T cell ALL, may show a mediastinal mass due to thymic enlargement. This form of ALL is common in adolescent boys. Bone X-rays are not infrequently abnormal and the typical abnormality is of radiolucent bands in the metaphyseal region. Diffuse demineralization also occurs, and discrete osteolytic lesions.

Biochemical investigation may show a raised uric acid due to rapid proliferation and death of leukaemic cells. A lumbar puncture may show leukaemic cells even though there may be no clinical evidence of disease in the CNS.

Remission induction and consolidation (Fig. 28.3)

Haematological and clinical remission is induced with vincristine, prednisolone and doxorubicin (or daunorubicin). Vigorous hydration, allopurinol and urinary alkalinization are necessary in the induction period. With this regimen 75% of patients remit within 3 weeks and the remission is achieved with little toxicity and recovery of normal haematopoiesis.

Following the induction of complete or partial remission, the treatment is intensified by using drugs such as asparaginase, an anthracycline (daunorubicin or doxorubicin), cytosine arabinoside and cyclophosphamide. Methotrexate in high dose may add to the durability of remission. These drugs are myelosuppressive but at this stage the bone marrow has recovered following the elimination of most of the leukaemic population.

Prophylaxis of CNS disease

The importance of CNS prophylaxis was demonstrated in the early 1970s. Before that time, infiltration of the meninges by leukaemic cells was responsible for relapse in half of all cases. The lymphoblasts infiltrate the meninges diffusely and extend to the spinal meninges and sheaths of cranial nerves. Clinical presentation is with symptoms of raised intracranial pressure: headache, nausea and vomiting, with a stiff neck and papilloedema. Convulsions may occur and cranial nerve palsies (particularly VII, VI and III) often develop, and may be the first sign. The diagnosis is made on lumbar puncture when leukaemic blasts are found. The risk of coning from the lumbar puncture is small.

Prophylactic treatment greatly diminishes the frequency of CNS relapse. Nowadays the usual regimen is cranial irradiation (18 Gy, 1800 rad, in 8–10 fractions over 2 weeks) together with intrathecal methotrexate ($10 \, mg/m^2 \times 4$ over the same period). Established CNS disease (which now occurs in 5–10% of cases) is treated by intrathecal methotrexate twice weekly with cranial irradiation to a higher dose (often 24 Gy, 2400 rad, over 2–3 weeks), together with or followed by spinal irradiation. Lasting control of CNS disease is, however, unusual. Intrathecal cytosine arabinoside is also used in patients who are thought to be resistant to methotrexate.

Treatment and prophylaxis of testicular disease

Relapse in the testis is common and is one reason for the worse prognosis of ALL in boys. Testicular relapse may be less frequent in regimens including high-dose methotrexate. It occurs in about 25% of prepubertal boys but is less common in older children. Relapse may not be clinically apparent at first — swelling and

Fig. 28.3 Outline of management of acute lymphoblastic leukaemia in childhood.

hardness being late signs. It is usually bilateral, and testicular biopsy shows peritubular leukaemic infiltration. Treatment is by testicular irradiation, generally to a dose of the order of 24 Gy (2400 rad) in 2–3 weeks. The role of prophylactic testicular irradiation is still undecided.

Maintenance therapy

The duration of 'maintenance' chemotherapy has not been defined. With more intensive induction and consolidation regimens it seems probable that prolonged maintenance therapy will be less necessary. At present the consensus of opinion is that maintenance therapy should be continued for at least 2 years. 6MP and methotrexate are the most widely used drugs, often in conjunction with vincristine and prednisolone. In cases with poor prognostic features (Table 28.4) more aggressive regimens have been used as intermittent pulsed therapy. At the end of treatment a testicular biopsy is sometimes performed, if prophylactic irradiation has not been given, to detect occult disease. Relapse at any site is unusual beyond 1 year after treatment has stopped.

Table 28.5 Adverse prognostic features in childhood ALL

1 Cytogenetics
2 CNS disease at presentation
3 Early marrow relapse
4 Testicular relapse
5 T cell phenotype

Treatment on relapse

If children relapse during initial or maintenance treatment or up to 1 year after cessation of therapy, the outlook is poor and bone marrow transplantation (BMT) is considered (see below). Following later relapses remission can usually be re-induced by intensive therapy and may be durable. This may not be the case with modern more intensive regimens, which would then imply that BMT will need to be considered for this group as well [7].

Allogeneic BMT has been used in an attempt to improve results in childhood ALL when the prognosis is poor. The procedure does not have a proven survival advantage over chemotherapy. The following clinical situations have been regarded as indications for consideration of allogeneic BMT in childhood ALL:

• second or third remission especially if relapse occurred while on maintenance therapy; and
• poor prognosis cases such as those with t(4; 11) AUL, t(8; 14) B cell ALL, Ph' +ve ALL. These children may benefit from BMT in first remission.

Results of BMT in first remission have been promising with 55% 3-year relapse-free survival. In standard risk cases in second remission 65% 5-year relapse-free survival is reported. The results depend greatly on the factors used to select patients [7]. Autologous BMT has, in general, been rather less impressive than allogeneic possibly because of marrow contamination but also because some high dose regimens have not included total body irradiation (TBI). Newer treatment regimens of combined chemotherapy and TBI (possibly with purging of the harvested marrow) may improve results of autologous BMT. The relative efficacies are difficult to assess in the absence of randomized comparison. Allogeneic BMT has a greater mortality than autologous partly because of graft-versus-host disease (GVHD). On the other hand GVHD may have an antileukaemic effect.

If relapse occurs in the CNS despite prophylaxis, a further remission may be obtained with more intrathecal methotrexate or craniospinal irradiation. Methotrexate can also be given through an Ommaya or Rickham reservoir which allows direct delivery of the drug into the cerebral ventricular system. Systemic relapse is inevitable, and further systemic treatment is usually given.

Prognosis

The important prognostic features are given in Table 28.5. Survival is better in girls than in boys and is shown in Fig. 28.4.

ACUTE LYMPHOBLASTIC LEUKAEMIA IN ADULTS [8]

The clinical features are similar to those in children except for the greater percentage of patients with a mediastinal mass. Above the age of 12 years, ALL has a significantly worse prognosis. More cases (20%) are Ph' +ve and at least some cases represent chronic granulocyte leukaemia presenting in the acute phase. Only 30% are common ALL, 12% are B cell ALL, 8% T cell ALL, and 30% of cases are unclassifiable (null cell ALL). Although the prognosis appears to be as poor as in adult AML, adult ALL is usually regarded separately because CNS relapse is as common as in childhood ALL.

The treatment of adult ALL is similar to the childhood disease with the following modifications.

• Induction treatment is more intense with regimens which include anthracyclines and asparaginase.
• More intensive 'consolidation' therapy with cytosine arabinoside and anthracyclines, and recently temposide.
• Testicular relapse is less frequent and prophylactic treatment is not given.

Currently, intensive induction regimens in unselected cases in 70−80% of cases with 40% in remission at 3 years [8]. Poor prognostic factors include: age over 40, Ph' +ve, T or B cell phenotype. CNS prophylaxis may, in the future, be avoided for some patients since the high risk of CNS relapse is in patients with B cell

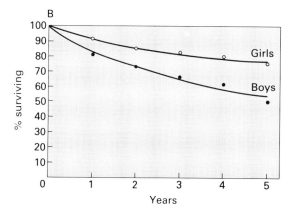

Fig. 28.4 Relapse-free survival (A) and overall survival in acute lymphoblastic leukaemia in children.

ALL, elevated LDH or alkaline phosphatase and a high proliferative fraction.

As in childhood leukaemia there may be a place for allogeneic or autologous BMT in the high risk groups defined above. Some centres would consider all first remission ALL over the age of 21 as an indication for BMT on the grounds that the prognosis is worse in adults than in children.

ACUTE MYELOBLASTIC LEUKAEMIA (AML)

In most cases the history and physical findings are similar to those in ALL (see above). Bone pain and radiological evidence of bone infil-

tration are less common in AML, and CNS disease is very unusual at presentation. Lymph node enlargement is also less frequently found than in ALL.

In myelomonocytic (M_4, Table 28.1) and monocytic (M_5) leukaemia, gum infiltration is common leading to gum 'hypertrophy'. Skin infiltrates are common in these forms and associated features are a high total WBC and high serum and urinary lysozyme which is liberated from the tumour.

Pallor, hepatosplenomegaly, purpura and bone tenderness are the most common physical signs. The white count is often elevated with myeloblasts usually demonstrable. Confirmation of the diagnosis is made by bone marrow examination and the use of special stains when appropriate (Table 28.2).

Treatment: remission induction (note the management of acute promyelocytic leukaemia is discussed separately)

The aim is to induce a complete marrow and clinical remission. To do this, intensive therapy is normally needed with blood, platelet and antibiotic support during the period of hypoplasia which is the inevitable accompaniment of the chemotherapy (see Chapter 8). Combinations of cytosine arabinoside, daunorubicin and 6-thioguanine are used (Fig. 28.5). The blast count usually falls rapidly in the blood and bone marrow with suppression of normal haematopoiesis. The mortality of this stage is now about 10% when skilled support is available. During the hypoplastic period further cytotoxic therapy is often needed if the marrow still shows disease, and this intensifies the hypoplasia and increases the risk. Regular bone marrow examination is therefore essential.

The induction of remission is therefore a highly skilled procedure, best carried out in a unit where the nursing and medical staff are experienced in the problems of bone marrow failure. Careful attention to fluid and electrolyte problems is essential as is prompt diagnosis and treatment of infection (see Chapter 8).

REMISSION INDUCTION	MAINTENANCE THERAPY
Cytosine arabinoside Daunorubicin 6-thioguanine Intensive supportive care	Drugs for remission with other agents Etoposide 6MP 5-azacytidine
	? late intensification

Fig. 28.5 Outline of management of acute myeloblastic leukaemia.

Prophylactic treatment of the CNS is not usually given.

Supportive care

Blood product support is essential during the intensive phase of remission induction. As discussed in Chapter 8, platelet transfusion has been a major advance in prevention of death from haemorrhage. The indications for platelet transfusion are discussed on p. 140. A falling platelet count below $20 \times 10^9/l$ is an indication for transfusion, as are haemorrhagic manifestations with counts below $40 \times 10^9/l$.

Blood transfusions are essential for anaemia but should be avoided if possible if the white blood count is very high (over $100 \times 10^9/l$) because leucostasis in cerebral vessels may occur. Chemotherapy and, if necessary, leucaphoresis, should be used to reduce the white count before transfusion. The use of haemopoietic growth factors is described in Chapter 8, p. 141. During intensive treatment an indwelling subcutaneously tunnelled intravenous line (Hickman line) running subcutaneously may be of great help, particularly in children and in adults with difficult veins.

During the period of remission induction several steps are taken to try to prevent infection. Patients should be instructed to wash carefully with particular attention to the perineal region. Dental and oral sepsis should be treated promptly. Food should be cooked and clean — fresh salads are best avoided. Regular examination of the mouth, skin and perineum are essential and swabs should be taken from these sites regularly to detect pathogens such as klebsiella or pseudomonas. Co-trimoxazole is given prophylactically in some units, and has the advantage that it gives considerable protection against the opportunistic pathogen *Pneumocystis carinii*.

Most patients will develop fever at some stage during the period of neutropenia. The management of infection in the neutropenic patient is discussed in Chapter 8. Often no bacteriological diagnosis is made. Most fatal infections are from gram-negative organisms. Infections occur around Hickman lines particularly with skin commensals such as *Staphylococcus epidermidis* or *Staphylococcus aureus*. Vancomycin and teicoplanin are very useful antibiotics for treatment of this complication.

Fungal infections may occur. They are very dangerous and can be extremely difficult to diagnose. Opportunistic infections cause considerable diagnostic difficulty in a patient with fever and pulmonary infiltration (see Chapter 8). Fungal infection, *Pneumocystis carinii* and, less commonly, cytomegalovirus and other viral infections must be considered.

After blood cultures have been taken at the onset of fever, broad-spectrum intravenous antibiotic therapy is begun. Such regimens usually include an aminoglycoside and a cephalosporin, and metronidazole is often added particularly if there is clinical deterioration after 24 hours. If there are pulmonary infiltrates, treatment with high-dose co-trimoxazole for pneumocystis, amphotericin B for fungal infection and acyclovir for herpes simplex, should be considered.

Maintenance therapy [9]

Although continued cytotoxic therapy probably prolongs the duration of remission, it is uncertain if it contributes to survival. Nevertheless, most regimens include a period of maintenance therapy. The agents used are cyclophosphamide, cytosine arabinoside, methotrexate, 6MP, daunorubicin, 5 azacytidine and etoposide (see Fig. 28.5).

Results of treatment

Currently about 70% of patients have a complete remission (higher in patients less than 30 years). Mitozantrone, etoposide and higher dose cytosine arabinoside appear to improve remission rates and are incorporated into most recent protocols. More intensive maintenance regimens are also under investigation and may prolong remission duration. Worse outcome occurs in patients over 30 years, those with a high WBC and poor performance status. Cytogenetic changes are prognostically important: t(g;11), 5q, inv3, are adverse and t(8;21) is favourable (Table 28.4). Overall, 10-year disease-free survival is about 25%.

Although the results of intensive conventional chemotherapy in AML have improved to some degree the long-term outlook is still poor for most patients. AML is mainly a disease of the elderly so approaches using BMT (especially allogeneic) are not appropriate for many patients. BMT is usually carried out in first CR, and, in historical comparisons with conventional treatment, seems to reduce leukaemic relapse by 20%. Against this must be set the acute mortality especially from allogeneic BMT. It seems that autologous BMT may be less effective, but the procedure is of course more widely applicable than allogeneic BMT, since matched donors are not needed. In allogeneic BMT high dose cyclophosphamide and TBI are usually used. In autologous BMT, regimens may be based on chemotherapy alone (e.g. busulphan and cyclophosphamide) [10].

Treatment of relapse

Although induction of a second remission is possible in patients who have relapsed after treatment has been discontinued, these remissions are usually short-lived. Patients who relapse while on treatment may have a worse prognosis, but an attempt at remission induction is usually made.

CNS relapse is treated in a similar fashion to ALL (see above).

Treatment of acute promyelocytic leukaemia (APL, M₃)

APL accounts for 10% of AML. Induction of remission is complicated by disseminated intravascular coagulation (DIC) when cytotoxic chemotherapy is given. This seems to be due to release of a procoagulant (cysteine proteinase). A very exciting recent observation is that the cells differentiate *in vitro* in response to all-*trans*-retinoic acid (ATRA). When patients with APL are treated with ATRA the bone marrow slowly (over 2 months) returns to normal (with loss of the typical t(15;17) karyotype), and DIC does not occur. Side-effects include dry skin, headache and potentially fatal hyperleucocytosis (which may cause pulmonary oedema). Patients relapse after 6 months. New trials will assess whether chemotherapy in addition to ATRA will improve results. Interestingly, the breakpoint of t(15;17) is near the gene for the retinoic acid α receptor.

Myelodysplastic syndromes (MDS)

These include a range of disorders, usually of unknown aetiology, characterized by one or more peripheral cytopenias, with a cellular marrow showing morphological evidence of disordered haematopoiesis. This may include ring sideroblasts, hypogranular polymorphs with abnormally segmented nuclei, and increased numbers of early myeloid cells. MDS have an inherent tendency to progress to acute leukaemia and for this reason the syndromes were often referred to as preleukaemia.

Myelodysplastic syndromes are classified according to the major abnormality present, but it should be appreciated that there is often more than one abnormality and that precise categorization may be difficult and arbitrary. When ring sideroblasts are the prominent abnormality a diagnosis of sideroblastic anaemia is usually made, and when blast cells are present in modest numbers the disease is labelled as refractory anaemia with an excess of blasts. This has a particular propensity to develop into acute leukaemia and it is synonymous with the term smouldering leukaemia.

Most MDS are treated with supportive measures only and chemotherapy is deferred until the development of overt acute leukaemia.

THE CHRONIC LEUKAEMIAS

There are two main forms of chronic leukaemia: chronic lymphocytic (lymphatic) leukaemia (CLL) and chronic granulocytic (myeloid) leukaemia (CGL). CLL is exceptionally rare below 40 years of age, whilst CGL can occur at any age, although it is commoner in middle and old age.

Chronic lymphocytic leukaemia

This disease is nearly always a chronic neoplastic proliferation of small B lymphocytes. These B cells are probably early in the B cell differentiation pathway. The immunoglobulin classes IgM and IgD are present in small amounts on the cell membrane but no cytoplasmic Ig can be detected. Nevertheless at some stage in the disease, free light chains can be found in the urine in many patients. Since the tumour is a clonal proliferation each cell bears the same immunoglobulin molecule with the same type of light chain. Although clonal, B cell CLL may not be a homogeneous disease. Chromosomal abnormalities (Table 28.4) include trisomy 12 and deletion of 13q14 (the retinoblastoma gene). Both are adverse prognostically [11].

About 5% of cases are of T cell type, usually a suppressor T cell phenotype (CD8). The condition is indolent and differs from B cell CLL in being associated with less peripheral node en-

largement and less suppression of normal immunoglobulin synthesis.

CLINICAL FEATURES

Over 25% of patients have no symptoms at the time of diagnosis. The disease is discovered because of lymphocytosis noted on a blood count taken for another reason, or because enlargement of lymph nodes or spleen is detected on routine physical examination. In other patients the symptoms are due to noticeably enlarged lymph nodes in the neck or elsewhere, fatigue and malaise due to mild anaemia, infection due to immunosuppression, pain from an enlarged spleen or bruising and bleeding due to thrombocytopenia.

Physical examination reveals painless enlarged lymph nodes which are rubbery and mobile. Many node groups are affected (unlike most lymphomas) and the spleen is often palpable. Massive splenomegaly is unusual at presentation and splenic infarction is less frequent than in CGL.

The diagnosis is made on the blood count. This shows a raised total white count which may even be as high as $500-1000 \times 10^9/l$ but is more usually below $100 \times 10^9/l$. The diagnosis must be considered when the lymphocyte count is above $10 \times 10^9/l$. The differential count shows a great excess of small lymphocytes which usually have a normal morphology but which are sometimes larger with less mature-looking nuclei. Cleaved nuclei suggest the diagnosis of follicular-centre cell lymphoma rather than CLL (see Chapter 26). Prolymphocytic leukaemia cells (see p. 561) are larger with more cytoplasm and a distinct prominent nucleolus. Hairy cells (see p. 561) are usually easily distinguished. If the diagnosis is in doubt it may be necessary to undertake a lymph node biopsy which in CLL shows diffuse infiltration with small well-differentiated lymphocytes, or a marrow aspiration and biopsy which may show focal collections of lymphoma cells in follicular lymphoma but which shows a marked diffuse increase in small well-differentiated lymphocytes in CLL. A blood film is all that is necessary for diagnosis in the great majority of cases.

Occasionally the lymphocytosis is slight and it is then not clear if the patient has a reactive lymphocytosis or CLL. This problem can now often be solved by examining the cell surface for light chain restriction, and the presence of CD5. In CLL all the cells are identical and are restricted to one light chain type (κ or λ), while both light chain types are represented in a reactive lymphocytosis.

Anaemia is variable and when present indicates extensive marrow infiltration. Autoimmune haemolytic anaemia sometimes occurs. The platelet count may be low as a result of marrow infiltration, hypersplenism, chemotherapy and occasionally autoimmune thrombocytopenia. There is suppression of immunoglobulin synthesis in many patients, with marked hypogammaglobulinaemia which leads to increased susceptibility to infection.

STAGING

It may seem contradictory to stage a leukaemia (see Chapter 4). However, it has been shown that a simple staging classification, based on clinical findings and blood count, has prognostic value. This staging notation is shown in Table 28.6. The worse prognostic categories (III—IV) have greater degrees of marrow failure at presentation.

TREATMENT

There is no cure for CLL and it is not even clear if treatment greatly influences survival. The careful use of treatment undoubtedly produces symptomatic benefit. This comes from reduction of the leukaemia mass and consequent improvement in marrow function. Asymptomatic patients should not be treated. Clear indications for treatment include troublesome symptoms of fatigue, greatly enlarged nodes especially if causing pressure, splenic discomfort and marrow failure causing anaemia and thrombocytopenia. Most patients requiring treatment will have Stages II—IV disease.

Drug treatment

Alkylating agents (especially chlorambucil and cyclophosphamide) and steroids are the mainstay of treatment. Steroids (usually prednisolone) are useful in patients developing marrow failure (anaemia, thrombocytopenia) since they do not suppress haemopoiesis. In a patient with anaemia, prednisolone 30—40 mg can be given daily by mouth for 2—3 weeks followed by an alkylating agent. Chlorambucil is given either as a low dose (2—4 mg/day) continuously, or intermittently at a dose of about 10 mg daily 2 weeks on, 2 weeks off. The treatment is continued until the symptoms and signs of the disease have regressed to a considerable extent,

Table 28.6 Staging of chronic lymphocytic leukaemia

Stage		Definition	Median survival (months)
0	A	No enlarged nodes or spleen, Hb >11 g/dl, platelets >100 × 10^9/l, lymphocytes <15 × 10^9/l	150
I	B	As stage 0 with enlarged nodes	100
II		As stage 0 with enlargement of spleen or liver	70
III	C	As 0, I or II; Hb <11 g/dl	20
IV		As 0, II, or III; platelets <100 × 10^9/l	20

The staging notation 0—IV was introduced by Rai *et al.* in 1975, and A—C by Binet *et al.* in 1981.

and then discontinued. A prolonged period of stable disease may then follow before progression which will then require further treatment. Repeated chemotherapy will ultimately contribute to bone marrow failure.

A few agents have recently been found to be effective. Fludarabine, a nucleoside analogue, produces responses in 60% of patients with 40% complete responses. The response rates are higher when the drug is combined with prednisolone. The drug adds to the immunosuppression which is present in these patients. 2-Chlorodeoxyadenosine also produces responses, but is myelosuppressive, and so does pentostatin. Further exploration of the use of these drugs, alone and in combination, is in progress.

Radiotherapy

Splenic irradiation is sometimes used, often to a dose of 10 Gy (1000 rad) in 6–8 fractions over 2 weeks. The lymphocyte count falls and the spleen shrinks. Peripheral nodes may diminish in size. The treatment may produce temporary control of the disease, but myelosuppression can be troublesome particularly if the spleen (and therefore the treatment field) is very large. If there are painful enlarged lymph nodes these can also be treated effectively by irradiation. Whole-body irradiation, given as small doses to a total of 1.0–1.5 Gy (100–150 rad) in 10–20 fractions has also been used for CLL, but is very myelosuppressive and responses are often not maintained.

Treatment of infection

The hypogammaglobulinaemia renders patients highly susceptible to bacterial infection. Febrile illnesses such as upper respiratory infections should be treated promptly with antibiotics and patients warned of their susceptibility. Immune globulin is sometimes given prophylactically to patients who have recurrent infections. Penicillin is usually given prophylactically to patients who have been splenectomized or who have had an episode of pneumococcal infection.

PROGNOSIS

In this elderly population death frequently occurs from other causes. Infection contributes to mortality and as the disease progresses, marrow failure develops, increasing the likelihood of infection and bleeding. A median survival of 5 years has been noted in several series, and there is little evidence that it is improving. Survival is closely related to initial stage of disease (Table 28.6).

Second cancers are possibly more common in CLL than in the general population. A small proportion of patients die from an aggressive malignant transformation with fever, weight loss, and rapidly increasing tumour containing large undifferentiated cells. This syndrome (Richter's syndrome) is unusual and most patients do not develop a transformation of the disease as a terminal event, unlike CGL (see below).

Prolymphocytic leukaemia

This uncommon disease occurs in the elderly. The presentation is like CLL but without much lymph node enlargement and with marked splenomegaly. The white count is high ($>100 \times 10^9/1$). The white cells are larger than CLL cells, with more cytoplasm and a single prominent nucleolus. The cells are B cells with bright staining for surface immunoglobulin, although occasional T cell variants have been described.

Treatment is with chemotherapy and splenic irradiation. Combination chemotherapy is usually used with regimens similar to those used in high-grade non-Hodgkin's lymphoma (see Chapter 26).

Hairy cell leukaemia (HCL) [12]

The disease occurs more commonly in men (M:F 4:1) aged 50–70 years and is characterized by anaemia, thrombocytopenia and

Chapter 28

neutropenia, splenomegaly and the presence of cells in the blood which have unusual cytoplasmic villi — so-called hairy cells. There is little enlargement of lymph nodes and constitutional symptoms (fever, night sweats) are very unusual unless there is an intercurrent infection due to the neutropenia. Pyrexia may be caused by intercurrent mycobacterial infection which is related to neutropenia.

There has been considerable debate as to the nature of the hairy cell. B cell markers (surface Ig) are usually present and the current view is that the cell is an activated clonal B lymphocyte. The cells contain tartrate-resistant acid phosphatase.

Treatment of HCL is changing [12]. Splenectomy was the mainstay of treatment since it may help reverse the cytopenia which is the major clinical problem. Splenectomy will only be beneficial if splenic sequestration is a major source of cytopenia. It does not benefit patients without splenomegaly or with heavy marrow infiltration. It is especially indicated in massive splenomegaly, splenic infarction and in life-threatening thrombocytopenia.

Interferon (IFN) is effective. Both recombinant α-2a and α-2b have been used. The schedules have varied in frequency (daily or twice weekly), duration (6–18 months) and dose. The CR rate is about 8% and PR rate 75%. IFN should be given for about 1 year. There are increasing reports of second malignancies. Pentostatin and 2-chlorodeoxyadenosine (2-CdA) have been shown to be effective [13]. The response rates have been very high with up to 70% complete remissions. The durability of remission and outcome is not yet clear. 2-CdA may become the drug of first choice in the disease [13].

Chronic myelogenous leukaemia (CML)

Chronic myelogenous leukaemia is a disease of great interest to oncologists because in the majority of patients it is associated with a specific acquired chromosomal defect, and because after a period of slow progression

the disease transforms into a more malignant variety of leukaemia.

The chromosomal characteristics of CML have been outlined on p. 551.

CLINICAL FEATURES

These are shown in Table 28.7. The patient may be asymptomatic and the diagnosis made on a routine blood count, but fatigue, anaemia, weight loss and splenic pain eventually occur. Bruising and bleeding may develop. Abdominal pain may be due to stretching of the splenic capsule or may be acute and pleuritic if there has been splenic infarction. Peptic ulceration is 10 times more common than in the general population.

On examination there is usually splenomegaly and often sternal tenderness. The spleen is often considerably enlarged with a splenic 'notch' palpable. Hepatomegaly and purpura

Table 28.7 Clinical and laboratory findings in CML

	Frequency	
Symptoms and signs		
Malaise and fatigue	80	⎫
Weight loss	60	⎪
Bruising and bleeding	40	⎪
Abdominal discomfort	40	⎬ cases (%)
Splenomegaly	95	⎪
Bone tenderness	70	⎪
Hepatomegaly	50	⎪
Purpura	25	⎭
Typical laboratory findings		
Anaemia	$9-12\,g/dl$	
WBC	$25-1000 \times 10^9/l$	
Granulocytes	40%	
Metamyelocytes	10%	
Myelocytes	30%	
Promyelocytes	5%	
Myeloblasts	3%	
Platelets		
$<150 \times 10^9/l$	10	⎫
$150-400 \times 10^9/l$	40	⎬ cases (%)
$>400 \times 10^9/l$	50	⎭

may be present and retinal haemorrhages are not infrequent.

INVESTIGATION

The white blood count is grossly elevated with an increase in all stages of the granulocyte series, particularly myelocytes. Promyelocytes and myeloblasts are present in smaller numbers than myelocytes unless the presentation of the disease is with acute transformation ('blast crisis'). There is a variable degree of anaemia and the platelet count may be high, because of excess production of abnormal platelets, or low, because of hypersplenism or marrow failure. Thrombocytopenia is an indication that blastic transformation may have occurred. The diagnosis can usually be made from the blood film, and the bone marrow examination (although usually performed) does not contribute to diagnosis. It shows an expanded hypercellular marrow with an increase in the myeloid series, with an excess of early forms.

Leucocyte alkaline phosphatase is low or absent, and the Ph' chromosome can be demonstrated in metaphases in cultured marrow cells. The greatly increased turnover of myeloid cells leads to hyperuricaemia.

Patients who are Ph' −ve usually show more anaemia, a less high WBC, more numerous monocytes in the blood and more abnormal myeloid forms.

THE EVOLUTION OF CML (Fig. 28.6)

As the leukaemic mass increases, the spleen enlarges and the patient becomes progressively more anaemic. The WBC doubles every 3−12 months. With treatment (see below) the WBC falls and a stable 'plateau' may then be reached with the patient off treatment. Eventually the WBC will rise again and with treatment will improve. Gradually the 'remissions' become shorter and the recurrences more rapid. Finally an aggressive disease develops with drug resistant splenomegaly or rising WBC showing blastic transformation (Fig. 28.6C). The clinical picture is now dominated by an acute leukaemia which responds poorly to treatment and with a fatal outcome in a few months.

The transformation is usually accompanied by malaise, splenic enlargement, skin deposits, bone pain which may be localized, and a rising blast count. It may be more insidious, the disease showing only a progressive loss of control from chemotherapy and sometimes with features of myelosclerosis. This progressive change is known as 'terminal metamorphosis'. In practical terms it is defined as the time when, for whatever reason, the primary form of treatment has to be abandoned.

The transformation is usually into AML but recently it has become clear that 20% of cases show transformation into ALL in which the blast cells are Ph' +ve. The ALL is of the CALLA phenotype (see p. 550). About 20% of cases of adult ALL are Ph' +ve.

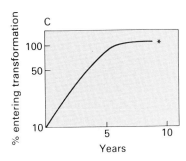

Fig. 28.6 Survival in chronic granulocytic leukaemia. (A) Overall survival; (B) survival after transformation (months); (C) percentage entering transformation.

(Fig. 28.7)

Several drugs are effective in the chronic phase. Busulphan is widely used, and is given by mouth. It is given at a dose of 0.07 mg/kg (4–5 mg) daily until the WBC falls to about $20 \times 10^9/1$. It is important to stop treatment at this point because the myelosuppressive effect of busulphan is delayed so the WBC may fall further, until it begins to rise again later. The rise in count may be very slow and treatment may not need to be restarted for months or even years. Some physicians prefer to give larger doses of busulphan (60–100 mg) as a single dose at 6-week intervals. Although the WBC usually falls slowly with busulphan, in some patients there is a more rapid reduction and they may even become pancytopenic.

With repeated treatments the recovery of the WBC becomes more rapid and the duration of the plateau, or 'remission', shorter. Side-effects of busulphan (see Chapter 6) include skin pigmentation and pulmonary fibrosis.

Hydroxyurea is used as an alternative to busulphan and has the advantage of not causing the long-term side-effects. α-Interferon (IFN) is now widely used. About 80% of patients show blood remission and 20% have a decrease in marrow Ph' +ve cells. The blood counts may remain stable for many months after IFN has been discontinued. Both progression-free survival and overall survival are improved.

Drug treatment produces symptomatic and haematological improvement in almost all patients. The leukaemic mass is reduced with a fall in WBC, reduction in spleen size, improvement in marrow function with a rise in haemoglobin, and a consequent amelioration of symptoms of fatigue and malaise. In spite of this, the cells in the marrow remain Ph' +ve and the transformation of the disease is not prevented. Indeed the extent to which survival is improved by chemotherapy is not clear.

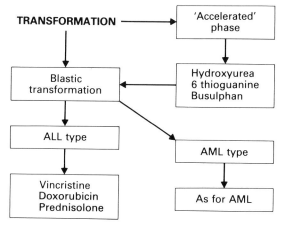

Fig. 28.7 Outline of management of chronic granulocytic leukaemia.

TREATMENT OF ACCELERATED
AND TRANSFORMED CGL

As the speed of relapse increases the spleen usually starts to enlarge and marrow failure, due both to the disease and its treatment, becomes apparent. Changing from busulphan to hydroxyurea (1–2 g/day) may produce temporary benefit. If there is massive splenomegaly which is thought to contribute to anaemia and thrombocytopenia, splenectomy may be helpful provided that blastic transformation has not yet occurred.

Blastic transformation is usually to AML and is often treated as such unless the patient is infirm or elderly. In those cases where ALL supervenes, treatment is as for adult ALL. In both cases the prognosis is very bad. Remissions may be obtained but median survival is only 3 months (Fig. 28.7).

BONE MARROW TRANSPLANTATION
IN CGL [14]

Allogeneic BMT has been used in both blastic transformation and in chronic phase. The results of BMT in blastic transformation are usually disappointing although occasional patients have had a return of normal Ph' −ve hasemopoiesis. Allogeneic BMT has been more successful when carried out in chronic phase, and sustained remissions have been achieved with Ph' −ve haemopoiesis.

Allogeneic BMT should be carried out in chronic phase for patients aged less than 50 and who have a matched donor [14]. The cure rate appears to be about 40%. The high-dose regimen is either cyclophosphamide and TBI or a chemotherapy regimen containing busulphan. If no matched donor is available a haplotype − mismatched marrow − might be used, but the graft-versus-host disease is more severe.

PROGNOSIS OF CGL

Less than 5% of patients survive 5 years (Fig. 28.6). The long-term survival of patients undergoing allogeneic BMT in chronic phase remains to be determined.

PH' −VE CGL

These patients differ from Ph' +ve CGL in having a greater degree of splenomegaly at presentation, more profound anaemia and a lower WBC. The blood film reveals more abnormal neutrophils and monocytes, and fewer myelocytes. The disease appears to run a more rapid course than Ph' +ve CGL with a median survival of only 18 months in some series. Treatment is along the same lines as Ph' +ve CGL.

Eosinophilic leukaemia

This disease is characterized by eosinophilia sometimes accompanied by anaemia, neutropenia and thrombocytopenia. There may be cough associated with transient pulmonary infiltration, and non-bacterial endocarditis occurs leading to heart failure.

The disease may be difficult to distinguish from other forms of chronic eosinophilia and the diagnosis of leukaemia may be hard to establish. Acute blastic transformation of the disease occurs in some patients and the response to treatment is poor.

Chronic myelomonocytic leukaemia

This is a disease of the elderly. The onset is insidious with bruising or bleeding, fleeting urticarial skin rash, slight splenomegaly and a history of infections. There is a monocytosis with abnormal forms and abnormal granulocyte morphology. Bone marrow shows left-shifted granulocytoparesis with abnormal nuclear morphology of a monocyte type. Chromosome 3 may show karyotypic abnormalities [t(3;16)]. The clinical course is slow and intensive treatment is usually inappropriate because of the patient's age and the slow course of the disease.

REFERENCES

1 Sandler O.P. Epidemiology and etiology of leukaemia. *Current Opinion in Oncology* 1990; **2**: 3−9.
2 Kaldor J.M., Day N.E. *et al.* Leukaemia following chemotherapy for ovarian cancer. *New England Journal of Medicine* 1990; **322**: 1−6. (See also the accompanying paper (*New England Journal of Medicine* 1990; **322**: 7−13) describing risk for Hodgkin's disease).
3 Bain B.J. *Leukaemia diagnosis. A guide to the FAB Classification.* Philadelphia: J.B. Lippincott, 1990.
4 MIC Study Group Morphologic, immunologic and cytogenetic (MIC) working classification of the acute

myeloid leukaemias. *British Journal of Haematology* 1988; **68**: 487–94.

5 Clark S.S., Crist W.M., Witte O.N. Molecular pathogenesis of Ph-positive leukaemia. *Annual Review of Medicine* 1989; **40**: 113–22.

6 Champlin R., Gale R.P. Acute lymphoblastic leukaemia: recent advances in biology and therapy. *Blood* 1989; **73**: 2051–66.

7 Barrett A.J., Horowitz M.M., Gale R.P. *et al.* Marrow transplantation for acute lymphoblastic leukaemia; factors affecting relapse and survival. *Blood* 1989; **74**: 862–71.

8 Hussein K.K., Dahlberg S., Head D. *et al.* Treatment of acute lymphoblastic leukaemia in adults with intensive induction, consolidation, and maintenance chemotherapy. *Blood* 1989; **73**: 57–63.

9 Dutcher J.P., Wiernik P.H., Markus S. *et al.* Intensive maintenance therapy improves survival in adult acute myelogenous leukaemia: an eight-year follow-up.

Leukaemia 1988; **2**: 413–19.

10 Chopra R., Goldstone A.H. Modern trends in bone marrow transplantation for acute myeloid and acute lymphoblastic leukaemia. *Current Opinion in Oncology* 1992; **4**: 247–58.

11 Juliusson G., Oscier D.G., Fitchett M. *et al.* Prognostic subgroups in B-cell chronic lymphocytic leukaemia defined by specific chromosomal abnormalities. *New England Journal of Medicine* 1990; **323**: 720–25.

12 Treatment of hairy cell leukaemia *Lancet* 1990; (leading article) **326**: 149–50.

13 Piro L.O., Carrera C.J., Carson D.A., Beutler E. Lasting remission in hairy cell leukaemia induced by a single infusion of 2-chlorodeoxyadenosine. *New England Journal of Medicine* 1990; **332**: 1117–21.

14 Thomas E.D., Clift R.A. Perspectives — indications for marrow transplantation in chronic myelogenous leukaemia. *Blood* 1989; **73**: 861–65.

Index

Page numbers in *italic* refer to figures and/or tables

ABCM regimen
  in myeloma 539, *540*
abdomino-perineal resection *312*
abl oncogene 33, *35*
AMT *see* autologous bone
    marrow transplantation
ABVD regimen
  and gonadal function 112
  in Hodgkin's disease *494, 495*
AC regimen
  in breast cancer *266*
  in ovarian carcinoma *339*
acanthosis nigricans *167, 168,* 283
achalasia 273
acid phosphatase 59, 367
acid reflux in oesophageal
    carcinoma 275
acinar cell tumour, exocrine
    pancreas 295
acinic cell tumour, salivary glands
    193
ACM regimen
  in soft tissue sarcoma *451*
acoustic neuroma 206, 216
acrocyanosis 543
acromegaly 162, 167, 205
ACTH 59
  ectopic production 161–2, 234,
    396
  production by pituitary tumours
    205
actinomycin D 83, 85, 105
  in choriocarcinoma 348
  in Ewing's sarcoma 444
  in Kaposi's sarcoma 430
  in malignant melanoma *426*
  in nephroblastoma 464, 465
  in neuroblastoma 460, *461*
  in osteosarcoma 439
  in rhabdomyosarcoma 469
  in soft tissue sarcoma 450, *451,*
    452
  in testicular germ cell tumours
    387, *388*
actuarial survival curve 16–17
acute lymphoblastic leukaemia
    (ALL)

adult 555–6
  childhood 553–5, *556*
  chromosome abnormalities in
    552
  classification *549*
  doubling time *87*
  incidence *547, 548*
  maintenance therapy 92
  pathology 549–50, *551*
  radiosensitivity 69
acute myeloblastic leukaemia (AML)
    556
  chromosome abnormalities in
    551–2
  classification *549*
  incidence *547, 548*
  maintenance therapy 557–8
  melphalan-induced 539
  pathology 549–50, *551*
  remission induction 556–7
  results of treatment 558
  supportive care 557
  treatment of relapse 558
acute myelo-monocytic leukaemia
    551–2, 556
acute non-lymphocytic leukaemia,
    following Hodgkin's disease
    500
acute promyelocytic leukaemia
    164, 558
acute renal failure 149, 150
addresses *136–7*
adenoacanthoma 328
adenocarcinoma
  age-specific incidence 12–13
  cervix 319
  endometrium 328
  exocrine pancreas 295
  leuco-erythroblastic anaemia in
    49
  lungs 231
  metastatic from unknown primary
    411
  oesophagus 273–4
  prostate 365
  small bowel 305, 306
adenoid cystic carcinoma 193

adenolymphoma 193
adenoma
  acidophil 205
  chromophobe 205, 215
  development to carcinoma *308*
  pleomorphic *192–3*
  villous 308
adenomatous polyps, association
    with large bowel cancer 308
ADH *see* antidiuretic hormone
adrenal gland
  adrenocortical carcinoma 402–3
  medullary tumours 403–4
adrenalectomy 115
  medical 263, 264–5
  surgical 263, 264, 265
adriamycin *see* doxorubicin
adult progeria 167
adult T cell leukaemia/lymphoma
    504
aesthesioneuroblastoma 457–8
aflatoxin 27, 28, 33, 289–90
AFP *see* alphafetoprotein
agammaglobulinaemia
  sex-linked 36
  Swiss-type 505
age-adjusted expected survival
    curve 14
age-related survival rates 14, *15*
AIDS
  and Kaposi's sarcoma 429–30,
    448
  and non-Hodgkin's
    lymphoma 503, *504,* 505,
    517, 525
  and primary cerebral lymphoma
    201, 206
AIHA *see* autoimmune haemolytic
    anaemia
alcohol, and head and neck cancer
    171
aleukaemic leukaemia 553
alkaline phosphatase *59*
  in Hodgkin's disease 487
  in non-Hodgkin's lymphoma
    512
  in osteosarcoma 435, 437

567

Alkeran *see* melphalan
alkylating agents 93−8
  in chronic lymphocytic leukaemia
    560
  and gonadal function 112
  in malignant melanoma *426*
  in myeloma 539−40
  in ovarian cancer 337
  in pancreatic cancer *297*
  phase specificity *88*
  in soft tissue sarcoma 450, 451
  teratogenicity 157
  see also specific agents
All *see* acute lymphoblastic
    leukaemia
all-*trans*-retinoic acid 558
allogeneic bone marrow
    transplantation (BMT) 69,
    74, 547
  in acute myeloblastic leukaemia
    558
  in childhood ALL 555
  in chronic granulocytic/
    myelogenous leukaemia 565
allopurinol 102, 150
alopecia 168
alpha heavy chain disease 522, 524,
    544
alpha particles 64
alphafetoprotein (AFP) 59−60
  in extra-gonadal germ cell
    tumours 206, 216
  in hepatoblastoma 292, 475
  in hepatocellular carcinoma 291
  in metastases from unknown
    primary *409*
  in ovarian germ cell tumours 340
  in testicular germ cell tumours
    382−3
alternative therapies 134−6
alveolar rhabdomyosarcoma 447,
    467
amenorrhoea following
    chemotherapy 499
amethopterin *see* methotrexate
aminoglutethimide 115
  in adrenocortical carcinoma 403
  in breast cancer 263, 264−5
  in ectopic ACTH secretion 162
  in metastases from unknown
    primary site 411
aminopterin 85, 98, 99
AML *see* acute myeloblastic
    leukaemia
amphetamines in terminal care 133
ampulla of Vater, carcinoma 293
amputation 125−6
  in osteosarcoma 438
  in soft tissue sarcoma 449
amyloid deposition in myeloma
    536
anabolic steroids in breast cancer
    265
anaemia 163

autoimmune haemolytic 163,
    483, 486
  in chemotherapy 140
  in chronic lymphocytic leukaemia
    560
  Fanconi's 36, *167*, 549
  in Hodgkin's disease 484, 486
  iron deficiency 283, 310
  microangiopathic haemolytic
    164
  in myeloma 537
  in non-Hodgkin's lymphoma
    512
  pernicious 280−1
  refractory with excess of blasts
    559
  sideroblastic 559
  and staging 49
analgesics in pain relief 128−31
anaplastic carcinoma 42
  salivary glands 193
  thyroid *394, 395, 397, 399,* 401,
    402
androgens
  in adrenocortical carcinoma 402
  therapy in renal cell
    adenocarcinoma 356
  total blockage 371
angioendotheliomatosis, malignant
    527
angiogenesis, tumours 42−3
angiography
  in brain tumour 208−9
  in hepatocellular carcinoma 291
angiosarcoma
  bone *433,* 446
  liver 289, 292
  soft tissue 448
aniline dyes 11, 357
aniridia 455, 461, 462
ANL, following Hodgkin's disease
    500
Ann Arbor staging
  gastric carcinoma 521, *522*
  Hodgkin's disease *486*
anorexia 146, *160*
  in stomach cancer 283
  in terminal cancer 132−3
anoxia, effect on cytotoxicity of
    X-rays 70−1
anti-androgen therapy in prostatic
    cancer 370−1
antibiotics
  antitumour 105−7
  in bloodstream infections 143
antidiuretic hormone (ADH) *59,* 60
  inappropriate secretion *160, 161,*
    234
anti-emetics 110−11, 133
antigen-presenting cells 481, 507
anti-idiotype antibodies 45−6
antimetabolites
  folic acid antagonists 98−100
  purine antagonists 101−2

pyrimidine antagonists 100−1
anti-oestrogens 115−16
anti-oncogenes 34−5
antitumour antibiotics 105−7
anus, carcinoma 315−16
anxiety in terminal cancer 133
APC gene 308
APL 164, 558
apoptosis 39
appendiceal tumours 298, 306
APUD system 300
ara-C *see* cytosine arabinoside
argentaffinoma 298
aromatic amines in carcinogenesis
    27, 28
arrhenoblastoma 341
arsenicals, carcionogenicity *27,*
    414, 415
asbestos 10−11, *27*
  and lung cancer 228
  and mesothelioma 247
ascites 152
  malignant 283
Askin's tumour 434, 442
L-asparaginase 107−8
  in acute lymphoblastic leukaemia
    553
  hepatic toxicity *112*
Aspergillus, pulmonary infection
    144
Aspergillus flavus 28, 289−90
aspermia 385
astrocytoma 202−3, *204,* 403
  management 209−11
  spinal cord 220
ataxia telangiectasia *36, 167,*
    505
  and risk of leukaemia 549
atmospheric pollution 10, *228*
atom bomb 10, 28, 547, *548*
atrophic gastritis and stomach
    cancer 280−1
atypical teratoma syndrome 391
Auer rods 549
autoimmune haemolytic anaemia
    (AIHA) 163
  in Hodgkin's disese 483, 486
autoimmune thyroiditis 398
autologous bone marrow
    transplantation (ABMT)
    547
  in acute myeloblastic leukaemia
    558
  in childhood ALL 555
  in non-Hodgkin's lymphoma
    516−17
avian leukaemia virus 31
avian leukosis virus 32
azathioprine *101, 102, 112*
azo dyes *27, 28*
azoospermia
  following chemotherapy
    499−500
  in testicular cancer 382

B cell lymphoma
  cell origins 508
  childhood 518–19
  in HIV infection 32
  management 512–17
  sclerosing 246
B cells, differentiation 506–7
bacteraemia 143
barium studies
  in Hodgkin's disease 490
  in large bowel cancer 310, *311*
  in oesophageal carcinoma 275, *276*
  in pancreatic cancer 296
  in small bowel cancer 305–6
  in stomach cancer 283, *284*
Barrett's oesophagus 273
basal cell carcinoma 416–17
  age-specific incidence *416*
  eyelid 197
  management 418–21
  pinna 190
BCG 46
  in bladder cancer 361
  in lung cancer 243
  in malignant melanoma 427
bcl-2 gene 39, 506
BCNU 97
  in glioma 211
  in large bowel cancer 313
  in malignant melanoma 426
Beckwith's syndrome 36
Bence-Jones protein 533, 543
benign macroglobulinaemia 543
benign monoclonal gammopathy 534, 542–3
benzanthracene 28
benzene 547
benzidine 11, *27*, 28
benzodiazepines 111, 133
3:4-benzpyrene 10, *27*, 28, 413
BEP regimen in testicular cancer 388
β-naphthylamine *27*, 28, 357
beta particles 64
βHCG *see* human chorionic gonadotrophin
bilharzia 271
biliary bypass 297
biliary tract cancer 292–4
bilirubin
  in Hodgkin's disease 486–7
  in non-Hodgkin's lymphoma 512
biology of cancer 27–46
biopsy
  CT scan guided 52
  liver 291
  in non-Hodgkin's lymphoma 511
  percutaneous in Hodgkin's disease 490
  in soft tissue sarcoma 449
  thyroid 398

BIP regimen in carcinoma of the cervix 326
biphosphonates 149
bitemporal hemianopia 205
BJP 533, 543
bladder cancer
  aetiology 357–8
  clinical features 359–60
  incidence *352*, 357–8
  life-time risk of development 3
  lyonization 37
  management 360–4
  pathology 358–9
  prognosis 364
  screening for 358
  staging 358–9
blast crisis in chronic granulocytic leukaemia 563
bleeding
  rectal 310, 311
  vaginal 320, 330, 344
bleomycin 106–7
  in ascites 152
  and bone marrow depression 139
  in head and neck squamous carcinoma 190–1
  in Hodgkin's disease *494*
  in Kaposi's sarcoma 430
  in nephroblastoma 466
  in osteosarcoma 439
  in ovarian germ cell tumours 341
  in pleural effusion 151
  and pulmonary fibrosis 112
  in testicular germ cell tumours 387–8
  in thyroid cancer 402
Blom–Singer valve in laryngectomy 179
blood–brain barrier 219
blood transfusion
  in acute myeloblastic leukaemia 557
  in anaemia 163
  in bone marrow suppression 140
Bloom's syndrome *36*, *167*, *505*, 549
BMT *see* allogeneic bone marrow transplantation
BOLD regimen in melanoma 427
bombesin 230
bone
  angiosarcoma *433*, 446
  fibrosarcoma *433*, 445
  giant cell tumour *433*, 445
  haemangioendothelioma *433*, 445
  haemangiopericytoma *433*, 445
  isotope scanning 56
    in Hodgkin's disease 490
    in osteosarcoma 437
  malignant fibrous histiocytoma *433*, 445
  metastases
    diagnosis 56, 57

  and hypercalcaemia 148
  radiotherapy 157
  non-Hodgkin's lymphoma *433*, 446, 524
  primary malignant tumour types *433*
  radiosensitivity 76–7
bone marrow
  aspiration in neuroblastoma 458
  biopsy in Hodgkin's disease 490
  effects of chemotherapy on 139–40, 498–9
  examination and staging 49
  failure 139–41
  involvement in Hodgkin's disease 484
  radiosensitivity 73–4
  see also allogeneic bone marrow transplantation; autologous bone marrow transplantation
boron neutron capture therapy 428
botryoidal rhabdomyosarcoma 447, 467
Bowen's disease 372, 415
brachial plexus block 131
brachytherapy 66
  in brain tumours 210
  in retinoblastoma 472
bradykinin in carcinoid syndrome 298, 300
Bragg effect 69
brain
  isotope scanning 57
  radiation damage 223
  radiosensitivity 74
  tumours 201
    cellular biology 201–2
    in childhood *455*
    clinical features 207–8
    diagnosis 208–9
    magnetic resonance imaging 54, *55*
    management 209–16
    management on relapse 216–17
    metastatic 57, 217–19, 242
    non-Hodgkin's lymphoma 201, 206, 216, 525–6
    pathological classification 202–7
    prognosis *210*, 217
brain stem tumours 203, 206, 212
breast
  biopsy 254
  cancer
    aetiology 251
    age-related survival rate *15*
    clinical features 253–4
    confirmation of diagnosis 254
    doubling time *87*
    epidemiology 251
    hormonal manipulation in 263–5

hormone receptors in   114—15,
    255—6, 264
incidence   251
    age-related 13, *252*
    in Japanese immigrants   *9*
    life-time risk of development   *3*
    male   *252*, 271
    management
        adjuvant systemic therapy
        268—70
        advanced primary tumour
        261—3
        complications   262—3
        early primary tumour
        256—61
        metastatic disease   263—8
    mode of spread   252--3
    pathology   251—2
    pre-operative investigation
    254
    prognosis   *49*, 270—1
    screening   23, 24, 256
    staging   *49*, 254—5
    survival curves   17—18
    treatment trials   20—1
carcinoma *in situ*   252
cysts, aspiration   254
lumps   253
prostheses   125
self-examination   256
surgical reconstruction   257, 262
ultrasound investigation   50
Breast Cancer Care   *136, 137*
British Testicular Tumour Panel
    classification   *378*
bromocriptine   215
bromodeoxyuridine   201
bronchioalveolar carcinoma   231
bronchoscopy   234
bronchospasm, in carcinoid
        syndrome   298—9, 300
bronchus   *see* lungs, carcinoma
Brown—Séquard syndrome   220,
    223
Budd—Chiari syndrome   290
BUdR   201
bullous eruptions   *167, 168*
buprenorphine   128, 129
Burkitt's lymphoma   9, 37, 516,
    518—19
    chromosome abnormalities   33,
    505—6
    doubling time   *87*
    Epstein—Barr virus in   33, 503
    geographical distribution   503
    management   521
    staging   *518*
busulphan   97
    and bone marrow suppression
    139
    in chronic granulocytic/
        myelogenous leukaemia   564
    and pulmonary fibrosis   112

structure   95, *96*
buthionine sulfoximine   91
butyrophenones   111

C-*abl* oncongene   33
C-*erb*B-1 oncongene   34
C-*erb*B-2 oncogene, in breast cancer
    271
C-*fms* oncogene, in leukaemia   552
C-*myc* oncogene   33, 201, 505—6
CA 19—9   60
Ca-125   59, 60
    in ovarian carcinoma   332
cachectin   118
cachexia   145—7, *160*
cadmium   27
caesium
    needle   65
    radioactive isotope   *65*
calcitonin   59, 149, 396
CALLA   516, *550*
cancer *en cuirasse*   253
Cancer Relief Macmillan Fund   *136,
    137*
candidiasis
    gastrointestinal   145
    oral   144—5
    pulmonary   144
CAP regimen in ovarian cancer
    339
carboplatin   107
    in ovarian cancer   338
    in rhabdomyosarcoma   469
    in small cell lung cancer   *241*
carcinoembryonic antigen (CEA)
    59—60
    in large bowel cancer   310—11,
    315
    in pancreatic cancer   296
    in stomach cancer   283—4
carcinogenesis
    in childhood   454—5
    epidemiological studies   9—12
    initiators   29
    physicochemical   27—30
    promoters   29
    recessive genetic mechanisms in
    34—5
    transplacental   455
    viral   11—12, 30—5
carcinogens   9—11, 27—8
carcinoid syndrome   298—9, 340
carcinoid tumours   297, 305
    appendix   306
    clinical features   298—9
    diagnosis   299
    ectopic ACTH production   161,
    162
    management   299—300, 306
    pathology   298
    thymus   245
carcinomatous myelopathy   165
carmustine   *see* BCNU

carotid body tumour   190
carpal tunnel syndrome   537
case—control studies   7
cataract, radiation-induced   76
catecholamine secretion
    by neuroblastoma   458
    by phaeochromocytoma   403—4
'cats eye reflex'   471
cauda equina syndrome   154—5,
    220
CCNU   97, 98
    and bone marrow suppression
    139
    in glioma   211, *214*
    in large bowel cancer   313
    in renal cell adenocarcinoma   356
    in small cell lung cancer   *241*
CD markers
    in leukaemia   *551, 552*
    in T cell lymphoma   518, 519
CEA   *see* carcinoembryonic antigen
Celestin endo-oesophageal tube
    278
cell-mediated immunity   143
    in Hodgkin's disease   482—3, 499
cell rests   390
cells
    cycle   38—9, 86, *87*
        and cytotoxic drug effects
        87—8
    death   39, 90—1
    differentiation   41
    susceptibility to cytotoxic drugs
    87—8
cellular oncogenes   *see* oncogenes
cellular proto-oncogenes   31
cellulitis   262
central nervous system
    in Hodgkin's disease   484—5
    non-Hodgkin's lymphoma   201,
    206, 216, 525—6
    prophylaxis in acute
        lymphoblastic leukaemia
        553—4
    radiosensitivity   74—5
    tumours   201—23
    see also brain; spinal cord
centroblasts   507, 508, *509*
centrocytes   507, 508
cerebellar ataxia   403
cerebellar degeneration   *160*, 165
    subacute   485
cerebellar lesions   208
cerebral oedema   218
cerebrospinal fluid in central
        nervous system lymphoma
        525—6
Cerubidin   *see* daunorubicin
cervical intraepithelial neoplasia
    319, 321
cervix
    carcinoma
        aetiology   32, 33, 317—19

clinical features 320
computed tomography 52, *53*
exophytic lesions 320
geographical variation in
 incidence 8
incidence 2, 12–13, 317–19
infiltrative 320
life-time risk of development 3
management 321–6
mortality 2
pathology 319
in pregnancy 327
prognosis 326–7
recurrent 326
screening 23, 24, 319, 326
spread 319
staging 320–1
carcinoma *in situ* 319
cone biopsy 321
CGL *see* chronic granulocytic/
 myelogenous leukaemia
CHAP regimen *339*
Chediak–Higashi syndrome *167,*
 504, *505*
chemodectoma 190, 247
chemosurgery 418–19
chemotherapy 1–2, 85
 acute lymphoblastic leukaemia
  553–4
 acute myeoloblastic leukaemia
  556, *557*, 558
 adjuvant 82–4, 92–3
  in anal carcinoma 316
  in breast cancer 268–70
  combination 191
  in Ewing's sarcoma 444
  in large bowel cancer 314
  in osteosarcoma 438–9
  in stomach cancer 286–7
  treatment trials in breast cancer
   20–1
 administration 108–9
 adrenocortical carcinoma 403
 in ascites 152
 basal/squamous cell skin
  carcinoma 420
 biliary tract cancer 294
 bladder cancer 361, 363–4
 breast cancer 265–7, 268–70
 Burkitt's lymphoma 516, 521
 carcinoid tumour 300
 cerebral metastases 219
 cervical carcinoma 326
 choriocarcinoma 347–8
 chronic granulocytic/myelogenous
  leukaemia 564–5
 chronic lymphocytic leukaemia
  560–1
 combination 89
  adjuvant 191
 contribution to cancer cure 93, *94*
 effect on bone marrow 139–40,
  498–9

effect on gonadal function
 476–7
effect on growth 476
Ewing's sarcoma 444
glioma 210–11
head and neck carcinoma 190–2
hepatic metastases 153
hepatoblastoma 292, 475
hepatocellular carcinoma 291
high dose 438–9, 440, 460
Hodgkin's disease 493–5, 496–7
hybrid regimens 494–5
integration with radiotherapy
 82–4
prostatic cancer 371
regional limb perfusion 427
renal cell adenocarcinoma 356
rhabdomyosarcoma 468–9
small cell lung cancer 240–2
soft tissue sarcoma 450–1, *452*
stomach cancer 286
superior vena caval obstruction
 156
testicular germ cell tumours
 387–9
thyroid cancer 402
topical 420
toxicity 498–9
treatment trials 86
uterine carcinoma 331
vomiting induced by 109–11
childhood cancer
 aetiology 454–6
 approach to 453–4
 incidence 454–6
 late sequelae of treatment 476–7
 survival *455*
 see also specific types
chlorambucil 96, 97
 in choriocarcinoma 348
 intra-arterial infusion 440
 intravenous infusion 286, 291,
  297, 314–15
 Kaposi's sarcoma 430
 large bowel cancer 313–15
 long-term complications
  112–13, 499–500
 maintenance 92, 554–5
 malignant melanoma 426–7
 medulloblastoma 214
 metastases from unknown
  primary site 411
 myeloma 539–41
 neoadjuvant 326, 363, 364,
  439–40
  in breast cancer 270
  in non-small cell lung cancer
   239–40
 nephroblastoma 464–6
 neuroblastoma 460, *461*
 non-Hodgkin's lymphoma
  513–16, 519–21
 non-small cell lung cancer

239–40
oesophageal cancer 278
osteosarcoma 438–40
ovarian cancer 337–9
ovarian germ cell tumours 341
pancreatic endocrine tumours
 303
pancreatic exocrine tumours 297
pericardial effusion 151
pleural effusion 151
in pregnancy 157
principles 86–93
in chronic lymphocytic leukaemia
 560
in Hodgkin's disease 494
in ovarian cancer 337
and second cancers 113
in testicular germ cell tumours
 387
chlorethylnitrosourea *94*
2-chlorodeoxyadenosine
 in chronic lymphocytic leukaemia
  561
 in hairy cell leukaemia 562
chlorozotocin in pancreatic cancer
 303
chlorpromazine 111
ChLVPP regimen 494, 495, 496
cholangiocarcinoma 289, 290
cholelithiasis, association with gall
 bladder cancer 292
chondrosarcoma 433, 441
 incidence *435*
 mesenchymal *433*, 441–2
CHOP regimen in non-Hodgkin's
 lymphoma 514, *515*
chordoma 206–7
 management 216
 mediastinal 247
choriocarcinoma
 ovarian 341
 testicular *379*, 380–1
 uterine 346–8
chromogranin 231
chromophobe tumours *204*, 205
chromosome abnormalities
 and bone sarcoma 433–4
 and brain tumours 202, 206
 and Burkitt's lymphoma 33,
  505–6
 and leukaemia 547–8, 551–2,
  559
 and nephroblastoma 461–2
 and non-Hodgkin's lymphoma
  505–6
 and retinoblastoma 470
 and small cell lung cancer 230–1
 and testicular cancer 380
chronic granulocytic/myelogenous
 leukaemia (CGL/CML) 33,
 37, 559, 562
  chromosome abnormalities 551,
  552

clinical features 562–3
evolution 563
incidence 547
investigation 563
management 564–5
Ph'–ve 565
prognosis 565
terminal metamorphosis 563
chronic lymphocytic leukaemia
552, 559–61
chronic myelomonocytic leukaemia
565
cigarette smoking *see* tobacco,
smoking
CIN in cervical carcinoma 319, 321
circumcision, male
and cervical carcinoma 317
and penile cancer 372
cirrhosis, association with
hepatocellular carcinoma
33, 289
cis-diammine dichloroplatinum
see cisplatin
cisplatin 107
in adrenocortical carcinoma 403
in bladder cancer 363, 364
in choriocarcinoma 348
in glioma 211, 212, *214*
in head and neck squamous
carcinoma 191
in hepatoblastoma 292, 475
in malignant melanoma 426, 427
in nephroblastoma 465
in neuroblastoma 460, *461*
in non-small cell lung cancer *239*
in osteosarcoma 439, 440
in ovarian cancer *337*, 338
in ovarian germ cell tumours 341
phase specificity *88*
in rhabdomyosarcoma 469
in small cell lung cancer *241*
in soft tissue sarcoma *451*
in stomach cancer 286
in testicular germ cell tumours
387–8
citrovorum factor 98, 100, 313, *314*
CLA *409*, 442–3
CLL 552, 559–61
clodronate 149
Clonorchis sinensis 292
CMF regimen *266*, 267
CML *see* chronic granulocytic/
myelogenous leukaemia
CMV *see* cytomegalovirus
coal tar 414
cobalt-60 64, *65*, 66
codeine 128, *129*
Codman's triangle 436, *437*
coeliac disease, association with
non-Hodgkin's lymphoma
505, 522, 524
coeliac plexus block 131, *132*, 297
cohort studies 7

cold agglutinin disease 543
cold sore 145
colloid cysts 207
colon, tumours *see* large bowel
tumours
colonic interposition 276, *277*
colonoscopy 310
colony stimulating factors 141–2
colostomy 125, 312, 315
colposcopy 320–1
common acute lymphoblastic
leukaemia antigen 516, *550*
common leucocyte antigen *409*,
442–3
communication with patients 4–5,
121–4
COMP regimen in lymphoblastic
leukaemia 520–1
compartmentectomy 449–50, 468
computed tomography
adrenocortical carcinoma 402–3
bladder cancer 360, *361*
brain tumours 207, *208*
head and neck cancer 174, *176*,
195
hepatocellular carcinoma 291
Hodgkin's disease *488*, 489–90
lung cancer 235
mesothelioma *248*
nephroblastoma 463
non-Hodgkin's lymphoma 512
oesophageal carcinoma 276
osteosarcoma 437, *438*
pancreatic cancer 296
renal cell adenocarcinoma 353,
354
soft tissue sarcoma 449
and tumour staging 50–3, *54*
condylomata acuminata 372
conjunctiva
non-Hodgkin's lymphoma 527
tumours 197–8
connective tissue, radiosensitivity
77
Conn's syndrome 402
constrictive pericarditis 499
corpus uteri *see* uterus
Corynebacterium parvum
in lung cancer 243
in malignant melanoma 427
cough
in lung cancer 233
in oesophageal carcinoma 275
cranial nerves
involvement in nasopharyngeal
carcinoma 181
palsies 208
tumours 206, 216
craniopharyngioma 205, 215
craniospinal irradiation 211–12,
213–14
Crasnitine *see* L-asparaginase
crocidolite 247

crude incidence rates 7
crude prevalence rates 7
CRUSE *136*
cryosurgery
basal/squamous cell skin
carcinoma 418
bladder cancer 361
CIN 3 321
retinoblastoma 472
Cryptococcus neoformans 145
cryptorchidism 377
CSFs 141–2
CT scanning *see* computed
tomography
cure, determination of 13–17
Cushing's syndrome *160*, 161–2,
205
in adrenocortical carcinoma 402,
403
in carcinoid of the thymus 245
cyclophosphamide 95–6
activation 92
in acute lymphoblastic leukaemia
553
in acute myeloblastic
leukaemia 558
in aetiology of bladder cancer
358
in bladder cancer 363
in breast cancer *266*, 268
in carcinoid tumours 300
in choriocarcinoma 348
in chronic lymphocytic leukaemia
560
in Ewing's sarcoma 444
and granulocytopenia 130
in head and neck squamous
carcinoma *191*
in Hodgkin's disease *494*
and hyponatraemia 161
in myeloma 539
in nephroblastoma *465*
in neuroblastoma 460, *461*
in non-small cell lung cancer *239*
in osteosarcoma 439
in ovarian cancer 337
in renal cell adenocarcinoma 356
in rhabdomyosarcoma 469
in small cell lung cancer *241*
in soft tissue sarcoma 450, 451,
452
cylindroma 193
cyproheptadine 299–300
cyproterone acetate 116
in prostatic cancer 371
cystadenocarcinoma 295
cystectomy 361–3
cysteine proteinase 558
cystodiathermy in bladder cancer
361
cystoscopy 359–60
cytarabine *see* cytosine
arabinoside

cytokeratins *409*
cytokines 46, 116−18
cytomegalovirus (CMV)
   in Kaposi's sarcoma 33
   pulmonary infection 144
cytosine arabinoside 101
   activation 92
   in acute lymphoblastic leukaemia 553
   in acute myeloblastic leukaemia 556, *557*, 558
   in malignant melanoma *426*
   phase specificity *88*
   in progressive multifocal leucoencephalopathy 166
   structure *100*
cytotoxic drugs 93−109
   activation 92
   administration 108−9
   carcinogenic effects 27, 28
   and cell cycle 87−8
   in combination 89
   development and trials 85−6
   history 85
   kinetics of cell killing 88−9
   predicting sensitivity to 93
   resistance to 89−92
   teratogenicity 157
   see also chemotherapy *and individual drugs*
cytotrophoblast *379*, 380
Cytoxan *see* cyclophosphamide
CYVADACT regimen *451*
CYVADIC regimen *451*, *452*

dacarbazine 98
   in Hodgkin's disease *494*
   in Kaposi's sarcoma 430
   in malignant melanoma 426, 427
   in soft tissue sarcoma 451
   structure 95
dactinomycin *see* actinomycin D
danazol 162
Darier−Pautrier abscess 528
data bases in treatment trials 23
daunorubicin 105−6
   in acute lymphoblastic leukaemia 553
   in acute myeloblastic leukaemia 556, *557*, 558
DCC gene 308
o, p′-DDD in adrenal carcinoma 403
DDP *see* cisplatin
DDT 547
de Quervain's subacute thyroiditis 398
Deca-Durabolin 265
demeclocycline 161
dendritic cells 481, 507
dense core granules *409*
2-deoxycoformycin 102, 562
depression in terminal cancer 133

dermatitis, radiation 415
dermatitis herpetiformis 168
dermatofibrosarcoma protruberans 429, 447
dermatomyositis *160*, 166, *167*
desmin *409*
dexamethasone *111*
   in cerebral metastases 218
   in recurrent brain tumour 217
   in spinal cord compression 155
   in superior vena cava obstruction 156
   suppression of ectopic ACTH production 162
   in terminal care 133
dextromoramide 128, *129*
dextropropoxyphene 128
diabetes mellitus
   and pancreatic carcinoma 296
   and uterine carcinoma 328
diamorphine 128−30, 131
diarrhoea
   in carcinoid syndrome 298, 299−300
   in gastrinoma 302
   in large bowel tumours 310
1:2,5:6 dibenzpyrene 27
DIC *160*, 164, 558
diet
   and cancer incidence 11
   and large bowel tumours 307
diethylstilboestrol 344, 455
dihydrocodeine *129*
dihydrofolate reductase 91
dimethylamino azobenzene 27, 28
dimethylnitrosamine 27, 28
dimethyltriazenoimidazole carboxamide *see* dacarbazine
dipipanone 128, *129*
disease-free survival curve 14
disseminated intravascular coagulation *160*, 164, 558
distal sensory and motor neuropathy 164
Dixon and Moore classification *378*
DNA, repair 30, 91−2
DNA viruses 32−3
Dobbie applicator 346
docetaxel 104
dorsal root block 131, *132*
Down's syndrome *36*, 549
doxorubicin 83, 105−6
   in acute lymphoblastic leukaemia 553
   in bladder cancer 363
   and bone marrow failure 139
   in breast cancer 266, 267
   in carcinoid tumours 300
   in Ewing's sarcoma 444
   in head and neck squamous carcinoma *191*
   in hepatoblastoma 292, 475

   in hepatocellular carcinoma 291
   in Hodgkin's disease *494*
   in metastases from unknown primary site 411
   in nephroblastoma 464, 465
   in neuroblastoma 460, *461*
   in non-small cell lung cancer *239*
   in osteosarcoma 439
   in ovarian cancer *337*, 338
   in pancreatic cancer *297*, 303
   in pleural effusion 151
   in renal cell adenocarcinoma 356
   in rhabdomyosarcoma 469
   in small cell lung cancer *241*
   in soft tissue sarcoma 450, 451, *452*
   in stomach cancer 286
   in thyroid cancer 402
DT-diaphorase 92
DTIC *see* dacarbazine
Dukes staging system *309*
dumb-bell tumours 246, 459
duodenum *see* small bowel tumours
dye workers 27, 357
dying, care of 127−34
dysgerminoma 340
dyspareunia in cervical cancer 320
dyspepsia, in oesophageal carcinoma 275
dysphagia
   in laryngeal cancer 176
   in lung cancer 233
   in oesophageal carcinoma 274−5
   in stomach cancer 283
dysplastic naevus syndrome 422
dyspnoea
   in laryngeal cancer 176
   in lung cancer 233
   in mesothelioma 248

ear tumours *171*, 189−90
early gastric cancer 281, 282
   diagnosis 284−5
   see also stomach, carcinoma
EBV *see* Epstein−Barr virus
edatrexate 99−100
edrophonium 166
EGFR 34, 202
Eldisine *see* vindesine
electrocautery 418
electromagnetic spectrum 63, *64*
electron therapy 68
   in mycosis fungoides 528
Elspar *see* L-asparaginase
EMA *409*
embryonal carcinoma
   ovarian 340
   testicular *379*, 380
embryonal rhabdomyosarcoma 447, 450, 466−7
endodermal sinus tumour 340, *379*, 475−6

endometrium
  carcinoma *see* uterus, carcinoma
  hyperplasia 328
endoprostheses in osteosarcoma
    438, *439*
endoscopic retrograde
    cholangiopancreatography
    293, 296
endoscopy in stomach cancer 283
Endoxana *see* cyclophosphamide
enteral feeding 147
enucleation 472
env gene 504
eosinophilic granuloma 474
eosinophilic leukaemia 565
ependymoblastoma 203
ependymoma 203, *204*
  management 211–12
  metastasis 208
  spinal cord 220
epidemiology
  and causation 9–12
  terminology and methods 7–8
epidermal growth factor receptor
    34, 202
epidermodysplasia verruciformis
    414, 415
epididymo-orchitis 382
epidural pain relief 131–2
epiglottic tumours 177
epilation 75
epilepsy 206
epipodophyllotoxin derivatives
    85, 104–5, 341
epirubicin
  in soft tissue sarcoma 451
  in stomach cancer 286
epithelial membrane antigen *409*
epithelioid
    haemangioendothelioma
    292
EPO 142, 163
Epstein–Barr virus (EBV) 12, 32
  and Burkitt's lymphoma 33, 503
  and Hodgkin's disease 480
  and nasopharyngeal carcinoma
    33, 171–72
  and non-Hodgkin's lymphoma
    504
ER *see* oestrogen receptor
erb oncogenes 31, 34, *35*, 201
ERCP 293, 296
erythema *167*
erythroblasts 549
erythrocyte sedimentation rate
  in Hodgkin's disease 486
  in myeloma 537
erythrocytosis *160*, 163
erythroderma *167*, 168
erythroleukaemia 549
erythroplasia of Queyrat 372,
    415–16
erythropoietin 142, 163

Escherichia coli 143
etidronate 149
etoposide *27*, 104–5
  in acute myeloblastic leukaemia
    558
  in adrenocortical carcinoma 403
  in choriocarcinoma 348
  in Ewing's sarcoma 444
  in nephroblastoma *465*, 466
  in neuroblastoma 460, *461*
  in non-small cell lung cancer *239*
  in rhabdomyosarcoma 469
  in small cell lung cancer *241*
  in testicular germ cell tumours
    388
Ewing's sarcoma *433*
  aetiology 434
  in childhood *455*
  clinical features 442
  incidence *435*, 442
  investigation 443
  management 443–5
  pathology 442–3
  prognosis 444–5
exhaust fumes 10
external auditory canal carcinoma
    190
eye
  metastases 156
  radiosensitivity 75–6, 197
  tumours 197–8, 527
eyelid tumours 197–8

faecal occult blood testing 315
fallopian tube carcinoma 341–2
FAM regimen 286
familial adenomatous polyposis coli
    36, 307–8
Fanconi syndrome, acquired 536
Fanconi's anaemia *36, 167*
  and risk of leukaemia 549
fat, dietary 11
fat necrosis *167*
fentanyl 131
fertility
  effects of chemotherapy on 112,
    499–500
  effects of childhood therapy on
    476
  effects of radiotherapy on 74, 499
fever 159–60
  in Hodgkin's disease 483
  in non-Hodgkin's lymphoma
    510
  in renal cell adenocarcinoma 352
fibre, dietary 11
fibreoptic bronchoscopy 234
fibrolamellar carcinoma 290
fibrosarcoma 447
  bone *433*, 445
  incidence *435*
FIGO staging 47
  cervical carcinoma 320–1

ovarian carcinoma 332–3
  uterine carcinoma 329–30
  vaginal carcinoma 345
  vulval carcinoma 343
finger clubbing in lung cancer 233
flow cytometry, brain tumours 201
fludarabine 561
5-fluorouracil (5-FU) 100–1
  activation 92
  in anal carcinoma 316
  in basal/squamous cell skin
    carcinoma 420
  in biliary tract cancer 294
  in bladder cancer 363
  in breast cancer *266*
  in carcinoid tumours 300
  in head and neck squamous
    carcinoma 191
  in hepatic metastases 153
  in hepatocellular carcinoma *291*
  in large bowel cancer 313,
    314–15
  in ovarian cancer 337, 338
  in pancreatic cancer *297*, 303
  in stomach cancer 286
  topical 420
flushing in carcinoid syndrome
    298, 300
flutamide 116
  in prostatic cancer 370–1
  in renal cell adenocarcinoma 356
folic acid 99
  antagonists 98–100
folinic acid 98, 100, 313, *314*
follicle-centre cell lymphoma 506,
    509
follicle-stimulating hormone 476
fotemustine 426
fractional cell kill hypothesis 88–9
frusemide 149, 152
FSH 476
5-FU *see* 5-fluorouracil
fungal infection
  in acute myeloblastic leukaemia
    557
  pulmonary 144

G6PD 37
G-CSF 141, 142, 429
G-protein 33, 34
gag gene 504
galactorrhoea 162
gall bladder cancer 290, 292–4
gallium scanning in Hodgkin's
    disease 490
gamma-heavy chain disease 544
gamma rays 64, 66
ganglioglioma 206
ganglioneuroblastoma 247
ganglioneuroma 206
  adrenal medulla 403
  mediastinal 246
Gardner's syndrome *36, 167*

gastrectomy 285–6
gastrin-releasing peptide 230
gastrinoma 302–3
gastrointestinal system
　in Hodgkin's disease 485
　infection 144–5
　non-Hodgkin's lymphoma
　　521–4
　radiosensitivity 76
　tumours 273–87, 305–16
gastrostomy 276
gelatinases 42
gene amplification, and resistance to
　cytotoxic drug 91
genetic counselling in
　retinoblastoma 470, 471
genital carcinoma *in situ* 372,
　415–16
genito-urinary cancer 351–74,
　377–91
geographical variations in cancer
　incidence 8–9, 455, 503–4
germ cell tumours
　childhood 455, 475–6
　extra-gonadal 206, 215–16,
　　245–6, 390–1, 475
　metastases from 407
　ovaries 340–1, 476
　sacrococcygeal 475
　testes 377–90, 475–6
germinoma, pineal 206, 215–16,
　390
gestational trophoblastic tumour
　347
gigantism 205
glioblastoma multiforme 203, 204,
　206, 209–11
glioma 202–3, 204, 205, 209–14
glomerulonephritis 169
glomus jugulare tumours 190
glomus tumour 433, 445, 448
glottis, carcinoma 177–8
glucagonoma 303
glucocorticoids
　in adrenocortical carcinoma 402
　in breast cancer 265
glucose 6-phosphate dehydrogenase
　37
glutathione in drug resistance 91
glutathione transferase 91
glycerine 218
GM-CSF 141, 142
goitre 396, 397
gold
　mining 11
　radioactive isotopes 65, 151, 337
gonadal function
　effects of chemotherapy on 112,
　　499–500
　effects of childhood therapy on
　　476–7
　effects of radiotherapy on 74, 499
gonadoblastoma 340, 476

Gorlin's syndrome 414
goserelin 115
　in breast cancer 263, 264
　in prostatic cancer 370
graft-versus-host disease 555
granisetron 110, 111
granulocyte colony stimulating
　factor 141, 142, 429
granulocyte-macrophage colony
　stimulating factor 141, 142
granulocyte transfusion 141
granulocytopenia 139, 140
granulosa cell tumours 341
Grawitz' tumour *see* renal cell
　adenocarcinoma
growth, effect of cancer therapy on
　476
GSH 91
guaiac test 315
guanidine hydrochloride 166
Guillain–Barré syndrome 165, 485
GVHD 555
gynaecological cancer 317–48
gynaecomastia 160, 162, 382

H-*ras* oncogene 34, 42
haemangioendothelioma 433, 445
haemangiopericytoma 433, 445,
　448
haematemesis 275
haematite mining 11
haematuria
　in bladder cancer 359
　in nephroblastoma 463
　occult 358
　in renal cell adenocarcinoma 352
haemochromatosis 289
haemolytic-uraemic syndrome 164
haemopoietic cell maturation in
　relation to leukaemia 550
haemopoietic growth factors
　141–2
haemoptysis 233
hairy cell leukaemia 504, 561–2
haloperidol 111
Hand–Schüller–Christian disease
　474
Hashimoto's thyroiditis 393, 528
HBLV 505
　HCG *see* human chorionic
　　gonadotrophin
HCL 504, 561–2
head and neck
　cancer
　　aetiology 171–3
　　chemotherapy 190–2
　　childhood germ cell tumours
　　　475
　　computed tomography 51–2
　　epidemiology 171–3
　　investigation 174–5, 176
　　pathology 173
　　secondary prevention 24–5

staging 173–5, 177, 182
　see also specific sites
　lymphatic drainage 180
head shell, use in radiotherapy
　planning 82
headache 207
heavy chain diseases 522, 524, 544
heavy chains 532
Helicobacter pylori infection 281,
　522
hemi-body irradiation 74, 81
　in myeloma 541
　in small cell lung cancer 243
hemicolectomy 306, 312
hemihypertrophy 36, 455
hemithyroidectomy 398
hepatic artery ligation/embolization
　153, 291, 299
hepatitis B virus 12, 28, 33
　association with hepatocellular
　　carcinoma 289, 290
hepatitis C virus 289, 290
hepatoblastoma 289, 292, 475
hepatocellular carcinoma
　(hepatoma)
　aetiology 33, 289–90
　clinical features 290
　diagnosis 290–1
　incidence 289, 290
　management 291
　pathology 290
　prognosis 291–2
herpes simplex infection 33, 145
herpes zoster infection 500
Hexa-CAF regimen in ovarian
　cancer 339
hexamethylmelamine 108, 337, 338
5HIAA 298, 299
Hickman line 557
histamine 404
histiocytes 473, 507
histiocytic lymphoma 206, 216, 508
histiocytoses 473–4
histiocytosis X 473, 474
histocompatibility antigens in
　Hodgkin's disease 479
historical control 23
HIV infection 12, 32
　and non-Hodgkin's lymphoma
　　505, 517
HLA associations in Hodgkin's
　disease 479
hoarseness
　in laryngeal cancer 175–6
　in lung cancer 233
　in oesophageal carcinoma 275
Hodgkin's cell 481, 490
Hodgkin's disease 479
　abnormal immunity in 482–3
　aetiology 479–80
　bone involvement 484
　bone marrow involvement 484
　central nervous system

involvement 484–5
childhood *455*, 497–8
classification 481–2
clinical features 483–5
cutaneous/subcutaneous 484
differential diagnosis 482
endobronchial 484
epidemiology 479
fever in 159
glomerulonephritis in 169
gut involvement 485
incidence 479, *480*
investigation 486–90
lymphocyte depleted 482
lymphocyte predominant 481
management 492–5
  problems in 497
  in relapse 495
  and stage 495–7
mediastinal 246
mixed cellularity 482
nodular sclerosing 481–2
pathology 480–2
patterns of spread 485
percutaneous biopsy in 490
in pregnancy 498
pruritus in 169
pulmonary involvement 484,
  487–8
second malignancies 113, 500,
  547
staging 485–6, *487*
staging laparotomy and
  splenectomy 491–2
thymic tissue 244
toxicity of treatment 498–500
urinary tract involvement 485
Hodgkin's Disease Association
  136
home care 133
homovanillic acid 458
hormone receptors 113–14
  assays 114–15
  in breast cancer 114–15, 255–6,
    264
  tamoxifen binding with 116
hormone therapy 113–16
  in breast cancer 263–5, 268
  and endometrial carcinoma 328
  in metastases from unknown
    primary site 411
  in prostatic cancer 370–1
  in renal cell adenocarcinoma 356
  in uterine carcinoma 330–1
hormomes
  ectopic production syndromes
    160–3, 230, 234, 396
  production by adrenocortical
    carcinoma 402
Horner's syndrome 235
hospice care 133–4
Hospice Information Service *136*
hospital care in terminal illness

134
5HT₃ antagonists 110, *111*, 338
5HT 298, 299, 396
HTLV2 504
human B cell lymphotropic virus
  505
human chorionic gonadotrophin
  (HCG) 59–60
  in choriocarcinoma 346, 347
  ectopic production 162
  in extra-gonadal germ cell
    tumours 206, 216
  in metastases from unknown
    primary *409*
  in testicular germ cell tumours
    382–3
human herpes virus 6 505
human immunodeficiency virus
  see HIV infection
human papilloma viruses 33
  and cervical carcinoma 318
  an skin cancer 414
human T cell leukaemia lymphoma
  virus 32, 504
humoral hypercalcaemia of
  malignancy 148
humoral immunity 143
Hutchinson's melanotic freckle
  422–3
HVA 458
hydatidiform mole 346, 347
Hydrea *see* hydroxyurea
hydrocortisone 149
5-hydroxyindoleacetic acid 298,
  299
5-hydroxytryptamine 298, 299, 396
hydroxyurea 108
  in chronic granulocytic/
    myelogenous leukaemia 564
  in head and neck squamous
    carcinoma 191
  in malignant melanoma *426*
  phase specificity *88*
  in renal cell adenocarcinoma 356
hypercalcaemia 49–50, 148–9, *160*
  in hepatocellular carcinoma 290
  in lung cancer 233–4
  in myeloma 537–8
hypergranular promyelocytic
  leukaemia 549
hyperkalaemia 149
hypernephroma *see* renal cell
  adenocarcinoma
hyperparathyroidism 149, 405
hyperphosphataemia 149
hyperpigmentation *160*, 167
hyperprolactinaemia 162
hypertension and uterine carcinoma
  328
hypertrichosis *167*, 168
hypertrophic pulmonary
  osteoarthropathy 166–7
hyperuricaemia 149, 150

hyperviscosity syndrome, in
  myeloma 537
hypoalbuminaemia 152
hypocorticism 208
hypogammaglobulinaemia,
  common variable *505*
hypoglycaemia *160*, 162, 208
hypogonadism 208
hypokalaemia 148
hyponatraemia 161
hypoparathyroidism following
  thyroidectomy 398
hypopharynx
  anatomy 180
  carcinoma *172*, 174, 183–4
hypophysectomy 115, 263, 265, 371
hypopituitarism 208
hypothalamic tumours 205, 208
hypothyroidism 208, 499
hypoxanthine-guanine
  phosphoribosyltransferase
  101–2
hypoxia
  effect on cytotoxicity of
    X-rays 70–1
  and resistance to cytotoxic
    drugs 90
hysterectomy
  in cervical carcinoma 321–2
  in choriocarcinoma 347
  in CIN 3 321
  in ovarian carcinoma 334
  radical/Wertheim 321–2
  in uterine carcinoma 330
Hysterectomy Support Network
  136

ibuprofen 128, *129*
ichthyosis 168
ifosfamide 96
  in Ewing's sarcoma 444
  in malignant melanoma 427
  in neuroblastoma 460
  in non-small cell lung cancer *239*
  in osteosarcoma 439
  in rhabdomyosarcoma 469
  in small cell lung cancer 241
  in soft tissue sarcoma 450, 451
  in testicular germ cell tumours
    388
IFs *see* interferon therapy
IgA 532
  deficiency *36*
  in myeloma 533
  properties 533
IgD 532
  in chronic lymphocytic leukaemia
    559
  in myeloma 533
IgE 532
  in myeloma 533
IgG 532
  in myeloma 533

IgM 532
  in chronic lymphocytic leukaemia
    559
  in cold agglutinin disease 543
  in myeloma 533
  properties 533
ileal conduit 361−2, 363
ileostomy 125, 362
Ileostomy Association 125
ileum *see* small bowel tumours
imaging techniques 4
immune defence mechanisms 143
  in Hodgkin's disease 482−3, 499
immune proliferative small intestine
    disease 540, 522, 524
immunoblasts 508
immunodeficiency
  infection in 142−5
  non-Hodgkin's lymphoma in
    505
immunoglobulins
  abnormalities in myeloma 531−
    4
  monoclonal production *534*
  production by neoplasms 37, *532*
  structure 532−3
immunosuppression
  chemotherapy-induced 499
  and risk of cancer 12, 414
immunotherapy 45−6
  in lung cancer 243
  in malignant melanoma 427
impotence following treatment for
    prostatic cancer 370
Imuran *101*, 102, *122*
incidence
  age-specific *1, 2*, 12−13
  definition 7
  geographical variations in 8−9
  and migration 9
  and mortality *1, 2*
  temporal changes in 9
indomethanic 128, *129*, 300
infection
  in acute myeloblastic leukaemia
    557
  in aetiology of Hodgkin's disease
    480
  in chronic lymphocytic leukaemia
    561
  cytomegalovirus 33, 144
  fungal 144, 557
  Helicobacter pylori 281, 522
  herpes simplex 33, 145
  herpes zoster 500
  HIV 12, 23, 505, 517
  in immunocompromised patient
    142−5
  urinary tract 144, 358
infectious mononucleosis
  association with Hodgkin's
    disease 480
  in X-linked lymphoproliferative

syndrome 504
infertility
  following chemotherapy 112,
    499−500
  following radiotherapy 74, 499
  following therapy in childhood
    476−7
  male 382
informed consent in treatment trials
    22
inheritance of cancer 35−6, 455
insertional mutagenesis 32
insulinoma 301−2
interferon therapy 46, 117
  in bladder cancer 361
  in carcinoid tumours 300
  in chronic granulocytic/
    myelogenous leukaemia 564
  in hairy cell leukaemia 562
  in lung cancer 243
  in malignant melanoma 427−8
  in myeloma 539
  in pancreatic cancer 303
  in renal cell adenocarcinoma 356
interleukin 1 *117, 141*
interleukin 2 *46*, 117−18
  in malignant melanoma 428
  in renal cell adenocarcinoma 356
interleukin 4 *117*, 118
interleukin 5 *117*
interleukin 6 *117*, 118, 141, 534
intermediate filaments *409*
intracranial pressure, raised 207
intraocular tumours 198
  metastatic 156
intravenous urography
  in bladder cancer 360
  in cervical carcinoma 321
  in renal cell adenocarcinoma
    352, *353*
  in ureteric carcinoma 357
iodine-131 65, 399−401
ionizing radiation 63
  background 10
  biological properties 69−72
  carcinogenicity 10, 28−9, 77−8
    bone sarcoma 433
    in childhood 455
    leukaemia 547
    myeloma 531
    skin cancer 414
  fractionation 71−2
  late sequelae 77−8
  mutagenicity 78
  sources and production 63−9
  teratogenicity 78, 157
  tissue responses to 72−7
  tumour sensitivity to 69−71
iron deficiency anaemia
  in large bowel tumours 310
  in stomach cancer 283
isotope scanning
  in Hodgkin's disease 490

in osteosarcoma 437
in thyroid cancer 397
in tumour staging 56−7
isotretinoin 25

Japanese immigrants, cancer
    incidence *9*
jaundice 153
  obstructive 293, 296
jejunum *see* small bowel tumours

K-*ras*-2 34
Kaposi's sarcoma 429−30, 448
  and cytomegalovirus infection
    33
  and HIV infection 32
keratoacanthoma 417
keratoconjunctivitis sicca 76
keratoses
  arsenical 415
  solar 413, 415
Kernohan grades 203
  and management 209−11
  and prognosis *210*, 217
kidney
  involvement in myeloma 535−6
  radiosensitivity 76
  transplantation, and cancer risk
    414
  tumours 35, 46, 159, 163, 351−7,
    461−6, *467*
  ultrasound investigation 50
Klinefelter's syndrome 36
  and extra-gonadal germ cell
    tumours 245, 390
  and male breast cancer 271
  and non-Hodgkin's lymphoma
    505
Krukenberg tumour 283
Kupffer cells 473

lachrymal gland tumours 196−7
lactate dehydrogenase *59*, 383
laetrile 135
LAK cells 46, 118, 356
Lambert−Eaton syndrome *160*,
    166
laminectomy, decompressive 155
Langerhans' cell histiocytosis 473,
    474
lanuginosa acquisita *167*, 168
laparotomy
  in Hodgkin's disease 491−2
  in ovarian carcinoma 334−5
  second look 339
large bowel tumours
  aetiology 307−8
  clinical features 310−11
  diagnosis 310−11
  doubling time 87
  geographical variation in
    incidence 8
  incidence *2*, 13, 307−8

in Japanese immigrants 9
life-time risk of development 3
management 312–15
mortality 2
pathology 309
prognostic factors 311
screening for 23, 24, 308–9, 315
staging 309–10
ultrasound 50
large cell carcinoma, lungs 231
laryngectomy
conservative techniques 178–9
rehabilitation following 125, 179
laryngopharynx
anatomy 180
carcinoma 172, 174, 183–4
laryngoscopy, indirect 175
larynx
anatomy 175, *176*
artificial 125
carcinoma 175–9
age-specific incidence *172*
investigation 174
mortality *171*
laser surgery, in CIN 3 321
laser therapy
in bladder cancer 361
in oesophageal carcinoma 278
laxatives 130
leiomyoma 447
leiomyosarcoma 447–8
incidence *435*
small bowel 305, 306
uterus 328
lentaron 265
lentigo maligna 422–3
LET 69
Letterer–Siwe disease 474
leucopenia 145
leucoplakia
oral cavity 185, 415
penile 372
syphilitic 171
leucovorin 98, 100, 313, *314*
leukaemia 547
aleukaemic 553
in childhood *455*
chromosome abnormalities
in 547–8, 551–2, 559
eosinophilic 565
immunological phenotype in
550, *551*
incidence and aetiology 2, 547–9
life-time risk of development 3
mortality 2
oncogene products 552–3
pathology and classification
549–50, *551*
as second malignancy 477
smouldering 559
see also specific types
Leukaemia Care Society *136*

leukaemic blasts 549
Leukeran *see* chlorambucil
leuprorelin 115
levamisole 100
in large bowel cancer 314
in lung cancer 243
in malignant melanoma 427
in myeloma 539
Leydig cell tumours 391, 476
Leydig cells, radiosensitivity 74
Lhermitte's syndrome 75, 223, 499
LHRH 115, *116*, 263, 264
analogues 115, *116*, 370
Li–Fraumeni syndrome 35, 434,
446, 455, 466
life-style and cancer incidence 11
light chains 532–3, 559
limb
amputation 125–6, 438, 449
preservation in osteosarcoma
438, *439*
limbic encephalitis 165
linear accelerator 67
linear energy transfer 69
linitis plastica 282
lip, carcinoma *171, 172*, 187–8
liposarcoma *435*, 447
liver
angiosarcoma 289, 292
biopsy
in hepatocellular carcinoma
291
in Hodgkin's disease 490
computed tomography 53
effects of chemotherapy on 112–
13
enzymes
in Hodgkin's disease 486–7
in non-Hodgkin's lymphoma
512
and staging 49
geographical variations in cancer
incidence 8
hepatoblastoma 289, 292, 475
isotope scanning 57
metastases
diagnosis 50, *51*, 57
management 152–3
scan, in Hodgkin's disease 490
see also hepatocellular carcinoma
liver flukes 292
LMP-1 gene 39
lobectomy 236, 237
log-rank test 18
lomustine *see* CCNU
LOPP/EVAP hybrid regimen 494
lorazepam 111
LSA$_2$L$_2$ regimen in lymphoblastic
lymphoma 516, 520
Lukes–Butler classification 481–2
lumbar puncture in central nervous
system lymphoma 525
lumpectomy 261

lungs
carcinoma
aetiology 227, *229*
age-related survival rate *15*
clinical features 233–4
computed tomography *51, 52*
doubling time *87*
geographical variation in
incidence 8
histological types 230–1
hypertrophic pulmonary
osteoarthropathy in 166–7
immunotherapy 243
incidence 2
investigation 234–6
life-time risk of development 3
local invasion 232
management 236–43
metastasis 232
mortality 2
pathology 230–2
staging 48, 234–6
see also small cell lung cancer
collapse 157
effects of chemotherapy on 112
infection 143–4
involvement in Hodgkin's disease
484, 487–8
metastases
diagnosis 53, 57
from osteosarcoma 440
non-Hodgkin's lymphoma 527
wedge/segmental resection 236
luteinizing hormone releasing
hormone 115, *116*, 263, 264
analogues 115, *116*, 370
lymph nodes
biopsy in non-Hodgkin's
lymphoma 511
CT scanning 52–3
enlargement
in Hodgkin's disease 483, 484
in non-Hodgkin's lymphoma
510–11
involvement and staging 48, 49
and spread of cancer 43
structure *507*
lymphadenectomy
in cervical carcinoma 322
in malignant melanoma 425–6
in testicular teratoma 385
lymphangiography in soft tissue
sarcoma 449
lymphangiosarcoma 448
lymphoblastic lymphoma
adult 515–16
childhood 519
lymphoblasts 508
lymphocytosis in chronic
lymphocytic leukaemia
559–60
lymphoedema 257, 262
lymphography

in Hodgkin's disease 488−9
in non-Hodgkin's lymphoma 512
in tumour staging 53, 54−6, 321
lymphoid cell maturation in relation to leukaemia *550*
lymphokine activated killer cells 46, 118, 356
lymphomatoid granulomatosis 527
lymphomatoid papulosis 519
lymphomatous polyposis 524
lymphopenia 73, 143, 499
lymphoplasmacytic cells 508
lymphotoxin 118, 534

M-BACOD regimen in non-Hodgkin's lymphoma *515*
M-CSF 141, 142
M-M-M regimen in breast cancer *266*
M-protein 533
mABs 44−5, 118−19, 410
MACOP-B regimen in non-Hodgkin's lymphoma *515*
macroglobulinaemia 543
macrophage colony stimulating factor 141, 142
macrophage tumours 508
macrophages 507
magnetic resonance imaging (MRI)
  in brain tumours *207, 208*
  in Hodgkin's disease 490
  in osteosarcoma 437, *438*
  in soft tissue sarcoma 449
  in spinal cord compression 154, *155*
  in tumour staging 53−4, *55*
malaria and Burkitt's lymphoma 503
malignant angioendotheliomatosis 527
malignant fibrous histiocytoma *433, 445, 447*
malignant melanoma 46
  choroidal 198
  clinical and pathological features 422−3
  conjunctiva 197−8
  epidemiology 421−2
  management 424−8
  nasal cavity 188
  pathogenesis 421−2
  pinna 190
  prognosis 428−9
  staging 48, 423−4
  uveal tract 198
  vagina 344
malignant mixed tumour 193
malignant teratoma intermediate *379, 380*
malignant teratoma trophoblastic *379*, 380−1
malignant teratoma undifferentiated

379, 380
malnutrition 146−7
mammography 254
  screening 256
management 1−5
  psychological aspects 121−4
  and quality of life 126−7
mannitol 218
mantle-zone lymphoma 513
marginal excision 449
Marie Curie Cancer Care *136*
Marjolin's ulcer 418
mastectomy 257
  adjuvant systemic therapy 268−70
  combined with radiotherapy 257−61
  complications following 262−3
  counselling 125
  male 271
  psychological disturbance following 262−3
  radical 257, 258−9, *260*
  toilet 261
Mastectomy Association 125
matrix metalloproteinases 42
mechlorethamine *see* nitrogen mustard
mediastinoscopy 235
mediastinum
  anatomy 243, *244*
  tumours 243−7, *390, 391*
medical problems 139−53
medroxyprogesterone acetate (MPA) 116
  in breast cancer 265
  in endometrial carcinoma 331
  in renal cell adenocarcinoma 356
medulloblastoma 203, *204*, 205
  management 212−14
  metastasis 208
megestrol acetate (Megace) 116, 265
melaena
  in large bowel tumours 310
  in oesophageal carcinoma 275
melphalan 27, 96
  and bone marrow suppression 139
  in breast cancer 266, 269
  in malignant melanoma 427
  in myeloma 539−40
  in neuroblastoma *461*
  in ovarian cancer 337
  and second cancers 113
MEN I 301, 396
MEN II 301, 396−7
MEN III 301
meningioma 205−6
  malignant 206, 215
  management 215
  monosomy 22 in 202
  spinal cord 220

meningiosarcoma 206, 215
meningitis
  carcinomatous/lymphomatous 152, 219, 485, 525−6
  in immunocompromised patient 145
menopause
  artificial 263, 264, 267
  late 328
6-mercaptopurine (6MP) 85, 101−2, 150
  in acute lymphoblastic leukaemia 554
  in acute myeloblastic leukaemia 558
  hepatic toxicity *112*
  phase specificity *88*
Merkel cell tumours 430
mesenchymal chondrosarcoma *433*, 441−2
mesoblastic nephroma 462
mesothelioma 10−11, 247−9
metabolic disturbances 148−50
meta-iodo-benzylguanidone 458
metastases
  bone 56, 57
    and hypercalcaemia 148
    radiotherapy 157
  cerebral 57, 217−19, 242
  cutaneous 430−1
  diagnosis 57
  from breast cancer 252−3, 263−8
  from bronchial carcinoma 232
  from cervical carcinoma 319
  from Hodgkin's disease 485
  from nephroblastoma 463
  from nervous system tumours 208
  from neuroblastoma 456−7
  from oesophageal cancer 274, *275*
  from osteosarcoma 440
  from ovarian carcinoma 333
  from stomach cancer 282−3
  from testicular germ cell tumours 381
  from uterine carcinoma 328−9
  from vaginal carcinoma 344−5
  hepatic 50, *51*, 57
    diagnosis 50, *51*, 57
    management 152−3
  oral cavity 185
  orbital/intra-ocular 156
  pulmonary 53, 57
  and staging 48−9
  unknown primary site 407
    investigation 409−10
    management 410−11
    prognosis 408−9
    site of origin 407−8
    site of presentation 407, *408*
methadone 128, *129*
methotrexate 98−100

in acute lymphoblastic leukaemia 553, 554
in acute myeloblastic leukaemia 558
in bladder cancer 363
in breast cancer *266*
in choriocarcinoma 347, 348
development 85
in Ewing's sarcoma 444
in head and neck squamous carcinoma 190, 191
hepatic toxicity *112*
high dose 439, 440
in malignant melanoma *426*
in medulloblastoma 214
in non-small cell lung cancer *239*
in osteosarcoma 438–9, 440
in ovarian cancer *337*, 338
phase specificity *88*
in rhabdomyosarcoma 469
in small cell lung cancer *241*
in soft tissue sarcoma 450, *451, 452*
teratogenicity 157
in testicular germ cell tumours 387, *388*
very high dose 438–9
methyl CCNU *97*
in large bowel cancer 313, 314
methyldopa 300
methysergide 299
metoclopramide 111
metyrapone
in adrenocortical carcinoma 403
in ectopic ACTH secretion 162
microglioma 206, 216
middle ear tumours *171*, 189–90
Middle East, non-Hodgkin's lymphoma in 504
migration, and cancer incidence 9
migratory thrombophlebitis 163, *167, 296*
mineralocorticoids in adrenocortical carcinoma 402
mithramycin 106, 149
in testicular germ cell tumours 387
mitomycin C
in anal carcinoma 316
in bladder cancer 363
in breast cancer *266*
in head and neck squamous carcinoma 191
in large bowel cancer 313, *314*
in malignant melanoma *426*
in non-small cell lung cancer *239*
in pancreatic cancer *297*
and pulmonary fibrosis *112*
in rhabdomyosarcoma *469*
in stomach cancer 286
mitosis
mitotane in adrenocortical carcinoma 403

mitozantrone 106
in acute myeloblastic leukaemia 558
in breast cancer *266*
mixed germ cell tumour 340
mixed salivary tumour 192–3
monoclonal antibodies 44–5, 118–19, 410
monoclonal gammopathy of unknown significance 534, 542–3
monocytes 507
monocytic leukaemia 549, 556
mononuclear phagocytes 507
monosomy 22 202, 206
MOPP regimen
and gonadal function 112, 477
in Hodgkin's disease 493, 494, 495, 496
morphine 128–9
and hyponatraemia 161
long-acting 129–30
mortality, and cancer incidence 1, *2*
mosaicism *36*
motor cortex lesions 208
mourning, anticipatory 454
6MP *see* 6-mercaptopurine
MPA *see* medroxyprogesterone acetate
MRI *see* magnetic resonance imaging
μ-heavy chain disease 544
mucoepidermoid carcinoma 193
mucosa, barrier function 143
mucosal neuroma syndrome 301
multi-drug resistance 91
multiple enchondromatosis *36*, 441
multiple endocrine neoplasia 301, 396–7, 403
multiple myeloma *see* myeloma
multiple neurofibromatosis *36*, 222–3, 446, 455
multiple thromboses *160*, 163
murine leukaemia virus 480
muscle
fatigue 166
radiosensitivity *77*
mustine *see* nitrogen mustard
MVPP regimen *494*
myasthenia gravis 244
myc oncogenes 201
in myeloma 534
in neuroblastoma 456
in non-Hodgkin's lymphoma 505–6
in small cell lung cancer 230
mycosis fungoides *32*, 527–8
myeloblasts 549, 563
myelocytes 563
myelodysplastic syndromes 549, 558–9
myelography 154, 221, *222*

myeloma
clinical features 536–8
diagnosis 538
incidence and aetiology 531
management 538–41
non-secretors 533
pathogenesis 531–6
prognosis 533–4, 541–2
myeloma cells 535
myeloma protein 533
myelomatosis *see* myeloma
myelopathy, carcinomatous 165
Myleran *see* busulphan

N-*myc* oncogene 33, 201
N-*ras* oncogene 34, 201
naevi
benign melanocytic 422
compound 422
dysplastic 422
intradermal 422
junctional 422
and malignant melanoma 421
naevoid basal cell carcinoma syndrome 414
nandrolone decanoate 265
2-naphthylamine 11
nasal cavity tumours 176, 188–9
age-specific incidence *172*
mortality *171*
nasendoscopy 173, 175
nasopharynx
anatomy 179, *180*
carcinoma 180–2
age-specific incidence *172*
and Epstein–Barr virus 33, 171–72
geographical variation in incidence *8*
pathology 173
racial factors in 171
staging *174*
non-Hodgkin's lymphoma 183, 526–7
National Association of Laryngectomee Clubs 125, *136*
National Cancer Alliance *136*
Natulan *see* procarbazine
natural killer cells 43, 143
nausea
in brain tumour 207
in stomach cancer 283
in terminal cancer 132–3
NCAM
in neuroblastoma 456
in small cell lung cancer 230, 231
neck *see* head and neck
nephrectomy 354, 465
nephritis, acute radiation 76
nephroblastoma 351, *455*
aniridia 455, 461, 462
clinical features 462–3

genetics 35
incidence and aetiology 461–2
investigation and staging 463–4
management 464–6
pathology 462
prognosis 466
nephrotic syndrome *160*, 169, 485
nephro-ureterectomy 354, 357
nerve blocks 131, *132*
neural-cell adhesion molecule 230,
    231, 456
neuroblastoma 402, 403, *455*, 456
    clinical features 457–8
    diagnosis and investigation 458
    differential diagnosis 458–9
    management 460, *461*
    mediastinal 246
    pathology 456–7
    staging 459–60
Neuroblastoma Society *136*
neuroepithelioma 222–3
neurofibroma, mediastinal 247
neurofibromatosis *167*, 403
neurofibrosarcoma 222, 246
neuron-specific enolase 231
neurosecretory granules
    in metastases from unknown
        primary 411
    in small cell lung cancer 230, *231*
neutron beam therapy 68, 194
neutropenia 139
NHL *see* non-Hodgkin's
    lymphoma
nickel 11, *27*
nitrogen mustard 27, 85, 93–4, 95
    in ascites 152
    in Hodgkin's disease 494
    in pleural effusion 151
nitrosamines 27, 28
nitrosoureas 27, 94, 95, 97–8
    effects on gonadal function 476
    in Ewing's sarcoma 444
    in hepatocellular carcinoma *291*
    in large bowel cancer 313, *314*
    in malignant melanoma 426
    in pancreatic cancer 297
    phase specificity *88*
    in stomach cancer 286
NK cells 43, 143
node of Rouvière 180
nodular melanoma 423
nominal standard dose 72
non-Hodgkin's lymphoma (NHL)
    AIDS-related 503, *504*, 505,
        517, 525
    bone 433, 446, 524
    bone marrow transplantation in
        516–17
    central nervous system 201, 206,
        216, 525–6
    childhood *455*
        diagnosis and investigation
        519

incidence and aetiology 517
management 519–21
pathology 517–19
staging *518*
classification 508–10
cutaneous 527–8
diffuse 509–10, 514–15
doubling time *87*
extra-nodal presentation 521–9
follicular 509–10
    management 512–14
gastro-intestinal 521–4
head and neck 173, 183, 510,
    526–7
in immune deficiency states 505
incidence and aetiology 503–5
lungs 527
lymphography 55
mediastinal 246
in the Middle East 504
molecular genetics 505–6
nodal
    clinical features 510–11
    diagnosis and investigation
        511–12
    management 512–17
ocular 195–6, 527
ovaries 529
pathology 506–10
salivary glands 193
small bowel 305, 306
staging 511–12
testis 377, 391, 529
thyroid 394, 397, 399, 401–2,
    528–9
non-small cell lung cancer (NSCLC)
    investigation and staging 234–6
    management 236–40
non-steroidal anti-inflammatory
    drugs 128, *129*
NSCLC *see* non-small cell lung
    cancer
nuclear power establishments and
    leukaemia incidence 547
nursing staff 5
nutritional support 147–8

obesity 11
    and uterine carcinoma 328
occupational factors in cancer
        incidence 10–11, 27, 414
octreotide
    in carcinoid tumours 300
    in pancreatic cancer 303
ocular melanosis 197
oesophagectomy 276, *277*
oesophagitis, radiation 278
oesophago-gastric anastomosis
    276
oesophagoscopy 275
oesophagus
    carcinoma
        aetiology 273

clinical features 274–5
geographical variation in
    incidence 8
incidence 2, 273, 274
investigation 275, *276*
life-time risk of development
    3
management 276–8
mortality 2
palliative treatment 278
pathology 273–4, *275*
prognosis 278–9
spread 274, *275*
staging 276
fibrosis/scarring 278
oestrogen receptor (ER) *114*
    in breast cancer 114–15, 255–6,
        264
    tamoxifen binding with 116
oestrogen therapy 116
    in breast cancer 263
    in prostatic cancer 370
    and risk of uterine cancer 328
oestrogens
    production in adrenocortical
        carcinoma 402
    synthesis 115
oligodendroblastoma 212
oligodendroglioma 203, *204*, 212
oligospermia 476
Ollier's disease 36, 441
oncogenes 30–2, 33–4, *35*, 42
    in bladder cancer 359
    in brain tumours 201–2
    in breast cancer 271
    in dysplastic naevi 422
    in leukaemia 552–3
    in myeloma 534
    in neuroblastoma 456
    in small cell lung cancer 230
Oncovin *see* vincristine
ondansetron 110, *111*
    in ovarian cancer 338
oophorectomy 113, 115
    in breast cancer 263, 264
    in cervical carcinoma 321
oophoropexy 491, 499
OPEC regimen in neuroblastoma
    461
ophthalmoplegia 195
Opisthorcis felineus 292
optic nerve glioma 203, 212
oral cavity tumours 184–5
    age-specific incidence *172*
    management 185–7
    mortality *171*
    staging *182*
orbit
    metastases 156
    pseudotumour 196
    tumours *176*, 195–7, 527
orchidectomy 113, 115
    in male breast cancer 271

in prostatic cancer 370
radical inguinal 384
trans-scrotal 384
orchioblastoma 475
orchitis, mumps 378
oropharynx
anatomy 179—80
cancer 172, 182—3
non-Hodgkin's lymphoma 526—7
orthopantomogram 185
osteitis fibrosa cystica 405
osteoclast activating factor 538
osteoclastoma 433, 445
osteosarcoma 433
aetiology 433—4
in childhood 455
clinical features 436
incidence 434—5
investigation 437, 438
juxtacortical/parosteal 435, 437, 440—1
management 438—40
metastases from 440
pathology 435—6
periosteal 436, 437, 440—1
radiological appearances 436—7
as second malignancy 477
staging 435
ovaries
benign dermoid cysts 340
carcinoma
aetiology 331
clinical features 331—2
incidence 2, 9, 12, 13, 318
life-time risk of development 3
management 333—9
mortality 2
pathology 332
prognosis 332—3
screening 24
second malignancies 113
staging 332—3
survival curves 14, 16, 17
choriocarcinoma 341
conservation in treatment of cervical carcinoma 321—2
effects of chemotherapy on 112
germ cell tumours 340—1, 476
granulosa cell tumours 341
irradiation 263, 264, 267, 268
non-Hodgkin's lymphoma 529
radiosensitivity 74
Sertoli—Leydig cell tumours 341
oxycodone 128, 129

p53 gene 38, 39
and large bowel cancer 308
and leukaemia 553
and small cell lung cancer 231
ultraviolet damage to 29
p-glycoprotein 91

P-staging, bladder cancer 358—9
paclitaxel 104, 337, 338, 339
Paget's disease 372
chondrosarcoma in 441
extra-mammary 430
pain
alcohol-induced in Hodgkin's disease 483
in bladder cancer 359
in cervical cancer 320
in large bowel tumours 310
in lung cancer 233
in myeloma 536
in pancreatic cancer 296
in spinal cord tumours 220
pain relief
analgesic 128—31
epidural 131—2
guidelines in terminal care 130—1
nerve blocks 131, 132
surgical 131, 132
palliative treatment 4, 127—34
oesophageal carcinoma 278
pancreatic cancer 297
pamidronate 149
Pancoast tumour 232, 233
management 237, 239
pancreatectomy
partial 302
total 294, 297
pancreatic cancer
age-related survival rate 15
age-specific incidence 2, 13
endocrine 295, 300—3
exocrine 294—7
life-time risk of development 3
migratory thrombophlebitis in 163
mortality 2
ultrasound investigation 50
pancreatic oncofetal antigen 59
pancreaticoduodenectomy 306
radical 294, 297
pancytopenia 140
panhypopituitarism 208
panophthalmitis 144, 195
papaveretum 128
papilloedema 207
papova viruses 165
paracentesis 152
paracetamol 128, 129
parachlorophenylalanine 300
paraganglioma 190, 247
paralysis, acute ascending 164
paranasal sinus tumours 52, 176, 188—9
age-specific incidence 172
mortality 171
paraneoplastic syndromes 159—69, 233—4, 485
paraparesis 220
paraproteinaemias 531—44

parathyroid gland cancer 405
parathyroid hormone 405
parathyroid hormone-related protein 148
parotid gland 192
tumours 192—5
parotidectomy 193—4
Paterson—Kelly syndrome 171, 273
patients
communication with 4—5, 121—4
counselling 126
organizations 136—7
support of 5, 124—6
PBSC support 516—17
PCB regimen in multiple myeloma 540
PCV regimen in brain tumours 211, 212
PDT see photodynamic therapy
peau d'orange 251—2
Pel—Ebstein fever 159, 483
pelvic exenteration 326
penile cancer 372—4
pentazocine 128, 129
Pentostating 102, 562
peptic ulcer in gastrinoma 302
percutaneous transhepatic cholangiography 293, 296
perianal infection 145
pericardectomy 151
pericardial effusion 151, 499
pericytes 448
peripheral blood stem cell support 516—17
peripheral nerve tumours 222—3
peripheral neuropathy 160, 164—5, 499
peritoneo-venous shunt 152
pernicious anaemia and stomach cancer 280—1
perphenazine 111
pethidine 128, 129
Peutz—Jeghers syndrome 36, 167, 331
Peyer's patches 521
phaeochromocytoma
adrenal medulla 403—5
mediastinal 247
in MEN II 396
phagocyte function 143
pharynx
anatomy 179—80
carcinoma 180—4
age-specific incidence 172
histological classification 174
mortality 171
non-Hodgkin's lymphoma 183, 526—7
phenothiazines 300
phenoxybenzamine 404
phentolamine 300, 404
Philadelphia chromosome 551

phimosis and penile cancer   372
phosphate therapy   149
phosphorus-32   65, 151, 337, 371
photocoagulation in retinoblastoma
    472
photodynamic therapy (PDT)   82
  in bladder cancer   361
  in oesophageal carcinoma   278
pi-meson irradiation   69
pineal tumours   206, 215–16, 390
pinealoblastoma   206, 216
pinealocytoma   206
pinna carcinoma   190
piperazine phenothiazines   111
pituitary apoplexy   208
pituitary tumours   *204, 205*
  clinical features   208
  management   215
placental alkaline phosphatase
    (PLAP)   *59,* 60–1
  in metastases from unknown
      primary   *409*
  in testicular germ cell tumours
      383
placental lactogen   *59*
PLAP   *see* placental alkaline
      phosphatase
plasma cell myeloma   *see* myeloma
plasma cells   507, 508
  malignant   535
platelet transfusion   140–1, 557
pleomorphic adenocarcinoma   193
pleomorphic adenoma   192–3
pleomorphic rhabdomyosarcoma
    447, 467
pleural effusion   150–1
pleurectomy   151
Plummer–Vinson syndrome   171,
    273
Pneumocystis, pulmonary infection
    144
pneumonectomy   236–7
pneumonitis, radiation   278, 499
podophyllotoxins   85, 104–5, 341
pol gene   504
Polya partial gastrectomy, and
    stomach cancer   280, 281
polyarthritis   *160,* 167
polycyclic hydrocarbons   10, 27–8
polycythaemia   163
polycythaemia rubra vera   163
polymorphonuclear leucocytosis in
    Hodgkin's disease   486
polymyositis   166
polyvinylchloride, exposure to
    292, 446
prednisolone
  in acute lymphoblastic leukaemia
      553, 554
  in chronic lymphocytic leukaemia
      560
  in hepatic metastases   153
  in Hodgkin's disease   *494*

in hypercalcaemia   149
  in myeloma   539–40
pregnancy
  cancer in   78, 157
  cervical carcinoma in   327
  following breast cancer   271
  Hodgkin's disease in   498
  malignant melanoma in   427
premelanosomes   *409*
prevalence, definition   7
primary cutaneous neuroendocrine
      tumours   430
primitive neuroectodermal tumour
      203, 212–14, 442
procarbazine   108
  effects on gonadal function   112,
      476
  in glioma   211
  in Hodgkin's disease   *494*
  phase specificity   *88*
prochlorperazine   111
proctocolectomy   307–8
progesterone receptor in breast
      cancer   115, 256, 264
progestogen therapy   116
  in metastases from unknown
      primary site   411
  in renal cell adenocarcinoma   356
  in uterine carcinoma   330–1
progressive multifocal
      leucoencephalopathy   165–
      6, 485
prolactinoma   215
prolymphocytic leukaemia   561
ProMACE-CytaBOM regimen in
      non-Hodgkin's lymphoma
      515
promazine   111
prophylactic cranial irradiation
      242
proptosis   195, 527
prostaglandins, ectopic production
      396
prostate-specific antigen   365, 367
prostatectomy   368, 369–70
prostatic acid phosphatase   *59*
prostatic cancer
  aetiology   365
  age-related survival rate   *15*
  clinical features   367
  incidence   *2, 9, 352,* 365
  investigation   367
  life-time risk of development   *3*
  management   367–71
  mortality   *2*
  pathology   365–7
  staging   365–7
prostheses   125–6
protected environment   145
proton irradiation   69
  Provera   *see*
      medroxyprogesterone acetate
pruritus   153, *167,* 168–9

in Hodgkin's disease   483
psammoma bodies   394, 398
Pseudomonas aeruginosa   143
pseudomyxoma peritonei   306
pseudotumour, orbital   196
psychological aspects of
      management   121–4
pulmonary fibrosis following
      chemotherapy   112
purine antagonists   101–2
Purkinje cells, antibodies to   165
pUVA   413–14
PVB regimen
  and gonadal function   112
  in testicular germ cell tumours
      387, *388*
PVC, exposure to   292, 446
pyoderma gangrenosum   *167,* 168
pyrexia   *see* fever
pyrimidine antagonists   100–1
pyrrolozidium   27

quackery   134–6
quadrantectomy   259
quality of life and cancer treatment
      126–7

racial factors
  in cervical carcinoma   317
  in childhood cancer   455
  in nasopharyngeal carcinoma
      171
radical treatment   127
radioactive isotopes   63–6
radiography
  chest
    in head and neck cancer   174
    in Hodgkin's disease   487–8
    in mesothelioma   248
    in neuroblastoma   458
    in non-Hodgkin's lymphoma
        511
    in oesophageal carcinoma   275
    in osteosarcoma   437
    in renal cell adenocarcinoma
        353
    in soft tissue sarcoma   449
    in thymic tumour   245
    in tumour staging   49
  in chondrosarcoma   441
  in Ewing's sarcoma   443
  in neuroblastoma   458
  in osteosarcoma   436–7
  in spinal cord compression   154
  in superior vena cava obstruction
      156
radio-iodine   65, 399–401
radionuclides   64
radiotherapy   1–2, 63
  in acute spinal cord/cauda equina
      compression   155
  adjuvant   83
  adverse effects

bone   433
brain and spinal cord   223
skin   415
thyroid   393
applied dose   80
ascites   152
basal/squamous cell skin
        carcinoma   419–20
biliary tract cancer   294
bladder cancer   361–63, *364*
bone metastases   157
breast cancer
    advanced primary   261
    early primary   257–61
    metastatic   267–8
cerebral metastases   218–19
cervical carcinoma   322–6
chronic lymphocytic leukaemia
        561
conformational   82
continuous hyperfractionated   72
craniospinal   211–12, 213–14
department   78–9
depth dose   67, 68, 80
effects on gonadal function   476,
        499
effects on growth   476
emergency   153–7
Ewing's sarcoma   443–4
fractionated   71–2, 80
gliomas   209–10, 211–14
hepatic metastases   153
hepatocellular carcinoma   291
Hodgkin's disease   492–3, 496–7
immobilization devices   81–2
integration with chemotherapy
        82–4
isotopes   63–6
large bowel cancer   313
laryngeal cancer   177–8
laryngopharyngeal carcinoma
        184
late sequelae   77–8, 499
lip carcinoma   187–8
low dose whole lung   440
malignant melanoma   426, 428
maximum dose   80
midplane dose   80
minimum dose   80
modal dose   80
myeloma   541
nasopharyngeal cancer   181
nephroblastoma   465–6
neuroblastoma   460
nominal standard dose   72
non-Hodgkin's lymphoma   513
non-small cell lung cancer   238–9
oesophageal carcinoma   276–8
open/direct field   80
oral cavity tumours   186
orbital tumours   156, 197
oropharyngeal carcinoma   183
osteosarcoma   440

ovarian carcinoma   335–7
palliative   428
pancreatic cancer   297
parallel opposed fields   80, *81*
penile cancer, 373–4
penumbra   66
pericardial effusion   151
pineal tumours 215–16
pituitary tumours   215
pleural effusion   151
in pregnancy   78, 157
prophylactic in acute
        lymphoblastic leukaemia
        554
prostatic cancer   368–70
recurrence after   70
recurrent brain tumours   216–17
renal cell adenocarcinoma   355
retinoblastoma   472–3
salivary gland tumours   194
sealed/unsealed sources   65
shrinking field technique   80–1
small cell lung cancer   240, 241–3
soft tissue sarcoma   449–50
spinal cord tumours   222
stomach cancer   286
superior vena caval obstruction
        156
systemic   *see* hemi-body
        irradiation; total body
        irradiation
techniques   79–82
teletherapy   65–6
testicular germ cell tumours
        385–7
thyroid cancer   399–401
tissue responses to   72–7
treatment prescription   80
treatment volume   80
tumour sensitivity to   69–71
urine carcinoma   330
vaginal carcinoma   345–6
wedged field   80
X-ray and particle production
        66–9
radium   63, 64
    isotopes   *65*
    needle   65
randomized consent   22
ras oncogenes   34, *35*, 39, 42
    in brain tumours   201
    in dysplastic naevus syndrome
        422
    in myeloma   534
recall phenomena   465, 469
rectum
    bleeding from   310, 311
    radiosensitivity   76
    tumour   *see* large bowel tumours
red cell aplasia   *160*, 164, 244
Reed–Sternberg cell   480–1
registries   12
relapsing panniculitis   296

remission induction and
        maintenance   92
renal arteriography   *354*
renal artery occlusion   355
renal cell adenocarcinoma   46, 351
    aetiology   351
    clinical features   352–3, *354*
    erythrocytosis in   163
    fever in   159
    management   354–6
    pathology   351–2
    prognosis   356
    staging   352
renal pelvis tumours   351, 356–7
respiratory infection   143–4
reticuloendothelial function   143
retinal/cerebellar angiomatosis   *36*
retinoblastoma   433, *455*
    clinical features   471
    genetics   34, 455, 470, *471*
    incidence   470
    investigation   471
    management   472–3
    pathology   470–1
    prognosis   473
    staging   471, *472*
Retinoblastoma Society   *136–137*
13-*cis*-retinoic acid   25
retinoids   11, 25, 184–5
retrograde pyelography   357
retroperitoneum, germ cell tumours
        390
retroviruses   30, 480
rhabdomyosarcoma   196, 447, 450
    childhood   466–70
rheumatoid arthritis   *505*
Richter's syndrome   561
RNA viruses   30–2, 480
rodent ulcer   *see* basal cell
        carcinoma
Rous sarcoma virus   30–1
RS cell   480–1
RSV   30–1

S100 proteins   *409*
saddle anaesthesia   154
salivary glands
    anatomy   192
    tumours   *172*, 192–5
salpingo-oophorectomy   330, 334
sarcoma
    alveolar soft part   448
    bone   *see* osteosarcoma
    classification   *433*, *434*
    clear cell   448
    epitheloid   448
    exocrine pancreas   295
    small bowel   305
    soft tissue   *see* soft tissue
        sarcoma
    synovial   448, 451
    uterus   331
sarcoma botryoides   447, 467

scalp, epilation 75
Schiller—Duval body in testicular
      germ cell tumours *379*
schistosomiasis 357
Schwannoma 220, 222, 246
SCLC *see* small cell lung cancer
screening 23—4
    for bladder cancer 358
    for breast cancer 23, 24, 256
    for cervical carcinoma 23, 24,
      319, 326
    for large bowel tumours 308—9,
      315
    for stomach cancer 284—5
sebaceous gland cancer 418
second malignancies
    following chemotherapy 113
    following Hodgkin's disease 500
    following therapy in childhood
      477
    leukaemia as 547
    prevention 24—5
self-help organizations *136—7*
seminoma 377, 378
    chemotherapy 389
    doubling time *87*
    extra-gonadal 206, 390—1
    histology *379*
    pathology 380
    prognosis 389—90
    radiotherapy 385—7
    surgery 385
sensory neuropathy 164—5
septicaemia 143
serotonin 298, 299, 396
Sertoli cell tumours 391, 476
Sertoli—Leydig cell tumours 341
sex-linked agammaglobulinaemia
    36
sexual activity in aetiology of
    cervical carcinoma 317
Sézary's syndrome 528
sheep dip 11
shingles 145
shoulder stiffness following
    mastectomy 262
SIADH *160*, 161, 234
sigmoidoscopy 310, 315
Sipple syndrome 301, 396—7
sis oncogene 31, *35*
Sjögren's syndrome *505*
skin
    barrier function 143
    cancer
      aetiology 413—16
      age-related survival rate *15*
      geographical variation in
        incidence *8*
      incidence *2*
      life-time risk of development
        3
      mortality *2*
      pathogenesis 413—16

screening 24
    see also specific types
infection 145
    involvement in Hodgkin's disease
      484
    manifestations of malignancy
      167—9
    metastatic carcinoma 430—1
    non-Hodgkin's lymphoma
      527—8
    premalignant lesions 414—16
    radiosensitivity 75
small bowel tumours
    aetiology 305
    clinical features 305
    diagnosis 305—6
    incidence 305, *306*
    lymphoma 522—4
    management 306
    pathology 305
    prognosis 306
small cell lung cancer (SCLC)
    doubling time *87*
    ectopic ACTH production
      161—2, 230
    ectopic ADH production 161
    histology 230—1
    investigation and staging 236
    Lambert—Eaton syndrome 166
    management 240—3
    metastasis 232
    prognosis 241, *242*
    survival curves 16
small non-cleaved cell lymphoma
    516
smear test 23, 24, 319, 326
smoking *see* tobacco, smoking
social class and cervical carcinoma
    317, *318*
soft tissue sarcoma 446
    aetiology 446
    in childhood *455*, 466—70
    classification *434*
    incidence *435*
    investigation and staging 448—9
    magnetic resonance imaging *55*
    management 449—51, *452*
    pathology and clinical features
      446—8
    prognosis 451—2
    staging *449*
solar keratoses 413, 415
solitary plasmacytoma 542
somatostatinoma 303
somnolence syndrome 223
speech therapy in laryngectomy
    179
spermatogonia, radiosensitivity 74
sphincter function loss 220
spinal cord
    compression 154—5, *221*, 526
    involvement in Hodgkin's disease
      484

irradiation 211—12, 213—14
lymphoma 525—6
magnetic resonance imaging 54
non-Hodgkin's lymphoma
    525—6
radiation damage 223
radiosensitivity 74—5
tumours 220—2
spindle cell tumours *433*, 445
spinothalamic tractotomy 131, *132*
spironolactone 152
splenectomy 143
    in hairy cell leukaemia 562
    in Hodgkin's disease 491—2
squamous cell carcinoma
    bladder 358
    cervix 319
    conjunctiva 197—8
    eyelid 197
    growth of *40*
    lungs 230
    oesophagus 273
    skin *416*, 417—21
src oncogene 30—1, *35*
staging 47
    bladder cancer 358—9
    breast cancer 254—5
    Burkitt's lymphoma *518*
    cervical carcinoma 320—1
    choriocarcinoma 347
    chronic lymphocytic leukaemia
      560
    effect on treatment and prognosis
      58—9
    gastric lymphoma 521, *522*
    head and neck cancer 173—5,
      177, 182
    Hodgkin's disease 485—6, *487*
    large bowel tumours 309—10
    lung cancer 48, 234—6
    malignant melanoma 48, 423—4
    mesothelioma *247*
    nasopharyngeal cancer *174*
    nephroblastoma 463—4
    neuroblastoma 459—60
    non-Hodgkin's lymphoma
      511—12, *518*
    notation 47—9
    oesophageal carcinoma 276
    osteosarcoma *435*
    ovarian carcinoma 332—3
    penile cancer 373
    prostatic carcinoma 365—7
    renal cell carcinoma 352
    retinoblastoma 471, *472*
    rhabdomyosarcoma *468*
    role of surgery 57—8
    stomach cancer *284*
    and survival *58*
    techniques 49—57
    testicular germ cell tumours
      383—4
    uterine carcinoma 329—30

vaginal carcinoma 345
vulval carcinoma 343
standardized populations 7
Staphylococcus epidermidis 143
steatorrhoea 153
stem cells 39, 41
Sternberg's sarcoma 246
steroid suppression test 149
Stewart—Treves syndrome 446
stoma care 125
stomach
  carcinoma
    aetiology 279—81
    clinical features 283
    diagnosis 283—5
    incidence *2, 13,* 279—81
      geographical variation in *8*
      in Japanese immigrants *9*
    life-time risk of development
      3
    management 285—7
    mortality *2*
    pathology 281—3
    screening for 24, 284—5
    staging *284*
    survival curves 16
  mobilization 277, 278
  non-Hodgkin's lymphoma
    521—2
  polyps 281
  ulcer 281
stratification, in treatment trials 19
streptozotocin
  in carcinoid tumours 300
  in pancreatic cancer *297,* 303
stridor in lung cancer 233
stromelysins 42
struma ovarii 340
Sturge—Weber syndrome 403
subglottic carcinoma 177, 178
sublingual gland 192
  tumours 192—5
submandibular gland 192
  tumours 192—5
sulphor-rhadamine B assay 86
sunlight and skin cancer 413—14,
  421
superficial spreading melanoma
  423
superior vena cava obstruction
  155—6, 233
supportive care teams 134
supraglottic carcinoma 177, 178
suprasellar germ cell tumours 390
surgery 1
  basal/squamous cell skin
    carcinoma 419
  breast cancer 256—61
  cerebral metastases 219
  debulking
    in small cell lung cancer 243
    in testicular germ cell tumours
      389

hepatic metastases 153
large bowel cancer 312—13
malignant melanoma 424—6
non-small cell lung cancer 236—8
oral cavity 186—7
oropharyngeal carcinoma 183
osteosarcoma 438, *439*
ovarian cancer 333—5
pituitary tumours 215
role in diagnosis and staging
  57—8
salvage 127
soft tissue sarcoma 449—50
testicular germ cell tumours
  384—5
thyroid cancer 398—9
vulval carcinoma 343—4
see also specific procedures
survival
  curves 14—17
  data 13—17
  mean 18
  median 18, *19*
  rates 85
sweat gland carcinoma 418
sweating in Hodgkin's disease 483
Swiss-type agammaglobulinaemia
  505
symptom support team 5
syncytiotrophoblast *379,* 380
syndrome of inappropriate ADH
  secretion *160,* 161, 234
syphilitic leukoplakia 171
systemic therapy 85—119

T cell convoluted lymphoblastic
  diffuse lymphoma 246
T cell growth factors *see*
  interleukin 2
T cell lymphoma
  cell origins 508
  childhood 519
  enteropathy-associated 524
  management 514—17
  peripheral 508, *509*
T cells
  cytotoxicity 44, 143
  differentiation 506, *507*
  see also T cell lymphoma
tamoxifen 114, 115—16
  adjuvant 268, 270
  in breast cancer 20—21, 261—2,
    263—5
  and endometrial carcinoma 268,
    328
  in malignant melanoma 427
  in metastases from unknown
    primary site 411
  in renal cell adenocarcinoma 356
taste, alterations in 146, *160*
taxanes 85
Taxol 104, *337, 338,* 339
Taxotere 104

Teilum tumour 475
teletherapy 65—6
temozalamide 211
temporal distribution of cancer 9
temporal lobe lesions 208
tendons, radiosensitivity 77
Tenovus Cancer Information Centre
  137
teratocarcinoma *379,* 380
teratoma
  childhood 475—6
  differentiated *379,* 380
  extra-gonadal 206, 216, 390—1
  immature 340
  monomorphic/monodermal 340
  testis 377, 378
    histology *379*
    management 385, 387
    pathology 380—1
    prognosis 389—90
terminal care 127—34
testes
  atrophy 378, 382
  carcinoma *in situ* 378, *379*—80
  effects of chemotherapy on 112
  germ cell tumours
    aetiology 377—8
    childhood 475—6
    classification 378—81
    clinical features 381—2
    incidence 377—8
    management 384—9
    pathology 378—81
    patterns of metastases 381
    prognosis 389—90
    staging 383—4
    tumour markers 382—3
  life-time risk of cancer
    development *3*
  non-germ cell tumours 391
  non-Hodgkin's lymphoma 377,
    391, 529
  radiosensitivity 74
  relapse of acute lymphoblastic
    leukaemia in 554
  trauma to 378
  ultrasound investigation 50
tetany 149
tetracycline 151
thalamic tumours 206, 212
6-thioguanine *101,* 102, 556, *557*
thiotepa 95
  in ascites 152
  in bladder cancer 361
third ventricle tumours 206
thoracocentesis 150
thoracoscopy 151
thorotrast 292
thrombocytopenia 139, 140, 483
thrombophlebitis *167*
  migratory 163, *167,* 296
thymidine 100, 201
thymoma 164, 243—5

thymus
  carcinoid 245
  carcinoma 244
  lymphoma 508
thyroglobulin 59, 397–8, 401, *409*
thyroid
  biopsy 398
  cancer 393
    aetiology 393
    anaplastic *394*, 395, 397, 399,
      401, 402
    clinical characteristics *394*
    diagnosis and investigation
      397–8
    follicular *394*, 395–6, 398–9,
      401
    incidence 393, *394*
    lymphoma *394*, 397, 399,
      401–2, 528–9
    management 398–401
    medullary *394*, 395, 396–7,
      399, 401
    papillary 393–5, 398, 399, 401
    pathology 393–7
    prognosis *394*, 401–2
    small cell *394*, 397, 399, 401
    ultrasound 50
thyroid-stimulating hormone 399,
    400
thyroidectomy 398–9
thyroiditis
  autoimmune 398
  de Quervain's subacute 398
thyrotoxicosis 393
thyroxine 399, 400
tissue inhibitors of
      metalloproteinases (TIMPS)
      42
TNFs *117*, 118, 146, 534
TNI *see* total nodal irradiation
TNM staging 47–9
  bladder cancer 358–9
  breast cancer 255
  gastric lymphoma 521, *522*
  head and neck cancer *173*, *174*,
    175, *177*, *182*
  lung cancer 234
  penile cancer 373
  prostatic carcinoma 365–6
  renal cell adenocarcinoma *352*
  stomach cancer *284*
  testicular germ cell tumours *384*
tobacco
  chewing 171
  smoking 9–10, 171
    and bladder cancer 357–8
    and laryngeal cancer 175
    and leukaemia 548–9
    and lung cancer 227–8, *229*
    and renal cell carcinoma 351
tongue cancer *171*, 182–3, 184–7
tonsillar tumours 182–3
total body irradiation 81

in childhood ALL 555
in small cell lung cancer 242–3
total nodal irradiation (TNI)
  in Hodgkin's disease 496
  in non-Hodgkin's lymphoma
    513
total parenteral nutrition 147–8
transitional cell carcinoma
  bladder 358
  prostate 365
transplantation antigens 44
treatment trials 3, 17
  chemotherapy 86
  and informed consent 22
  non-randomized 23
  randomized 17–22
tri-iodothyronine 399–400
trimetrexate 99–100
trisomy 21 *36*, 549
tropisetrom 110
TSTA 44
tuberous sclerosis *36*, *167*, 403
tubulin 104
tumour antigens 44, 45–6
tumour lysis syndrome 149–50,
    529
tumour markers 42, 59–61
  choriocarcinoma 346, 347
  extra-gonadal germ cell tumours
    206, 216
  hepatoblastoma 292, 475
  hepatocellular carcinoma 291
  large bowel cancer 310–11, 315
  osteosarcoma 435, 437
  ovarian carcinoma 332
  ovarian germ cell tumours 340
  pancreatic cancer 296
  prostatic carcinoma 365, 367
  stomach cancer 283–4
  testicular germ cell tumours
    382–3
  thyroid carcinoma 396
tumour necrosis factors *117*, 118,
    146, 534
tumour specific transplantation
    antigens 44
tumour suppressor genes 34–5
tumours
  anaplasia 36
  angiogenesis 42–3
  characteristics 36–7
  differentiation in 41–2
  doubling times 40–1, *87*
  enzyme secretion 42
  factors in staging 47–8
  Gompertzian growth 41
  growth 38–41, 86–7
  growth fraction 39, 87
  heterogeneity 38
  immunology 44–6
  invasion and metastasis 36,
    42–4
  lifespan *41*

monoclonality 37–8
radiosensitivity 69–71
undifferentiated 41–2
tylosis palmaris *36*, *167*, 168, 273
tyramine 404

ulcerative colitis
  and bile duct cancer 292
  and large bowel cancer 307
Ulster Cancer Foundation *137*
ultrasound
  endoscopic 50, 276
  in hepatocellular carcinoma 291
  in Hodgkin's disease 489
  in oesophageal cancer 276
  in pancreatic cancer 296
  in renal cell adenocarcinoma
    352–3
  in thyroid cancer 397
  in tumour staging 50, *51*
ultraviolet radiation 10, 29
  and skin cancer 413–14, 421
urate nephropathy 149
ureter
  carcinoma 357
  diversion 361–2, *363*
urethral cancer
  female 372
  male 371–2
urinary diversion 361–2
urinary exfoliative cytology 360
urinary tract
  in Hodgkin's disease 485
  infection 144
    and bladder cancer 358
Urostomy Association *137*
uterus
  carcinoma
    aetiology 327–8
    clinical features 330
    incidence 12, *13*, 318
    life-time risk of development
      3
    management 330–1
    pathology 328–9
    prognosis 331
    screening 24
    staging 329–30
  sarcoma 331

v-*erb* B gene 31
v-*sis* gene 31
v-*src* gene 30–1
VAC regimen *451*
VAC regimen *461*
VAC II regimen *461*
VAD regimen 540
VADIC regimen *451*
vagina
  bleeding from 320, 330, 344
  carcinoma
    aetiology 344
    clinical features 344–5

diagnosis 345
incidence 12, *13*, *318*, 344
management 345−6
spread 344−5
staging 345
discharge from 320
vaginal intraepithelial neoplasia
       (VAIN) 345
vanillyl mandelic acid (VMA)
   in adrenal medullary tumours
       404
   in neuroblastoma 458
VAP regimen *266*, 267
Varicella zoster 145
vasectomy 377−8
VBMCP regimen in multiple
       myeloma *540*
Velbe *see* vinblastine
ventriculo-atrial shunt 209
ventriculo-peritoneal shunt 209
vepesid 104−5, 211
Verner−Morrison syndrome 303
vimentin *409*, 456
VIN 342
vinblastine 104
   in Hodgkin's disease *494*
   in nephroblastoma 465−6
   in ovarian germ cell tumours 341
   in renal cell adenocarcinoma 356
   in testicular germ cell tumours
       387, *388*
vinca alkaloids 103−4
   phase specificity *88*
   see also specific drugs
vincristine 103−4
   in acute lymphoblastic leukaemia
       553, 554
   and bone marrow failure 139
   in breast cancer *266*
   in Ewing's sarcoma 444
   in glioma 211
   in Hodgkin's disease *494*

and hyponatraemia 161
   in large bowel cancer *314*
   in malignant melanoma *426*
   in medulloblastoma *214*
   in nephroblastoma 464, 465
   in neuroblastoma 460, *461*
   in non-small cell lung cancer *239*
   in rhabdomyosarcoma 469
   in small cell lung cancer *241*
   in soft tissue sarcoma 450, 451
vindesine 104
   in breast cancer *266*
   in malignant melanoma *426*
   in non-small cell lung cancer *239*
vinorelbine 104
VIP, ectopic production 396
VIP regimen 388
VIPoma 303
Virchow's node 283
viruses
   in cancer induction 11−12, 30−5
   see also specific viruses
visual pathway disturbances 208
vitamin A analogues 11, 25, 184−5
vitamin C therapy 135
VM26 104−5, 211
VMA *see* vanillyl mandelic acid
VMCP-VBAP regimen in multiple
       myeloma *540*
vomiting
   in brain tumours 207
   chemotherapy-induced 109−11
   in stomach cancer 283
   in terminal cancer 132−3
Von Hippel−Lindau syndrome *36*,
       351, 403
Von Recklinghausen's
       neurofibromatosis *36*, 222−
       3, 446, 455
VP-16213 85, 104−5, 341
vulval carcinoma *318*, 342−4

vulval intraepithelial neoplasia 342

Waldenström's macroglobulinaemia
       543
Waldeyer's ring, non-Hodgkin's
       lymphoma 173, 510, 526−7
Warthin's tumour 193
Weber−Christian disease 296
weight loss 145−7
   in Hodgkin's disease 483
   in oesophageal carcinoma 274
   in pancreatic cancer 296
welders 547
Wermer's syndrome 301, 396
Werner's syndrome *167*
wheeze in lung cancer 157, 233
Wilms' syndrome *36*
Wilms' tumour *see*
       nephroblastoma
Wiskott−Aldrich syndrome *36*,
       167, 504, *505*
Women's Nationwide Cancer
       Control Campaign *137*

X-linked lymphoproliferative
       syndrome *36*, 504, *505*
X-rays
   artificial production 66−9
   carcinogenic effects 10, 414
   megavoltage 67
   orthovoltage 67
   see also radiography
xeroderma pigmentosum 35, 414
XLR *36*, 504, *505*
47 XXY *see* Klinefelter's syndrome

yolk sac tumour 340, *379*, 475−6

Zoladex *see* goserelin
Zollinger−Ellison syndrome 302−
       3